Oxford Handbook of
Anaesthesia

Second edition

Edited by

Keith G. Allman

Consultant Anaesthetist,
Royal Devon and Exeter Healthcare NHS Trust,
UK

and

Iain H. Wilson

Consultant Anaesthetist,
Royal Devon and Exeter Healthcare NHS Trust,
UK

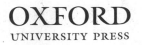

OXFORD
UNIVERSITY PRESS

OXFORD
UNIVERSITY PRESS

Great Clarendon Street, Oxford OX2 6DP

Oxford University Press is a department of the University of Oxford.
It furthers the University's objective of excellence in research, scholarship,
and education by publishing worldwide in

Oxford New York

Auckland Cape Town Dar es Salaam Hong Kong Karachi
Kuala Lumpur Madrid Melbourne Mexico City Nairobi
New Delhi Shanghai Taipei Toronto

With offices in

Argentina Austria Brazil Chile Czech Republic France Greece
Guatemala Hungary Italy Japan Poland Portugal Singapore
South Korea Switzerland Thailand Turkey Ukraine Vietnam

Oxford is a registered trade mark of Oxford University Press
in the UK and in certain other countries

Published in the United States
by Oxford University Press Inc., New York

British Library Cataloguing in Publication Data
Data available

Library of Congress Cataloging in Publication Data
Data available

Typeset by Newgen Imaging Systems (P) Ltd., Chennai, India
Printed in China through Phoenix Offset Ltd.

ISBN 978–0–19–856609–0

10 9 8 7 6 5

Preface

Welcome to the second edition of the *Oxford Handbook of Anaesthesia*. We were delighted with the success of the first editon, and hope that this edition will be as well received.

The second edition contains many changes to take account of the feedback obtained from readers and reviewers. We have involved new authors in around a third of the book so that the material remains up-to-date and reflects a balanced set of views. In our opinion, each author is an established expert in their field and, more importantly, a good clinical anaesthetist.

The book describes the preparation of the patient for anaesthesia, and now includes a comprehensive account of consent and anaesthetic risk. The implications of many concurrent diseases on anaesthesia are detailed and the general principles of anaesthetic practice for different subspecialties are reviewed. Appropriate techniques are suggested where possible. There are detailed chapters on obstetric and paediatric anaesthesia, and also emergencies. A comprehensive drug formulary is included.

The *Oxford Handbook of Anaesthesia* remains a practical guide to anaesthesia written for those who have mastered basic anaesthetic techniques, but need advice for the many common problems encountered in clinical practice.

The first edition of the *Oxford Handbook of Anaesthesia* has proved popular in many countries throughout the world. A low cost edition is available in India, Pakistan, and Bangladesh, but not as yet in Africa. The World Federation of Societies of Anaesthesiologists Publications Committee has names and addresses of anaesthetists without literature working in the developing world who would be grateful for a copy of either edition of the *Oxford Handbook of Anaesthesia*. If you are willing to make a donation of your existing copy or new copy, please email iain.wilson@rdehc-tr.swest.nhs.uk and we shall supply a name and address of someone who will be thrilled to receive a book.

We are particularly grateful for the expert proof reading skills of Dr Aidan O'Donnell who has provided invaluable support during the preparation of this edition. Despite all our efforts it is possible that an occasional error exists, please be careful. We hope that you will enjoy this latest edition of the *Oxford Handbook of Anaesthesia*. Please email us your criticisms and suggestions, so that we can keep improving the book.

Many thanks to our understanding families, authors, and the landlord of the Artichoke Inn, Christow for support during editorial meetings.

Keep well,

Keith and Iain
iain.wilson@rdeft.nhs.uk
2006

Contents

Contributors

Barry Baker
Nuffield Professor of Anaesthesia,
Sydney, Australia

Anna Batchelor
Consultant Anaesthetist,
Newcastle, UK

Mark Bellamy
Professor of Critical Care and
Anaesthesia, Leeds, UK

Simon Berg
Consultant Paediatric
Anaesthetist,
Oxford, UK

Colin Berry
Consultant Anaesthetist,
Exeter, UK

Hannah Blanshard
Specialist Registrar,
Bristol, UK

Andrew Bodenham
Consultant Anaesthetist,
Leeds, UK

Bruce Campbell
Professor of Vascular Surgery,
Exeter, UK

John Carlisle
Consultant anaesthetist,
Torquay, UK

Tracey Clayton
Consultant Anaesthetist,
Gloucester, UK

David Conn
Consultant Anaesthetist,
Exeter, UK

Tim Cook
Consultant Anaesthetist,
Bath, UK

Julius Cranshaw
Consultant Anaesthetist,
Bournemouth, UK

Adrian Dashfield
Consultant Anaesthetist,
Plymouth, UK

Peter Davies
Consultant Anaesthetist,
Plymouth, UK

John Dean
Consultant Cardiologist,
Exeter, UK

James Eldridge
Consultant Anaesthetist,
Portsmouth, UK

Rhys Evans
Clinical Reader in Anaesthesia,
Oxford, UK

Andrew Farmery
Consultant Anaesthetist,
Oxford, UK

Simon Galloway
Specialist Registrar, Leeds, UK

Richard Griffiths
Consultant Anaesthetist,
Peterborough, UK

Carl Gwinnutt
Consultant Anaesthetist,
Salford, UK

Jane Halsall
Associate Specialist MH Unit,
Leeds, UK

Mark Hamilton
Research Fellow,
London, UK

Jeffrey Handel
Consultant Anaesthetist,
Bath, UK

Paul Harvey
Consultant Anaesthetist,
Plymouth, UK

Graham Hocking
Consultant Anaesthetist,
Perth, Australia

Kath Jenkins
Consultant Anaesthetist,
Bristol, UK

Gavin Kenny
Professor of Anaesthesia,
Glasgow, UK

Bruce McCormick
Consultant Anaesthetist,
Exeter, UK

Andrew McIndoe
Consultant Anaesthetist,
Bristol, UK

Alexander Manara
Consultant Neuroanaesthesia,
Bristol, UK

Paul Marshall
Consultant Anaesthetist,
Exeter, UK

Alan Merry
Professor of Anaesthesiology,
Auckland, New Zealand

Quentin Milner
Consultant Anaesthetist,
Exeter, UK

Julia Munn
Consultant Anaesthetist,
Exeter, UK

Peter Murphy
Consultant Paediatric Anaesthetist,
Bristol, UK

Monty Mythen
Portex Professor of Anaesthesia,
London, UK

Barry Nicholls
Consultant Anaesthetist,
Taunton, UK

Richard Nickalls
Consultant Anaesthetist,
Nottingham, UK

Jerry Nolan
Consultant Anaesthetist,
Bath, UK

Aidan O'Donnell
Specialist Registrar,
Edinburgh, UK

Jonathan Purday
Consultant Anaesthetist,
Exeter, UK

Fred Roberts
Consultant Anaesthetist,
Exeter, UK

Anne Rossiter
Consultant Occupational Physician,
Exeter, UK

Matt Rucklidge
Consultant Anaesthetist,
Exeter, UK

John Saddler
Consultant Anaesthetist,
Exeter, UK

David Sanders
Consultant Anaesthetist,
Exeter, UK

Babinder Sandhar
Consultant Anaesthetist,
Exeter, UK

Robert Self
Research Fellow,
London, UK

Peter Shirley
Consultant Anaesthetist,
London, UK

Paul Sice
Specialist Registrar,
Exeter, UK

Michael Sinclair
Consultant Cardiac Anaesthetist,
Oxford, UK

Mark Stoneham
Consultant Anaesthetist,
Oxford, UK

James Szymankiewicz
Senior House Officer,
Exeter, UK

Andrew Teasdale
Consultant Anaesthetist,
Exeter, UK

Richard Telford
Consultant Anaesthetist,
Exeter, UK

Stephen Townley
Senior Registrar,
Perth, Western Australia

Anne Troy
Consultant Anaesthetist,
Chester, UK

David Walker
Research Fellow,
London, UK

Jon Warwick
Consultant Anaesthetist,
Oxford, UK

Gavin Werrett
Specialist Registrar,
Exeter, UK

David Wilkinson
Anaesthetic Practitioner,
Exeter, UK

Ralph Worms
Specialist Registrar,
Leicester, UK

Gordon Yuill
Specialist Registrar,
Salford, UK

Abbreviations

A&E	accident and emergency
AAA	abdominal aortic aneurysm
AADR	anaesthetic adverse drug reactions
AAGBI	Association of Anaesthetists of Great Britain and Ireland
AAS	atlantoaxial sublimation
ABC	airway, breathing, circulation
ABG	arterial blood gas
ACE	angiotensin-converting enzyme
ACT	activated clotting time
ACTH	adrenocorticotrophic hormone
ADH	antidiuretic hormone
AF	atrial fibrillation
AFOI	awake fibreoptic intubation
AICD	automatic implantable cardioverter defibrillator
AIDS	acquired immunodeficiency syndrome
ALS	advanced life support
ALT	alanine aminotransferase
ANH	acute normovolaemic haemodilution
AP	anteroposterior
APL	adjustable pressure limiting (valve)
APTR	activated partial thromboplastin ratio
APTT	activated partial thromboplastin time
AR	aortic regurgitation
ARDS	acute respiratory distress syndrome
ARF	acute renal failure
AS	aortic stenosis
ASA	American Society of Anesthesiologists
ASD	atrial septal defect
ASRA	American Society of Regional Anesthesia and Pain Medicine
AST	aspartate transaminase
ATLS	advanced trauma life support
ATP	adenosine triphosphate

AV	atrioventricular
AVM	arteriovenous malformation
AVSD	atrioventricular septal defect
BBV	blood born virus
bd	twice daily *(bis diem)*
BiPAP	biphasic positive airways pressure
BLS	basic life support
BMI	body mass index
BNF	British National Formulary
BP	blood pressure
bpm	beats per minute
BSS	balanced salt solution
BURP	backward upward and rightwards pressure
C&S	culture and sensitivity
CABG	coronary arterial bypass graft
CBF	cerebral blood flow
CC	creatinine clearance
CCF	congestive cardiac failure
CCU	coronary care unit
Ch	Charrère (French) gauge (also FG or Fr)
CHD	congenital heart disease
CJD	Creutzfeldt–Jacob disease
CK	creatine kinase
CMV	cytomegalovirus
CNS	central nervous system
COAD	chronic obstructive airways disease
COETT	cuffed oral endotracheal tube
COHb	carboxyhaemoglobin
COPA	cuffed oropharyngeal airway
COPD	chronic obstructive pulmonary disease
COX	cyclo-oxygenase
CPAP	continuous positive airway pressure
CPB	cardiopulmonary bypass
CPDA	citrate phosphate dextrose adenine
CPK	creatine (phospho) kinase
CPP	cerebral perfusion pressure

CPR	cardiopulmonary resuscitation
CPX	cardiopulmonary exercise testing
CRF	chronic renal failure
CRP	C-reactive protein
CSE	combined spinal/epidural
CSF	cerebrospinal fluid
CT	computed tomogaphy
CVA	cerebrovascular accident
CVE	cerebrovascular episode/event
CVP	central venous pressure
CVS	cardiovascular system
CXR	chest X-ray
DCR	dacrocystorhinostomy
DDAVP	desmopressin
DIC	disseminated intravascular coagulation
DLT	double lumen [endobronchial] tube
DMARD	disease modifying antirheumatoid drug
DVT	deep vein thrombosis
ECF	extracellular fluid
ECG	electrocardiogram
ECM	external cardiac massage
ECT	electroconvulsive therapy
EDD	estimated date of delivery
EEG	electroencephalogram
EF	ejection fraction
EMD	electromechanical dissociation
EMG	electromyograph
EMLA	eutectic mixture of local anaesthetic
ENT	ear, nose, and throat
EPO	erythropoietin
ERCP	endoscopic retrograde cholangio-pancreatography
ERPC	evacuation of retained products of conception
ESR	erythrocyte sedimentation rate
$ETCO_2$	end tidal carbon dioxide
ETT/ET	endotracheal tube
EUA	examination under anaesthetic

FB	foreign body
FBC	full blood count
FES	fat embolism syndrome
FEV_1	forced expiration in 1 s
FFP	fresh frozen plasma
FG	French gauge (also Fr or Ch)
FGF	fresh gas flow
FiO_2	fractional inspired oxygen content
FM	face mask
Fr	French gauge (also FG or Ch)
FRC	functional residual capacity
FTSG	full thickness skin graft
FVC	forced vital capacity
G	Gauge (standard wire gauge)
G&S	group and save
G-6-PD	glucose-6-phosphate dehydrogenase
GA	general anaesthetic
GCS	Glasgow coma score
GEB	gum elastic bougie
GFR	glomerular filtration rate
GI(T)	gastrointestinal (tract)
GTN	glyceryl trinitrate
HAS	human albumin solution
HbC/HbD/ HbF/HbS	haemoglobin C/D/F/S
HBV/HCV	hepatitis B/C virus
Hct	haematocrit
HDU	high-dependency unit
HELLP	haemolysis, elevated liver enzymes, low platelets
HES	hydroxyethyl starches
HFO	high frequency oscillation
HIB	*Haemophilus influenzae B*
HIT	heparin-induced thrombocytopenia
HME	heat and moisture exchanger
HOCM	hypertrophic obstructive cardiomyopathy
HR	heart rate

HRS(UK)	Heart Rhythm Society (UK)
HRT	hormone replacement therapy
I:E ratio	inspired:expired ratio
IABP	intra-aortic balloon pump
ICP	intracranial pressure
ICU	intensive care unit
ID	internal diameter
IDDM	insulin-dependent diabetes mellitus
IDT	intradermal testing
IHD	ischaemic heart disease
ILMA	intubating laryngeal mask airway
IM	intra-muscular
INR	international normalised ratio
IO	intra-osseous
IOP	intra-ocular pressure
IPPV	intermittent positive pressure ventilation
ITU	intensive therapy unit
ITP	idiopathic thrombocytopenic purpura
IV	intravenous(ly)
IVC	inferior vena cava
IVCT	*in vitro* muscle contracture test
IVH	intraventricular haemorrhage
IVI	intravenous infusion
IVRA	intravenous regional anaesthesia
JVP	jugular venous pressure
LA	local anaesthetic
LCNT	lateral cutaneous nerve of thigh
LFT	liver function test
LMA	laryngeal mask airway
LMWH	low-molecular-weight heparin
LP	lumbar puncture
LSCS	lower segment Caesarean section
LSD	lysergic acid diethylamide
LV	left ventricle/ventricular
LVEDP	left ventricular end diastolic pressure

LVF	left ventricular failure
LVH	left ventricular hypertrophy
MAC	minimum alveolar concentration
MAO	monoamine oxidase
MAOB	monoamine oxidase B
MAOI	monoamine oxidase inhibitor
MAP	mean arterial pressure
MCV	mean corpuscular volume
MEAC	minimum effective analgesic concentration
MEN	multiple endocrine neoplasia
MH	malignant hyperthermia
MI	myocardial infarction
MIBG	*meta*-iodobenzylguanidine
MR	mitral regurgitation
MRI	magnetic resonance imaging
MRSA	methicillin-resistant *Staphylococcus aureus*
MST	morphine sulphate
MUA	manipulation under anaesthesia
MUGA	multigated acquisition scan
MW	molecular weight
NCA	nurse-controlled analgesia
NCEPOD	National Confidential Enquiry into Patient Outcome and Death
NG	nasogastric
NIBP	non-invasive blood pressure
NICE	National Institute for Clinical Excellence
NIDDM	non-insulin-dependent diabetes mellitus
NIPPV	non-invasive positive pressure ventilation
NMB	neuromuscular blockade
NMBD	neuromuscular blocking drugs
NMDA	*N*-methyl-D-aspartate
nocte	at night
NOF	Fractured Neck of Femur
NR	not recommended
NSAID	non-steroidal anti-inflammatory drug
OCP	oral contraceptive pill
od	once daily

OLEM	optimal external laryngeal manipulation
OLV	one-lung ventilation
ORIF	open reduction internal fixation
OSA	obstructive sleep apnoea
$P\bar{v}O_2$	mixed venous partial pressure of oxygen
PA	pulmonary artery/arterial
$PaCO_2$	arterial partial pressure of carbon dioxide
PAFC	pulmonary artery flotation catheter
PaO_2	arterial partial pressure of oxygen
PAO_2	alveolar partial pressure of oxygen
PAOP	pulmonary artery occlusion pressure
PAP	pulmonary artery pressure
P_{AW}	airway pressure
PAWP	pulmonary artery wedge pressure
PCA	patient-controlled analgesia
PCEA	patient-controlled epidural analgesia
PCI	percutaneous coronary intervention
PCWP	pulmonary capillary wedge pressure
PDA	patent ductus arteriosus
PE	pulmonary embolism
PEA	pulseless electrical activity
PEEP	positive end expiratory pressure
PEFR	peak expiratory flow rate
PEP	post-exposure prophylaxis
PICU	paediatric intensive care unit
PND	paroxysmal nocturnal dyspnoea
PO	*per os* (oral)
PONV	postoperative nausea and vomiting
POP	plaster of paris
PR	per rectum
prn/PRN	as required (*pro re nata*)
PS	pulmonary stenosis
PT	prothrombin time
PTH	parathyroid hormone
PVC	polyvinyl chloride
PVR	pulmonary vascular resistance

qds	four times daily (*quater die sumendus*)
RA	rheumatoid arthritis
RAE	Ring, Adair, and Elwyn [tube]
RAST	radioallergosorbent test
rEPO	recombinant erythropoietin
RIMA	reversible inhibitor of monoamine oxidase A
ROSC	restoration of a spontaneous circulation
RS	respiratory system
RSI	rapid sequence induction
RTA	road traffic accident
RV	right ventricle/ventricular
rVIIa	recombinant factor VIIa
$S\bar{v}O_2$	mixed venous oxygen saturation
SA	sinoatrial
SAH	subarachnoid haemorrhage
SaO_2	arterial oxygen saturation
SBE	subacute bacterial endocarditis
SC	subcutaneous
SCBU	special care baby unit
$ScvO_2$	central venous oxygen saturation
SEA	spinal epidural abscess
SHOT	Serious Hazards of Transfusion
SIADH	syndrome of inappropriate antidiuretic hormone
SIRS	systemic inflammatory response syndrome
SjO_2	jugular venous oxygen saturation
SL	sublingual
SLE	systemic lupus erythematosus
SLT	single lumen tube
SMR	submucous resection
SNP	sodium nitroprusside
SpO_2	peripheral oxygen saturation
SPT	skin-pricking test
SSG	split skin graft
SSRI	selective serotonin reuptake inhibitor
STEMI	ST elevation myocardial infarction
(S)TOP	(suction) termination of pregnancy

SV	spontaneous ventilation
SVC	superior vena cava
SVR	systemic vascular resistance
SVT	supraventricular tachycardia
TB	tuberculosis
TBSA	total body surface area
TBW	total body water
TCA	tricyclic antidepressant
TCI	target-controlled infusion
tds	three times daily (*ter die sumendus*)
TEDS	thromboembolism stockings
TEG	thrombelastograph
TENS	transcutaneous electric nerve stimulation
TFT	thyroid function tests
THR	total hip replacement
TIA	transient ischaemic attack
TIPS	transjugular intrahepatic portal-systemic shunt procedure
TIVA	total intravenous anaesthesia
TKR	total knee replacement
TMJ	temporomandibular joint
TNF	tumour necrosis factor
TNS	transient neurologic symptom
TOE	transoesophageal echocardiography
TOF	train of four
TPN	total parenteral nutrition
TRALI	transfusion-related acute lung injury
TRAM	transverse rectus abdominis muscle
TTI	transfusion-transmitted infection
TTP	thrombotic thrombocytopenic purpura
TURP	transurethral resection of the prostate
TUVP	transurethral vaporisation of the prostate
U&E	urea and electrolytes
UPPP	uvulopalatopharyngoplasty
URTI	upper respiratory tract infection
V/Q	ventilation/perfusion
VAE	venous air embolism

VATS	video-assisted thoracoscopic surgery
VF	ventricular fibrillation
VIP	vasoactive intestinal peptide
VP	venous pressure
VR	ventricular rate
VSD	ventricular septal defect
VT	ventricular tachycardia
V_t or V_T	tidal volume
VWF	Von Willebrand factor
WBC	white blood cell count
WPW	Wolff–Parkinson–White
X-match	crossmatch

General considerations

Good practice

Making anaesthesia safe

- Pay attention to detail.
- Prepare properly and don't rush.
- Read the notes.
- Correct patient, correct surgery?
- Assess patient personally—check airway and allergies.
- Check drugs and apparatus.
- Always have a Plan B.
- Never leave an anaesthetised patient unattended.
- When ventilating, check the chest is moving.
- Hypotension needs an explanation.
- If in trouble, ask for help.
- Failed intubation—ventilate and oxygenate.
- Difficult ventilation—equipment or patient?
- If in doubt, take it out.
- Never assume.
- Don't panic—remember ABC.
- The anaesthetist, surgeon, and staff are on the same team.
- Know your limits.

Preoperative tests

Every department should have local protocols for preoperative testing based as the following NICE guidelines. A test should be done only if the results will affect patient treatment and outcomes. Tests should be preceded by a valid consenting process.
- Start with tests based on surgical grade and age.
- Add tests not yet done as indicated by disease severity.
- Local protocols determine whether to undertake a shaded 'NO' (no consensus from NICE).
- Offer pregnancy tests to all women who say they may be pregnant.
- Sickle cell test: African or Afro-Caribbean; Middle Eastern; Asian; East Mediterranean.
- Consider CXR if worsening lung, heart, or renal disease, or postoperative Level 2 or 3 care expected.
- For dynamic CVS testing see p992.

Surgical grades	Examples
Grade 1 (minor)	Excision skin lesion; drainage breast abscess
Grade 2 (intermediate)	Inguinal hernia; varicose vein(s); tonsillectomy; arthroscopy
Grade 3 (major)	Hysterectomy; TURP; lumbar discectomy; thyroidectomy
Grade 4 (major+)	Joint replacement; thoracic operations; colonic resection; radical neck dissection

For **ASA grading** (see p1168)

Preoperative tests by surgical grade and age

Surgery grade	Age (yr)	CXR	ECG	FBC	INR/APTT	U&Es creat	Random glucose	Urine	Total
One	<16	NO	NO	NO	NO	NO	NO	NO	0
One	16–60	NO	NO	NO	NO	NO	NO	NO	0
One	61–80	NO	NO	NO	NO	NO	NO	NO	0
One	>80	NO	YES	NO	NO	NO	NO	NO	1
Two	<16	NO	NO	NO	NO	NO	NO	NO	0
Two	16–60	NO	NO	NO	NO	NO	NO	NO	0
Two	61–80	NO	NO	YES	NO	NO	NO	NO	1
Two	>80	NO	YES	YES	NO	NO	NO	NO	2
Three	<16	NO	NO	NO	NO	NO	NO	NO	0
Three	16–60	NO	NO	YES	NO	NO	NO	NO	1
Three	61–80	NO	YES	YES	NO	YES	NO	NO	3
Three	>80	NO	YES	YES	NO	YES	NO	NO	3
Four	<16	NO	NO	NO	NO	NO	NO	NO	0
Four	16–60	NO	NO	YES	NO	YES	NO	NO	2
Four	61–80	NO	YES	YES	NO	YES	NO	NO	3
Four	>80	NO	YES	YES	NO	YES	NO	NO	3

Preoperative tests by disease status (shaded 'NO' should be determined by local protocols)

Disease	ASA	CXR	ECG	FBC	INR/APTT	U&Es creat	Blood gases	Lung function	Total
CVS	2	NO	YES	NO	NO	NO	NO	NO	1
CVS	3	NO	YES	NO	NO	YES	NO	NO	2
Lung	2	NO	NO	NO	NO	NO	NO	NO	0
Lung	3	NO	NO	NO	NO	NO	NO	NO	0
Renal	2	NO	NO	NO	NO	YES	NO	NO	1
Renal	3	NO	YES	YES	NO	YES	NO	NO	3

Premedication drugs

See also paediatric premedication—p773.

It is well recognised that a clear explanation of anticipated events and a rapport with the anaesthetic team provide more effective anxiolysis than drugs. Premedication is much less commonly prescribed than a few years ago but is still indicated in anxious patients and those in whom there is an increased risk of gastro-oesophageal reflux. Suitable drugs are listed below. Many patients benefit from sedation the night before surgery.

Sedatives: 1hr preoperatively unless otherwise indicated			
Benzodiazepines	Lormetazepam	PO	0.5–1.5mg
	Temazepam		10–30mg
	Lorazepam (2hr preop)		1.0–2.5mg
	Midazolam (40min preop)		10–30mg
	Midazolam (20–40min preop)	IM	2–10mg
Non-benzodiazepines	Zopiclone	PO	7.5–15mg

Gastric pH increasing drugs			
H₂ antagonists	Ranitidine	PO	150–300mg night before and 2hr preop
		Slow IV or IM	50mg 2hr preop
Proton pump inhibitors	Omeprazole	PO	40mg night before and 2hr preop
		IV infusion	40mg over 30min
Antacid	Sodium citrate (0.3M)	PO	30ml 10min preop

Analgesic drugs			
Opioids	Morphine	IM or SC	10–15mg
	Pethidine	IM	50–100mg
NSAIDs	Diclofenac	PO	50–100mg
		PR	100mg
	Paracetamol	PO or PR	1g

Prokinetic drugs		
Metoclopramide	PO, IV, IM	10mg

Fasting

Background

Pulmonary aspiration of gastric contents, even 30–40ml, is associated with significant morbidity and mortality. Factors predisposing to regurgitation and pulmonary aspiration include inadequate anaesthesia, pregnancy, obesity, difficult airway, emergency surgery, full stomach, and altered gastrointestinal motility.

Fasting before anaesthesia aims to reduce the volume of gastric contents and hence the risk should aspiration occur.

Gastric physiology

- Clear fluids (water, fruit juices without pulp, clear tea, and black coffee) are emptied from the stomach in an exponential manner with a half-life of 10–20min. This results in complete clearance within 2hr of ingestion.
- Gastric emptying of solids is much slower than for fluids and is more variable. Foods with a high fat or meat content require 8hr or longer to be emptied from the stomach, whereas a light meal such as toast is usually cleared in 4hr. Milk is considered a solid because when mixed with gastric juice, it thickens and congeals. Cow's milk takes up to 5hr to empty from the stomach. Human breast milk has a lower fat and protein content and is emptied at a faster rate.

Fasting guidelines

Recommendations on preoperative fasting in elective, healthy patients were issued by the American Society of Anesthesiologists (ASA) in 1999, followed by similar guidance from the Association of Anaesthetists of Great Britain and Ireland (AAGBI).

Ingested material	Minimum fast
Clear liquids	2hr
Breast milk	4hr
Light meal, infant formula, and other milk	6hr

Delayed gastric emptying

- Delayed gastric emptying due to metabolic causes (e.g. poorly controlled diabetes mellitus, renal failure, sepsis), decreased gastric motility (e.g. head injury), or pyloric obstruction (e.g. pyloric stenosis) will primarily affect emptying of solids, particularly high-cellulose foods such as vegetables. Gastric emptying of clear fluids is affected only in the advanced stages.
- Gastro-oesophageal reflux may be associated with delayed gastric emptying of solids, but emptying of liquids is not affected.
- Raised intra-abdominal pressure (e.g. pregnancy, obesity) predisposes to passive regurgitation.

- Opioids cause marked delays in gastric emptying.
- Trauma delays gastric emptying. The time interval between the last oral intake and the injury is considered as the fasting period and a rapid sequence induction should be used if this interval is short. The time taken to return to normal gastric emptying after trauma has not been established and varies depending upon the degree of trauma and the level of pain. The best indicators are probably signs of normal gastric motility such as normal bowel sounds and patient hunger.
- Anxiety has not been shown to have any consistent effect on gastric emptying.
- Oral premedication given 1hr before surgery is without adverse effect on gastric volume on induction of anaesthesia. Studies on premedication with oral midazolam 30min preoperatively have not reported any link with gastric regurgitation or aspiration.

Chemical control of gastric acidity and volume

- Antacids can be used to neutralise acid in the stomach, thereby reducing the risk of damage should aspiration occur. Particulate antacids are not recommended. Sodium citrate solution administered shortly before induction is the agent of choice in high-risk cases (e.g. pregnancy).
- H_2 blockers/proton pump inhibitors decrease secretion of acid in the stomach and should be used for high-risk patients. Ideally, these agents should be administered on the evening before surgery (or early morning for an afternoon list) and a second dose given 2hr preoperatively.
- Gastric motility enhancing agents such as metoclopramide increase gastric emptying in healthy patients, but a clear benefit in trauma patients has not been demonstrated. Metoclopramide is more effective IV than PO.
- Anticholinergic agents do not have a significant effect and are not routinely recommended.
- Pregnant patients should be given ranitidine 150mg on the evening before elective surgery (or at 0700hr for an afternoon list) and again 2hr preoperatively. During labour, high-risk patients should be given oral ranitidine, 150mg 6-hourly. For emergency cases, ranitidine 50mg IV should be given at the earliest opportunity. In addition, 30ml of 0.3M sodium citrate should be given to neutralise any residual gastric acid.
- The ASA does not recommend routine use of these agents in healthy, elective patients.

Further reading

Maltby R (1993). New guidelines for preoperative fasting. *Canadian Journal of Anaesthesia*, **40**, R113–R117.
Practice guidelines for preoperative fasting and the use of pharmacological agents for the prevention of pulmonary aspiration: application to healthy patients undergoing elective procedures (1999). *Anesthesiology*, **90**, 896–905.
The Cochrane database of systematic reviews 2003(4), P: CD004423, Refs: 87, ISSN 1469-493X.

Prophylaxis of venous thromboembolism

Pulmonary embolism (PE) is responsible for 10% of all hospital deaths. Without prophylaxis, 40–80% of high-risk patients develop detectable DVT and up to 10% die from PE. Most PEs result from DVTs which start in the venous plexuses of the legs and which then extend proximally. Calf vein DVT is detectable in up to 10% of low-risk patients but seldom extends into proximal veins.

Increased risk of venous thromboembolism perioperatively is due to
- Hypercoagulability caused by surgery, cancer, or hormone therapy
- Stasis of blood in the venous plexuses of the legs during surgery and postoperatively
- Interference with venous return (pregnancy, pelvic surgery, pneumoperitoneum)
- Dehydration
- Poor cardiac output

Any patient confined to bed is at risk of venous thromboembolism. Sick, elderly patients may need prophylaxis from the time of admission.

Risk factors for venous thromboembolism

Patients can be divided into three categories of risk—low, medium, or high—dependent upon the type of operation, patient factors, and associated diseases.

- Duration and type of operation
  - Operations lasting <30min are considered minor (low risk) and >30min, major (higher risk).
  - Particularly high-risk procedures include major joint replacements (hip and knee) and surgery to the abdomen and pelvis.
- Patient factors
  - Previous history of DVT or PE, thrombophilia
  - Pregnancy, puerperium, oestrogen therapy (contraceptive pill, HRT)
  - Age >40yr (risk increases with age)
  - Obesity and immobility
  - Varicose veins (in abdominal and pelvic surgery)
- Associated diseases
  - Malignancy (especially metastatic or in abdomen/pelvis)
  - Trauma (especially spinal cord injury and lower limb fractures)
  - Heart failure, recent myocardial infarction
  - Systemic infection
  - Lower limb paralysis (e.g. after stroke)
  - Haematological diseases (polycythaemia, leukaemia, paraproteinaemia)
  - Other diseases, including nephrotic syndrome and inflammatory bowel disease.

For example, a fit patient >40yr having minor surgery is low risk, whereas a fit patient <40yr having major abdominal surgery is moderate risk; and an elderly patient having pelvic surgery for cancer is high risk for thromboembolism.

Methods of prophylaxis

Every hospital should have a policy detailing local practice. General measures which seem logical include
- Avoidance of prolonged immobility (encourage early mobilisation)
- Avoidance of dehydration

SC heparin

SC heparin reduces the incidence of DVT and fatal PE by about two-thirds. Unfractionated (ordinary) heparin has been largely replaced by the newer low-molecular-weight heparins (LMWHs), which may be more effective and cause fewer bleeding complications. They have the added advantage of less frequent administration but are more expensive.

Low-dose unfractionated heparin

- Start 2hr before operation in fit patients, and on admission if unfit or immobile.
- Dose is 5000U 12-hourly (8-hourly administration may give greater protection and should be used for very high risk patients).

LMWHs

- Start on admission or evening before surgery.
- Daily doses are certoparin 3000U, dalteparin 2500U, enoxaparin 2000U, reviparin 1432U, tinzaparin 3500U.
- Risk of epidural haematoma can be minimised by giving LMWH on the evening before surgery, so that 12hr or more has elapsed before central neuraxial blockade (LMWH plasma half-life is 4hr) or starting prophylaxis postoperatively (see also p1058).

Graduated compression stockings (anti-embolism stockings)

- These reduce the risk of DVT but are not proven to reduce PE.
- They may give enhanced protection when used in combination with SC heparin.
- Below-the-knee stockings are probably as effective as above-the-knee stockings, but this is controversial.
- Stockings are probably advisable for all patients having laparoscopic procedures.
- Fit with care and monitor for pressure damage: stockings should be avoided in patients with severe arterial disease of the legs (check ankle systolic pressure if in doubt).

Intermittent pneumatic compression devices

- These devices compress the leg (35–40mmHg) for about 10s every minute, promoting venous flow.
- They are as effective as heparin in reducing the incidence of DVT.
- They are used particularly in orthopaedic practice to avoid the bleeding risks of heparin, or in combination with heparin.
- Foot pumps are similar and promote blood flow by compressing the venous plexuses of the feet.

Warfarin, dextran, and aspirin

- Warfarin is used most often in orthopaedic practice, where there is good evidence of its efficacy in relation to hip operations. It may be given either as a fixed low dose (2mg/day) or as a monitored dose (target INR 2.0–3.0).
- Dextran (Dextran 70/40) is as effective as SC heparin in preventing DVT and PE but is not often used because it requires IV infusion. Fluid overload is a risk and anaphylaxis can occasionally occur.
- Aspirin provides some protection against venous thromboembolism but is less effective than other methods.

Choice of anaesthetic

- Local anaesthesia eliminates lower limb immobility associated with general anaesthesia.
- Regional anaesthesia (spinal/epidural) appears to be protective in certain kinds of surgery, especially hip/knee replacement.

Oral contraceptive pills (OCPs) and venous thromboembolism

- The risk of spontaneous venous thrombosis is increased in women taking combined OCPs, particularly third-generation pills containing desogestrel or gestodene.
- OCPs may increase the risk of perioperative thromboembolism by up to 3–4 times, but the evidence is not compelling.
- The risk may decrease the longer an individual takes a combined OCP.
- Progestogen-only OCPs (and injectable progestogens) do not increase the risk of DVT or PE.

Advice on perioperative management is conflicting. Manufacturers and the British National Formulary (2005) recommend stopping oestrogen containing OCPs 4wk before major operations and restarting only after the menstrual period at least 2wk following full mobilisation. By contrast, specialist groups advise that the OCP should not routinely be stopped, because of insufficient evidence and the danger of unwanted pregnancy.

A reasonable policy is as follows:

- There is no need to stop progestogen-only contraceptives for any operation.
- There is no need to stop combined OCPs for minor operations.
- For patients on combined OCPs facing major elective surgery, the decision should be made on an individual basis, balancing the risk of thromboembolism (consider other risks factors such as obesity), the possibility of unwanted pregnancy, and the preferences of the patient.
- Patients having intermediate or major surgery when taking the combined OCP should receive SC LMWH and wear anti-embolism stockings.
- There is no possibility of stopping any contraceptives for emergency surgery.
- Always record decisions about contraceptives in the case notes, including a record about discussion with the patient.

- If the OCP is stopped, advice must be given about alternative contraceptive measures. In selected cases, consider a change to depot progestogen injections
- Consider a pregnancy test before operation if there is a possibility of 0unprotected intercourse having taken place.

Hormone replacement therapy (HRT) and venous thromboembolism

- HRT increases the incidence of spontaneous venous thromboembolism, but there are no good data on perioperative risk.
- Stopping HRT may cause recurrence of troublesome menopausal symptoms.
- The British National Formulary (2005) suggests that 'it may be prudent to stop HRT' 4–6wk before major surgery, but it is common practice to continue HRT and to use prophylaxis (heparin and stockings).

Further reading

Drugs in the perioperative period: 3—hormonal contraceptives and hormone replacement therapy (1999). *Drugs and Therapeutics Bulletin*, **37**, 78–80.

Geerts WH, Heit JA, Clagett GP, Pineo GF, Colwell CW, Anderson FA, Wheeler HB (2002). Prevention of venous thromboembolism. *Chest*, **121**, 132S–175S.

Low molecular weight heparins for venous thromboembolism (1998). *Drugs and Therapeutics Bulletin*, **36**, 25–32.

Thromboembolic Risk Factors (THRIFT) Consensus Group (1992). Risk of and prophylaxis for venous thromboembolism in hospital patients. *British Medical Journal*, **305**, 567–574.

Perioperative guidelines for body piercing jewellery

The prevalence of body piercing has been increasing in recent years. Often patients are reluctant to remove such jewellery owing to difficulties with reinsertion postoperatively. The following are general recommendations.

All body piercing should be **removed** prior to anaesthesia and surgery in the following situations:

- All tongue and lip jewellery should be removed prior to *any* general anaesthetic. Such items may cause airway obstruction or enter the tracheo-bronchial tree if dislodged.
- Any nasal septum, nose, or ear piercing should be removed prior to ENT surgery.
- Body piercing jewellery should also be removed if
  - It is at risk of being caught or ripped out, e.g. by ECG leads, surgical drapes, surgical instruments, or towel clips.
  - If there is any risk of pressure damage, e.g. chin or lip piercing (pressure from a face mask), nipple piercing (if patient is to be positioned prone).
  - If the piercing is in close proximity to the surgical site.
- Any piercing with signs of infection around the site should also be removed due to possible focus of infection. This may also preclude some types of 'clean' surgery.

Body piercing does not always have to be removed for

- Male catheterisation in a patient with penile piercing—the ring can often be pulled to one side
- Surgery distant from the site of female/male genital piercing

If body piercing jewellery is to be left in situ:

- It should be taped over preoperatively—if possible.
- The site and nature of piercing should be documented on the preoperative checklist.
- A check should be performed to ensure the item is still in situ postoperatively.

Further reading

Perioperative guidelines for principles of safe practice with reference to surgical patients with body piercing (1999). *British Journal of Theatre Nursing*, **9**, 469.

Chapter 2

Consent and anaesthetic risk

Barry Baker and Kath Jenkins

Gavin Werrett

Consent

- 'It is a legal and ethical principle that valid consent must be obtained before starting treatment, physical investigation, or providing personal care for a patient.'[1] Health professionals who carry out procedures without valid consent are liable to legal action by the patient and investigation by the General Medical Council or equivalent professional bodies.
- Valid consent implies it is given voluntarily by a competent and informed person. To have capacity for consent, the patient must be able to comprehend and remember the information provided, weigh up the risks and benefits of the proposed procedure, and consider the consequences of not having the procedure in order to make a balanced decision.
- Case law on provision of information to patients has evolved over the last 10yr. Consent is a process rather than just a form to be signed. Patients should understand the nature and purpose of the procedure and be informed of any material or significant risks associated with the procedure, alternative treatments, and risks of doing nothing. It is the responsibility of the doctor to inform a patient of 'a significant risk which would affect the judgement of a reasonable patient'.[2]
- 'Known risks should be disclosed when an adverse outcome is common even though the detriment is slight, or when an adverse outcome is severe even though its occurrence is rare . . . Complex interventions require more information, as do interventions where the patient has no illness'.[3]
- Consent should be taken within the context of each patient's individual experiences, i.e. their values, background, and culture. However, in the current medico-legal climate it will be rare that patients should have detailed information withheld about the risks of anaesthesia or surgery on the grounds that they are likely to suffer adversely from such information.
- 'If an adult with capacity makes a voluntary and appropriately informed decision to refuse treatment this decision must be respected. This is the case even when this may result in death of the patient and/or the death of an unborn child, whatever stage of the pregnancy.'[1]
- Advance directives: advance refusal of treatment or 'living wills' written by competent individuals in case of future incapacity are normally valid and if so are legally binding.
- Young adults: competent young adults over the age of 16yr can give consent for any treatment without obtaining separate consent from a parent or guardian.
- Children: those under 16yr who demonstrate the ability to fully appreciate the risks and benefits of the intervention planned can be considered competent to give consent.[4]
- Refusal of treatment: children and young adults who refuse treatment may have their decision overridden by a parent or the court, but the treatment should proceed only if in the child's 'best interests'. When a child lacks capacity for consent, parental consent should be sought. If such a child refuses treatment, judgement needs to be exercised by the parent and the doctor as to the level of restraint that is acceptable,

depending on the urgency of the case. It may be better to postpone the case until adequate premedication can be given.

- In an emergency, verbal consent by telephone is adequate, and essential treatment can be started in the absence of parental authorisation if necessary. Where the child or parent refuses essential treatment, a ward of court order can be obtained (contact duty manager for the hospital), but this should not delay the emergency management. This enables the doctor to proceed with the treatment lawfully.

- Treatment without consent: in an emergency, consent is not necessary for life-saving procedures. Unconscious patients may be given essential treatment without consent. It is good practice to consult with the next of kin, but they cannot give or refuse consent for adult patients. Patients who are 'incompetent' may be given treatment provided it is in their 'best interests'. Electroconvulsive therapy requires patient's consent or the second opinion of an authorised medical practitioner.

- Restricted consent: patients may consent to treatment in general but refuse certain aspects of this treatment, e.g. Jehovah's Witness patients who refuse blood transfusion. This must be discussed in full with the patient so that they are fully aware of the implications of withholding the treatment. The details of the restriction should be carefully documented on the consent form. A competent patient's wishes must be respected at all times.

- Research and teaching: the same legal principles apply when seeking consent from patients for research or teaching. All clinical research requires ethics committee approval. As research may not have direct benefits for the patients involved, they must receive the fullest possible information about the proposed study, not be pressurised into taking part, and advised they can withdraw at any time without their care being affected. Incompetent patients can be included only in therapeutic research that is considered to be in their best interests. Competent children may give consent for clinical research associated with minimal risk. Students should obtain a patient's consent to undertake clinical procedures.

- Documentation: after discussion with the patient in an appropriate environment, the agreed anaesthetic and postoperative plan should be documented, including a list of risks explained. Written consent is obtained as part of the overall surgical consent form; separate anaesthetic consent forms are not currently deemed necessary[5] though they exist in some jurisdictions.

1 Department of Health (2001). *Reference guide to consent for examination or treatment.* http://www.doh.gov.uk/consent.
2 *Pearce* v. *United Bristol Healthcare NHS Trust* (1999). **48** *British Medical Law Reports* 118.
3 National Health and Medical Research Council (1993). *General Guidelines for Medical Practitioners on Providing Information to Patients.* Canberra: Australian Government Publishing Service.
4 *Gillick* v. *West Norfolk and Wisbech Area Health Authority* (1986). Appeal Court 112. http://www.swarb.co.uk/c/hl/1985gillick.html.
5 Association of Anaesthetists of Great Britain and Ireland (1999). *Information and consent for anaesthesia.* www.aagbi.org

Anaesthetic risk

The perception of risk is modified by a number of factors:
- Probability of occurrence—true incidence requires a large population sample and may be susceptible to
  - Regional bias—geographical variation in techniques
  - Exposure bias—catastrophic or dramatic over-publicity
  - Compression/expansion bias—underestimation of large risks, overestimation of small risks

Both patients' and anaesthetists' perceptions will contribute to the discussion of risks. Anaesthetists should recognise that their bias may frame the presentation of anaesthetic risk and that 'informed consent' may suffer as a consequence.

- Severity—high-severity risks such as death, paraplegia, and permanent organ failure, even though of very low probability, are perceived as higher overall risks than more common complications.
- Vulnerability—denial/optimism and a feeling of 'immunity' or 'invincibility' allow us to ignore daily risks.
- Controllability—loss of conscious choice with a feeling of loss of control increases vulnerability. Informed consent with a choice of clinical alternatives is important, as patients who perceive they have had adequate and realistic information with a choice of different anaesthetic options will be less resentful of any subsequent complications.
- Certainty/uncertainty—uncertainty, particularly about the facts, and fear of the uncertain or unknown upset the balance between rational and irrational decisions.
- Familiarity—patients who have had many anaesthetic procedures before will be less worried about any inherent risks, even though these risks may increase with progression of disease. Conversely, patients having their first anaesthetic will be more worried.
- Acceptability/dread—anaesthetists fear patient paraplegia more than patient death, stroke, or major myocardial infarction. Cultural or regional expectations may alter these perceptions, e.g. variations in use of local anaesthetic techniques.
- Framing or presentation—particularly when relative risks are discussed with patients, positive framing is better than negative framing: '90% survival' rather than '10% mortality', or outcomes are 'twice as good' with one management regimen than with another although the actual differences may only be between 0.005% and 0.01% mortality! Such 'bias' should not, however, impede discussion of the true incidence or real clinical significance with patients.

The mnemonic BRAN offers a useful approach when assessing the risks of a course of action: benefits, risks, alternatives, and what would happen if nothing were done.

Remember, whatever choice is made for or by any one patient, it will never be known what would have happened if another option had been chosen.

Risk level (ratio)	Verbal scale	Anaesthetic/medical examples	Example
1:1–9 Single digits	Very common	Pain 1:2 (day surgery) Transient ptosis after eye block 1:2 at 24hr (1:5 at 1 month) Sore throat 1:2 (ETT), 1:5 (LMA) Delirium after #NOF 1:2 PONV 1:4 Transient diplopia after eye block 1:4 Postop cognitive dysfunction (>60yr) 1:4 at 1wk Dizziness 1:5 Headache 1:5 Backache 1:5 (surgery <1hr), 1:2 (surgery >4hr) Transient arterial occlusion following cannulation 1:5 Transient deafness after spinal 1:7	Heads or tails coin toss 1:2 No pair (poker) 1:2 One pair (poker) 1:2.5 Rolling a six on a dice 1:6
1:10–99 Double digits	Common	Thrombophlebitis 1:10 Severe pain (major surgery) 1:10 Dural puncture headache 1:10 (day surgery) Postop cognitive dysfunction (>60yr) 1:10 at 3month Pneumothorax 1:20 (supraclavicular block) Transient blurred vision after GA 1:20 All oral trauma following intubation 1:20 Myocardial re-infarction 1:20 <3 months post-infarction (1:40 at 4–6 months) CVA or death 1:15 (symptomatic) for carotid endarterectomy CVA or death 1:25 (asymptomatic) for carotid endarterectomy Disabling CVA or death 1:50 (all) for carotid endarterectomy CVA 1:50 if previous stroke Arterial puncture at internal jugular vein cannulation 1:35	Getting 3 balls in UK National Lottery 1:11 Two pairs (poker) 1:20 Rolling a double six on a dice 1:36 Three of a kind (poker) 1:50 Dying in next 12 mth (men 55–64 yrs) 1:74

Table contd.

Risk level (ratio)	Verbal scale	Anaesthetic/medical examples	Example
		Emergency surgery death 1:40 (at 1 month)	
		Difficult intubation 1:50	
		Brachial plexus neurapraxia 1:50 (regional block)	
		Urinary dysfunction 1:50 (spinal/epidural)	
		Coronary stenting (death) 1:70	
1:100–999 Hundreds	Moderately common	CVA 1:100 (general surgery)	Dying of any cause in the next year 1:100
		Loss of vision (cardiac surgery) 1:100	
		Permanent postop cognitive dysfunction (>60yr) 1:100	
		Dural puncture headache following spinal 1:100	
		Permanent complications of arterial cannulation 1:100	Getting 4 balls in UK National Lottery 1:206
		Dental damage 1:100	
		Arterial puncture at subclavian vein cannulation 1:200	
		Periop death 1:200 (at 1 month) or 1:500 (at 2 days)	
		Awareness without pain 1:300	Flush (poker) 1:500
		Ulnar neuropathy 1:300 (GA)	Full house (poker) 1:700
		Awareness (TIVA) 1:500	
		Failure to intubate 1:500	
		Cerebral seizures 1:500 (brachial plexus block)	
		Brainstem anaesthesia following ophthalmic block 1:700	
1:1000–9999 Thousands	Less common	Corneal abrasion (GA) 1:1000	Exercise stress test death 1:2000
		Neuropathy (other than ulnar) 1:1000	
		Systemic LA toxicity 1:1500 (regional blocks)	
		Cerebral seizures 1:4000 (IV regional LA)	Four of a kind (poker) 1:4000
		Pulmonary artery perforation 1:2000	
		Awareness with pain 1:3000	Road traffic death in the next year 1:8000
		Aspiration pneumonitis 1:3000	
		Cardiac arrest 1:1500 (spinal) or 1:3000 (LA)	
		Permanent neuropathy at epidural 1:2000	

Category / frequency	Anaesthetic risk	Comparison
	Permanent neuropathy at epidural 1:2000 Permanent neuropathy at spinal 1:5000 Permanent neuropathy at peripheral nerve block 1:5000 Retrobulbar haemorrhage following eye block 1:5000 Epidural abscess after epidural catheter 1:5000 Failure to intubate/ventilate 1:5000 Death related to anaesthesia 1:5000 (ASA 3/4)	Accidental death at home 1:11 000
Rare 1:10 000–99 999 Tens of thousands	Anaphylaxis 1:10 000 Systemic LA toxicity 1:10 000 (epidural) Spontaneous epidural abscess 1:10 000 Globe perforation at eye block 1:10 000 Idiopathic deafness (GA) 1:10 000 Cardiac arrest 1:10 000 (epidural or regional block) Spontaneous sensorineural hearing loss (no anaesthesia) 1:10 000 (GA even rarer) Cardiac arrest 1:15 000 (GA)—with 15% death rate Death (related to anaesthesia) 1:50 000 Cranial nerve palsies (spinal) 1:50 000—commonest abducens	Getting 5 balls in UK National Lottery 1:11 098 Straight flush (poker) 1:70 000 Death hang gliding per flight 1:80 000
Very rare 1:100 000–999 999 Hundreds of thousands	Death (related to anaesthesia) 1:100 000 (ASA 1/2) Paraplegia (spinal/epidural) 1:100 000 Loss of vision (GA) 1:125 000 Epidural haematoma 1:150 000 (epidural), 1:200 000 (spinal) Death due solely to anaesthesia 1:180 000 Cranial subdural haematoma (after spinal) 1:500 000	Rail accident death 1:500 000 Royal straight flush (poker) 1:650 000
Excessively rare 1:1 000 000–9 999 999 Millions	Spontaneous epidural haematoma (no anaesthesia) 1:1 000 000	Getting 6 balls in UK National Lottery 1:2 796 763
Exceptional >1:10 000 000 Tens of millions or billions		Lightning strike 1:10 000 000

Perioperative mortality

- Overall mortality figures (UK) for *all* patients 1 month after
  - Elective surgery 1:177 (~1:200)
  - Emergency surgery 1:34 (~1:40)[1]
- Adult mortality rate within 30d of surgery
  - 1.2% total
  - 2.2% for age 60–69yr
  - 2.9% for age 70–79yr
  - 5.8–6.2% age for 80–89yr
  - 8.4% for age >90yr

Major surgery doubles these risks.[2]

- Incidence of death associated with anaesthesia in adult ASA 1 and 2 patients is approximately 1:100 000, with risk increased 5–10 times for high-risk patients (ASA 3–4) and/or emergency surgery.
- Anaesthetic paediatric mortality is 1:50 000.
- National studies of mortality that assess the quality of delivery of care continue to highlight factors that contribute to anaesthetic related mortality:
  - Inadequate preoperative assessment
  - Inadequate preparation and resuscitation
  - Inappropriate anaesthetic technique
  - Inadequate perioperative monitoring
  - Lack of supervision
  - Poor postoperative care
- Death rate associated with anaesthesia for Caesarean section is approximately 1:10 000, particularly due to difficult/failed endotracheal intubation.

1 Department of Health. NHS performance indicators. http://www.doh.gov.uk/nhsperformanceindicators.
2 Jin F, Chung F (2001). Minimizing perioperative adverse events in the elderly. *British Journal of Anaesthesia*, **87**, 608–624.

Perioperative morbidity

Cardiovascular

(See also p40.)

- The commonest causes for anaesthesia-related cardiac arrest include drug-related events, hypovolaemia, and failure of airway management.
- Beware restrictive cardiac output syndromes—aortic stenosis, mitral stenosis, constrictive pericarditis.
- Major cardiac complication rates are approximately halved when β-blockers are administered prophylactically for patients with more than two risk factors.
- Preoperative predictors of CVS risk in non-cardiac surgery are
  - High-risk surgery
  - History of ischaemic heart disease
  - History of congestive cardiac failure
  - History of cerebrovascular disease
  - Preoperative treatment with insulin
  - Preoperative serum creatinine >150μmol/l (or >2mg/dl).

Cardiac risk factors[1]		
Number of simple cardiac risk factors present	**Cardiac risk index**	**Approximate rate of cardiac complications (incl. death)(%)**
0	Class I	~0.5
1	Class II	~1.0
2	Class III	~5.0
3	Class IV	~10.0
4	Class V	~15.00

High-risk surgery (cardiac risk >5%)	**Intermediate-risk (cardiac risk 1–5%)**	**Low-risk surgery (cardiac risk <1%)**
Emergency major operations (particularly elderly patients)	Carotid endarterectomy	Endoscopic procedures
	Head and neck surgery	Superficial procedures
	Intraperitoneal surgery	Cataract surgery
Major vascular surgery	Intrathoracic surgery	Breast surgery
Peripheral vascular sugery	Orthopaedic surgery	
	Prostatic surgery	
Prolonged surgery with large fluid shifts		

Respiratory

See also p93.

- Postoperative respiratory complications (pneumonia/respiratory arrest) remain a major cause of surgical morbidity and mortality—poor postoperative analgesia may often contribute to the aetiology. Other major patient factors are FVC <1.5l or FEV_1/FVC <50%.[2]

Neurological

See p30.

Minor

- Incidences of relatively minor morbidity, such as pain and postoperative nausea and vomiting, have not changed significantly over the last 30yr despite improvements in anaesthetic drugs and techniques.
- Minor sequelae following surgery often have significant impact on patient recovery, leading to decreased function and slower resumption of daily activities following discharge.
- More than 50% of patients assume that pain is a normal part of the postoperative course/healing process and are prepared to suffer rather than complain.
- PONV has a multifactorial aetiology including type/duration of anaesthesia, drug therapy, type of surgery, and patient characteristics (particularly young, overweight, non-smoking females with a history of motion sickness/previous PONV) (see p1049).
- Identified patient risk factors associated with postoperative headache include a daily caffeine consumption of >400mg/d, a preoperative headache, a longer duration of fasting, and those who normally experience two or more headaches per month.

Further reading

Adams A (2002). The meaning of risk. In: McConachie I, ed. *Anaesthesia for the High Risk Patient*. London: Greenwich Medical Media, 239–247.

Association of Anaesthetists of Great Britain and Ireland (1999). Information and consent for anaesthesia. www.aagbi.org

Department of Health (2001). Reference guide to consent for examination or treatment. http://www.doh.gov.uk/consent.

General Medical Council, London (1998). Seeking patients' consent: the ethical considerations. http://www.gmc-uk.org.

Jenkins K, Baker AB (2003). Consent and anaesthetic risk. *Anaesthesia*, **58**, 962–984.

---

1 Eagle KA *et al.* (2002). ACC/AHA guideline update. http://www.acc.org/clinical/guidelines.
2 Gass GD, Olsen GN (1986). Preoperative pulmonary function testing to predict postoperative morbidity and mortality. *Chest*, **89**, 127–135.

Mortality and morbidity	Incidence	Comments
Total perioperative deaths within 30 days (UK)	1:200 elective surgery 1:40 emergency surgery	
Death		
Related to anaesthesia	1:50 000	1:100 000 (ASA 1–2)
CVS		
Cardiac arrest (GA)	1:10 000–1:20 000	Mortality 1:15 000 – 1:150 000
Cardiac arrest (LA)	1:3000	
Cardiac arrest (spinal)	1:1500	25% fatal
Myocardial reinfarction		
(0–3 months post-MI)	1:20	
(4–6 months post-MI)	1:40	
Respiratory		
Aspiration (GA)	1:3000	x4 in emergencies, x3 in obstetrics
Mortality due to aspiration	1:60 000	
Difficult intubation	1:50	
Failure to intubate	1:500	1:250 in obstetrics
Failure to intubate and ventilate	1:5000	

Neurological

Postop cognitive dysfunction (>60yr)	1:4 at 1 week 1:10 at 1 month 1:100 permanent	Irrespective of regional/general anaesthesia
Postoperative delirium	1:7 general surgery (up to 1:2 elderly #NOF)	
Cerebrovascular accident	1:50 if previous stroke 1:100 general surgery 1:20 head and neck surgery 1:20 carotid surgery	1:700 in non-surgical population
Awareness with pain	1:3000	
Awareness without pain	1:300	

Miscellaneous

Anaphylaxis	1:10 000	
Pain after major surgery	1:10 severe 1:3 moderate	
Pain after day surgery	1:2	
Nausea and vomiting (PONV)	1:4	Female:male 3:1
Sore throat	1:2 tracheal tube 1:5 laryngeal mask 1:10 facemask	
Drowsiness	1:2	
Dizziness	1:5	
Headache	1:5	

Table contd.

Mortality and morbidity	Incidence	Comments
Dental damage	1:100 overall	
	(1:5000 requiring intervention)	
All oral trauma post-intubation	1:20	
Deafness	1:10 000 GA	
	1:7 spinal (transient)	
Loss of vision	1:125 000 GA	
	1:100 cardiac surgery	
Peripheral nerve injury (GA)	1:300 ulnar neuropathy	
	1:1000 other nerves	
Regional		
Paraplegia after neuraxial block	1:100 000	
Permanent nerve injury (spinal)	1–3:10 000	
Permanent nerve injury (epidural)	0.3–10:10 000	
Permanent nerve injury (peripheral block)	1:5000	
Transient nerve injury (spinal)	1:125–1:2500	
Transient nerve injury (epidural)	1:1000–1:10 000	
Transient radicular irritation (spinal)	up to 1:3 (lidocaine/mepivacaine)	
Epidural haematoma	1:150 000 epidural	
	1:200 000 spinal	
	(1:1 000 000 spontaneous)	

Epidural abscess	1:2000–1:7500
	(1:10 000 spontaneous)
Cardiac arrest (spinal)	1:1500
Cardiac arrest (epidural)	1:10 000
Cardiac arrest (regional block)	1:10 000
Cardiac arrest (LA)	1:3000
Post-dural puncture headache (PDPH)	1:100
PDPH in day surgery	1:10
Backache	1:5 if <1hr surgery
	1:2 if >4hr surgery
Systemic LA toxicity	1:10 000 epidural
	1:1500 regional blocks
Eye blocks	
Retrobulbar haemorrhage	1:250–1:20 000
Brainstem anaesthesia	1:700
Globe perforation	1:10 000
Ptosis (transient)	1:2 at 24hr
	1:5 at 1 month

Nerve injury

- Neurological complications following regional anaesthesia can be divided into two categories—those directly related to the technique and those that coincide temporally with the technique (more frequent).
- The ASA Closed Claims Project Database (1975–95)[1] is one of the most reliable sources of information about perioperative nerve damage. Nerve injury was the second most common claim in the entire database (16% of total claims). Specifically, the nerves affected were ulnar nerve (28%), brachial plexus (20%), lumbosacral root (16%), and spinal cord (13%). Less commonly affected nerves were the sciatic, median, radial and femoral nerves.
- Spinal cord injury claims increased in frequency over the period—many associated with coagulopathy.
- Many cases of perioperative nerve damage have no identifiable mechanism (91% of ulnar injuries). However, the mechanism for spinal cord injury is determined in 48% of claims, and a regional anaesthetic has been administered in 68% of cases of spinal cord injury.
- Studies indicate that patients wish to know about the frequency of severe complications such as permanent nerve damage during informed consent for regional techniques.

Mechanisms of injury

- Direct trauma by needles, sutures, and instruments.
- Neurotoxicity of local anaesthetic agents.
- Ischaemia either from compression (haematoma/abscess/tourniquet/ positioning) or as a result of hypotension or added vasoconstrictors
- Infection.

Predisposing factors

- Surgery itself, tourniquets, tight-fitting casts, and intra-operative positioning more commonly cause specific nerve injury than regional techniques.
- Patients with pre-existing generalised peripheral neuropathy are at increased risk. Take a careful history and document any pre-existing deficit preoperatively.
- Anaesthetic factors include direct needle damage during regional anaesthesia. This can be decreased with good anatomical knowledge, experience, and careful technique.
- Traumatic insult occurs less frequently with short-bevelled needles, but, when it does occur, it is likely to be more significant than with sharp needles.
- There is no convincing evidence to mandate one technique of nerve localisation over another (paraesthesia v. nerve stimulation v. ultrasound).
- Significant resistance or severe pain on injection is an indication to stop injection (likely intraneural or intrafascicular injection). In work by

Auroy[2] 63% of cases of radiculopathy after spinal anaesthesia and 100% of cases of radiculopathy following epidural or peripheral nerve blockade were associated with either a paraesthesia during needle insertion or pain on injection.

- Failure to announce such pain on injection when performing blocks 'asleep' implies that 'awake' blocks might be safer, although this remains contentious and no adequate prospective trial data exist. Studies in anaesthetised children have not shown an increase in complication rates.
- Coagulopathy and local infection predispose to haematoma and abscess, respectively (see p35–36).
- Minimise tourniquet times and always use pneumatic tourniquets.
- Solutions of local anaesthetics with preservatives should not be used for spinal or epidural block. Laboratory and clinical evidence suggests that LA solutions themselves are potentially neurotoxic especially in high concentrations and after prolonged exposure. Bupivacaine appears to be safer than lidocaine and certainly causes less TNS (see below). Isobaric solutions reduce non-uniform distribution. Avoid routine use of adrenaline mixtures when not required, especially when combined with lidocaine.[3]

Diagnosis

- Symptoms can occur within hours (likely extra- or intraneural haematoma/oedema) but may not present for 2–3wk (suggestive of tissue reaction or scar formation).
- The intensity and duration of symptoms vary with severity of injury, from numbness and mild paraesthesia lasting a few weeks to persistent painful paraesthesia, sensory loss, motor loss, or indeed progression to a complex regional pain syndrome (Type 2).
- Significance of injury depends on three factors: severity, duration, and the patient; i.e. mild motor weakness may be a nuisance to an elderly patient yet catastrophic for an athlete.
- Perform a thorough neurological examination and document carefully any abnormalities detected. Refer for specialist neurological advice early.
- A senior neurologist should be able to delineate clinically between a specific peripheral nerve root lesion and a radiculopathy. This can be confirmed with nerve conduction studies/EMG.
- Suspected central lesions need definitive localisation with MRI imaging.
- Any progressive pathology or suggestion of central damage needs immediate investigation (see below).
- In cases of neurological injury, consider commencing therapy early, aiming to reduce neuropathic pain states, e.g. tricyclic antidepressants (amitriptyline up to 150mg/day, starting at 25mg nocte) and anti-epileptics (gabapentin 300mg od increased to 600mg tds or carbamazepine 100mg od/bd increased to 200mg qds).

1 Cheney FW et al. (1999). Nerve injury associated with anaesthesia—a closed claims analysis. Anesthesiology, **90**, 1062–1069.
2 Auroy Y et al. (1997). Serious complications related to regional anesthesia: results of a prospective survey in France. Anesthesiology, **87**, 479–486.
3 Drasner K (1997). Lidocaine spinal anesthesia: a vanishing therapeutic index? Anesthesiology, **87**, 469–472.

Peripheral nerve injury

The ulnar nerve is the most commonly affected (see below). Other commonly affected nerves include the common peroneal (especially after prolonged lithotomy), radial, femoral, and the lateral cutaneous nerve of the thigh (meralgia paraesthetica—often wrongly attributed to regional anaesthesia). Neurological injury is especially common in obstetrics (20% transient dysfunction postpartum but only 1:500 significant in long term). Overall incidence for other nerves (excluding ulnar) is 1:1000. Symptoms will vary according to the site and severity of the lesion.

Ulnar neuropathy

- This is more common in males (3:1).
- Increased at extremes of weight and with prolonged hospital stay. Uncommon in young patients.
- Prospective studies indicate a frequency of ~1:200 patients acutely, but clinically significant lesions are much less common at 3 months.
- 85% of cases occur in association with GA; 15% occur after regional block (6% after spinal), indicating the unclear aetiology.
- Injuries occur at the superficial condylar groove of the elbow. Men appear to have less fat at this site and a narrower tunnel, possibly explaining the sex distribution.
- Additional padding was explicitly stated to have been used in 27% of closed claims!
- In 62% the onset was 'delayed' (i.e. >1d postoperatively).
- Abnormal nerve conduction is common in the contralateral, unaffected arm, indicating subclinical neuropathy that may have become symptomatic in the perioperative period.

Classification

- The degree of damage will determine the level of intervention required and the likelihood of recovery:
    - Neurapraxia—myelin damaged, axon intact. Recovery in weeks to months. Good prognosis.
    - Axonotmesis—axonal disruption. Prognosis and recovery variable.
    - Neurotmesis—nerve completely severed. Surgery may be required. Prognosis poor.

Brachial plexus injury

- Incidence varies from 1:25 000[1] to 1:250[2] for long-term complications.
- Causal factors include excessive stretch (arm abduction with lateral rotation of the head to the opposite side), compression (upward movement of the clavicle and sternal retraction), and associated regional block (only 16% of closed claims for brachial plexus injury).
- Pain or paraesthesia on injection was noted in 50% of claims associated with a regional technique.
- The long thoracic nerve was damaged in 13% of closed claims for brachial plexus injury (causing winging of the scapula). The mechanism was unknown.
- Lesions affecting the upper roots are more common.
- Catheter techniques do not appear to be associated with increased risk of injury.

Lumbosacral root injury (radiculopathy)

- There is an approximate incidence of 1:5000 for permanent damage.
- Over 90% occur in association with a regional technique (55% spinal, 37% epidural).
- Paraesthesia, pain during needle insertion, or pain on injection of drug is often reported. Postoperative radicular pain may persist in up to 0.2% of cases but will almost always resolve in weeks/months.
- Multiple unsuccessful attempts increase the likelihood of damage.
- Persisting paraesthesia, with or without motor symptoms, is the most common complaint.

Nerve root	Sensory loss	Motor weakness
L2	Upper anterior thigh	Hip flexion
L3	Lower anterior and medial thigh	Thigh adduction
L4	Lateral thigh, knee, medial leg	Leg extension
L5	Lateral leg, dorsum of foot	Ankle dorsi-flexion
S1	Lateral foot	Ankle plantar flexion

1 Pearce v. *United Bristol Healthcare NHS Trust* (1999). **48** *British Medical Law Reports* 118.
2 Borgeat A *et al.* (2001). Acute and nonacute complications associated with interscalene block and shoulder surgery. *Anesthesiology*, **95**, 875–880.

Spinal cord injury

General considerations

- 58% of cases were associated with regional anaesthesia in the closed claims data. See also p30.
- A definitive pathogenesis was implicated in ~50% of the cases—much higher than with other causes of nerve damage.
- The commonest mechanisms were epidural haematoma, chemical injury, anterior spinal artery syndrome, and meningitis, in that order.
- Lumbar epidural was the commonest regional technique implicated—*four times* more frequently than subarachnoid block. There is no evidence to suggest thoracic epidurals have a higher incidence of associated injury.
- Injury was more common in blocks performed for chronic pain management and in the presence of systemic anticoagulation (LMWH introduced to the United States in 1993).
- Significant delays in the diagnosis of cord or nerve compression were noted. Persistent weakness or numbness was often presumed to be secondary to epidural infusions.
- Motor blockade of the legs is not a feature of thoracic epidural with dilute solutions of LA and opioid. Regular assessment of motor function is essential and epidural analgesia should be stopped if patients have inappropriate motor blockade or neurological deficit in their limbs. If there is no improvement in 2hr, urgent MRI is required to exclude haematoma/abscess.
- Cases of spinal epidural abscess/haematoma are more frequently associated with epidural block, whereas cauda equina syndrome, radiculopathy, and meningitis are more often associated with a spinal technique.[1]
- As a rule, serious neurological complications occur much less frequently in the obstetric population—1 in 25 000 against 1 in 3600.[2]

Conus medullaris injury[3]

- Incidence about 1:20 000. Confirmed at MRI—often with a visible syrinx.
- Suggested by pain at needle insertion and subsequent sensory loss at L4/5. Urinary symptoms may or may not be present. Normal CSF flow and block do not exclude this pathology.
- Tip of conus medullaris usually lies at L1/2 although it may extend further. Tuffier's line (line joining the iliac crests) is an unreliable marker for identifying lumbar interspaces. Anaesthetists are poor at predicting lumbar interspaces—therefore, choose the lowest possible interspace.

Anterior spinal artery syndrome

- Blood supply to the cord is precarious, and systemic hypotension, with or without a regional block, can produce spinal cord ischaemia. There is theoretical evidence to suggest adrenaline-containing solutions increase the risk.
- Aortic surgery, thromboembolism, vasculitides, and vertebral surgery are other causes.

Cauda equina syndrome (CES)

- Incidence ~1:10 000.
- Small nerve fibres are most vulnerable to ischaemia/pressure/toxic compounds. Thus autonomic nerves of the cauda equina are often the first to be involved. Damage to S2–S4 sacral nerve roots leads to alteration in bladder and/or bowel habit, leading to urinary retention and absolute constipation in the untreated patient.
- Sensory alteration usually occurs in the perineum.
- Leg weakness will be lower motor neurone and may progress upwards.
- CES has most commonly been related to use of microcatheters and 5% lidocaine. Microcatheters thinner than 24G have been banned in the USA since 1992.

Transient neurological symptoms (TNS)

- Defined as pain or dysaesthesia in the legs or buttocks starting within 24hr of, but after recovery from, spinal anaesthesia.
- There is typically no demonstrable motor or sensory defect. NCS/EMG will be normal. Symptoms typically resolve within days.
- Incidence is markedly increased with use of lidocaine solutions. Lithotomy and knee flexion positions possibly increase the incidence.
- Clinical significance/genuine aetiology is unknown—possibly represents the origin of toxicity on a continuum to irreversible CES.

Spinal epidural abscess (SEA)

- Spontaneous SEA (i.e. unrelated to any regional technique) has an incidence of ~1:10 000.
- Epidural abscess related to a neuraxial technique occurs between 1:2000[4] and 1:5000 blocks. In the obstetric population this risk is reduced to ~1:25 000.
- Proposed mechanisms of infection include haematogenous spread, invasion of skin bacteria via needle track, contaminated syringes or LA solutions, and breaches in sterile technique.
- Chlorhexidine in 80% ethanol is superior to povidone iodine at decontamination as it penetrates into hair follicles and stratum corneum.
- Handwashing, gloves, gowns, hats, and probably masks should be used (clusters of streptococcal meningitis have been reported following catheter placement by an infected anaesthetist).
- The classic triad of symptoms is fever, backache, and neurological deficits. However, prognosis for recovery is very poor once neurological signs have been present for >24hr.
- Incidence is higher with catheters inserted for >2d, in IV drug users, the immunocompromised (including chronic renal failure, alcoholism, and diabetes) and in anticoagulated patients. Perioperative antibiotics may provide some protection from SEA.

1 Moen V et al. (2004). Severe neurological complications after central neuraxial blockade in Sweden 1990–1999. Anesthesiology, 101, 950–959.
2 Association of Anaesthetists of Great Britain and Ireland (1999). Information and consent for anaesthesia. www.aagbi.org
3 Reynolds F (2001). Damage to the conus medullaris following spinal anaesthesia. Anaesthesia, 56, 235–247.
4 Wang LP et al. (1999). Incidence of spinal epidural abscess after epidural analgesia: a national 1-year survey. Anesthesiology, 91, 1928–1936.

- Suspect SEA in patients with fever and back pain or those with unexplained pyrexia and a history of spinal intervention. Pus at the site of needle track, erythema extending >1cm around the injection site, and local tenderness are all worrying signs. Neurological examination may be normal in up to two-thirds of cases in the early stages. Bladder/bowel dysfunction is a very late sign.
- CRP is the best blood marker (>40mg/l) and can be used to monitor therapy in patients with no serious neurological deficits who may not need to undergo decompressive surgery. WCC and ESR are both usually also raised. Early MRI is the definitive investigation.
- All patients should have blood cultures taken, skin swab and epidural catheter tips sent for bacterial culture. The commonest organism is *Staphylococcus aureus* (~60%). Start broad-spectrum antibiotics immediately at diagnosis being sure to cover staphylococci. IV antibiotics will be modified when organisms detected. Minimum 3wk IV therapy and subsequently oral therapy for 8wk if CRP/MRI show improvement.
- Immediate neurosurgical referral is mandatory and prompt surgical decompression is vital if there is a significant neurological deficit—recovery is related to the duration of neurological symptoms. Patients treated after 36hr of severe deficits are unlikely to improve. Diagnosis to surgery should be under 8hr.
- Patients with evidence of systemic infection may safely undergo spinal anaesthesia only if antibiotic therapy has been initiated earlier and there has been a response to therapy, e.g. reduction in fever. Indwelling catheters in this group remain controversial. Careful selection, close monitoring (for SEA and meningitis), and early removal of epidural catheter is paramount. Avoid entirely if local infection present.

Arachnoiditis

- This may present weeks or even months after regional anaesthesia.
- There is progressive weakness and sensory loss, sometimes leading to paraplegia and death.
- It carries a poor prognosis and may be caused by haemorrhage, meningitis, spinal surgery, or toxic substances inadvertently introduced into the spinal or epidural space.

Spinal/epidural haematoma

- Most spinal haematomas originate in the epidural space from the venous plexus.
- In a patient with normal clotting and free of medication affecting clotting, the incidence of haematoma is estimated to be 1:150 000 for epidurals and 1:220 000 for spinals. Incidence is increased with age, female sex, renal disease, and hepatic disease. Decreased weight may predispose to relative overdose of 'prophylactic' LMWH.
- However, many patients receiving a neuraxial technique will have a degree of coagulopathy that is either iatrogenic or a result of their medical condition.
- The incidence increases markedly (1:3000) for epidural-induced haematoma in the presence of high-dose LMWH therapy.

- Despite being a procoagulant state, haematoma has also been reported in obstetrics, but at a frequency of 1:200 000[1].
- If suspected—stop epidural infusion, do not remove catheter, and if neurology is unchanged at 2hr, arrange urgent MRI scan. Discuss positive findings with a senior neurosurgeon.

Neuraxial blockade in the anticoagulated patient
See p1054.

Clinical features of spinal syndromes

	Spinal/epidural abscess	Spinal haematoma	Anterior spinal artery syndrome
Age	Any	Majority over 50yr	Elderly
History	Infection, immuno-compromised	Abnormal clotting	Atheroma, peripheral vascular disease, hypotension
Onset	1–3 days	Hours	Sudden
General symptoms	Malaise, fever, back-ache, meningism	Sharp back pain. Radicular	None
Sensory signs	None or paraesthesia	Variable, late	Minor
Motor signs	Flaccid, later spastic	Flaccid	Flaccid
Scan	Compression	Compression	Normal
CSF	Infected	Normal	Normal
Blood	CRP, WCC, ESR raised	Coagulopathy	Normal

Further reading
Horlocker TT (2004). What`s a nice patient like you doing with a complication like this? Diagnosis, prognosis and prevention of spinal haematoma. *Canadian Journal of Anaesthesia*, **51**, 527–534.
Horlocker TT et al. (2000). Neurologic complications of spinal and epidural anesthesia. *Regional Anesthesia and Pain Medicine*, **25**, 83–99.

1 Association of Anaesthetists of Great Britain and Ireland (1999). Information and consent for anaesthesia. www.aagbi.org

Cardiovascular disease

Richard Telford

Peter Murphy

Ischaemic heart disease

Ischaemic heart disease (IHD) is one of the main contributory factors to postoperative morbidity and mortality. Up to 20% of patients undergoing surgery have preoperative evidence of myocardial ischaemia. The overall rate for perioperative myocardial infarction (MI) is 0.7% for general surgery, increasing to 3% for vascular surgery.

Perioperative risk

The key to reducing perioperative cardiovascular morbidity is to identify high-risk patients beforehand. Cardiovascular risk is influenced by patient factors (including functional capacity), and by the nature of the planned surgery. See also p24.

Patient factors

Major risk predictors (markers of unstable coronary artery disease)	Recent MI (<1 month prior to planned surgery) Unstable or severe angina Ongoing ischaemia after MI (clinical symptoms or non-invasive testing) Decompensated heart failure Significant arrhythmias (high grade AV block, symptomatic arrhythmias or supraventricular arrhythmias with uncontrolled ventricular rate) Severe valvular heart disease (aortic, mitral stenosis) CABG/PTCA (<6wk)
Intermediate risk predictors (markers of stable coronary artery disease)	Prior MI (>1 month prior to planned surgery) Stable mild angina Compensated heart failure Abnormal renal function Diabetes
Minor risk predictors (increased probability of heart disease)	Advanced (physiological) age Abnormal ECG Rhythm other than sinus Low functional capacity Previous stroke Uncontrolled systemic hypertension

Functional capacity

Exercise tolerance is a major predictor of perioperative risk. The physiological response to surgery increases oxygen demand, requiring a subsequent increase in cardiac output. Ability to exercise is an excellent indicator of 'cardiovascular fitness'. It is usually expressed in metabolic equivalents (METs) on a scale defined by the Duke Activity Status Index. Patients who cannot sustain 4 METs of physical activity frequently have adverse outcomes following high risk surgery (see also p42 'Cardiopulmonary exercise testing').

1–4 METs	• Eating, dressing, dishwashing, and walking around the house
4–10 METs	• Climbing a flight of stairs, walking on level ground at >6km/hr, running briefly, playing golf
>10 METs	• Strenuous sports: swimming, singles tennis, football

Surgical factors

High risk: >5% death/non-fatal MI	Major emergency surgery (esp. in elderly) Aortic/major vascular surgery Prolonged surgery with large fluid shifts
Intermediate risk: <5% death/non-fatal MI	Carotid endarterectomy Head and neck surgery Intraperitoneal and intrathoracic surgery Orthopaedic surgery Prostatic surgery
Low risk: <1% death/non-fatal MI	Minimally invasive endoscopic surgery Cataract extraction Superficial surgery (incl. breast)

Special investigations

12-lead ECG

- All patients over 60yr undergoing major surgery, and anyone with risk factors for IHD should have a preoperative ECG.
- Arrhythmias and cardiac conduction abnormalities require careful evaluation for underlying cardiopulmonary disease, drug toxicity, or metabolic abnormality.
- Many patients with underlying IHD have a normal resting ECG.

Exercise testing

- Exercise ECG: test of choice in ambulatory patients. Provides an estimate of functional capacity and detects myocardial ischaemia. ST segment depression is suggestive of myocardial ischaemia. Tachyarrhythmias or significant falls in systolic blood pressure are also highly suggestive of impaired oxygen delivery to the myocardium. Those patients who are unable to exercise or have pre-existing ECG abnormalities (e.g. left bundle branch block, ventricular hypertrophy/ strain, digitalis effect) should have a pharmacological stress test.
- Cardiopulmonary exercise testing: usually performed on a bicycle ergometer using respiratory gas analysis and an ECG. An arm ergometer is available for those patients who cannot cycle. Under exercise conditions oxygen consumption is a linear function of cardiac output, thus aerobic capacity is a surrogate measurement of ventricular function. An aerobic threshold of >11ml/min/kg appears to predict survival after major abdominal surgery with high sensitivity and specificity—see also p992.

Pharmacological stress testing

- Dipyridamole thallium scintography: uses a coronary vasodilator (dipyridamole) and a radio isotope (thallium) which is taken up by perfused heart muscle. It shows up areas of impaired perfusion as reversible perfusion defects caused by dipyridamole induced 'steal'. Areas of non-perfused myocardium show up as permanent perfusion defects.
- Dobutamine stress echocardiography: utilises an increasing dose of dobutamine (to a maximum of 40µg/kg/min) with simultaneous 2D precordial echocardiography to look for new or worsening wall motion abnormalities as an indicator of impaired perfusion. It is a complex, time-consuming test requiring expertise.

Coronary arteriography

Patients who have positive stress tests should be referred for coronary arteriography. Indications for coronary revascularisation prior to noncardiac surgery are identical to those for coronary artery bypass grafts on prognostic grounds, i.e. left main stem disease, severe triple vessel disease, proximal left anterior descending disease, and impaired left ventricular function. Following cardiac surgery subsequent surgery should be delayed for 3 months.

Percutaneous coronary intervention

There is no indication for PCI prior to elective surgery. PCI causes trauma to the vessel wall rendering the endoluminal surface thrombogenic until the stent has re endothelialised. Dual antiplatelet medication (aspirin/clopidogrel) is necessary to prevent local coronary thrombosis—aspirin for life, clopidogrel for 6 weeks (bare metal stents) or up to 12 months (drug eluting stents). Stopping antiplatelet medication perioperatively is associated with a very high cardiac complication rate. Drug eluting stent thrombosis has been reported as late as 1yr after stent insertion when antiplatelet medications have been stopped for surgery. In most patients the antiplatelet regime should be continued perioperatively as the risk of stent thrombosis is greater than the risk of bleeding. If a patient taking dual antiplatelet therapy post PCI needs an operation where bleeding may be problematic, consider briefly stopping clopidogrel (<3 days) and adding heparin by infusion (APTR >1.5) or low molecular weight heparin (enoxaparin 1mg/kg/day).

Only life saving operations should be performed within 6–12 weeks of PCI, irrespective of the antiplatelet regime, as there is a very high risk of cardiac complications (up to 45%).[1]

Choice of perioperative testing

Evaluation of patients with IHD depends on the planned surgery, facilities, and time available. Precise recommendations remain controversial, but careful history, examination, and practical application of preoperative screening tests is important. Little advantage is gained from complex examinations which will not alter management. The positive predictive value of most tests is low. Close liaison with both cardiological and surgical colleagues is required. At times investigations will indicate the need to consider an alternative less invasive surgical procedure.

Cardiological referral

Exercise tolerance	Any	<4 METs	>4 METs	<4 METs	>4 METs
	Cardiac risk				
Surgical risk	Major	Intermediate		Minor	
High	Refer	Refer	Refer	Refer	Operate
Intermediate	Refer	Refer	Operate	Operate	Operate
Low	Refer	Operate	Operate	Operate	Operate

See p41 for definition of METs and surgical risk.

1 Spahn DR, Howell SJ, Delebays A, Chassot PG (2006). Coronary stents and perioperative antiplatelet regimen: dilemma of bleeding and stent thrombosis. *British Journal of Anaesthesia* **96**, 675–677.

Perioperative medical therapy

Continue medical therapy perioperatively to protect against ischaemic stresses. Drugs should be given IV where possible if GI absorption is impaired.

- Small prospective randomised trials have shown benefit if patients are treated with a β-blocker in the perioperative period. This should be considered in high risk patients, particularly before major vascular surgery. Ideally the patient should be established on a β-blocker for a week preoperatively, but IV loading may be beneficial in emergency patients. β-blockers should continue for at least a week postoperatively.[1,2]
- Randomised trials have shown α₂ agonists to be beneficial and represent an alternative to β-blockers.[3] Clonidine is the most widely available (up to 300µg daily).
- Nitrates should be continued perioperatively—IV or transdermally if necessary. There is no evidence that prophylactic administration decreases the risk of perioperative cardiac complications.
- Calcium channel blockers should be continued preoperatively and resumed as soon as possible postoperatively. They have never been shown to confer protection against perioperative cardiac complications. The dihydropyridine group (especially nifedipine) may add to the risk of acute MI.
- ACE inhibitors improve survival in patients with left ventricular dysfunction and offer major benefits to patients with vascular disease or diabetes and normal left ventricular function. In the perioperative period they may increase the risk of hypotension, requiring more invasive haemodynamic monitoring for major surgery. Some anaesthetists routinely stop administration in the perioperative period—if stopped for several days restart at a reduced dose.
- Perioperative statin administration has been shown to improve both short term and long term cardiac outcome following non cardiac and coronary bypass surgery. Statins enhance plaque stability making plaque rupture less likely[4].

Anaesthetic considerations

- In addition to standard monitoring, invasive cardiovascular monitoring (arterial line, CVP ± cardiac output monitoring) should be used for high/intermediate-risk patients undergoing major surgery. ECG monitoring should be CM5 configuration or similar.
- There is no evidence that any particular technique is superior. Avoid tachycardia, hypotension/hypertension to minimise myocardial ischaemia.
- Good analgesia is important since uncontrolled pain is a potent cause of tachycardia: regional blocks can be very effective. Central neuraxial blocks ameliorate the hypercoagulable state seen following anaesthesia and surgery.

- Haemoglobin levels should be kept >9g/dl.
- Myocardial ischaemia may occur during emergence and extubation. Hypertension and tachycardia should be anticipated and avoided. The use of a short-acting β-blocker, e.g. esmolol, should be considered.
- Consider admission to HDU postoperatively for close monitoring.
- Following major surgery, all patients at risk should have supplemental oxygen for 3–4d.

1 Mangano DT, Layug EL, Wallace A, Tateo I for the Multicenter Study of Perioperative Ischemia Research Group (1996). Effect of atenolol in mortality and cardiovascular morbidity after non-cardiac surgery. New England Journal of Medicine, 335, 1713–1720.
2 Poldermans D, Boersma E, Baxx JJ, et al. (1999). The effect of bisoprolol on perioperative mortality and myocardial infarction in high risk patients undergoing vascular surgery. Dutch Echocardiographic Cardiac Risk Evaluation Applying Stress Echocardiography Study Group. New England Journal of Medicine, 341, 1789–1794.
3 Wijeysundera DN, Naik JS, Beattie WS (2003). Alpha 2 agonists to prevent perioperative cardiovascular complications: a metanalysis. American Journal of Medicine, 114, 742–752.
4 Biccard BM, Sear JW, Foex P. (2005). Statin therapy: a potentially useful perioperative intervention in patients with cardiovascular disease. Anaesthesia 60, 1106–1114

Perioperative acute myocardial infarction

Perioperative myocardial infarction usually occurs in the 3–4d following surgery. The majority are preceded by episodes of ST segment depression. Acute plaque rupture and haemorrhage is common, but the severity of underlying stenosis does not necessarily predict infarct territory. The best markers of myocardial injury are the cardiac troponins T and I. These are highly sensitive and specific for myocardial damage.

• Rapid treatment is essential. Move patients to an HDU.
• All patients should receive supplemental oxygen.
• Patients should be given SL glyceryl trinitrate and IV morphine to relieve any chest pain.
• Pulmonary oedema if present should be treated with upright posture, IV furosemide (40mg), and IV nitrates. CPAP should be considered.
• Other therapeutic options are reduced postoperatively. Acute thrombolysis is relatively contraindicated by recent surgery. Aspirin (150mg od) should be used and β-blockade instituted if possible (atenolol 5mg IV followed by 50–100mg PO daily). If available, acute angioplasty should be considered—close liaison with a cardiologist is essential.

Further reading

Mukherjee D, Eagle KA (2003). Perioperative cardiac assessment for noncardiac surgery: eight steps to the best possible outcome. *Circulation*, **107**, 2771–2774.

Eagle KA, Berger PB, Calkins H, *et al.* (2002). ACC/AHA Guideline Update for Perioperative Cardiovascular Evaluation for Non Cardiac Surgery. A Report of the American College of Cardiology/American Heart Association Task Force on Practice Guidelines (Committee to Update the 1996 Guidelines on Perioperative Cardiovascular Evaluation for Non Cardiac Surgery). *Circulation*, **105**, 1257–1267.

Chassot PG, Delabays A, Spahn DR (2002). Preoperative evaluation of patients with, or at risk of, coronary artery disease undergoing coronary artery surgery. *British Journal of Anaesthesia*, **89**, 747–759.

Heart failure

Heart failure is the commonest cause of admission to hospital in those aged >65yr. Incidence rises with increasing age. It has ~50% 5yr mortality. Characterised by

- Fatigue
- Exercise intolerance
- Orthopnoea
- Exertional dyspnoea
- High incidence of ventricular arrhythmias
- Shortened life expectancy

Perioperatively heart failure is associated with a substantially increased risk of mortality/morbidity. A patient with uncontrolled heart failure undergoing an emergency laparotomy has a mortality risk of 20–30%.

Medical management

- Diuretics reduce peripheral and pulmonary congestion. Spironolactone improves mortality when used in conjunction with ACE inhibitors in patients with severe heart failure (EF <25%)
- Vasodilators decrease preload and afterload. ACE inhibitors, and to a lesser extent angiotensin-II receptor antagonists, improve survival. Nitrates are also used.
- β-blockers (carvedilol, bisoprolol) are indicated to reduce heart rate and myocardial oxygen demand. Studies show improved survival but cardiological input is required.
- Inotropes: digoxin improves symptoms and may be used to control the ventricular rate in atrial fibrillation and in patients in sinus rhythm with severe or worsening heart failure.
- Anticoagulation: indicated for atrial fibrillation and for those with a history of thromboembolism, left ventricular aneurysm, or with evidence of intracardiac thrombus on echo.
- Some patients with intractable heart failure may have atrial synchronous biventricular pacing devices inserted in an attempt to improve functional capacity and quality of life.
- Some patients with severely impaired ventricular performance and a history of ventricular tachycardia/ventricular fibrillation will have biventricular automatic implantable cardioverter defibrillators (AICDs) inserted for secondary prevention of arrhythmic death—see p90.

Preoperative assessment
- History and examination should identify present or recent episodes of decompensated heart failure (any within 6 months adversely affects risk).
- Optimise medical therapy to minimise symptoms of left ventricular dysfunction and maximise functional capacity.
- Continue anti-failure therapy in the preoperative period.
- Consider a period of preoperative 'optimisation' in the ICU/HDU.
- Treat metabolic abnormalities.
- Treat symptomatic arrhythmias and attempt to optimise heart rate to around 80bpm. Rhythms other than sinus are poorly tolerated (especially AF), as properly timed atrial contractions contribute up to 30% of ventricular filling.

Special investigations

Blood tests (to evaluate aggravating factors)
- FBC, U&Es, LFT, thyroid function tests, fasting lipids, and glucose

12-lead ECG
- Check for arrhythmias. AF may worsen heart failure by reducing cardiac filling time.

CXR
- Prominent upper lobe veins (upper lobe diversion), engorged peripheral lymphatics (Kerley B lines), alveolar oedema ('bats' wings')
- Pleural effusions, cardiomegaly

Transthoracic echocardiography
- Most useful test particularly when coupled with Doppler flow studies. Will determine whether the primary abnormality is pericardial/myocardial/valvular, systolic/diastolic, segmental/global. Echo also allows quantitative assessment of the ventricles, atria, pericardium, valves, and vascular structures.
- Alternatives include transoesophageal echocardiography, radionuclide imaging, or cardiac magnetic resonance imaging
- Modern echo machines generate values for ejection fraction (normal range 60–80%) and fractional shortening (normal range 28–44%) which define the degree of left ventricular (LV) impairment.

Ejection fraction 40–50 %	—	mild LV impairment
Ejection fraction 30–40%	—	moderate LV impairment
Ejection fraction <30%	—	severe LV impairment

Cardiac catheterisation
- Is sometimes performed if significant coronary or valvular heart disease is suspected as a cause of heart failure. Ventricular performance may sometimes be improved if there are areas of ventricular muscle whose contractility may be improved if the blood supply is restored—'hibernating myocardium'.

Perioperative management

- Some patients may be deemed unfit for the proposed surgery. Patients with severe heart failure (EF <30%) are dependent on preload to maintain ventricular filling. Many also rely on increased sympathetic tone. Such patients are living 'on a knife edge' and are exquisitely sensitive to small alterations in their physiology.
- Use local or regional techniques for peripheral procedures.
- There is little conclusive evidence of the benefits of general versus regional anaesthesia for more major surgery.
- Patients should receive all their anti-failure medications on the morning of surgery.
- Digoxin should be given IV postoperatively if the patient is in AF but if in sinus rhythm it can usually be omitted until eating resumes. Nitrates can be given transdermally while nil by mouth.
- ACE inhibitors should be resumed as soon as possible postoperatively. If omitted for 3d or more they should be reintroduced at a low dose to minimise first-dose hypotension.
- Whichever anaesthetic technique is chosen minimise negative inotropy, tachycardia, diastolic hypotension, and systolic hypertension. Careful monitoring of fluid balance is essential. Invasive cardiovascular monitoring, including measurement of cardiac output should be considered for all major surgery.
- Patients who decompensate in the perioperative period may require treatment with inotropes such as dobutamine or phosphodiesterase inhibitors.
- Renal perfusion is easily compromised due to markedly impaired glomerular filtration rates and patients are susceptible to renal failure perioperatively. If urine output falls, hypovolaemia should be excluded and adequate perfusion pressure and cardiac output ensured before diuretics are used. NSAIDs are a potent renal insult in these patients and their use requires care.
- All patients should have supplemental oxygen following surgery.
- Good postoperative analgesia is essential to minimise detrimental effects of catecholamine release in response to pain.
- Have a low threshold for admission to ICU/HDU in the postoperative period.

Further reading

Magner JJ, Royston D (2004). Heart failure. *British Journal of Anaesthesia*, **91**, 74–85.

Hypertension

15% of patients are hypertensive (systolic >140mmHg, diastolic >90mmHg). The link between elevated arterial pressure and cardiovascular disease is well established, with the greatest risk associated with the highest arterial pressures.

Traditionally many patients have had anaesthesia and surgery deferred to allow hypertension to be treated. Evidence that moderately elevated blood pressure is associated with increased perioperative risk is limited, although increased cardiovascular lability under anaesthesia ('alpine anaesthesia') frequently occurs. However, the association of hypertension with end-organ damage (ischaemic heart disease, heart failure, renal failure) contributes significantly to the likelihood of perioperative cardiovascular complications.

Preoperative evaluation

- Is hypertension primary or secondary? Consider the rare possibility of phaeochromocytoma, hyperaldosteronism, renal parenchymal hypertension, or renovascular hypertension. These will have individual anaesthetic implications.
- Is the hypertension severe? Patients with Stage 3 hypertension (systolic >180mmHg, diastolic >110mmHg) should ideally have this treated prior to elective surgery.
- Is there evidence of end-organ involvement? The presence of coronary or cerebrovascular disease, impairment of renal function, signs of left ventricular hypertrophy, or heart failure puts patients in a high-risk category. These conditions may require further investigation and/or treatment in addition to control of elevated blood pressure.

Perioperative management

Few guidelines exist as to which patients should be cancelled to allow hypertension to be treated or the duration of such treatment prior to surgery. There is little evidence for an association between admission arterial pressures of <180mmHg systolic or <110mmHg diastolic and perioperative cardiovascular complications. A recent meta analysis of 30 papers involving 12 995 perioperative patients demonstrated an odds ratio for the association between hypertensive disease and cardiovascular complications of 1.35, which is not clinically significant.[1]

- Do not defer surgery on the basis of a single blood pressure reading on admission to hospital. Obtain several further readings after admission. The GP may have a record of previous readings.
- Continue preoperative antihypertensive treatment during the perioperative period.
- **Stage 1** (systolic 140–159mmHg, diastolic 90–99mmHg) and **Stage 2** (systolic 160–179mmHg, diastolic 100–109mmHg) hypertension is not an independent risk factor for perioperative cardiovascular complications. Surgery should normally proceed in these patients.

- If a patient has **Stage 3** hypertension (systolic >180mmHg, diastolic >110mmHg), with evidence of damage to the heart or kidneys, defer surgery to allow blood pressure to be controlled and the aetiology investigated. There is, however, no level-one evidence as to how long the operation should be delayed (>4wk is often recommended) or that this strategy reduces perioperative risk.
- Patients with **Stage 3** hypertension considered fit for surgery in other respects and with no evidence of end-organ involvement should not be deferred simply on the grounds of elevated blood pressure. Attempt to ensure cardiovascular stability, using invasive monitoring where indicated and actively control excursions in mean arterial pressure greater than 20% from baseline.
- Patients undergoing major surgery or who are unstable perioperatively should be monitored closely in ICU/HDU.
- Perioperative β-blockade may be used. These drugs are known to reduce perioperative myocardial ischaemia and cardiovascular complications in high risk patients.
- Other sympatholytic therapies such as α_2 agonists (clonidine) and thoracic epidural blockade may have a role but also carry risks of hypotension postoperatively.
- Relate perioperative BP readings to the underlying norm—a systolic <100mmHg may represent hypotension in a normally hypertensive patient.

1 Howell SJ, Sear JW, Foex P (2004). Hypertension, hypertensive heart disease and perioperative cardiac risk. *British Journal of Anaesthesia*, **92**, 570–583.

Valvular heart disease

Found in 4% of patients over the age of 65yr. Patients with a known valve problem may already be under a cardiologist. Sometimes a murmur may be picked up during preoperative assessment. In each case:

• Assess the significance of the cardiac lesion for the proposed surgery.
• Plan anaesthesia according to the haemodynamic picture.
• Remember to administer antibiotic prophylaxis—see p1163.

2D echocardiography indicates abnormal valvular motion and morphology, but does not indicate the severity of stenosis or regurgitation except in mitral stenosis. Doppler echocardiography identifies increased velocity of flow across stenotic valves from which pressure gradients and severity may be estimated. Doppler flow imaging can also provide estimates of the severity of regurgitant valve disease.

Aortic stenosis (see also p332)

- Occasionally congenital (abnormal bicuspid valve in 2%), mostly due to calcification and rheumatic heart disease. Anatomic obstruction to ejection leads to concentric hypertrophy of left ventricular heart muscle resulting in decreased diastolic compliance.
- Elevated filling pressures and sinus rhythm are required to fill the non-compliant left ventricle. 'Normal' left ventricular end diastolic pressure may reflect hypovolaemia.
- Properly timed atrial contractions contribute as much as 40% to left ventricular preload in patients with aortic stenosis (normal = 20–30% Arrhythmia may produce a critical reduction in cardiac output.
- High risk of myocardial ischaemia due to increased oxygen demand and wall tension in the hypertrophied left ventricle. 30% of patients who have aortic stenosis with normal coronary arteries have angina. Sub-endocardial ischaemia may exist as coronary blood supply does not increase in proportion to the muscular hypertrophy. Tachycardia is detrimental as it may produce ischaemia. Maintenance of diastolic blood pressure is crucial to maintain coronary perfusion.

Aortic valve area reduction

Normal	$2.6–3.5cm^2$
Mild	$1.2–1.8cm^2$
Moderate	$0.8–1.2cm^2$
Significant	$0.6–0.8cm^2$
Critical	$<0.6cm^2$

LV-aortic gradient

Mild	12–25mmHg
Moderate	25–40mmHg
Significant	40–50mmHg
Critical	>50mmHg

History

- Angina, breathlessness, syncope

Symptoms do not correlate well to the severity of stenosis; some patients with small valve areas can be asymptomatic.

Examination

- Slow rising pulse with narrow pulse pressure
- Ejection systolic murmur maximal at the 2nd intercostal space, right sternal edge radiating to the neck

Investigations

- ECG: left ventricular hypertrophy and strain (with secondary ST–T wave abnormalities)
- CXR: normal until the left ventricle begins to fail, post-stenotic dilatation of the aorta, calcified aortic annulus

- Echocardiogram: enables calculation of valve gradient (see table) and assessment of left ventricular performance
- Cardiac catheterisation is also used to estimate the gradient across the valve and to quantify any concurrent coronary artery disease

Perioperative care

- Symptomatic patients for elective non-cardiac surgery should have aortic valve replacement first as they are at great risk of sudden death perioperatively (untreated severe symptomatic stenosis has a 50% 1yr survival)—see also p332.
- Asymptomatic patients for major elective surgery associated with marked fluid shifts (thoracic, abdominal, major orthopaedic) with gradients across the valve >50mmHg should have valve replacement considered prior to surgery.
- Asymptomatic patients for intermediate or minor surgery generally do well if managed carefully.

Haemodynamic goals

- (Low) normal heart rate.
- Maintain sinus rhythm.
- Adequate volume loading.
- High normal systemic vascular resistance.

Patients with severe aortic stenosis have a fixed cardiac output. They cannot compensate for falls in systemic vascular resistance which result in severe hypotension, myocardial ischaemia, and a downward spiral of reduced contractility causing further falls in blood pressure and coronary perfusion.

The selected technique should maintain afterload and avoid tachycardia to maintain the balance between myocardial oxygen demand and supply. Titrate drugs carefully. Treat hypotension using direct acting α-agonists such as metaraminol or phenylephrine as these improve systolic and diastolic LV function. Careful fluid balance is essential, guided by invasive monitoring if required (CVP, oesophageal Doppler, transoesophageal echocardiography). Direct measurement of arterial blood pressure should be routine except for very short procedures.

Arrhythmias must be treated promptly or haemodynamic collapse may ensue. Effective analgesia avoids catecholamine-induced tachycardia and hypertension and the risk of cardiac ischaemia. However, central neuraxial blocks must be used with extreme caution because of the danger of hypotension due to afterload reduction. Limb blocks can be used alone or in conjunction with general anaesthesia.

Postoperative management

- Have a low threshold for admission to ICU/HDU.
- Meticulous attention must be paid to fluid balance and postoperative pain management.
- Infusions of vasoconstrictors may be required to maintain haemodynamic stability.

Aortic regurgitation (see also p334)

- Primary aortic regurgitation may result from rheumatic heart disease or endocarditis.
- Aortic dissection and connective tissue disorders that dilate the aortic root (tertiary syphilis, Marfan's Syndrome, ankylosing spondylitis) result in secondary aortic incompetence.
- Valvular regurgitation usually develops over many years allowing the heart to adapt to increased volume.
- Acute regurgitation secondary to endocarditis or aortic dissection presents with acute left heart failure and pulmonary oedema. Such patients require emergency valve surgery.

In patients who have chronic aortic regurgitation:

- Afterload and heart rate determine the degree of regurgitation. Lower aortic pressure decreases left ventricular afterload, augmenting forward flow.
- Vasodilators increase forward flow by lowering afterload, decrease left ventricular size, and enhance ejection fraction.
- Heart rates greater than 90bpm reduce diastolic 'regurgitation' time and degree of regurgitation.
- Aortic diastolic pressure is dependent on the aortic valve and decreases when the valve becomes incompetent.

History

- Dyspnoea, secondary to pulmonary congestion.
- Palpitations.

Examination

- Widened pulse pressure.
- Collapsing ('waterhammer') pulse. Corrigan's sign—visible neck pulsation. De Musset's sign—head nodding. Quincke's sign—visible capillary pulsations in the nail beds.
- Diastolic murmur 2nd intercostal space right sternal edge.

Investigations

- CXR: cardiomegaly, boot-shaped heart.
- ECG: non-specific LVH.
- Echocardiography gives qualitative analysis of the degree of regurgitation.

Perioperative care

Asymptomatic patients usually tolerate non-cardiac surgery well. Patients with poor functional capacity need to be considered for valve replacement surgery.

Haemodynamic goals

- High normal heart rate—around 90bpm.
- Adequate volume loading.
- Low systemic vascular resistance.
- Maintain contractility.

The selected anaesthetic should maintain afterload in the low normal range to maintain diastolic pressure. Spinal and epidural anaesthesia are well tolerated. Treat perioperative SVT/atrial fibrillation promptly with synchronised DC cardioversion (see p81, p82), particularly if associated with hypotension. Persistent bradycardia may need to be treated with β-agonists. Intra-arterial pressure monitoring is useful for major surgery. Oesophageal Doppler and other methods of cardiac output monitoring are inaccurate.

Mitral stenosis (see also p336)

- Rheumatic fever is the commonest cause. A minority have isolated stenosis; the majority have mixed mitral valve disease (stenosis and regurgitation). Mitral valve stenosis underfills the left ventricle and increases both pressure and volume upstream of the valve.
- The left ventricle functions normally but is small and poorly filled.
- Initially the left atrium dilates, keeping the pulmonary artery pressure low. As disease progresses pulmonary artery pressure increases and medial hypertrophy develops, resulting in chronic reactive pulmonary hypertension. The right heart hypertrophies to pump against a pressure overload, then fails. Secondary pulmonary/tricuspid regurgitation develops.
- The pressure gradient across the narrow mitral orifice increases with the square of cardiac output (NB pregnancy). Rapid heart rates, especially with atrial fibrillation, decrease diastolic filling time and markedly decrease cardiac output.
- LV filling is optimised by a slow heart rate.

Patients are frequently dyspnoeic due to fluid transudate in the lungs, which reduces lung compliance and increases the work of breathing. Pulmonary oedema may occur if the pulmonary venous pressure exceeds the plasma oncotic pressure. This is especially likely if a large fluid bolus, head-down position, or a uterine contraction raises pulmonary pressure suddenly.

Normal valve surface area	4–6cm^2
Symptom free until	1.5–2.5cm^2
Moderate stenosis	1–1.5cm^2
Critical stenosis	<1cm^2

History

- Dyspnoea, haemoptysis, recurrent bronchitis
- Fatigue
- Palpitations.

Examination

- Mitral facies—malar flush on cheeks.
- Peripheral cyanosis.
- Signs of right heart failure (elevated JVP, hepatomegaly, peripheral oedema, ascites).
- Tapping apex beat. Loud first heart sound, opening snap (if in sinus rhythm), and low-pitched diastolic murmur heard best at the apex (with the bell of the stethoscope).

Investigations

- ECG: P mitrale (left atrial enlargement) if sinus rhythm. Atrial fibrillation usual.
- CXR: valve calcification. Large left atrium (lateral film). Double shadow behind heart on PA film. Splaying of the carina. Kerley B lines indicating pulmonary congestion.
- Echocardiography: measures the gradient and valve area—see table.

Perioperative care

Asymptomatic patients usually tolerate non-cardiac surgery well. Patients with poor functional capacity need to be considered for mitral valve replacement.

Haemodynamic goals

- Low normal heart rate 50–70bpm. Treat tachycardia aggressively with β-blockers.
- Maintain sinus rhythm if possible. Immediate cardioversion if AF occurs perioperatively.
- Adequate preload.
- High normal systemic vascular resistance.
- Avoid hypercarbia, acidosis, and hypoxia, which may exacerbate pulmonary hypertension.

Anaesthesia—similar to aortic stenosis as there is a relatively fixed cardiac output. Maintain adequate afterload, slow heart rate, and avoid hypovolaemia. Measure CVP/PAOP and maintain an adequate preload. Spinal and epidural anaesthesia may be very hazardous.

Mitral regurgitation (see also p338)

- Mitral regurgitation (MR) results from leaflet, chordal, or papillary muscle abnormalities or is secondary to left ventricular dysfunction.
- Leaflet MR is a complication of endocarditis, rheumatic fever, or mitral valve prolapse.
- Chordal MR follows chordae rupture after acute myocardial infarction or after bacterial endocarditis.
- Papillary muscle MR results from ischaemic posterior papillary muscle dysfunction.
- Left ventricular failure leads to varying amounts of MR when the mitral annulus dilates.
- As much as 50% of the left ventricular volume flows into a massively dilated left atrium through the incompetent mitral valve before the aortic valve opens. Left ventricular ejection fraction is therefore supranormal.
- Pulmonary vascular congestion develops, followed by pulmonary hypertension.
- The degree of regurgitation is determined by the afterload, size of the regurgitant orifice, and the heart rate. A moderately increased heart rate (>90bpm) decreases the time for regurgitation in systole and decreases the time for diastolic filling, reducing LV overload.

History
- Fatigue, weakness
- Dyspnoea

Examination
- Displaced and forceful apex (the more severe the regurgitation, the larger the ventricle).
- Soft S_1, apical pansystolic murmur radiating to the axilla, loud S_3.
- Atrial fibrillation.

Investigations
- ECG: left atrial enlargement. Atrial fibrillation.
- CXR: left atrial and left ventricular enlargement. Mitral annular calcification.
- Echocardiography assesses the degree of regurgitation. (Trans-oesophageal echo particularly useful as mitral valve close to the oesophagus.)

Perioperative care
Asymptomatic patients usually tolerate non-cardiac surgery well. Patients with poor functional capacity need to be considered for valve replacement surgery.

Haemodynamic goals
- High normal heart rate
- Adequate preload
- Low systemic vascular resistance
- Low pulmonary vascular resistance.

Anaesthesia aims are similar to aortic regurgitation. Preload can be diffi-cult to estimate; for major non-cardiac surgery a pulmonary artery catheter may be useful. In advanced disease pulmonary hypertension is common—avoid factors that increase pulmonary artery pressure (hypoxia, hypercarbia, high inspiratory pressures, acidosis).

Mitral valve prolapse

- Common (incidental finding in 5% of population).
- Usually asymptomatic, but may be associated with atypical chest pain, palpitations, syncope, and emboli.
- Mid-systolic click and late diastolic murmur.
- Echocardiography shows enlarged redundant mitral valve leaflets prolapsing into the left atrium during mid- to late systole causing arrhythmias and regurgitation.
- Anti-arrhythmics must be continued perioperatively.
- SBE prophylaxis is mandatory.

Mixed valve lesions

- With mixed regurgitant/stenotic lesions manage the dominant lesion.

The patient with an undiagnosed murmur

Most heart murmurs do not signify cardiac disease. Many are related to physiological increases in blood flow. Assess functional capacity (Duke Activity Status Index, p41) and the presence or absence of symptoms. Many asymptomatic children and young adults with a murmur can safely undergo anaesthesia and surgery if they have good functional capacity and are asymptomatic.

Elderly asymptomatic patients may have an 'aortic' systolic murmur related to sclerotic aortic valve leaflets. Aortic sclerosis is now considered to be an early form of aortic stenosis, but should not cause clinical problems until progression to stenosis occurs. Factors which differentiate early asymptomatic sclerosis from stenosis include

• Good exercise tolerance (>4 METs)
• No history of angina/breathlessness/syncope
• Absence of slow rising pulse (normal pulse pressure)
• Absence of LVH/LV strain on ECG.

The volume of the murmur does not help.

Take a full history and examine the ECG/CXR. Patients able to manage 4 METs (able to climb a flight of stairs, walk at 6km/hr on the flat) with a normal ECG and CXR will tolerate minor and intermediate surgery but should have an echocardiogram prior to major surgery. Conversely poor functional capacity in association with an abnormal ECG (such as ventricular hypertrophy or a prior infarction) should be investigated by echocardiography.

Prosthetic valves

- Most patients will be under the surveillance of a cardiologist.
- Antibiotic prophylaxis is required—see p1163.
- Tissue valves do not require anticoagulation. Mechanical valve replacements require lifetime anticoagulation—see p216.
- The risk of thromboembolism if anticoagulation is stopped with a mechanical valve is small (8/100 patient yr). Most patients can be managed by stopping warfarin 3d prior to planned surgery. Aim for a target INR 2.
- For certain operations where there is a high risk of bleeding complications (neurosurgery) a period without anticoagulation is required. It takes ~4d after stopping warfarin for the INR to reach 1.5. Available evidence suggests that anticoagulation can be stopped for up to 7d with only a small risk of thrombotic complications from the mechanical valve. However some specialists will still advocate the administration of an IV infusion of heparin once the INR is less than 3. This can be stopped 2hr prior to surgery.
- Restart oral anticoagulation as soon as practically possible. If there is a delay, heparin should be continued either as an infusion or as LMWH SC.

Further reading

British Committee for Standards in Haematology. (1998). Guidelines on Oral Anticoagulation *British Journal of Haematology*, **101**, 374–387.

Pericardial disease

Acute pericarditis

- Usually a viral condition presenting with chest pain. Diagnosis is supported by widespread ST elevation on ECG.
- Frequently occurs with myocarditis which may increase the likelihood of arrhythmia and sudden death.
- Elective surgery should be postponed for at least 6wk.

Constrictive pericarditis

- This may be postinfective or secondary to an autoimmune disease such as SLE. The only effective treatment is pericardectomy which may be dramatically effective.
- Pulsus paradoxus may be evident—a fall in systolic blood pressure with inspiration. The normal maximum fall is 10mmHg.
- Systolic function of the myocardium is well maintained but diastolic function is severely impaired. When exercise tolerance is reduced general anaesthesia carries a significant risk.
- Bradycardia and reduced cardiac filling are poorly tolerated.
- Elevations in intrathoracic pressure, as occur during IPPV, can result in profound hypotension.
- If anaesthesia is unavoidable and regional block is not possible then a spontaneously breathing technique is preferable to IPPV. Preload should be maintained and tachycardia avoided.

Cardiomyopathy

Most patients have heart failure and have little reserve for surgery and anaesthesia.

Hypertrophic obstructive cardiomyopathy (HOCM)

- Causes dynamic obstruction of the left ventricular outflow during systole.
- Main feature is asymmetric hypertrophy of the interventricular septum, which obstructs the outflow tract when it contracts.
- Ventricular systole is associated with movement of the anterior mitral valve leaflet towards the septum ('systolic anterior motion'—SAM) and the outflow tract is further obstructed. In some patients this causes mitral regurgitation.
- As with aortic stenosis, HOCM results in a pressure overload of the left ventricle. Diastolic dysfunction is evident on echo.
- Sinus rhythm is crucial to maintain ventricular filling.

Aetiology is unknown but possibly inherited as an autosomal dominant condition in >50% of cases. Presents with symptoms similar to aortic stenosis—angina, dyspnoea, syncope, and palpitations. Sudden death is common. ECG is abnormal showing evidence of left ventricular hypertrophy.

Echocardiography is essential to estimate the degree of functional obstruction, asymmetric left ventricular hypertrophy, and SAM of the mitral valve.

Inotropes are contraindicated as left ventricular obstruction is exacerbated by increased myocardial contractility. Treatment is with β-blockers or verapamil as they are negatively inotropic. Patients are prone to arrhythmias which are refractory to medical treatment and may require dual chamber pacing.

Haemodynamic goals

Maintain a 'large ventricle' since dynamic obstruction is reduced.
- Low normal heart rate.
- Maintain sinus rhythm.
- Adequate volume loading.
- High normal systemic vascular resistance.
- Low ventricular contractility.

Invasive haemodynamic monitoring is indicated. Measurement of the CVP or use of oesophageal Doppler helps to guide volume resuscitation. Direct acting α-agonists such as metaraminol may be used in an emergency.

Restrictive cardiomyopathy

Rare condition. Commonest cause is myocardial infiltration by amyloid. Characterised by stiff ventricles that impair ventricular filling. Right heart failure often prominent. Echocardiography shows diastolic dysfunction.
- Anaesthesia is hazardous.
- Peripheral vasodilatation, myocardial depression, and reduced venous return may cause catastrophic cardiovascular decompensation and may precipitate cardiac arrest.

- Venous return may be further compromised by positive pressure ventilation. Wherever possible maintain spontaneous respiration.
- Ketamine may be useful as it increases myocardial contractility and peripheral resistance.
- Fluids should be given to maintain elevated right heart pressures.

Haemodynamic goals
- Maintain sinus rhythm.
- Adequate volume loading.
- High normal systemic vascular resistance.
- Avoid myocardial depression.

Dilated cardiomyopathy

- Manifests as cardiac failure with an enlarged poorly contractile heart. Stroke volume is initially preserved by dilatation and increased LV end diastolic volume. Functional mitral and tricuspid incompetence occurs commonly due to dilatation of the valve annulus, exacerbating heart failure.
- Commonest problems are heart failure, arrhythmias, and embolic phenomena.
- Heart failure is treated with diuretics, ACE inhibitors, and vasodilators. Amiodarone is the drug of choice for arrhythmias as it has least myocardial depressant effect. Patients are frequently anticoagulated. Synchronised dual chamber pacing may be used. Some patients may have a biventricular pacing/defibrillator (AICD) in place.
- Extensive cardiovascular monitoring is required during anaesthesia (arterial and pulmonary arterial catheters and non-invasive methods of cardiac output estimation, e.g. oesophageal Doppler, PiCCO, LiDCO).

Haemodynamic goals
- Maintain sinus rhythm.
- Adequate volume loading.
- Normal systemic vascular resistance.
- Avoid myocardial depression: inotropic support is frequently required with dobutamine or phosphodiesterase inhibitors.

Further reading

Bovill JG (2003). Anaesthesia for patients with impaired ventricular function. *Seminars in Cardiothoracic and Vascular Anesthesia,* **7**, 49–54.

Patients with a transplanted heart

(See also Anaesthesia after lung transplantation. 📖 p121)
Heart transplantation is increasing in frequency and patients may present
to a non-specialist centre for non-cardiac surgery. Anaesthesia requires
attention to:

- Altered physiology
- Effects of immunosuppression
- Medications
- Associated risk factors.

Altered physiology

- The heart is denervated; resting heart rates are usually around
  85–95bpm. Some patients may have experienced temporary
  bradyarrhythmias after transplantation. A pacemaker may be in situ.
- Normal autonomic system responses are lost (beat-to-beat variation in
  heart rate, response to Valsalva manoeuvre/carotid sinus massage).
- Contractility of the heart is close to normal, unless rejection is
  developing. In the absence of sympathetic innervation the age
  predicted maximal heart rate is reduced.
- Despite some evidence that reinervation can occur some years after
  transplantation the heart should be viewed as permanently
  denervated. This results in poor tolerance of acute hypovolaemia.
- If pharmacological manipulation is required then direct-acting agents
  should be used: atropine has no effect on the denervated heart, the
  effect of ephedrine is reduced and unpredictable, and hydralazine and
  phenylephrine produce no reflex tachy- or bradycardia in response
  to their primary action. Adrenaline, noradrenaline, isoprenaline, and
  β-blockers act as expected.

Immunosuppression

Three classes of drugs are used:

- Immunophilin binding drugs (ciclosporin A, tacrolimus) prevent
  cytokine-mediated T cell activation and proliferation.
- Nucleic acid synthesis inhibitors (azathioprine) block lymphocyte
  proliferation.
- Steroids block the production of inflammatory cytokines, lyse
  T lymphocytes, and alter the function of the remaining lymphocytes.

Anaemia and thrombocytopenia as well as leucopenia may result,
requiring treatment before surgery. Ciclosporin is associated with renal
dysfunction and is the most likely cause of hypertension that affects 40%
of heart–lung transplant recipients. It may also prolong the action of non-
depolarising muscle relaxants. Calcium antagonists increase ciclosporin
levels variably and are used in some centres to reduce ciclosporin dose
in an attempt to reduce side effects. The effect on blood concentrations
must be remembered if calcium antagonists are omitted for any reason
perioperatively. Renal dysfunction is also commonly caused by
tacrolimus. Steroid supplementation may be required if large doses of
prednisolone are being used.

Strict asepsis must be used with all invasive procedures.

Associated risk factors

- Previous and often repeated use of central and peripheral vessels can make IV and arterial access difficult.
- Cough may be impaired due to a combination of phrenic and recurrent laryngeal nerve palsies. This increases the risks of sputum retention and postoperative chest infection.
- Heart–lung recipients will have a tracheal anastomosis. It is desirable to avoid unnecessary intubation but if it is necessary use a short tube and carefully monitor tracheal cuff pressure. Disrupted lung lymphatic drainage increases the risk of pulmonary oedema.

Choice of technique

There is no evidence to support one anaesthetic technique above another.
- Peripheral surgery under regional block is likely to be well tolerated.
- Subarachnoid/epidural block may result in marked falls in blood pressure because of absent cardiac innervation.

Further reading

Toivonen HJ (2000). Anaesthesia for patients with a transplanted organ. *Acta Anaesthesiologica Scandinavica*, **44**, 812–833.

Congenital heart disease and non-cardiac surgery

Congenital heart disease (CHD) is common, 8:1000 births, with 85% of these children reaching adult life. Although most of these children will have undergone corrective surgery, many will have residual problems. Studies have reported a high incidence of adverse perioperative events in CHD patients undergoing non-cardiac surgical procedures.

General considerations

Operative procedures for CHD aim to improve the patient's haemo-dynamic status although complete cure is not always achieved. Paediatric cardiac surgical procedures can be divided as follows:

- Curative procedures: the patient is completely cured and life expectancy is normal (e.g. persistent ductus arteriosus and atrial septal defect closure).
- Corrective procedures: the patient's haemodynamic status is markedly improved but life expectancy may not be normal (e.g. tetralogy of Fallot repair).
- Palliative procedures: these patients may have abnormal circulations and physiology but avoid the consequences of untreated CHD. Life expectancy is not normal but many survive to adulthood (e.g. Fontan procedures).

Preoperative assessment

Aim to gain an understanding of the anatomy and pathophysiology of the patient's cardiac defect.

- History: define the nature and severity of the lesion. Ask about CCF—especially limitation of daily activities. Consider other associated abnormalities. Check current medication.
- Examination: check for cyanosis, peripheral oedema, hepato-splenomegaly, murmurs, and signs of infection/failure. Check peripheral pulses. Neurological examination for cyanosed patients.
- Investigations: CXR/ECG. Record baseline SpO_2 on air. Laboratory tests depend on the proposed surgery but most will require FBC, clotting screen, LFTs, and electrolytes. Some patients will need pulmonary function tests.
- Consult the patient's cardiologist—recent echocardiography report and catheter data should be available. Potential risk factors should be considered, along with potential treatment regimes, e.g. inotropes or vasodilators.
- Consider whether the proposed surgery is necessary, with regard to the potential risks, whether admission to ICU/HDU will be required, and whether the patient can or should be moved to a cardiac centre.

Factors indicative of high risk

- Recent worsening of CCF or symptoms of myocardial ischaemia
- Severe hypoxaemia with SpO_2 <75% on air
- Polycythaemia (haematocrit >60%)
- Unexplained dizziness/syncope/fever or recent CVA
- Severe aortic/pulmonary valve stenosis
- Uncorrected tetralogy of Fallot or Eisenmenger's syndrome
- Recent onset of arrhythmias

Specific problems

- Myocardial dysfunction/arrhythmias: may be due to underlying disease (e.g. hypoplastic left ventricle) or secondary (e.g. due to surgery or medication).
- Air emboli: all CHD patients are at risk from air embolism. Intravascular lines should be free of air.
- Cyanosis has many causes, e.g. shunting of blood from the right to left side of the heart (tetralogy of Fallot, Eisenmenger's syndrome) or due to intracardiac mixing (complete atrioventricular septal defect). Cyanosis results in polycythaemia and increased blood volume. Blood viscosity is increased, impairing tissue perfusion. There is often thrombocytopenia and fibrinogen deficiency leading to a bleeding tendency. An increase in tissue vascularity worsens bleeding problems. Cyanosis can also lead to renal/cerebral thrombosis and renal tubular atrophy.
- Anticoagulant treatment (aspirin or warfarin) is common in CHD patients.
- Antibiotic prophylaxis: required for all CHD patients except isolated secundum atrial septal defect repaired without a patch >6 months ago or persistent ductus arteriosus ligated >6 months ago.
- Myocardial ischaemia developing in a patient with CHD is significant and should be investigated.

Specific CHD lesions

There are over 100 forms of CHD, but 8 lesions account for 83% of all cardiac defects. These are ventricular septal defect (VSD), atrial septal defect (ASD), persistent ductus arteriosus (PDA), pulmonary stenosis (PS), tetralogy of Fallot (TOF), aortic stenosis (AS), coarctation of the aorta, and transposition of the great vessels (TOGV). Many of the other cardiac lesions are managed palliatively by producing a Fontan circulation.

ASD (secundum type)

- Patients are often asymptomatic.
- Usually results in a left-to-right shunt.
- Can be closed surgically or transcatheter.
- Danger of paradoxical emboli.

ASD (primum type)

- Endocardial cushion defect—may involve atrioventricular valves.
- More severe form, atrioventricular septal defect (AVSD), is associated with Down's syndrome and results in severe pulmonary hypertension.
- Surgical repair of these lesions may result in complete heart block.

VSD

- Commonest form of CHD.
- Clinical effects depend on size and number of VSDs.
- A small, single VSD may be asymptomatic with a small left-to-right shunt (pulmonary:systemic flow ratio < 1.5:1). In patients who have not had corrective surgery, prevent air emboli and fluid overload and remember antibiotic prophylaxis.
- Patients with a moderate sized, single VSD often present with mild CCF. They have increased pulmonary blood flow (pulmonary:systemic flow ratio 3:1). If the lesion is not treated they are at risk of pulmonary hypertension and shunt reversal.
- Patients with a large VSD have equal pressures in their right and left ventricles and present around 2 months of age with severe CCF. They require early operations. However, if they need anaesthesia for another procedure prior to definitive cardiac surgery they present severe problems. They should be intubated, for all but the most minor procedures, and increases in left to right shunt should be avoided (e.g. avoid hyperventilation and high FiO_2). Care should be taken with fluid administration, and inotropic support is often required.
- Patients with multiple VSDs often require pulmonary artery banding to protect the pulmonary circulation. This band tightens as the child grows, leading to cyanosis. VSDs often close spontaneously and then the band may be removed.

PDA

- Patients with PDA may have a moderate left-to-right shunt and this can result in an elevated pulmonary vascular resistance rather like a moderately sized VSD.
- Can be closed surgically or transcatheter.

Tetralogy of Fallot (TOF)

- Pulmonary stenosis, VSD, overriding aorta, and right ventricular hypertrophy.
- Prior to complete repair, TOF may be treated medically with β-blockade or surgically via a Blalock–Taussig (BT) shunt (subclavian to pulmonary artery).
- In patients without a BT shunt, and prior to definitive surgery, the ratio of SVR:PVR determines both the systemic blood flow and blood oxygen saturation. If they require anaesthesia at this stage they should be intubated and ventilated in order to maintain a low PVR. Cyanosis should be treated with hyperventilation, IV fluid, and systemic vaso-pressors such as phenylephrine.
- Total repair of TOF is undertaken around 3–8 months of age.

Eisenmenger's syndrome

- Associated with markedly increased morbidity and mortality.
- Abnormal and irreversible elevation in PVR resulting in cyanosis and right-to-left shunting. The degree of shunting depends on the PVR:SVR ratio. Increasing the SVR or decreasing the PVR leads to better arterial SpO_2, as in patients with TOF.
- Avoid reductions in SVR (epidural/spinal anaesthesia) and rises in PVR (hypoxia/hypercarbia/acidosis/cold).
- Desaturation episodes can be treated as for TOF above.
- Inotropic support may be required for the shortest of procedures and an ITU bed should be available.
- Manage patient in a specialist centre whenever possible.

Fontan repair

- Palliative procedure, classically for patients with tricuspid atresia, but can be performed for many different cardiac lesions including hypoplastic left heart syndrome. The Fontan procedure is not a specific operation but a class of operations that separate the pulmonary and systemic circulations in patients with an anatomical or physiological single ventricle. This separation is accomplished by ensuring that all superior and inferior vena caval blood flows directly into the pulmonary artery, bypassing the right ventricle and, usually, the right atrium. Thus, pulmonary blood flow is dependent solely on systemic venous pressure. SpO_2 should be normal.
- Leads to elevated systemic venous pressures, liver congestion, protein-losing enteropathy, tendency for fluid overload, ascites, pleural and pericardial effusions. Hypovolaemia can lead to hypoxia and cardiovascular collapse. Patients are anticoagulated with warfarin.
- In these patients intermittent positive pressure ventilation results in a fall in cardiac output and high ventilatory pressures result in poor pulmonary perfusion. Fluid overload is poorly tolerated, as is hypovolaemia.
- Central venous pressure monitoring is helpful and is best instituted via the femoral venous route.

Adults with congenital heart disease

Anything but the most straightforward situation should be discussed and referred to a cardiac centre.

Uncorrected disease

- VSD/ASDs may be small and have no symptoms and little haemodynamic effect. With the exception of endocarditis prophylaxis and the potential for paradoxical emboli, small defects present no anaesthetic problems.
- Lesions resulting in large left-to-right shunts will cause progressive pulmonary hypertension and eventual shunt reversal (Eisenmenger's syndrome). Once irreversible pulmonary hypertension has developed surgical correction is not possible. These patients are high risk. If surgery is absolutely necessary it should be performed in a specialist centre.

Corrected disease

- These patients have either had spontaneous resolution or a corrective procedure. They can generally be treated as normal.
- Best assessment of cardiovascular function is generally the exercise tolerance.
- Exclude surgical sequelae/continuing disease.
- Exclude any associated congenital abnormalities.

Palliated disease

- These patients have had operations that improve functional capacity and life expectancy but do not restore normal anatomy. Operations include Senning and Mustard for transposition of the great vessels (neonatal switch is now preferred) and Fontan for single ventricle syndromes (e.g. hypoplastic left heart and pulmonary atresia).
- An understanding of the underlying physiology is required to avoid disaster when anaesthetising these patients. At present, management is best provided in specialist cardiac centres.
- In patients with a Fontan circulation blood leaves a single ventricle, passes through the systemic circulation and then through the pulmonary circulation before returning to the heart. The consequences of this are that the CVP is high, providing a pressure gradient across the pulmonary circulation. Any pulmonary hypertension is poorly tolerated and results in reduced ventricular filling. The high venous pressure can result in life-threatening haemorrhage from mucosal procedures like adenoidectomy (or nasal intubation!).

Further reading

Nichols DG et al. (1995). *Critical Heart Disease in Infants and Children.* St Louis: Mosby.
Andropoulos DB et al. (2005). *Anesthesia for Congenital Heart Disease.* Cambridge, MA: Blackwell.

Chapter 4

Perioperative arrhythmias

John Dean

Perioperative arrhythmias (see also p866–869)

Perioperative cardiac arrhythmias are common and may be life threatening. Whenever possible they should be controlled preoperatively as surgery and anaesthesia can cause marked deterioration. Management is easier if the underlying problem has been recognised, investigated, and treated preoperatively. Never give an IV drug for any rhythm disturbance unless you are in a position to cardiovert immediately.

Practical diagnosis of arrhythmias

Ideally undertaken with a paper printout of the ECG and preferably in 12 lead format. In theatre this is often impractical—use the different leads available on the monitor to improve interpretation.

Determine

- What is the ventricular rate?
- Is the QRS complex of normal duration or widened?
- Is the QRS regular or irregular?
- Are P waves present and are they normally shaped?
- How is atrial activity related to ventricular activity?

Ventricular rate

- Calculate approximate ventricular rate (divide 300 by the number of large squares between each QRS complex).
- Tachyarrhythmia: rate > 100bpm. Bradyarrhythmia: rate < 60bpm.

QRS complex

- Supraventricular rhythms include nodal rhythms and arise from a focus above the ventricles. Since the ventricles still depolarise via the normal His/Purkinje system the QRS complexes are of normal width (<0.12s or 3 small squares) and are termed 'narrow complex rhythms'.
- Arrhythmias arising from the ventricles will be 'broad complex' with a QRS width of >0.12s. In the presence of AV or bundle branch block a supraventricular rhythm may have broad complexes (2%). This may be present on the 12 lead ECG or develop as a consequence of the arrhythmia—rate related aberrant conduction.

Regularity

- Irregular rhythm suggests ectopic beats (atrial or ventricular), atrial fibrillation, atrial flutter with variable block, or second-degree heart block with variable block.

P waves

- The presence of P waves indicates atrial depolarisation. Absent P waves with an irregular ventricular rhythm suggest atrial fibrillation, whereas a saw-toothed pattern is characteristic of atrial flutter.

Atrial/ventricular activity

- Normally there will be 1 P wave per QRS complex. Any change in this ratio indicates a block to conduction between atria and ventricles.

Narrow complex arrhythmias

Sinus arrhythmia

Irregular spacing of normal complexes associated with respiration. Constant P–R interval with beat-to-beat change in the R–R interval. Normal finding especially in young people.

Sinus tachycardia

Rate > 100bpm. Normal P–QRS–T complexes are evident. Causes include:
* Inadequate depth of anaesthesia, pain/surgical stimulation
* Fever/sepsis, hypovolaemia, anaemia, heart failure, thyrotoxicosis
* Drugs, e.g. atropine, ketamine, catecholamines

Correct the underlying cause where possible. β-blockers may be useful if tachycardia causes myocardial ischaemia but should be used with caution in patients with heart failure and avoided in asthma.

Sinus bradycardia

Rate < 60bpm. May be due to vagal stimulation or normal in athletic patients. Other causes include:
* Drugs, e.g. β-blockers, digoxin, anticholinesterases, halothane, suxamethonium
* Myocardial infarction, sick sinus syndrome
* Raised intracranial pressure, hypothyroidism, hypothermia

Unnecessary to correct in fit person unless there is haemodynamic compromise (usually when HR < 40–45bpm). However, consider:
* Correcting the underlying cause, e.g. stop surgical stimulus.
* Atropine up to 20μg/kg or glycopyrronium 10μg/kg IV.
* Patients on β-blockers may be resistant and an isoprenaline infusion is occasionally required (0.5–10μg/min)—adrenaline is an alternative. Glucagon (50–150μg/kg IV in 5% glucose) can be used—this is an unlicensed indication and dose.

Atrial ectopics

These are common and benign. May occur normally; other causes include:
* Ischaemia/hypoxia
* Light anaesthesia, sepsis, shock
* Anaesthetic drugs

Correct any underlying cause. Specific treatment unnecessary unless runs of atrial tachycardia occur.

Arrhythmias due to re-entry

These arrhythmias occur where there is an anatomical branching and re-joining of conduction pathways. If an impulse arrives at a time when the first pathway is no longer refractory, it can pass around the circuit repeatedly activating it. The classical example is Wolff–Parkinson–White syndrome, where an accessory conduction pathway exists between atria and ventricles. Other re-entry circuits occur with atrial flutter, atrial fibrillation, supraventricular tachycardia, and ventricular tachycardia.

Junctional/AV nodal/supraventricular tachycardia
- ECG usually shows a narrow complex (QRS < 0.12s) tachycardia, with a rate of 150–200bpm. A broad complex pattern may occur if antero-grade conduction occurs down an accessory pathway or if there is bundle branch block. May cause severe circulatory disturbance.
- If hypotensive, especially if anaesthetised, the first-line treatment is *synchronised* direct current cardioversion with 200 then 360J.
- Carotid sinus massage may slow the rate and reveal the underlying rhythm. It is helpful in differentiating SVT from atrial flutter and fast atrial fibrillation.
- Adenosine blocks AV nodal conduction and is especially useful for terminating re-entry SVT. Give 0.2mg/kg IV rapidly, followed by a saline flush. The effects of adenosine last only 10–15s. It should be avoided in asthma.
- β-blockers, e.g. esmolol by IV infusion at 50–200µg/kg/min, or metoprolol 3–5mg over 10min repeated 6-hourly.
- Verapamil 5–10mg IV slowly over 2min is useful in patients with SVT who relapse following adenosine. A further 5mg may be given after 10min if required. This may cause hypotension—avoid with β-blockers.
- Amiodarone is an alternative when first-line drugs have failed.
- Digoxin should be avoided—it facilitates conduction through the AV accessory pathway in Wolff–Parkinson–White syndrome and may worsen tachycardia. Atrial fibrillation in the presence of an accessory pathway may allow rapid conduction which can degenerate to ventricular fibrillation.

Atrial flutter/atrial tachycardia
Due to an ectopic focus the atria contract >150bpm; P waves can some-times be seen superimposed on T waves of the preceding beats. In atrial flutter there is no flat baseline between P waves and the typical saw-tooth pattern can be seen. Atrial tachycardia is uncommon in adults. Both may occur with any kind of block, e.g. 2:1, 3:1, etc. Same risk of thromboembolism as AF.
- Sensitive to synchronised DC cardioversion—nearly 100% conversion. In the anaesthetised patient with recent onset this should be the first line of treatment.
- Carotid sinus massage and adenosine will slow AV conduction and reveal the underlying rhythm and block where there is any doubt.
- Other drug treatment is as for atrial fibrillation.

Sick sinus syndrome
May coexist with AV nodal disease. Episodes of AV block, atrial tachy-cardia, atrial flutter, and atrial fibrillation may occur.
- Most common causes are congenital, ischaemic, rheumatic, hypertensive heart disease
- Can be asymptomatic, or present with dizziness syncope
- Permanent pacing required if symptomatic

Atrial fibrillation (AF)

Uncoordinated atrial activity with ventricular rate dependent on AV node transmission—commonly 120 –180bpm. Causes of AF include:

- Hypertension, myocardial ischaemia, or other disease
- Pericarditis/mediastinitis, thoracic surgery
- Mitral valve disease
- Electrolyte disturbance (especially hypokalaemia or hypomagnesaemia)
- Sepsis, thyrotoxicosis, alcohol—especially binge drinking

Atrial contraction contributes up to 30% of normal ventricular filling. The onset of AF (particularly fast AF) causes a reduction in ventricular filling and cardiac output. Ischaemia often results due to diastolic time reduction and hypotension.

Blood clots may form within the atria and embolise systemically. This risk is highest if there is a return to sinus rhythm after >48hr of AF. In stable AF the risk of CVE is 4%/yr at 75yr—halved by anticoagulation.

Treatment aims to restore sinus rhythm or control ventricular rate to <100bpm and prevent embolic complications. In acute AF (<48hr) restoration of sinus rhythm is often possible, whereas in longstanding AF control of the ventricular rate is the usual aim. Ideally the ventricular rate should be controlled by appropriate therapy preoperatively. Occasionally rapid control of the rate is required perioperatively.

Management of acute AF[1,2,3]

Correct precipitating factors where possible, especially electrolyte disturbances. When AF is secondary to sepsis or thoracic/oesophageal surgery, conversion to sinus rhythm is difficult until the underlying condition is controlled.

Onset <48hr

- Synchronised DC cardioversion at 200 then 360J (if practical).
- Flecainide 2mg/kg (max 150mg) over 30min IV is the best drug for converting AF to sinus rhythm. It should be used with caution in the presence of LV dysfunction and ventricular arrhythmias.

Onset >48hr

Conversion to sinus rhythm is associated with risk of arterial embolisation unless the patient is anticoagulated (at least 3wk)—aim for rate control unless haemodynamically compromised. Drugs include:

- Digoxin (if K^+ is normal). IV loading dose 500µg in 100ml saline over 20min, repeated at intervals of 4–8hr if necessary, to a total of 1–1.5mg. Lower doses are required for patients already taking digoxin. Digoxin does not convert AF to sinus rhythm, or prevent further episodes of paroxysmal AF.
- β-blockers (esmolol, sotalol, metoprolol) may be used to slow ventricular rate—caution with impaired myocardium, thyrotoxicosis and avoid with calcium channel blockers. β-blockers can be useful in theatre until other drugs have taken effect.

- Amiodarone slows rate and helps sustain sinus rhythm once regained. There are a number of concerns with long-term side effects which include pulmonary fibrosis. Useful in acute AF associated with critical illness and can be combined with digoxin or β-blockers. A loading dose of 300mg (in 5% dextrose) IV via a central vein is given over 1hr and followed by 900mg over 23hr. It may be given peripherally in an emergency, but extravasation is extremely serious. Well tolerated with LV impairment.
- Verapamil 5–10mg IV may be used to slow ventricular rate in patients unable to tolerate β-blockers. Avoid if there is impaired LV function, evidence of ischaemia, or in combination with β-blockers.

Uncontrolled chronic AF

Ventricular rates >100bpm should be slowed preoperatively to allow adequate time for ventricular filling/myocardial perfusion.

- Digitalisation if the patient is not already fully loaded with digoxin. This should usually be done over 1–2d preoperatively. Rapid IV digitalisation may be required when the surgery is urgent. Digoxin levels can be measured (therapeutic levels 0.8–2.0μg/l).
- Additional β-blocker (metoprolol, atenolol) or verapamil if good LV function.
- Amiodarone IV if poor LV.

1 Nathanson G (1998). Perioperative management of atrial fibrillation. *Anaesthesia*, **53**, 665–676.
2 Alboni P, Botto GL, Baldi N, *et al.* (2004). Outpatient treatment of recent-onset atrial fibrillation with the 'pill-in-the-pocket' approach. *New England Journal of Medicine*, **351**, 2384–2391.
3 Van Gelder IC, Hagens VE, Bosker HA (2002). A comparison of rate control and rhythm control in patients with recurrent persistent atrial fibrillation: the Rate Control versus Electrical Cardioversion for Persistent Atrial Fibrillation Study Group. *New England Journal of Medicine*, **347**, 1834–1840.

Broad complex arrhythmias

Ventricular ectopics

In the absence of structural heart disease, these are usually benign. May be provoked by hypokalaemia, dental procedures, or anal stretch, particularly in combination with halothane, raised CO_2, and light anaesthesia. In fit young patients, they are of little significance and respond readily to manipulation of the anaesthetic. Small doses of IV β-blocker are usually effective. Occasionally herald the onset of runs of ventricular tachycardia.

- Correct any contributing causes—ensuring adequate oxygenation, normocarbia, and analgesia.
- If the underlying sinus rate is slow (<50bpm), then 'ectopics' may be ventricular escape beats. Try increasing the rate using IV atropine/glycopyrronium.

Ventricular tachycardia

Focus in the ventricular muscle depolarises at high frequency resulting in wide QRS which may vary in shape. P waves may be seen if there is AV dissociation. This is a serious, potentially life-threatening arrhythmia. It may be triggered intra-operatively by

- Myocardial ischaemia, hypoxia, hypotension
- Fluid overload
- Electrolyte imbalance (low K^+, Mg^{2+}, etc.)
- Injection of adrenaline or other catecholamines

Management

- Synchronised DC cardioversion (200 then 360J) if the patient is haemodynamically unstable. Will restore sinus rhythm in virtually 100% of cases. If the VT is pulseless or very rapid, synchronisation is unnecessary. If the patient relapses into VT lidocaine or amiodarone may be given to sustain sinus rhythm.
- Lidocaine (100mg bolus) restores sinus rhythm in 30–40% and may be followed by a maintenance infusion of 4mg/min for 30min, then 2mg/min for 2hr, then 1mg/min.
- Drugs which may be used if lidocaine fails include
  - Amiodarone 300mg IV via central venous catheter over 1hr followed by 900mg over 23hr. Give peripherally if necessary.
  - Sotalol 100mg IV over 5min has been shown to be better than lidocaine for acute termination of VT.
  - Procainamide 100mg IV over 5min followed by one or two further boluses before commencing infusion at 3mg/min.

Supraventricular tachycardia with aberrant conduction

A supraventricular tachycardia (SVT) may be broad complex due to aberrant conduction between atria and ventricles. This may develop secondary to ischaemia and appear only at high heart rates (rate-related aberrant conduction). SVT caused by an abnormal or accessory pathway (e.g. Wolff–Parkinson–White syndrome) will be of normal width if conduction in the accessory pathway is retrograde (i.e. it is the normal pathway that initiates the QRS complex) but broad complex if conduction is anterograde in the accessory pathway. Adenosine may be used diagnostically to slow AV conduction and will often reveal the underlying rhythm. In the case of SVT it may also result in conversion to sinus rhythm. In practice, however, all broad complex tachycardias should be treated as ventricular tachycardia until proven otherwise.

Acute management of broad complex tachycardia

- If in doubt as to nature of rhythm assume it is ventricular rather than supraventricular tachycardia (98% will be, especially if there is a history of ischaemic heart disease).
- In the presence of hypotension/cardiovascular compromise—synchronised DC shock with 200 then 360J.
- Perform a 12-lead ECG—if possible both before and after correction, as this will help with retrospective diagnosis.
- If the patient is not acutely compromised, adenosine 0.2mg/kg rapidly IV will be both diagnostic and often curative if it is a supraventricular tachycardia.

Ventricular fibrillation

- This results in cardiac arrest. There is chaotic and disorganised contraction of ventricular muscle and no QRS complexes can be identified on the ECG.
- Immediate direct current cardioversion as per established resuscitation protocol (200, 200, thereafter 360J)—see p862.

Action plan in theatre when faced with an arrhythmia

- Assess vital signs—ABC.
- Determine whether the arrhythmia is serious (cardiovascular compromise—BP/CO/HR).

Is there a problem with the anaesthetic?

- Oxygenation?
- Ventilation—check end tidal CO_2.
- Anaesthesia too light—alter inspired volatile agent concentration and give a bolus of rapid acting analgesic e.g. alfentanil.
- Drug interaction/error?

Is there a problem with surgery?

- Vagal stimulation from traction on the eye or peritoneum
- Loss of cardiac output—air/fat embolism
- Unexpected blood loss
- Injection of adrenaline
- Mediastinal manipulation

Disturbances of conduction (heart block)

First-degree block

Delay in conduction from the SA node to the ventricles. Prolongation of the PR interval to >0.2s. Normally benign but may progress to second-degree block, usually Mobitz type I. First-degree heart block is not a problem during anaesthesia.

Second-degree block—Mobitz type I (Wenkebach)

Progressive lengthening of the PR interval and then failure of conduction of an atrial beat. This is followed by a conducted beat and the cycle repeats. This occurs commonly after inferior myocardial infarction and tends to be self-limiting. Asymptomatic patients do not normally require treatment perioperatively but may require long-term pacing as a 2:1 type block may develop with haemodynamic instability.

Second-degree block—Mobitz type II

Excitation intermittently fails to pass through the AV node or the bundle of His. Most beats are conducted normally but occasionally there is atrial contraction without a subsequent ventricular contraction. This often progresses to complete heart block.

Second-degree block—2:1 type

Alternately conducted and non-conducted beats, resulting in two P waves for every QRS complex. 3:1 block may also occur, with one conducted beat and two non-conducted beats. This may progress to complete heart block.

Third-degree block/complete heart block

Complete failure of conduction between atria and ventricles. Occasionally a transient phenomenon due to severe vagal stimulation, in which case it often responds to stopping stimulation and IV atropine. Very rarely it may be congenital.

Bundle branch block

If there is a delay in depolarisation of the right or left bundle branches, this will cause a delay in depolarisation of part of the ventricular muscle with subsequent QRS widening.

Right bundle branch block

Wide complexes with an 'RSR' in lead V1 (may appear 'M' shaped) and a small initial negative downward deflection followed by a larger upwards positive wave and then a second downward wave in V6. Often benign.

Left bundle branch block

Septal depolarisation is reversed so there is a change in the initial direction of the QRS complex in every lead. This may indicate heart disease and makes further interpretation of the ECG other than rate and rhythm difficult.

Bifascicular block

Combination of right bundle branch block and block of the left anterior or left posterior fascicle. Right bundle branch block with left anterior hemiblock is commoner and appears as an 'RSR' in V1 together with left-axis deviation. Right bundle branch block with left posterior hemiblock is less common and appears as right bundle branch block with an abnormal degree of right-axis deviation. However, other causes for right-axis deviation should be considered and it is a non-specific sign.

Trifascicular block

Sometimes used to indicate the presence of a prolonged PR interval together with bifascicular block.

Preoperative management
- First-degree heart block in the absence of symptoms is common. It needs no specific investigation or treatment.
- Second- or third-degree heart block may need pacemaker insertion. If surgery is urgent this may be achieved quickly by inserting a temporary transvenous wire prior to definitive insertion.
- Bundle branch, bifascicular, or trifascicular block (bifascicular with first-degree block) will rarely progress to complete heart block during anaesthesia and so it is not normal practice to insert a pacing wire unless there have been episodes of syncope.

Indications for preoperative pacing
- Symptomatic first-degree heart block
- Symptomatic second-degree (Mobitz I) heart block
- Second-degree (Mobitz II) heart block
- Third-degree heart block
- Symptomatic bifascicular block or symptomatic first-degree heart block plus bifascicular block (trifascicular block)
- Slow rates unresponsive to drugs

Intra-operative heart block

- Atropine is rarely effective but should be tried.
- If hypotension is profound then an isoprenaline infusion (alternative is adrenaline) can be used to temporise: 1–10µg/min.
    - dilute 0.2mg in 500ml of 5% glucose/dextrose–saline and titrate to effect (2–20ml/min).
    - dilute 1mg in 50ml 5% glucose/dextrose–saline and titrate to effect (1.5–30ml/hr).
- Transcutaneous pacing may be practical in theatre if electrodes can be placed. Oesophageal pacing is also effective. The electrode is passed into the oesophagus like a nasogastric tube and connected to the pulse generator. The position can be adjusted until there is ventricular capture.
- Transvenous pacing is both more reliable and effective and relatively easy. A Swan–Ganz sheath of adequate size to pass the wire is inserted into the internal jugular or subclavian vein (this can be done while other equipment is being collected).
    - Insert balloon-tipped pacing wire to the 20cm mark.
    - Inflate the balloon and connect pulse generator at 5V.
    - Advance until ventricular capture. When this happens deflate the balloon and insert a further 5cm of catheter.
    - If the 50cm mark is reached the catheter is coiling up or not entering the heart. Deflate the balloon, withdraw to the 20cm mark and try again.

Pacemakers and defibrillators

Pacemakers are usually used to treat bradyarrhythmias. However, biventricular systems are used to improve functional capacity and quality of life in selected patients with severe heart failure.

The Heart Rhythm Society (HRS) and Heart Rhythm Society UK (HRSUK) pacemaker codes are used to describe pacemaker types and function. The code consists of five letters or positions. The first three describe anti-bradycardia functions and are always stated. The fourth and fifth positions relate to additional functions and are often omitted.

Position 1: chamber paced (0/V/A/D—none, ventricle, atrium, dual)

Position 2: sensing chamber (0/V/A/D)

Position 3: response to sensing (0/T/I/D—none, triggered, inhibited, dual)

Position 4: programmability or rate modulation (0/P/M/R—none, simple programmable, multiprogrammable, rate modulation)

Position 5: anti-tachycardia functions (0/P/S/D—none, pacing, shock, dual)

Implications for anaesthesia and surgery

- Patients with pacemakers should attend follow-up clinics. The most recent visit should confirm adequate battery life and normal function of the pacemaker system. A preoperative ECG will provide confirmation of expected function, e.g. AV synchronicity, polarity of pacing and baseline rate.
- The main source of concern is electromagnetic interference (EMI). Possible responses include inappropriate triggering or inhibition of a paced output, asynchronous pacing, reprogramming (usually into a backup mode), and damage to device circuitry. Pacing wires may also act as aerials and cause heating where they contact the endocardium. Diathermy is the most common source of EMI found in the operating theatre.
- Bipolar diathermy is safe. If conventional diathermy is necessary, position the plate so that most of the current passes away from the pacemaker. In an emergency most pacemakers can be changed to asynchronous ventricular pacing (V00) by placing a magnet over the box. There is a theoretical risk of inducing ventricular fibrillation as the magnet induced asynchronous pacing may result in stimulation during a vulnerable period and induce an arrhythmia—'competitive pacing'. In modern pacemakers the switch to asynchronous pacing is coupled with the next cardiac event to avoid this.
- For patients with severe heart failure, where loss of AV synchrony may precipitate haemodynamic compromise, these should be a telemetric programmer and cardiac technician close at hand.

Implantable cardioverter defibrillators (ICDs)

- The National Institute for Clinical Excellence (NICE) has recently recommended that ICDs should be routinely considered for patients who have survived ventricular fibrillation or ventricular tachycardia with haemodynamic compromise.
- In addition they recommend these devices should be used as primary prevention for sudden cardiac death in patients with impaired ventricular function (ejection fraction <35%), non-sustained ventricular tachycardia on ambulatory 24hr monitoring, or inducible ventricular tachycardia at electrophysiological testing.
- These devices should be disabled for anaesthesia and surgery as diathermy signals may be interpreted as an arrhythmia and cause inappropriate discharge. Facilities for external defibrillation should be immediately available. If possible remote pads should be applied in suitable positions prior to surgery.

HRS/HRSUK codes to describe ICD type and function

Position 1: shock chamber (0/A/V/D—none, atrium, ventricle, dual).

Position 2: chamber to which anti-tachycardia pacing is delivered (0/A/V/D).

Position 3: means of detection of tachyarrhythmia (E/H—intracardiac electrogram, haemodynamic means).

Position 4: the three or five letter code for the pacemaker capability of the device (as above).

Further reading

Salukhe TV, Dob D, Sutton R (2004). Pacemaker and defibrillators: anaesthetic implications. *British Journal of Anaesthesia*, **93**, 95–104.

Chapter 5

Respiratory disease

Bruce McCormick

Effects of surgery and anaesthesia on respiratory function

Site of surgical incision

- Upper abdominal operations are associated with pulmonary complications in 20–40% of general surgical population.
- Incidence with lower abdominal surgery is 2–5%.
- Following upper abdominal or thoracic surgery, lung volume (FRC) and tidal volume fall, and coughing may be ineffective. The diaphragm moves less after abdominal surgery (vital capacity falls by 50% after cholecystectomy, even in healthy patients).
- Poor basal air entry and sputum retention often result, which may develop into atelectasis and/or infection. Effective postoperative analgesia, early mobilization, and physiotherapy may reduce incidence and severity.

Pre-existing respiratory dysfunction

- Patients with underlying respiratory disease are at increased risk of developing problems during and after surgery.[1]
- Complications are minimised if underlying condition is identified and optimally controlled preoperatively.
- All patients benefit from a review of their medical therapy, early mobilisation, and pre- and postoperative chest physiotherapy.
- Consider review by a respiratory physician.

Anaesthesia

- On induction of anaesthesia, functional residual capacity (FRC) decreases by 15–20% (~450ml): the diaphragm relaxes/moves cranially and the rib cage moves inward.
- FRC may be reduced by 50% of awake, supine value in morbidly obese patients. FRC is relatively maintained during ketamine anaesthesia.
- Under anaesthesia, closing capacity (the lung volume at which airway closure begins) encroaches upon FRC and airway closure occurs. This happens more readily in smokers, the elderly, and those with underlying lung disease.
- Chest CT shows atelectasis in the dependent zones of the lungs in >80% of anaesthetised subjects. At least 10% of pulmonary blood flow is shunted or goes to areas of low V/Q ratio.
- Intubation halves dead space by circumventing the upper airway.
- The response to hypercapnia is blunted and the acute responses to hypoxia and acidaemia almost abolished by anaesthetic vapours at concentrations as low as 0.1MAC.
- Most of these adverse changes are more marked in patients with lung disease but usually improve within a few hours postoperatively. After major surgery they may last several days.

---

1 Hall JC, Tarala RA, Tapper J, Hall J (1996). Prevention of respiratory complications after abdominal surgery: a randomised control trial. *British Medical Journal*, **312**, 148–152.

Predicting postoperative pulmonary complications[1,2]

- Preoperative identification of patients with pre-existing respiratory dysfunction reduces postoperative complications.
- Even for patients with severe pulmonary disease, surgery which does not involve the abdominal or chest cavities is inherently of very low risk for serious perioperative pulmonary complications.
- Abnormal findings on examination or an abnormal CXR may reflect significant lung disease and are independent predictors of pulmonary complications.
- Absence of symptoms or signs does not exclude significant pathology which will be unmasked by anaesthesia (e.g. sarcoidosis p120).
- Spirometry was formerly considered highly important in the assessment of surgical patients. Recent evidence suggests that preoperative spirometry does not predict individual risk of pulmonary complications and should not be used alone to determine operability for non-thoracic surgery.
- Large and rigorous studies to identify risk factors for pulmonary complications are lacking (in contrast to those identifying cardiac risk).

Factors shown to predict perioperative pulmonary complications

- Scoring systems which assess overall co-morbidity (ASA physical status grade, Goldman cardiac risk index, and Charlson co-morbidity index)
- Increasing age (>60yr)
- Smoking within 8wk
- History of malignancy
- Symptoms of chronic bronchitis
- Body mass index >27kg/m^2
- Upper abdominal and thoracic surgery
- Abnormal clinical signs in chest
- Abnormality on CXR
- $PaCO_2$ >6kPa (45mmHg)
- Impaired cognitive function
- Postoperative nasogastric intubation.

1 Lawrence VA, Dhanda R, Hilsenbeck SG, Page CP (1996). Risk of pulmonary complications following abdominal surgery. *Chest*, **110**, 744–750.
2 Zollinger A, Pasch T (1998). The pulmonary risk patient. *Bailliere's Clinical Anaesthesia*, **5**, 391–400.

Assessment of respiratory function[1,2,3]

History

- Ask about hospital admissions with respiratory disease, particularly admissions to intensive care.
- Determine patient's assessment of lung function and their compliance with treatment. Respiratory disease tends to fluctuate in severity and patients are usually best at determining their current state. Elective surgery should be performed when respiratory function is optimal.
- Note cough and sputum production (character and quantity). Send a sputum specimen for culture and sensitivity.
- Note past and present cigarette consumption, encouraging cessation.
- Assess current treatment, reversibility of symptoms with bronchodilators, and steroid intake.
- Note any respiratory symptoms suggestive of cardiac disease (orthopnoea, PND). Investigate and treat accordingly.
- Dyspnoea can be described using Roizen's classification. Undiagnosed dyspnoea of grade II or worse may require further investigation (see below).

Roizen's classification of dyspnoea

Grade 0:	No dyspnoea while walking on the level at normal pace
Grade I:	'I am able to walk as far as I like, provided I take my time'
Grade II:	Specific street block limitation—'I have to stop for a while after one or two blocks'
Grade III:	Dyspnoea on mild exertion—'I have to stop and rest going from the kitchen to the bathroom'
Grade IV:	Dyspnoea at rest

Examination

- Abnormal findings on clinical examination are predictive of pulmonary complications after abdominal surgery (see p95).
- Complications of respiratory disease (right heart failure) and its treatment (steroid effects) should be sought. Try to establish any contribution of cardiac disease to respiratory symptoms.
- A formal assessment of exercise tolerance such as stair climbing correlates well with pulmonary function tests and provides a reliable test of pulmonary function. However, it also reflects cardiovascular status, cooperation, and determination and is an impractical assessment for those with limited mobility.

---

1 Smetana GW (1999). Preoperative pulmonary evaluation. *New England Journal of Medicine*, **340**, 937–944.
2 Lawrence VA, Dhanda R, Hilsenbeck SG, Page CP (1996). Risk of pulmonary complications after elective abdominal surgery. *Chest*, **110**, 744–750.
3 Zollinger A, Pasch T (1998). The pulmonary risk patient. *Bailliere's Clinical Anaesthesia*, **5**, 391–400.

Respiratory investigations

Peak flow

- A useful test for COPD or asthma.
- Measured on ward using a peak flow meter (best of three attempts); technique is important. For normal values see p1170.
- The patient's daily record gives a good indication of current fitness.
- Coughing is ineffective if the peak flow is <200l/min.

Spirometry

- Useful to quantify severity of ventilatory dysfunction and to differentiate restrictive from obstructive defects. Measured in the respiratory function laboratory or at the bedside using a bellows device.
- Normally the forced vital capacity (FVC) is reported along with forced expiration in 1s (FEV_1), plus the ratio FEV_1/FVC (as a percentage). The results of these tests are given with normal values calculated for that individual. A normal FEV_1/FVC ratio is 70% (see p1170).
- Previously used to assess risk in patients with significant respiratory disease scheduled for major surgery. However, recent evidence suggests that spirometry does not predict pulmonary complications, even in patients with severe COPD.
- No spirometric values should be viewed as prohibitive for surgery. Despite poor preoperative spirometry, many series of patients undergoing thoracic and major non-thoracic surgery are being increasingly reported. An FEV_1 <1000ml indicates that postoperative coughing and secretion clearance will be poor and increases the likelihood of needing respiratory support following major surgery.
- Specific subgroups of patients who may benefit from spirometry are:
  - Those with equivocal clinical and radiological findings or unclear diagnosis.
  - Patients in whom functional ability cannot be assessed because of lower extremity disability.
- Spirometry also forms part of the assessment of patients for lung parenchymal resection (see p353).
- In those with an obstructive picture (low FEV_1/FVC ratio), reversibility with salbutamol should be tested. If time permits, the spirometry should be repeated after a course of steroids (prednisolone 20–40mg daily for 7d).

Flow volume loops

- Measured in the respiratory function department.
- Peak flows at different lung volumes are recorded. Although more complex to interpret, loops provide more accurate information regarding ventilatory function. They provide useful data about the severity of obstructive and restrictive respiratory disease.
- Used in assessment of airway obstruction from both extrinsic (e.g. thyroid) and intrinsic (e.g. bronchospasm) causes.

Transfer factor (diffusing capacity)

- Measures the diffusion of carbon monoxide into the lung, using a single breath of gas containing 0.3% CO and 10% helium held for 20s
- Reduced in lung fibrosis and other interstitial disease processes affecting gas transfer from alveolus to capillary
- Normal value: 17–25ml/min/mmHg

Arterial blood gases

- Measure baseline gases in air for any patient breathless on minimal exertion. Check for previous results in patients who have been hospitalised before.
- Detects CO_2 retention. A resting $PaCO_2$ > 6.0kPa (45mmHg) is predictive of pulmonary complications and suggests ventilatory failure.
- Demonstrates usual level of oxygenation, which indicates severity of disease and is useful to set realistic parameters postoperatively.

CXR

- Essential in patients scheduled for major surgery with significant chest disease or signs on examination. Try to obtain an erect PA film in the X-ray department.
- An abnormality predicts risk of pulmonary complications.
- Reveals lung pathology, cardiac size and outline, and provides a baseline should postoperative problems develop.

Chest CT

- Chest CT is required in a few patients with lung cysts/bullae to accurately assess the size and extent of their disease.
- Impingement of mass lesions on the major airways and likely extent of lung resection can be assessed.
- May demonstrate anterior or posterior pneumothorax and interstitial disease such as lung fibrosis, not seen on CXR.
- Spiral CT chest investigations can detect pulmonary embolus and dissecting aortic lesions.

V/Q scan

- Reports the likelihood of pulmonary embolism. Difficult to interpret in the presence of other pathology.
- Useful in assessment of patients for lung parenchymal resection to predict the effect of resection on overall pulmonary performance (resecting a non-ventilated/perfused lung will reduce shunt and should improve oxygenation).

Postoperative care

Early mobilisation and posture

- Respiratory performance, FRC, and clearance of secretions are improved when sitting or standing compared with the supine position.
- Early mobilisation reduces the incidence of thromboembolic disease.

Regular clinical review

- Respiratory deterioration may present in a non-specific way (confusion, tachycardia, fever, unwell). Regular review allows urgent investigation and aggressive therapy.
- Chart respiratory rate.
- Seek assessment and advice of intensive care/outreach team early if patient does not respond to initial treatment.

Physiotherapy

- Incentive spirometry, breathing exercises, and early physiotherapy aid clearance of secretions and reduce atelectasis.

Oxygen

- Anaesthetic agents exert a dose-dependent depression on the sensitivity of central chemoreceptors, reducing the stimulatory effect of CO_2.
- Depression of respiratory function can occur for up to 72hr postoperatively and is most common at night. Supplemental oxygen should be delivered for at least this period of time.
- Preoperative measurement of PaO_2/SaO_2 and $PaCO_2$ is essential to establish a realistic target for each patient.
- Patients who chronically retain CO_2 (advanced COPD) may be dependent on hypoxaemia as their main ventilatory drive due to down-regulation of central chemoreceptors. The concentration of delivered oxygen should be controlled (e.g. by Venturi mask) and titrated, in order to optimise oxygenation and prevent hypoventilation. Adequate monitoring should be available, ideally using serial ABG measurement (pulse oximetry shows only SaO_2).
- Humidification of oxygen aids physiotherapy and sputum clearance.

Fluid balance

- Accurate management and documentation of fluid balance is essential. Adequate intravascular filling is required to maintain adequate perfusion of organs such as the kidneys and gut.
- However, patients with lung disease are at increased risk of pulmonary oedema (a dilated right ventricle may mechanically compromise the function of the left ventricle). Fluid overload is poorly tolerated in these patients and a high index of suspicion should be maintained.
- Readings from central venous catheters may be misleading in the presence of pulmonary hypertension or right ventricular failure (cor pulmonale).

Pain management

- Good analgesia is essential for the maintenance of efficient respiratory function, compliance with physiotherapy, early mobilization, and minimising cardiac stress.
- Regular oral or rectal paracetamol and, where not contraindicated, NSAIDs should be prescribed. NSAIDs should be used with caution in the elderly as renal function may be compromised and they may induce fluid retention.
- Patients with lung dysfunction may benefit from local or regional anaesthesia. The sedative effects of systemic opioids can be avoided. The surgeon may be willing to place a catheter for regional anaesthesia at the time of operation (e.g. paravertebral catheter for thoracotomy).
- The benefits of opioid-based analgesia (patient control, mobility, and avoidance of catheterisation) should be weighed against the benefits of regional analgesia (avoidance of high-dose systemic opioids, preservation of respiratory function) and discussed with the patient preoperatively.
- Involve the pain management team early in the postoperative period, requesting at least daily reviews.

Postoperative admission to HDU/ICU

- Ideally admission to ICU or HDU should be planned preoperatively.
- Patients may require admission for ventilatory support (CPAP, BIPAP, invasive ventilation) or increased levels of monitoring and nursing care that are not available on the surgical ward.

The precipitating reasons for admission to ICU or HDU may be predictable or unpredictable:

Predictable	Unpredictable
Borderline or established failure of gas exchange preoperatively	Unexpected perioperative complications (e.g. fluid overload, haemorrhage, etc.)
Intercurrent respiratory infection (with urgent surgery)	Inadequate or ineffective regional analgesia with deterioration in respiratory function
Chest disease productive of large amounts of secretions (e.g. bronchiectasis)	Unexpectedly prolonged procedure
Major abdominal or thoracic surgery	Acidosis
Major surgery not amenable to regional analgesia and necessitating systemic opioids	Hypothermia
Long duration of surgery	Depressed conscious level/ slow recovery from anaesthetic/ poor cough

Indications for minitracheostomy

- 'Minitracheostomy' describes devices available for cricothyroidotomy and insertion of a tube (typically 4mm internal diameter) to facilitate tracheal suction via fine-bore catheters.
- Useful in patients with a poor cough or excessive secretions and enables more effective physiotherapy. Ineffective at removing more tenacious secretions and may partially occlude the airway.
- Insertion carries the risks of haemorrhage and surgical emphysema.
- Use of minitracheostomy is declining. A percutaneous tracheostomy cannula may be down-sized to minitracheostomy for bronchial toilet prior to complete decannulation.

Respiratory tract infection and elective surgery[1,2]

See p770 for paediatric implications.

- Patients who have respiratory tract infections producing fever and cough with or without chest signs on auscultation should not undergo elective surgery under general anaesthesia due to the increased risk of postoperative pulmonary complications.
- Adult patients with simple coryza are not at significantly increased risk of developing postoperative pulmonary problems, unless they have pre-existing respiratory disease or are having major abdominal or thoracic surgery.
- Laryngospasm may be more likely in patients with a recent history of upper respiratory tract symptoms who are asymptomatic at the time of surgery.
- Compared with asymptomatic children, children with symptoms of acute or recent upper respiratory tract infection are more likely to suffer transient postoperative hypoxaemia (SaO_2 <93%). This is most marked when intubation is necessary.

1 Fennelly ME, Hall GM (1990). Anaesthesia and upper airway respiratory tract infections—a non-existent hazard? *British Journal of Anaesthesia*, **64**, 535–536.
2 Levy L, Pandit UA, Randel GI, Lewis IH, Tait AR (1992). Upper respiratory tract infections and general anaesthesia in children. *Anaesthesia*, **47**, 678–682.

Smoking[1,2]

- Cigarette smoke contains nicotine, a highly addictive substance, and at least 4700 other chemical compounds, of which 43 are known to be carcinogenic. Long-term smoking is associated with serious underlying problems such as COPD, lung neoplasm, ischaemic heart disease, and vascular disorders.
- Respiratory tract mucus is produced in greater quantities, but mucociliary clearance is less efficient. Smokers are more susceptible to respiratory events during anaesthesia and to postoperative atelectasis/pneumonia. Abdominal or thoracic surgery and obesity increase these risks.
- Carboxyhaemoglobin (COHb) levels may reach 5–15% in heavy smokers, causing reduced oxygen carriage by the blood. COHb has a similar absorption spectrum to oxyhaemoglobin and will cause falsely high oxygen saturation readings.
- Increased airway irritability increases coughing, laryngospasm, and desaturation during induction and airway manipulation (laryngeal mask insertion). Avoid by using a less irritant volatile (e.g. sevoflurane) and deepening anaesthesia slowly.
- Maintaining spontaneous breathing via an ETT or LMA may be awkward due to airway irritation—try local anaesthesia to the vocal cords, opioids, relaxants, and IPPV.

Risk reduction

- Abstinence from smoking for 8wk is required to decrease morbidity from respiratory complications to a rate similar to that of non-smokers.
- Smokers unwilling to stop preoperatively will still benefit by refraining from smoking for 12hr before surgery. During this time the effects of nicotine (activation of the sympathoadrenergic system with raised coronary vascular resistance) and COHb will decrease.

1 Nel MR, Morgan M (1996). Smoking and anaesthesia revisited (editorial). *Anaesthesia*, **51**, 309–311.
2 Schwilk B, Bothner U, Schraag S, Georgieff M (1997). Perioperative respiratory events in smokers and non-smokers undergoing general anaesthesia. *Acta Anaesthesiologica Scandinavica*, **41**, 348–355.

Asthma[1,2,3]

Asthma is reversible airflow obstruction due to constriction of smooth muscle in the airways. Bronchial wall inflammation is a fundamental component and results in mucus hypersecretion and epithelial damage as well as an increased tendency for airways to constrict. Bronchoconstriction may be triggered by a number of different mechanisms.

Symptoms of asthma are most frequently a combination of shortness of breath, wheeze, cough, and sputum production. Asthma can be differentiated from COPD by the presence of childhood symptoms, diurnal variation, specific trigger factors (especially allergic), absence of smoking history, and response to previous treatments.

General considerations

- Most well-controlled asthmatics tolerate anaesthesia and surgery well.
- The incidence of perioperative bronchospasm and laryngospasm in asthmatic patients undergoing routine surgery is <2%, especially if routine medication is continued.
- The frequency of complications is increased in patients >50yr and in those with active disease.
- Poorly controlled asthmatics are at risk of perioperative problems (bronchospasm, sputum retention, atelectasis, infection, respiratory failure).
- Do not anaesthetise patients for elective surgery unless the patient's asthma is optimally controlled.

Preoperative assessment

- Patients and doctors frequently underestimate the severity of asthma, especially if it is longstanding.
- Assess exercise tolerance (e.g. breathless when climbing stairs, walking on level ground, or undressing) and general activity levels.
- Document any allergies/drug sensitivities, especially the effect of aspirin/NSAIDs. The prevalence of aspirin-induced asthma (measured by oral provocation) is 21% in adult asthmatics and 5% in paediatric asthmatics. Much lower rates are quoted if verbal history is used to assess prevalence (3% and 2%, respectively).
- Examination is often unremarkable but may reveal chest hyperinflation, prolonged expiratory phase, and wheeze. The presence or absence of wheeze does not correlate with severity of underlying asthma.
- For patients with severe asthma, consider additional medication or treatment with systemic steroids.
- Patients with mild asthma (peak flow >80% predicted and minimal symptoms) rarely require extra treatment prior to surgery.
- Emphasise benefits of good compliance with treatment prior to surgery. Consider doubling dose of inhaled steroids 1wk prior to surgery if there is evidence of poor control (>20% variability in PEFR). If control is very poor, consider review by chest physician and a 1wk course of oral prednisolone (20–40mg daily).

- Viral infections are potent triggers of asthma, so postpone elective surgery if symptoms suggest URTI.
- Association with nasal polyps in atopic patients.

Investigations

- Serial measurements of peak flow are more informative than a single reading. Measure response to bronchodilators and look for 'early morning dip' in peak flow (suggests control is not optimal).
- Spirometry gives a more accurate assessment. Results of peak flow and spirometry are compared with predicted values based on age, sex, and height (see p1170).
- Blood gases are only necessary in assessing patients with severe asthma (poorly controlled, frequent hospital admissions, previous ICU admission), particularly prior to major surgery.

Perioperative recommendations for asthma medications

Class of drug	Examples	Perioperative recommendation	Notes
β_2 agonists	Salbutamol, terbutaline, salmeterol	Convert to nebulised preparation	High doses may lower K^+. Causes tachycardia and tremor
Anticholinergic drugs	Ipratropium	Convert to nebulised form	
Inhaled steroids	Beclomethasone, budesonide, fluticasone	Continue inhaled formulation	If >1500µg/d of beclomethasone, adrenal suppression may be present
Oral steroids	Prednisolone	Continue as IV hydrocortisone until taking orally	If >10mg/d, adrenal suppression likely (p166)
Leukotriene inhibitor (anti-inflammatory effect)	Montelukast, zafirlukast	Restart when taking oral medications	
Mast cell stabiliser	Disodium cromoglycate	Continue by inhaler	
Phosphodiesterase inhibitor	Aminophylline	Continue where possible	In severe asthma consider converting to an infusion perioperatively

1 *British Guideline on the Management of Asthma.* A national clinical guideline. British Thoracic Society. Revised edition April 2004 http://www.brit-thoracic.org.uk
2 Hirshman CA (1991). Perioperative management of the asthmatic patient. *Canadian Journal of Anaesthesia*, **38**, R26–R32.
3 Warner DO et al. (1996). Perioperative respiratory complications in patients with asthma. Anesthesiology, **85**, 460–467.

Conduct of anaesthesia

- For major surgery start chest physiotherapy preoperatively.
- Add nebulised salbutamol 2.5mg to premedication.
- Avoid histamine-releasing drugs or use with care (morphine, D-tubocurarine, atracurium, mivacurium).
- Intubation may provoke bronchospasm—consider potent opioid cover (alfentanil). LA to the cords may help.
- When asthma is poorly controlled, regional techniques are ideal for peripheral surgery. Spinal anaesthesia or plexus/nerve blocks are generally safe, provided the patient is able to lie flat comfortably.
- Where general anaesthesia is necessary, use short acting anaesthetic agents. Short-acting opioid analgesics (e.g. alfentanil, remifentanil) are appropriate for procedures with minimal postoperative pain or when a reliable regional block is present.
- Patients with severe asthma (previous ICU admissions, brittle disease) undergoing major abdominal or thoracic surgery should be admitted to HDU/ICU for postoperative observation.
- Extubate and recover in sitting position.

Drugs considered safe for asthmatics

Induction	Propofol, etomidate, ketamine, midazolam
Opioids	Pethidine, fentanyl, alfentanil
Muscle relaxants	Vecuronium, suxamethonium, rocuronium, pancuronium
Volatile agents	Halothane, isoflurane, enflurane, sevoflurane

Severe bronchospasm during anaesthesia
See p884.

Postoperative care

- Ensure all usual medications are prescribed after surgery.
- Following major abdominal or thoracic surgery, good pain control is important and epidural analgesia is frequently the best choice, provided widespread intercostal blockade is avoided.
- For patient-controlled analgesia (PCA), consider pethidine if morphine has previously exacerbated bronchospasm.
- Prescribe oxygen for the duration of epidural or PCA.
- Prescribe regular nebuliser therapy with additional nebulised bronchodilators as needed.
- Review dose and route of administration of steroid daily.
- Regular NSAIDs can be used if tolerated in the past. Avoid in brittle and poorly controlled asthmatics.
- If there is increasing dyspnoea and wheeze following surgery, consider other possible contributing factors (left ventricular failure and pulmonary emboli are potent triggers of bronchospasm). Also consider fluid overload and pneumothorax (?recent central line).

Chronic obs~~~ disease (C~~~

• COPD enc~~~ronchitis and emphysema. Chronic bronchiti~~~ a history of a productive cough on most winter ~~~cutive years. Emphysema is a histological diag~~~tion and destruction of the airways distal to the te~~~nchioles.

• ~~~ajority of patients with COPD have been tobacco smokers for a ~~~nificant period of their lives. Other factors associated with COPD include occupational exposure to dusts and atmospheric pollution, poor socio-economic status, repeated viral infections, α1-antitrypsin deficiency and regional variation.

• Patients with predominantly emphysema may be thin, tachypnoeic, breathless at rest, and, although hypoxic, develop CO_2 retention only as a late or terminal event. Patients with predominantly chronic bronchitis are frequently overweight with marked peripheral oedema, poor respiratory effort, and CO_2 retention. These classical stereotyped pictures of 'pink puffer' or 'blue bloater' are infrequently seen compared with the majority of patients, who have a combination of features.

General considerations

• Principal problems in COPD are development of airflow obstruction and mucus hypersecretion exacerbated by repeated viral and bacterial infections. Many patients have an element of reversible airflow obstruction. If this can be demonstrated it is managed as asthma. Progressive airflow obstruction may lead to respiratory failure.

• Non-invasive ventilation via a full face or nasal mask (BIPAP) is increasingly used to treat acute severe exacerbations of COPD. This technique may be used to assist severely affected patients through the postoperative phase of major surgery. Preoperative training is essential in conjunction with a respiratory unit or HDU.

Preoperative assessment

• Symptoms of COPD usually start after the age of about 55yr. The commonest symptom is shortness of breath but cough, wheeze, and sputum production are also often present. Symptoms are frequently severe by the time medical help is sought. Repeated infective exacerbations of respiratory symptoms are common during the winter months.

• Establish exercise tolerance—ask specifically about hills and stairs. A formal assessment of exercise tolerance such as stair climbing correlates well with pulmonary function tests.

- Ensure any element of reversible airflow obstruction (asthma) is optimally treated. Consider a trial of oral prednisolone, combined with review by a respiratory physician.
- Pulmonary hypertension and right ventricular failure may follow severe or chronic pulmonary disease—optimise treatment of heart failure if present.
- Change to nebulised bronchodilators prior to surgery and continue for 24–48hr afterwards.

Investigations

- Check spirometry to clarify diagnosis and assess severity (this is much more informative than peak flow in COPD).
- Check ABGs if the patient has difficulty climbing one flight of stairs, is cyanosed, has SaO_2 <95% on air, or has peripheral oedema.
- ECG may reveal right heart disease (right ventricular hypertrophy or strain). Consider echocardiography.
- CXR is useful to exclude active infection and other pathology (e.g. bronchial carcinoma).

Conduct of anaesthesia

- See guidelines under 'Asthma' (p106).
- If patients have severe COPD (exercise tolerance less than one flight of stairs or CO_2 retention), postoperative respiratory failure is likely after abdominal or thoracic surgery. Plan for elective HDU/ICU admission.
- Avoid intubation where possible—however some patients (particularly those who are obese, breathless, and require long operations) are unsuitable for a spontaneously breathing technique. Patients with heavy sputum production may benefit from ETT toilet.
- Be vigilant for pneumothorax.

Postoperative care

- Extubate and recover in sitting position.
- Mobilise as early as possible.
- Regular physiotherapy to prevent atelectasis and encourage sputum clearance.
- Give oxygen as appropriate.
- If the patient becomes pyrexial with more copious or purulent sputum send a sample for culture and start antibiotics. Oral amoxycillin or clarithromycin are usually sufficient for mild exacerbations. If the patient becomes systemically unwell treat as pneumonia.
- Continue with nebulised salbutamol (2.5mg qds) and ipratropium (500µg qds) until fully mobile. Change back to inhalers at least 24hr before discharge.
- If the patient is slow to mobilise consider referral to a pulmonary rehabilitation programme.

1 Wong DH, Weber EC, Schell MJ, Wong AB, Anderson CT, Barker SJ (1995). Factors associated with postoperative pulmonary complications in patients with severe chronic obstructive pulmonary disease. *Anesthesia and Analgesia*, **80**, 276–284.

Bronchiectasis

Bronchiectasis may be caused by genetic factors, e.g. cystic fibrosis, or acquired following damage to the lower respiratory tract, especially in severe early childhood infections. Most patients have a chronic productive cough, which may be present throughout the year. There is frequently a component of asthma associated with chronic inflammatory changes in the airways. Cystic fibrosis is also associated with malabsorption due to pancreatic insufficiency, so appropriate dietary advice and pancreatic supplements are essential. See also p114.

General considerations

- Patients with bronchiectasis need to be as fit as possible before undergoing any major surgery which will inhibit coughing and impair respiratory function. For elective surgery this may mean a planned admission for IV antibiotics and physiotherapy prior to surgery.
- Once established, bacterial infections can be difficult or impossible to eradicate. *Pseudomonas aeruginosa* is a common pathogen that may be present for many years and be associated with intermittent exacerbations of respiratory symptoms.
- The mainstay of treatment for bronchiectasis is regular physiotherapy, frequent courses of appropriate antibiotics, and treatment of any asthmatic symptoms.

Preoperative assessment

- Before elective surgery the patient should be as fit as possible.
- Consultation with their chest physician is essential.
- Send sputum sample for culture before surgery. A course of IV antibiotics and physiotherapy for 3–10d immediately prior to surgery may be necessary. Prior to major surgery, consider starting IV antibiotics on admission. Use current or most recent sputum culture to guide appropriate prescribing. If in doubt assume that the patient has *Pseudomonas aeruginosa* and use a combination such as ceftazidime and gentamicin, or imipenem and gentamicin.
- Maximise bronchodilation by converting to nebulised bronchodilators.
- Increase dose of prednisolone by 5–10mg/day if on long-term oral steroids.
- Postpone elective surgery if the patient has more respiratory symptoms than usual.

Investigations

- In patients with severe disease check spirometry and blood gases.
- Send sputum sample for culture.

Conduct of anaesthesia
- Chose regional above general anaesthesia where possible.
- Although it is desirable to avoid intubation, this will be necessary for all but the shortest operations to facilitate intra-operative removal of secretions.
- Use short-acting anaesthetic and analgesic agents where postoperative pain is minimal or regional analgesia can be used.
- Extubate and recover in sitting position.
- Ensure that the patient will receive physiotherapy immediately postoperatively. Contact on-call physiotherapist if necessary.

Postoperative care
- Ensure that regular physiotherapy is available: three times daily and at night if severely affected.
- Monitor SaO_2, giving supplemental oxygen to achieve adequate oxygenation (guided by preoperative value).
- Continue appropriate IV antibiotics for at least 3d postoperatively or until discharged.
- Maintain adequate nutrition, especially if any malabsorption.
- Refer to respiratory physician early if there is any deterioration in respiratory symptoms.

Cystic fibrosis[1]

Basic defect is an abnormal epithelial chloride and sodium transport system encoded on chromosome 7. Patients experience chronic sinusitis, nasal polyps in 50% (polypectomy is a leading reason for anaesthesia in this group), and respiratory, cardiovascular, and gastrointestinal disease.

General considerations
- Neonates may present for surgical treatment of meconium ileus.
- In the lung, viscid mucus causes plugging, atelectasis, and frequent chest infection (particularly *Pseudomonas*). Treatment is primarily clearance of secretions by postural drainage and antibiotic treatment of infections.
- Heart–lung transplant was first performed in 1985 and early series show a 78% 1yr survival.
- The perioperative complication rate in cystic fibrosis is ~10% (mostly pulmonary).

Preoperative assessment
- Exclude or treat active chest infection.
- Clinical signs can be misleading.

Investigations
- Perform a CXR looking for bullae and pneumothorax. CT clarifies the extent of bullous disease and detects anterior pneumothoraces.
- Spirometry: FEV_1 may be prognostic.

Conduct of anaesthesia
- Almost all patients with cystic fibrosis have symptoms of bronchiectasis and will require treatment—see p112.
- Always inform the patient's physician of an admission to a surgical ward.
- Intubation allows bronchial toilet. Monitor for pneumothorax.

Postoperative care
- As for bronchiectasis.
- 80% of cystic fibrosis patients have pancreatic malabsorption. Maintaining adequate nutrition after surgery is essential and the advice of an experienced dietician is essential.

1 Walsh TS, Young CH (1995). Anaesthesia and cystic fibrosis. *Anaesthesia*, **50**, 614–622.

Restrictive pulmonary disease

Intrinsic parenchymal lung disease

• Results in decreased lung compliance and impaired gas exchange.
• An initial inflammatory reaction centred on the alveoli impairs gas exchange. This is followed by collagen deposition and fibrosis, resulting in lungs that are smaller in volume and less compliant to inflation.
• Causes of pulmonary fibrosis include autoimmune disorders (e.g. rheumatoid arthritis, scleroderma), exposure to inhaled dusts (e.g. asbestos), allergenic substances (bird fancier's and farmer's lung), ingested substances (especially drugs such as amiodarone, chemotherapy agents, paraquat poisoning), and fibrosis after acute respiratory distress syndrome.
• Pulmonary infections rarely trigger a fibrotic response.
• Treatment is usually with oral steroids but other immunosuppressive therapy may be used and young patients may be considered for lung transplantation if severely affected.

Extrinsic conditions of the chest wall

• Failure of the respiratory mechanical structures to provide or allow adequate ventilation, e.g. disease of the chest wall (kyphoscoliosis, ankylosing spondylitis, severe obesity), abdominal pathology producing significant splinting of the diaphragm.

General considerations

• Work of respiration is optimised by rapid shallow breaths and is easier in the sitting position.
• Many patients are stable and only slowly deteriorate over some years. These patients may tolerate surgery relatively well.

Preoperative assessment

• Discuss seriously affected patients with a respiratory physician.

Investigations

• Check ABGs—often remain normal until late. Reduced PaO_2 reflects significant disease and CO_2 retention is a late sign, implying impending ventilatory failure.
• Obtain lung function tests including spirometry, lung volumes (all are reduced), and gas transfer if these have not been done within previous 6–8wk.
• CXR changes will be according to the underlying condition.

Conduct of anaesthesia

• As for other pathologies, consider regional techniques and minimise positive pressure ventilation and airway instrumentation as far as possible. Spinal disease may preclude subarachnoid or epidural blocks.
• Where IPPV is necessary, minimise peak airway pressure using pressure-controlled ventilation, with high rate and low tidal volume.
• For those on steroids, increase dose on day of surgery and continue an extra 5–10mg of prednisolone per day until the patient goes home.
• High index of suspicion for pneumothorax.

Postoperative care
- Consider postoperative ICU/HDU admission following major surgery. May be suitable for elective training in CPAP/NIPPV techniques preoperatively.
- Extubate in sitting position.
- Supplemental oxygen, maintain SaO_2 >92%.
- Good physiotherapy and analgesia are vital to achieve sputum clearance. With severe disease, minor respiratory complications may precipitate respiratory failure.
- Mobilise early.
- Treat respiratory infection vigorously.
- Ensure steroid cover continues in appropriate formulation.

Sleep apnoea syndrome[1,2]

See also p604.

Sleep apnoea is defined as cessation of airflow at the mouth and nose for at least 10s. Sufferers develop intermittent respiratory arrest and hypoxaemia during rapid eye movement (REM) sleep. Respiration resumes due to hypoxic stimulation. The majority of sufferers are overweight, middle-aged men, who present with complaints of snoring with periods of apnoea, disturbed sleep, excessive daytime drowsiness, and headache.

Two types of sleep apnoea are recognised (5% of patients have both types):

- Obstructive sleep apnoea (85%) results from obstruction of the upper airway.
- Central apnoea (10%) is due to intermittent loss of respiratory drive.

The condition is diagnosed in a sleep laboratory by monitoring oxygen saturation and nasal airflow. Additional tests including measurement of respiratory and abdominal muscle activity, EEG, and EMG activity (polysomnography) may be required in some cases.

General considerations

- The patient may develop systemic and pulmonary hypertension, right ventricular hypertrophy, congestive cardiac failure, and respiratory failure with CO_2 retention.
- Most patients are treated with CPAP applied overnight by a nasal mask.
- In children, obstructive sleep apnoea is most commonly associated with adenotonsillar hypertrophy, but the severity of obstructive sleep apnoea is not always proportional to the size of the tonsils and adenoids.
- Patients with sleep apnoea syndrome are at risk of perioperative airway obstruction and respiratory failure while under the effects of sedative drugs.

Preoperative assessment

- Ask about daytime hypersomnolence (falling asleep during daily activities, e.g. reading or driving).
- Ask partner about snoring and whether apnoeic spells have been noted at night (patient usually unaware).
- Obesity and a collar size of >17 inches (43cm) are risk factors for obstructive sleep apnoea—weight reduction is beneficial.
- Obstructive sleep apnoea should be considered in all children presenting for adenotonsillectomy.
- Ensure that management of associated conditions such as obstructive airway disease, hypertension, and cardiac failure is optimal.
- Consider a respiratory opinion in patients with peripheral oedema and oxygen saturation <92%.
- Ask patients to bring their own CPAP machine and mask for postoperative use. Ensure that ward staff are familiar with set-up and running of equipment.

Investigations

- In known obstructive sleep apnoea, perform full blood count (poly-cythaemia), pulse oximetry, and ECG (right heart strain).
- If ECG shows right ventricular strain (3% of children presenting for adenotonsillectomy) echocardiography is indicated to exclude right ventricular hypertrophy.
- Obtain baseline ABGs.

Conduct of anaesthesia

- If the patient is on inhalers, change to nebulised bronchodilators.
- Avoid night sedation or sedative premedication.
- Anticipate that mask ventilation and intubation may be difficult and prepare for this.
- Regional anaesthesia/analgesia and postoperative analgesia will avoid or minimise use of general anaesthetic agents and sedative opioid analgesics.
- Use short-acting anaesthetic/analgesic agents where postoperative pain is minimal.
- NSAIDs and paracetamol.

Postoperative care

- Extubate in sitting position and nurse sitting up whenever possible.
- Patients are best managed in the HDU or ICU.
- A few hours of postoperative ventilation may be required after major surgery.
- Continuous pulse oximetry should be used on the ward.
- Aim to maintain the oxygen saturation that the patient had preoperatively, titrating oxygen to the minimum required. A few patients may develop CO_2 retention with oxygen therapy. Serial blood gas analysis may be necessary in drowsy patients at risk of CO_2 retention.

1 Boushra NN (1996). Anaesthetic management of patients with sleep apnoea syndrome. *Canadian Journal of Anaesthesia*, **43**, 599–616.
2 Warwick JP, Mason DG (1998). Obstructive sleep apnoea syndrome in children. *Anaesthesia*, **53**, 571–579.

Sarcoidosis

A systemic disease characterised by formation of non-caseating granulomata, which occur in any body tissue and heal with fibrosis. It probably results from an abnormal response to several antigens and occurs at all ages, with the highest prevalence at 20–40yr. It is more common in black individuals in the USA.

General considerations

- Pulmonary changes occur in 50%. Pleural, peri-bronchial, and alveolar granulomata are replaced by fibrosis. Hilar lymphadenopathy may cause bronchial obstruction and distal atelectasis. Infiltration of the bronchial mucosa may cause stenosis. Mucosal infiltration of nose, nasopharynx, tonsils, palate, or larynx may occur.
- Cardiac effects (in 20%). Right ventricular failure secondary to lung disease. Myocardial and valvular granulomata are rare. Conduction abnormalities, VT, or sudden death is reported.
- Other effects include skin involvement, uveitis/iritis and hypercalcaemia.

Preoperative assessment

- Pulmonary and cardiac features most important.
- May have extensive pathology but only minor symptoms.
- Note steroid treatment or other immunosuppressive drugs.

Investigations

- Preoperative respiratory function tests may reveal a restrictive defect. Transfer factor (diffusion capacity) may be reduced. ABGs will determine the level of hypoxaemia.
- ECG may show right ventricular hypertrophy or arrhythmias.
- Check Ca^{2+}—hypercalcaemia (treat with systemic steroids).

Conduct of anaesthesia

- Consider avoidance of GA and use of local/regional anaesthesia where possible if respiratory function impaired clinically.
- Consider regional analgesia for abdominal surgery if significant respiratory disease.
- Give appropriate steroid cover if needed.

Postoperative care

- Sit up.
- Good postoperative analgesia.
- Chest physiotherapy/breathing exercises.

Anaesthesia after lung transplantation

See also p70, Patients with a transplanted heart.

Lung transplantation was first performed in 1963; outcomes have improved since the introduction of ciclosporin A in 1981. Surgery may be indicated for:

• Complications related to transplant
• Complications of immunosuppressive treatment
• The underlying condition (emphysema, α1-antitrypsin deficiency, pulmonary fibrosis, primary pulmonary hypertension, cystic fibrosis)
• Unrelated reasons

General considerations

• The transplanted lung is denervated—mucosal sensitivity and the cough reflex are suppressed below the anastomosis, and sputum clearance is impaired postoperatively.
• Hypoxic vasoconstriction is unimpaired.
• Lymphatic drainage is severed but then re-established 2–4wk post-transplantation. Transplanted lungs are at particular risk of pulmonary oedema, especially in the early postoperative period.
• In double lung transplant, the heart may be denervated and has a higher resting heart rate (90–100bpm). It may be more susceptible to arrhythmias.

Preoperative assessment

• Underlying disease may have effects on pulmonary function. There may be residual systemic disease.

Conduct of anaesthesia

• The interaction of immunosuppressive drugs (ciclosporin A, steroids, azathioprine) with anaesthetic drugs is more theoretical than clinical.
• Monitor neuromuscular function and avoid high doses of opioid in order to achieve early extubation.
• Intubation should be performed to leave the tube just through the cords and the cuff carefully inflated and checked intra-operatively to minimise the risk of damage to the tracheal/bronchial anastomosis. If a double lumen tube is required it should be placed under direct vision using a fibrescope.
• Strict attention to fluid balance is required.
• Aim for early return of pulmonary function and extubation.

Postoperative care

• Postoperative admission to ICU is only indicated when anaesthesia is complicated by inadequate recovery of respiratory function, the surgical condition, or the presence of rejection or infection.

Chapter 6

Renal disease

Quentin Milner

Patient with raised creatinine

Creatinine is a product of skeletal muscle metabolism. Little renal tubular secretion occurs normally, and creatinine clearance reflects glomerular filtration rate (GFR). Plasma creatinine shows a rectangular hyperbolic relationship with creatinine clearance. This means

- GFR must be reduced by 50% before serum creatinine starts to rise.
- Small changes in serum creatinine in the low (normal) range imply a large change in GFR, making the test very sensitive.
- GFR falls by 1% per annum after 30yr of age.
- Creatinine clearance (CC) can be more accurately estimated from the serum creatinine by using the Cockcroft Gault formula:

$$\text{Creatinine clearance (ml/min)} = \frac{(140 - \text{age}) \times \text{weight (kg)}}{0.814 \times \text{serum creatinine } (\mu\text{mol/l})} \; (\times\, 0.85 \text{ for women}).$$

Chronic renal failure

Chronic renal failure (CRF) is a multi-system disease. Patients have a complex medical history, take a multitude of drugs, and frequently have severe systemic complications from the causes and/or effects of CRF. A diagnosis of renal failure is made when the GFR falls below 35ml/min and dialysis is required in CRF when the GFR is <15ml/min. End-stage renal failure occurs when the GFR is <5ml/min.

Main causes of CRF	
Diabetes mellitus	30%
Hypertension	24%
Glomerulonephritis	17%
Chronic pyelonephritis	5%
Polycystic renal disease	4%
Unknown cause	20%

Preoperative

- Determine underlying cause, previous surgery including transplantation, and drug therapy.
- Check for hypertension, diabetes, and anaemia. Ischaemic heart disease is common and often silent, especially in diabetics. Incidence of calcific valvular heart disease and left ventricular failure is increased. Pericardial effusions are rare if dialysis is effective.
- Type of dialysis: peritoneal or haemodialysis—line or fistula.
- Determine residual urine output per day.
- Examine for fluid overload (dependent oedema, basal crepitations, dialysis record) or hypovolaemia (postural hypotension, JVP, thirst, skin turgor, urine output).
- Allow 4–6hr to elapse after haemodialysis before surgery. This allows fluid compartment equilibration and metabolism of residual heparin. Indications for urgent dialysis include hyperkalaemia, fluid overload, acute acidosis, and symptomatic uraemia.
- If major surgery, plan postoperative care with renal/ICU team.

Investigations

- FBC: usually well compensated normochromic normocytic anaemia due to decreased erythropoiesis, decreased red cell survival, and GI losses. Aim for Hb 8–10g/dl; transfusion can worsen hypertension and precipitate heart failure.
- Electrolytes: a recent serum K^+ is essential—if >6.0mmol/l dialysis will be required. Na^+ may be low due to water retention. Hypocalcaemia and hyperphosphataemia are common but rarely symptomatic. A mild metabolic acidosis is frequent.
- Coagulation: INR, APTT, and platelet count usually normal; uraemia affects platelet function and causes a prolonged bleeding time. Dialysis improves coagulation once heparin has worn off. Thrombocytopathy is not corrected by platelet transfusion but may be improved by cryoprecipitate or DDAVP (0.3μg/kg in 30ml saline over 30min).

Perioperative care

- Venous access and fistulae: many patients have an upper limb AV fistula. Avoid cannulation and NIBP in this arm. Wrap the fistula arm in padding for protection. Wherever possible cannulate the dorsum of the hand to avoid damage to veins in the forearm and antecubital fossa for future fistulae. Arterial lines should be used only when essential and the radial artery is preferred.
- Fluid and electrolyte balance must be carefully managed. Many patients have some residual renal function and urine output. Normovolaemia is ideal. Maintain normal renal blood flow with 0.9% saline and avoid hypotension.
- If large fluid shifts are likely, CVP or oesophageal Doppler monitoring is useful. These patients may have had multiple CVP lines—use ultrasound guidance.
- Avoid fluids containing K^+; generally use 0.9% saline or Gelofusine. Significant blood loss should be replaced.
- Suxamethonium elevates serum K^+ by 0.5mmol/l. Hyperkalaemia is also worsened by acidosis, so avoid hypoventilation and hypercarbia.
- Delayed gastric emptying (autonomic neuropathy) and increased gastric acidity make gastric reflux more likely. Most patients are on H_2 antagonists/proton pump inhibitors (cimetidine may cause confusion and should be avoided). In practice, rapid sequence induction is reserved for patients who have not fasted, have symptomatic reflux and a normal serum potassium.
- Immunity: sepsis is a leading cause of death in CRF. Inhibition of humoral and cell-mediated immunity occurs. Careful attention to asepsis is required for all invasive procedures.
- Hepatitis B and C are common. Staff must protect themselves from body fluids.

Postoperative

- Liaise carefully with the renal unit about the timing/need for dialysis postoperatively.
- Prescribe analgesics carefully (see below).
- Pay attention to fluid balance. In oliguria, hourly fluid maintenance should replace fluid losses (including urine output) plus 30ml/hr for insensible losses.
- Avoid nephrotoxic drugs and periods of hypotension.

Anaesthetic drugs in chronic renal failure

Most drugs are excreted by the kidneys, either unchanged or as metabolites. Loading doses of drugs are often unchanged but maintenance doses should be reduced or dosing interval prolonged. Hypoalbuminaemia and acidosis increase the free drug availability of highly protein bound drugs (e.g. induction agents). Most anaesthetic drugs and techniques reduce renal blood flow, GFR, and urine output.

- Analgesics: most opioids are excreted by the kidney and so have a prolonged duration of action in CRF. The long-acting morphine metabolite morphine-6-glucuronide has far greater potency than morphine itself. Avoid pethidine as norpethidine can cause convulsions. Fentanyl has inactive metabolites, but may accumulate with prolonged use. Alfentanil and remifentanil may be used in normal doses. Half-lives of codeine and dihydrocodeine are prolonged five times. Tramadol and its active metabolites are renally excreted. The manufacturer does not recommend its use in end-stage renal failure.
- PCA morphine or fentanyl ($20\mu g$ bolus, 6min lockout time) can be used but with caution. In theory the reduction in excretion increases plasma concentration causing negative feedback and thus reducing subsequent demand.
- Paracetamol is safe in normal doses. Avoid NSAIDs even in anuric patients.
- Induction agents: reduce doses of benzodiazepines, thiopental, etomidate, and propofol by ~30% because of changes in protein binding, volume of distribution, and cardiac function.
- The elimination of volatile anaesthetic agents is not dependent on renal function. Isoflurane, halothane, and desflurane are all safe. Sevoflurane is safe for induction but will produce inorganic fluoride ions with prolonged use, as will enflurane.
- Muscle relaxants: suxamethonium is discussed above; plasma cholinesterase activity is unchanged in CRF. Atracurium and cisatracurium are logical choices. Vecuronium and rocuronium can be used as single doses, but should not be infused. Always use a peripheral nerve stimulator.
- The excretion of neostigmine and glycopyrronium is prolonged in CRF.
- The duration of action of local anaesthetics is reduced. Reduce maximum doses by 25% because of decreased protein binding and a lower CNS seizure threshold. Epidurals and spinals work well but consider the increased risk of haemorrhage and spinal haematoma formation.
- Most antibiotics are excreted by the kidney. It is common to use a normal loading dose with reduced and/or delayed maintenance doses. If in doubt check in the BNF or with a microbiologist.

	Drugs safe in CRF	Drugs safe in limited or reduced doses	Drugs contra-indicated in CRF
Premedication	Lormetazepam, midazolam, temazepam		
Induction	Propofol, thiopental, etomidate	Ketamine	
Maintenance	Isoflurane, desflurane, halothane, propofol	Sevoflurane	Enflurane
Muscle relaxants	Suxamethonium, atracurium, cisatracurium	Vecuronium, rocuronium	Pancuronium
Opioids	Alfentanil, remifentanil	Fentanyl, morphine	Pethidine
Local anaesthetics	Bupivacaine, lidocaine		
Analgesics	Paracetamol		NSAIDs

Renal dialysis/renal transplant

Haemodialysis

- Haemodialysis patients undergo dialysis for several hours, 3 or 4 times a week.
- Normally patients have AV fistula which must be carefully protected. Use dialysis catheters for IV access only as a last resort, and remember that the dead space contains high dose heparin (at least 1000IU/ml).
- Haemodialysis should finish 4–6hr before surgery to allow fluid shifts to equilibrate and residual heparin to be metabolised. Patients will often be relatively hypovolaemic post-dialysis (deliberately).
- Perioperative cardiovascular instability is common. Replace fluid losses carefully using 0.9% saline or colloids to maintain normovolaemia. Excess fluid can be removed by dialysis.
- Delay postoperative haemodialysis for 1–2d if possible because of heparin-induced bleeding.
- Anaesthesia for AV fistula formation: ask the surgeon where the fistula is to be formed. Local infiltration works well for a brachiobasilic fistula. Axillary brachial plexus block or light GA is recommended for a brachiocephalic fistula. Avoid hypotension to prevent fistula thrombosis. The fistula may be used for dialysis after 3–4wk.

Peritoneal dialysis

- Peritoneal dialysis uses the large surface area of the peritoneum to exchange fluid and metabolites via temporary (hard) or permanent Tenchkoff (soft) catheters in the lower abdomen. This type of dialysis is inefficient but can run continuously. Catheter placement or removal usually requires a mini-laparotomy.
- Dialysis fluid should be drained before anaesthesia to prevent respiratory function compromise. Patients can usually omit 24–48hr of dialysis, but a period of haemodialysis may be needed if undergoing bowel surgery.

Anaesthesia in a patient with a renal transplant

- The serum creatinine may be normal but renal function and creatinine clearance are not normal. The transplanted kidney never works perfectly and has only half the number of nephrons. Immunosuppression decreases the function further.
- Patients are immunosuppressed and strict asepsis must be applied. Discuss immunosuppression with the nephrologist if the patient will be nil by mouth following surgery.
- Cardiovascular depression may compromise kidney function; avoid hypovolaemia and hypotension.
- Avoid nephrotoxic drugs if possible. Do not use NSAIDs, but paracetamol is safe in normal doses.
- The new kidney is placed superficially in the abdomen and can be damaged by patient positioning (i.e. prone) or supports.
- Rejection of the transplanted kidney is heralded by renewed hypertension, proteinuria, and worsening renal function.

Acute renal failure

Acute renal failure (ARF) developing in the perioperative period has a high mortality. It is diagnosed by oliguria and a rising serum creatinine. Occasionally ARF may occur with normal volumes of urine but poor creatinine clearance (high output ARF).

Risk factors for perioperative ARF

Pre-existing problem	Renal compromise, diabetes, advanced age
Perioperative	Sepsis, hypotension/hypovolaemia, dehydration
Drugs	Nephrotoxins: antibiotics, NSAIDs, ACE inhibitors, lithium, chemotherapy agents, radiological contrast media
Trauma	Rhabdomyolysis (myoglobinaemia from crush injuries)
Surgery	Biliary surgery in the presence of obstructive jaundice (hepatorenal syndrome)
	Renal and abdominal vascular surgery
Intra-abdominal hypertension	Any cause of abdominal distension
Urinary obstruction	

Assessment of renal function

- Measure hourly urine output (remember catheters can block). Urinary electrolytes may help differentiate hypoperfusion (Na^+ <20mmol/l, urine osmolality >500mosmol/kg) from acute tubular necrosis (Na^+ >20mmol/l, urine osmolality <500mosmol/kg). These results are meaningless if diuretics have been given.
- Serum creatinine is the main initial measurement. Serum urea is much less specific since it is increased in dehydration, GI bleeding, sepsis, and excessive diuretic use.
- Check electrolytes before surgery (especially serum K^+).
- Creatinine clearance is useful but requires a 24hr urine collection.
- Abdominal ultrasound will differentiate chronic causes (e.g. horseshoe kidney) from obstruction.

Perioperative considerations

- Aim to prevent further deterioration of renal function and maintain an adequate urine output (>1ml/kg/hr).
- Preoperative rehydration is essential, and any fluid deficit should be corrected before surgery. Invasive monitoring may be needed. ICU if possible.
- Remember that an adequate blood pressure is needed for renal perfusion. Aim for a mean arterial pressure >70mmHg (>85mmHg in hypertensives). Inotropes may be required.

- The outcome from polyuric ARF is better than oliguric ARF. There is no place for diuretics (furosemide) until adequate filling and arterial blood pressure have been achieved.
- Furosemide is given initially as an IV bolus of 20–40mg. In patients with established renal failure furosemide 250mg may be infused over 1hr.
- There is no evidence to support the use of low dose ('renal') dopamine; it may even be harmful.
- Mannitol (0.5g/kg IV) may improve urine flow.
- Check serum K^+ regularly.
- Seek advice from renal unit/ICU about postoperative care and need for dialysis.

Postoperative care

- Avoid NSAIDs in all patients at risk of renal failure.
- Avoid dehydration—consider CVP monitoring.
- Closely monitor hourly urine output. If oliguria occurs (<0.5ml/kg/hr) try a fluid challenge of 250–500ml 0.9% saline/Gelofusine, or mannitol (0.5–1g/kg IV).
- Intra-abdominal hypertension (pressure >20mmHg) is common following major abdominal surgery and can cause anuria by direct compression of the renal pelvis and reduced renal perfusion. It can be measured via the bladder using a transducer connected to the urinary catheter: instil 50ml saline into the bladder, clamp off the drainage port, and measure pressure via a needle inserted into the catheter lumen.

Emergency management of hyperkalaemia

See p178.

Further reading

Milner QJW (2003). Pathophysiology of chronic renal failure. *BJA CEPD Reviews*, **3**,130–133.

Sladen RN (2000). Anaesthetic considerations for the patient with renal failure. *Anaesthetic Clinics of North America*, **18**, 862–882.

Toivonen HJ (2000). Anaesthesia for patients with a transplanted organ. *Acta Anaesthesiologica Scandinavica*, **44**, 812–833.

Hepatic disease

Jonathan Purday

Complications of liver disease

There are numerous causes of hepatic disease. The most common in the Western world is cirrhosis secondary to viral hepatitis or alcoholism. Patients with underlying hepatic disease often present to the anaesthetist and surgeon. Problems include:

• Bleeding: the liver is responsible for the production of clotting factors. Prothrombin time is usually prolonged and can be improved by daily vitamin K injections (10mg IV slowly). Thrombocytopenia is also common, as is defective platelet function. Bleeding is more likely to be due to thrombocytopenia than clotting factor deficiency. Clotting studies and FBC must be carefully checked perioperatively and adequate provision must be made for the crossmatch of blood, fresh frozen plasma (FFP), and platelets.

• Encephalopathy: in severe liver failure toxic products build up (particularly ammonia, due to deranged amino acid metabolism) leading to a progressive encephalopathy. In cirrhosis this may be precipitated by sedatives, a high-protein diet (including GI bleed), infection, surgical operations, trauma, hypokalaemia, or constipation. A decreased level of consciousness may compromise the airway and intubation may be required if cerebral oedema develops.

Grades of hepatic encephalopathy

Grade 0	Alert and orientated
Grade I	Drowsy and orientated
Grade II	Drowsy and disorientated
Grade III	Rousable stupor, restlessness
Grade IV	Coma—unresponsive to deep pain

• Hypoglycaemia: the liver contains major stores of glycogen, a glucose precursor. Check blood glucose levels regularly. Give 10% dextrose infusions if <2mmol/l. Monitor plasma K^+.

• Ascites: fibrotic changes in the liver lead to portal hypertension, and in combination with salt/water retention and a low serum albumin, fluid accumulates in the peritoneal cavity. This can lead to respiratory failure due to pressure on the diaphragm.

• Infection: immune function is depressed and infections of the respiratory and urinary tract are common.

• Renal failure: this is often multifactorial. Combined liver and renal failure may result from:
  • A common pathomechanism (sepsis, toxic, immune, and genetic).
  • Secondary due to decreased circulating blood volume or increased renovascular resistance (prerenal), impaired renal tubular function, or hepatorenal failure. Hepatorenal failure is due to intrarenal arterial and arteriolar vasoconstriction and can be diagnosed only after exclusion of shock, sepsis, and nephrotoxic drugs. See p144.

Acute hepatic disease

Definition

- Hyperacute hepatic failure—within 7d
- Acute hepatic failure—7–28d
- Subacute hepatic failure—28d–6 months

Previously well patients with acute liver failure rarely present for anaesthesia and surgery (mortality rates of 10–100% have been described). More commonly, acute failure is due to decompensation of chronic liver disease. Hyperacute hepatic failure paradoxically has the best prognosis.

Causes of acute liver failure

- Viral hepatitis: types A–G, cytomegalovirus, herpes simplex/Epstein–Barr virus
- Drugs: paracetamol excess, idiosyncratic reactions, halothane
- Toxins: carbon tetrachloride, *Amanita phalloides* mushrooms
- Others: acute fatty infiltration of pregnancy, HELLP syndrome, Wilson's disease, Reye's syndrome.

Patients with acute liver disease and encephalopathy have severe coagulopathy, active fibrinolysis, high cardiac output/reduced systemic vascular resistance, hypoglycaemia/hypokalaemia, and metabolic acidosis. They are also at risk of raised intracranial pressure.

Management

- Due to the high perioperative mortality, patients should have all surgery postponed (unless true emergency) until at least 30d after liver function tests have returned to normal.
- Hepatitis B and C are highly contagious via parenteral inoculation to theatre personnel and universal precautions must be strictly followed.
- Patients with abnormal liver function tests and coagulopathy should be closely monitored.
- Patients with an encephalopathy, deteriorating INR, hypoglycaemia, or acidosis should be discussed with a specialist liver unit.
- Patients with grade III/IV encephalopathy need intubation to protect their airway.
- Hypovolaemia and hypotension should be treated with IV fluids and inotropes/vasopressors (noradrenaline first choice).
- Bicarbonate-buffered haemofiltration and intracranial pressure monitoring are often required.
- N-acetyl cysteine infusion (essential in paracetamol overdose) may be helpful.
- Orthotopic liver transplantation may be a definitive treatment in some cases.

Chronic hepatic disease

The commonest cause of chronic liver disease is cirrhosis, but chronic hepatitis is widespread, with an estimated 5% of the world's population being chronic hepatitis B carriers.

- Chronic hepatitis: any hepatitis lasting >6 months
- Cirrhosis: hepatic fibrosis with regeneration nodules

- Cirrhosis can be acquired (alcohol, viral hepatitis, drugs, secondary biliary, or veno-occlusive disease) or inherited (primary biliary, haemachromatosis, Wilson's, galactosaemia, sickle cell disease).
- Chronic hepatitis B develops in 3% of those infected. It is widespread in the Far East/Africa and infects 300 million people worldwide. Other high-risk groups include homosexuals, IV drug abusers, haemophiliacs, haemodialysis patients, and those in institutional care. It may progress to cirrhosis or hepatocellular carcinoma.
- Chronic hepatitis C develops in 75% of those infected. Risk groups are similar to hepatitis B/cirrhosis and hepatocellular carcinoma can develop. Blood products were previously responsible for many cases of hepatitis C, but now all donors are screened.
- Other causes of chronic hepatitis include alcohol, autoimmune, metabolic, and drugs (isoniazid, methyldopa).
- Assessment of risk factors for surgery and anaesthesia is described by Child's classification (excluding portal-systemic shunt procedures, e.g. transjugular intrahepatic portal-systemic shunt procedure (TIPSS)). Common causes of mortality in the perioperative period include sepsis, renal failure, bleeding, and worsening liver failure with encephalopathy.

Surgical risk assessment: Child's classification as modified by Pugh

Mortality	Minimal (<5%)	Modest (5–50%)	Marked (>50%)
Bilirubin (µmol/l)	<25	25–40	>40
Albumin (g/l)	>35	30–35	<30
PT (seconds prolonged)	1–4 (INR < 1.7)	4–6 (INR 1.7–2.3)	>6 (INR > 2.3)
Ascites	None	Moderate	Marked
Encephalopathy (p134)	None	Grades 1 and 2	Grades 3 and 4
Nutrition	Excellent	Good	Poor

PT = prothrombin time.
INR = international normalised ratio.

Drug metabolism and liver disease

- The vast majority of drugs, including anaesthetic drugs, are metabolised by the liver.
- Most drugs are initially metabolised by the cytochrome P450 system. In Phase I they are either oxidised or reduced and in Phase II they are conjugated with a glucuronide, glycine, or sulphate to enhance water solubility and excretion in bile or urine.
- In early alcoholic liver disease, the cytochrome P450 system is often induced, leading to rapid metabolism of drugs, whereas this is reversed in end-stage disease.
- The liver has a large functional reserve, so these functions are usually preserved until end-stage disease.
- Pharmacodynamics and the sensitivity of target organs for sedatives and anaesthetics may be altered, with coma easily induced in end-stage liver disease.
- Advanced liver disease may prolong the half-life and potentiate the clinical effects of alfentanil, morphine, vecuronium, rocuronium, mivacurium, and benzodiazepines.

Causes of altered drug pharmacokinetics in liver failure	
Liver problem	**Pharmacological effect**
Decreased portal blood flow in hepatic fibrosis	Decreased first pass metabolism
Hypoalbuminaemia	Increased free drug in plasma
Ascites and sodium and water retention	Increased volume of distribution
Biotransformation enzymes	Activity may increase or decrease
Reduced liver cell mass	Reduced activity
Obstructive jaundice	Decreased biliary excretion of drugs

Anaesthetic management of the patient with liver failure

Patients with liver disease have a high perioperative risk which is proportional to the degree of hepatic dysfunction.

Preoperative laboratory investigations

- Full blood count and clotting studies. Prothrombin time (PT) is a good marker of liver function.
- Electrolytes and creatinine. The urea is often falsely low due to decreased hepatic production.
- Glucose—hepatic stores of glycogen and glucose utilization are often affected.
- Liver function tests (see below).
- Arterial blood gases—hepatopulmonary syndrome (HPS), hypoxia related to intrapulmonary shunting is common in severe liver disease.[1]
- Urinalysis.
- Hepatitis screening (although universal precautions should always be observed).

Assessment of liver function

- Serum liver function tests are rarely specific but PT, albumin, and bilirubin are sensitive markers of overall liver function. Serial measurements are useful and indicate trends. Avoid giving FFP unless treating active bleeding, as the PT time is an excellent guide to overall liver function.
- Liver transaminases (aspartate transaminase (AST), alanine aminotransferase (ALT)) are sensitive to even mild liver damage and have no role in mortality prediction. Levels may decrease in severe disease.
- Alkaline phosphatase is raised with biliary obstruction.
- Immunological tests: antinuclear antibody is present in 75% of patients with chronic active hepatitis and smooth muscle antibody in nearly all cases of primary biliary cirrhosis. α-fetoprotein is a marker of hepatoma.
- Imaging techniques: ultrasound is the main initial investigation of obstructive jaundice. Other useful investigations include ERCP, CT, MRI cholangiograms.
- Liver function tests (LFTs) must always be interpreted alongside a careful history and examination. The liver has a large reserve function and can often withstand considerable damage before LFTs become deranged.

Liver function tests

Test	Normal range	Raised
Bilirubin	2–17µmol/l	Haemolysis Gilbert's syndrome Acute liver failure
Aspartate transaminase (AST)	0–35IU/l	Non-specific (found in liver, heart, muscle etc.) Hepatocellular injury
Alanine aminotransferase (ALT)	0–45IU/l	Specific Hepatocellular injury—alcohol, drugs, hepatitis, inherited liver diseases
Alkaline Phosphatase (ALP)	30–120IU/l	Physiological (pregnancy, adolescents, familial) Bile duct obstruction (stones, drugs, cancer) Primary biliary cirrhosis Metastatic liver disease Bone disease
Gamma-glutamyl transpeptidase (γ-GT)	0–30IU/l	Non-specific (found in heart, pancreas, kidneys) Useful to confirm hepatic source for ↑ALP or ↑AST or ↑ALT Alcoholic liver disease
Albumin	40–60g/l	Non-specific (affected by nutritional status, catabolism, and urinary and GI losses) Prognostic in chronic liver disease
Prothrombin time and international normalised ratio (INR)	10.9–12.5s (INR 1.0–1.2)	Non-specific (Vitamin K deficiency, warfarin therapy, DIC) However, best prognostic marker in acute liver failure

1 Mazzeo AT, Lucanto T, Santamaria LB (2004). Hepatopulmonary syndrome: a concern for the anaesthetist? Pre-operative evaluation of hypoxaemic patients with liver disease. *Acta Anaesthesiologica Scandinavica*, **48**, 178–186.

Perioperative considerations

- Proton pump inhibitors or H_2 antagonists should be used preoperatively. Rapid sequence induction will further reduce the risks of gastric aspiration.
- Even in severe liver disease the problem is usually one of exaggerated effects of drugs on the CNS, rather than poor liver metabolism.
- Hepatic blood flow is altered by anaesthetic drugs (including α and β agonists/antagonists), positive pressure ventilation, PEEP, and surgical technique.
- In most cases anaesthesia reduces liver blood flow, particularly if halothane is used. However, isoflurane may improve it.
- Regional techniques can be used as long as coagulation is not deranged, and it should be remembered that all local anaesthetics are metabolised by the liver.
- Isoflurane, sevoflurane, or desflurane are the preferred volatile agents as enflurane, and particularly halothane, have marked effects in decreasing hepatic blood flow and inhibiting drug metabolism.

Anaesthetic drugs in liver failure

	Drugs safe in liver failure	Drugs to be used with caution (may need reduced dosage)	Drugs contraindicated in liver failure
Premedication	Lorazepam	Midazolam, diazepam	
Induction	Propofol, thiopental, etomidate		
Maintenance	Desflurane, sevoflurane, isoflurane, nitrous oxide	Enflurane	Halothane (possibly)[a]
Muscle relaxants	Atracurium, cisatracurium	Pancuronium, vecuronium, suxamethonium	
Opioids	Remifentanil	Fentanyl, alfentanil, morphine, pethidine	
Analgesics	Paracetamol	NSAIDs, lidocaine, bupivacaine	

[a] Halothane has been rarely reported to cause hepatitis (see p143).

Physiological considerations
- Cardiovascular: liver disease causes various types of shunt, from cutaneous spider angioma to portosystemic shunts. These lead to an increase in cardiac output, often by 50%. This is combined with a reduction in systemic vascular resistance and an increase in extracellular fluid due to an activated renin–angiotensin system. In contrast, some alcoholics may have a decreased cardiac output secondary to cardiomyopathy.
- Ascites: a common manifestation of liver disease. Water and sodium retention may be treated with potassium-sparing diuretics, e.g. spironolactone. A careful check of electrolytes is essential. Removal of ascites at operation will be followed by postoperative reforming. This should be taken into account in fluid balance.
- Pulmonary: up to 50% of patients have intrapulmonary shunting and V/Q mismatch, pleural effusions, and respiratory splinting of the diaphragm by ascites causing a decrease in PaO_2 not improved by increasing the FiO_2. Diuretics or paracentesis may improve ascites.
- Bleeding and clotting problems: clotting factors and platelets are affected quantitatively and qualitatively. Coagulation should be carefully assessed preoperatively and adequate provision made for intra-operative blood products.

Anaesthesia for transjugular intrahepatic porto-systemic shunt procedure (TIPSS)
- Typically used in end-stage liver failure to decrease portal pressure and decrease complications such as variceal bleeding and ascites.
- A stent is positioned radiologically between the hepatic and portal veins, allowing blood to bypass the dilated oesophageal and gastric veins.
- Patients should be adequately resuscitated and variceal bleeding controlled with balloon tamponade.
- Complications of the procedure include pneumothorax (if the internal jugular route is used), cardiac arrhythmias, or massive bleeding secondary to hepatic artery puncture or hepatic capsular tear.
- Anaesthetic technique involves having a cardiovascularly stable patient with good IV access, invasive arterial line monitoring, and inotropes and blood products easily available.

Postoperative liver dysfunction or jaundice

Although postoperative jaundice is relatively common, significant liver dysfunction is relatively rare. Dysfunction has varied aetiology and often resolves without treatment. It should be remembered that hepatitis due to volatile agents is extremely rare and is largely a diagnosis of exclusion.

Causes of postoperative liver dysfunction or jaundice	
Bilirubin overload (haemolysis)	Blood transfusion
	Haematoma resorption
	Haemolytic anaemia (sickle cell, prosthetic heart valve, glucose-6-phosphatase deficiency)
Hepatocellular injury	Exacerbation of pre-existing liver disease
	Hepatic ischaemia: hypovolaemia, hypotension, cardiac failure
	Septicaemia
	Drug-induced (antibiotics, halothane)
	Hypoxia
	Viral hepatitis
Cholestasis	Intrahepatic (benign, infection, drug-induced, e.g. cephalosporins, carbamazepine, erythromycin)
	Extrahepatic (pancreatitis, gallstones, bile duct injury)
Congenital	Gilbert's syndrome

- Common causes include hepatic oxygen deprivation from intra- and postoperative hypoxia and hypotension.
- Benign postoperative intrahepatic cholestasis mimics biliary obstruction and usually occurs after major surgery associated with hypotension, hypoxaemia, or multiple transfusions.
- The surgical procedure should also be considered, and significant haematoma resolution is a common cause.

Halothane hepatitis

Halothane has been linked to postoperative liver dysfunction. Two syndromes are recognised:

- The first is associated with a transient rise in liver function tests and low morbidity, often after initial exposure.
- The second is thought to occur after repeated exposure and has an 'immune' mechanism with the development of fulminant hepatic failure (FHF) and high mortality. It is rare, with an incidence of 1:35 000 anaesthetics.
- Antibodies specific to FHF patients exposed to halothane are found in 70% of such patients. It is postulated that a halothane oxidative metabolite binds to liver cytochromes to form a hapten and induce a hypersensitivity reaction. All patients exposed to halothane have altered liver proteins but it is unknown why only a few develop liver failure.
- There does appear to be a genetic susceptibility, as shown by *in vitro* testing.
- Halothane has also been shown in several animal studies to significantly decrease liver blood flow, particularly during hypoxia.

Other inhalational anaesthetic agents

- The chance of an 'immune' reaction to a volatile agent occurring is thought to relate to the amount it is metabolised. Halothane is 20% metabolised.
- Enflurane is 2% metabolised and should therefore cause 10 times fewer reactions. Products of enflurane metabolism have been shown to alter liver proteins and there have been rare case reports linking enflurane with liver damage. There is a theoretical basis for cross-reactivity with previous halothane exposure.
- Isoflurane is 0.2% metabolised. There is, therefore, a theoretical risk of reaction, and indeed there have been a few case reports. These, however, have been contested and isoflurane is considered safe for use in patients at risk of hepatic failure.
- Sevoflurane and desflurane also appear to be safe in liver failure.

Renal failure and the hepatorenal syndrome

Hepatorenal syndrome and acute tubular necrosis are common in patients with liver disease. Maintenance of an adequate urinary output with fluids is the mainstay of prevention. Once renal failure occurs, mortality is close to 100%.

- The hepatorenal syndrome is a functional renal failure which occurs spontaneously, or more commonly due to fluid shifts particularly in patients with obstructive jaundice.
- The kidney is normal histologically and functions normally following a liver transplant or if transplanted into a recipient.
- All pathophysiological changes seen in ascites (renal sodium/water retention and plasma expansion) are present to an extreme form in the hepatorenal patient.
- Diagnostic criteria are
  - Urinary sodium <10mmol/l
  - Urine:plasma osmolarity and creatinine ratios >1
  - Normal CVP with no diuresis on central volume expansion
  - A patient with chronic liver disease and ascites.
- Worsening hepatorenal failure results in death, despite haemofiltration or dialysis, and can only be corrected by liver transplantation.

Prevention

- 8–12hr preoperatively an IV infusion of 0.9% saline should be commenced to avoid hypovolaemia.
- Renal blood flow must be optimised by monitoring CVP and correcting any hypovolaemia.
- Remember that tense ascites may cause compression of the right atrium and falsely high CVP measurements.
- Mannitol is often used prophylactically to maintain urine output (0.5g/kg over 30min).
- Hypotension should be avoided intra-operatively and mean BP should be maintained within 10–20% of preoperative levels—particularly in the hypertensive patient.
- An adequate urine output of at least 1ml/kg/hr must be achieved.
- Avoid the use of any nephrotoxic drugs such as NSAIDs, and gentamicin in repeated doses.

Portal hypertension and oesophageal varices

- Portal hypertension commonly occurs with cirrhosis but can arise in any condition where there is disruption of pre-, intra-, or posthepatic blood flow.
- Portal hypertension causes enlargement of the anastomoses between the portal and systemic circulation, leading to varices at the gastro-oesophageal junction, haemorrhoids, and dilated abdominal wall veins ('caput medusae').
- 30% of varices bleed and present as haematemesis or malaena.
- Mortality is up to 50% for the acute bleed, particularly in patients with advanced cirrhosis.

Treatment

- Initial management is to correct hypovolaemia, stop the bleeding, and reverse the coagulopathy.
- Two large-bore IVs and a CVP line should be inserted.
- Drugs that may cause or exacerbate the bleeding, e.g. aspirin, should be stopped.
- Early endoscopy is warranted to confirm the diagnosis and control bleeding. Band ligation appears more effective than sclerosant injection for variceal haemorrhage. Ulcers may be injected with adrenaline. However, 70% of patients will rebleed, most within 6wk. Occasionally, intubation may be necessary to protect the airway.
- Vasoactive drugs (terlipressin 2mg 6-hourly, vasopressin 0.2–0.4U/min for 24–48hr) constrict vessels in the mesenteric beds but may cause coronary constriction and angina. GTN patches or infusion may help. Terlipressin causes less angina than vasopressin.[1]
- Somatostatin (a hypothalamic hormone) 250µg/hr and octreotide (an analogue) 50µg/hr for 2–5d (as well as terlipressin/vasopressin) in combination with endoscopic therapy may be more effective than either alone and should be started while waiting for an experienced endoscopist.
- Balloon tamponade with an oesophageal and gastric balloon can provide temporary haemostasis but should be used only where endoscopic and drug treatments have failed. There is a high risk of fatal complications (aspiration, oesophageal tear/rupture, and airway obstruction) and therefore this should be used only in HDU/ICU.
- β-blockade (propranolol 40–160mg twice daily) can decrease portal pressure in the chronic situation and may decrease the rebleed rate from 70% to 50%, but may mask the early signs of hypovolaemia and exacerbate hypotension during rebleeding.
- Portal-systemic shunting is now rarely performed as an emergency due to high mortality. It can occasionally be performed after the first bleed, to lower portal pressure, but is contraindicated if there is any clinical or EEG evidence of encephalopathy.

- A transjugular intrahepatic portosystemic shunt (TIPSS) achieves shunting without the need for surgery with a lower morbidity and mortality and should be the treatment of choice (see p141).
- Oesophageal staple transection can be used if endoscopic therapy fails or TIPSS is unavailable. The effectiveness and mortality are similar to sclerotherapy. These patients are at increased anaesthetic risk from hypovolaemia, a full stomach, and liver impairment.

Further reading

Clarke P, Bellamy MC (2000). Anaesthesia for patients with liver disease. *The Royal College of Anaesthetists Bulletin*, **4**, 158–161.

Dagher L, Moore K (2001). The hepatorenal syndrome. *Gut*, **49**, 729–737.

Early management of bleeding oesophageal varices (2000). *Drug and Therapeutics Bulletin*, **38**, 37–40.

Hyde GM, Limdi JK (2003). Evaluation of abnormal liver function tests. *Postgraduate Medical Journal*, **79**, 307–312.

Lai WK, Murphy N (2004). Management of acute liver failure. *Continuing Education in Anaesthesia, Critical Care & Pain* (Supplement to *British Journal of Anaesthesia*), **4**, 40–42.

Lentschener C, Ozier Y (2003). What anaesthetists need to know about viral hepatitis. *Acta Anaesthesiologica Scandinavica*, **47**, 794–803.

---

1 Kam PCA, Williams S, Yoong FFY (2004). Vasopressin and terlipressin: pharmacology and clinical relevance. *Anaesthesia*, **59**, 993–1001.

Chapter 8

Endocrine and metabolic disease

Hannah Blanshard

Diabetes mellitus

Insulin is necessary, even when fasting, to maintain glucose homeostasis and balance stress hormones (e.g. adrenaline). It has two classes of action:
- Excitatory—stimulating glucose uptake and lipid synthesis
- Inhibitory (physiologically more important)—inhibits lipolysis, proteolysis, glycogenolysis, gluconeogenesis, and ketogenesis

Lack of insulin is associated with hyperglycaemia, osmotic diuresis, dehydration, hyperosmolarity, hyperviscosity predisposing to thrombosis, and increased rates of wound infection. Sustained hyperglycaemia is associated with an increased mortality, hospital stay, and complication rates.

Diabetes mellitus is present in 5% of the population.
- Type I diabetes (20%): immune mediated and leads to absolute insulin deficiency. Patients cannot tolerate prolonged periods without exogenous insulin. Glycogenolysis and gluconeogenesis occur, resulting in hyperglycaemia and ketosis.
- Type II diabetes (80%): a disease of adult onset, associated with insulin resistance. Patients produce some endogenous insulin and their metabolic state often improves with fasting.

General considerations

Many diabetic patients are well informed about their condition and have undergone previous surgery. Discuss management with them. Hospital diabetic teams can be useful for advice. The overall aims of perioperative diabetic management are to maintain physiological glucose levels of (above hypoglycaemic levels, but below those at which deleterious effects of hyperglycaemia become evident), prevent hypokalaemia, hypomagnesaemia, and hypophosphataemia.

Preoperative assessment

- Cardiovascular: the diabetic is prone to hypertension, ischaemic heart disease (may be 'silent'), cerebrovascular disease, myocardial infarction, and cardiomyopathy. Autonomic neuropathy can lead to tachy- or bradycardia and postural hypotension.
- Renal: 40% of diabetics develop microalbuminuria, which is associated with hypertension, ischaemic heart disease, and retinopathy. This may be reduced by treatment with ACE inhibitors.
- Respiratory: diabetics are prone to perioperative chest infections, especially if they are obese and smokers.
- Airway: thickening of soft tissues (glycosylation) occurs, especially in ligaments around joints—limited joint mobility syndrome. Intubation may be difficult if the neck is affected or there is insufficient mouth opening.
- Gastrointestinal: 50% have delayed gastric emptying and are prone to reflux.
- Diabetics are prone to infections.

Investigations

- Blood sugar.
- Test urine for ketones and glucose.
- Measure glycosylated haemoglobin (HbA1$_c$), a measure of recent glycaemic control (normal 3.8–6.4%). A value >9% suggests inadequate control.

Preoperative management

- Place patient first on operating list if possible.
- Stop long-acting oral hypoglycaemics, e.g. metformin and glibenclamide, 24hr before surgery. Chlorpropramide should ideally be stopped 3d before surgery because of its long action and substituted with a shorter-acting drug such as gliclazide. Its use is no longer recommended in the UK.

Perioperative management

- If the patient can be expected to eat and drink within 4hr classify the surgery as minor. All other surgery is major. If diabetic control is poor, i.e. a fasting blood glucose of >10mmol/l, they should be treated with an insulin/glucose regime.
- Glucose/insulin infusions should be administered through the same cannula to prevent accidental administration of insulin without glucose. Both infusions should be regulated by volumetric pumps, with an anti-reflux valve on the IV glucose line.
- Hartmann's solution is controversial as lactate converts rapidly to glucose in the fasted state. Saline may be a more appropriate choice.
- Check blood glucose hourly.
- Consider a rapid sequence induction if gastric stasis is suspected.
- Regional techniques may be useful for extremity surgery and to reduce the risk of undetected hypoglycaemia. Chart any pre-existing nerve damage.
- Autonomic dysfunction may exacerbate the hypotensive effect of spinals and epidurals.

Hypoglycaemia

- A blood glucose <4mmol/l is the main danger to diabetics perioperatively. Fasting, recent alcohol consumption, liver failure, and septicaemia commonly exacerbate this.
- Characteristic signs are tachycardia, light-headedness, sweating, and pallor. This may progress to confusion, restlessness, incomprehensible speech, double vision, convulsions, and coma. If untreated, permanent brain damage will occur, made worse by hypotension or hypoxia.
- Anaesthetised patients may not show any of these signs. Monitor blood sugar regularly and suspect hypoglycaemia with unexplained changes in the patient's condition.
- If hypoglycaemia occurs, give 50ml of 50% dextrose IV (or any glucose solution available) and repeat blood sugar measurement. Alternatively give 1mg of glucagon (IM or IV). 10–20g (2–4 teaspoons) of sugar by mouth or nasogastric tube is an alternative.

	Morning list *Fast from midnight*	**Afternoon list** *Early light breakfast before 07:00hr*
Type I (IDDM)		
Major procedure	Omit morning SC insulin Start IV insulin/glucose regime at 07:00hr	Give two-thirds normal morning dose of soluble insulin (e.g. Actrapid, Humulin S or Humalog) or one-third of normal dose of pre-mixed insulin (e.g. Mixtard or Humulin M_{1-5}) before breakfast Start IV insulin/glucose regime at 11:00hr
	When a light diet is tolerated, discontinue IV regime and commence qds SC regime (see p153)	
Minor procedure, good diabetic control	Omit morning SC insulin	Give normal SC insulin with breakfast Omit midday SC insulin
	Ensure IV access. Check blood glucose hourly until patient has eaten. When patient can eat give usual SC insulin	
Type II (NIDDM)		
Major procedure or poor diabetic control	Omit oral hypoglycaemics Start IV insulin/glucose regime at 07:00hr	Omit oral hypoglycaemics Start IV insulin/glucose at 12:00hr
	If patient can eat later that day and control is good, discontinue IV regime and recommence oral hypoglycaemics If IV > 24hr or control is poor, discontinue IV regime before first meal and commence qds SC regime	
Minor procedure	Omit tablets on day of procedure. If blood glucose <4mmol/l start 10% glucose at 100ml/hr. Measure blood glucose every 2hr until patient has eaten. Give a meal and tablets as soon as possible after return to ward	

Intravenous insulin/dextrose regime

- Start IV. Use 5% dextrose at 120ml/hr or 10% dextrose at 60ml/hr (prevents water overload, particularly in elderly). Dextrose 4.2%/saline 0.18% is acceptable.
- If K^+ <4.5mmol/l, add 10mmol KCl to each 500ml bag dextrose.
- Start IV insulin infusion using a syringe pump. Adjust according to sliding scale below. Test blood glucose hourly initially. Patients on >50U of insulin/day will need higher doses of insulin by infusion.

Blood glucose (mmol/l)	Insulin infusion rate (U/hr)	Insulin infusion rate if blood glucose not maintained <10mmol/l (U/hr)
<3.0	Stop for 30min and review	Stop for 30min and review
3.0–4.0	0.5	0.5
4.1–9.0	1	2
9.1–13.0	2	3
13.1–17.0	3	4
17.1–28.0	4	6
>28	6 (check infusion running and call doctor)	8 (check infusion running and call doctor)

QDS SC insulin regime

- Use when discontinuing IV insulin and glucose regime.
- Calculate total daily insulin requirement from the preceding 24hr or the usual daily amount. Divide by four and give each dose just before meals and at bedtime.
- Adjust doses as necessary.

Glucose potassium insulin regime (GKI or Alberti)[1]

This is an alternative, simpler regime which does not require infusion pumps, but may provide less accurate control of blood sugar. The original regime as described by Alberti consists of:

- 500ml of 10% dextrose.
- Add 10–15U actrapid, plus 10mmol potassium chloride per 500ml bag.
- Infuse at 100ml/hr.
- Provides insulin 2–3U/hr, potassium 2mmol/hr, and glucose 10g/hr.

Dextrose 10% is not always available, so the following regime with 5% dextrose can be used: infuse 5% dextrose (500ml bags) at the calculated rate for the patient's fluid maintenance requirements. Insulin and potassium should be added to each bag as per the table below. The bag may be changed according to 2-hourly blood glucose measurements.

Blood glucose (mmol/l)	Soluble insulin (U) to be added to each 500ml bag 5% dextrose	Blood potassium (mmol/l)	KCl (mmol) to be added to each 500ml bag 5% dextrose
<4	5	<3	20
4–6	10	3–5	10
6.1–10	15	>5	None
10.1–20	20		
>20	Review	If potassium level not available, add 10mmol KCl to each bag	

Further reading

Sonksen P, Sonksen J (2000). Insulin: understanding its action in health and disease. *British Journal of Anaesthesia*, **85**, 69–79.

McAnulty GR, Robertshaw HJ, Hall GM (2000). Anaesthetic management of patients with diabetes mellitus. *British Journal of Anaesthesia*, **85**, 80–90.

Rehman HU, Mohammed K (2003). Perioperative management of diabetic patients. *Current Surgery*, **60**, 607–611.

1 Alberti KGMM (1991). Diabetes and surgery. *Anesthesiology*, **74**, 209–211.

Acromegaly

A rare clinical syndrome caused by overproduction of growth hormone from the anterior pituitary. Patients may present for pituitary surgery (p398) or require surgery unrelated to their pituitary pathology.

Preoperative assessment

- Cardiovascular: cardiac assessment for hypertension (30%), ischaemic heart disease, cardiomyopathy, heart failure, and valvular disease.
- Airway: difficult airway management and intubation may occur—check for large jaw, head, tongue, lips, and general hypertrophy of the larynx and trachea. Also vocal cord thickening or strictures and chondrocalcinosis of the larynx. Consider direct/indirect laryngoscopy preoperatively if vocal cord or laryngeal pathology is suspected. Snoring and daytime somnolence may indicate sleep apnoea. Look for enlargement of the thyroid (25%) which may compress the trachea.
- Drugs: somatostatin analogues (octreotide, lanreotide) may cause vomiting and diarrhoea. Bromocriptine, a long-acting dopamine agonist, is often used to lower growth hormone levels. It can cause severe postural hypotension.
- Neurological: symptoms and signs of raised intracranial pressure.

Investigations

- ECG as routine
- CXR if cardiorespiratory problems
- Echo if patient symptomatic or has murmurs
- Blood sugar—25% are diabetic.

Conduct of anaesthesia

- Large face masks and long-bladed laryngoscopes may make airway management and intubation easier. Awake fibreoptic intubation is the technique of choice for patients with anticipated difficult intubation, but is seldom required. Elective tracheostomy should be considered in those with severe respiratory obstruction.
- The patient's size makes positioning difficult and a long table may be required.
- Nerve compression syndromes are common so take care to protect vulnerable areas (the ulnar nerve at the elbow, the median nerve at the wrist, and the common peroneal nerve below the knee).
- If evidence of sleep apnoea, extubate the patient awake and sitting up if possible.

Postoperative care

If major surgery, consider ventilating the patient with sleep apnoea for a few hours in ICU until they are stable to wean from the ventilator.

Further reading

Seidman PA, Kofke WA, Policare R, Young M (2000). Anaesthetic complications of acromegaly. *British Journal of Anaesthesia*, **84**, 179–182.

Smith M, Hirsch NP (2000). Pituitary disease and anaesthesia. *British Journal of Anaesthesia*, **85**, 3–14.

Thyroid disease

Patient may present for thyroidectomy (see p554) or for non-thyroid surgery.

General considerations for non-thyroid surgery

Hypothyroidism

- Commonly due to autoimmune thyroid destruction.
- Cardiovascular complications include decreased blood volume, cardiac output, and heart rate with a predisposition to hypotension and ischaemic heart disease. Pericardial effusions also occur.
- If clinical evidence of hypothyroidism, delay elective surgery to obtain euthyroid state. Liaise with endocrinologist. Suggest L-thyroxine (starting dose 50µg increasing to 100–200µg PO over several weeks). The elderly are susceptible to angina and heart failure with increasing cardiac work caused by thyroxine, so start with 25µg and increase by 25µg at 3–4-weekly intervals.
- If surgery is urgent then liothyronine (T_3) (50–100µg slow IV with ECG monitoring, followed by 25µg 8-hourly) can be used.

Hyperthyroidism (thyrotoxicosis)

- Typically presents with weight loss, hypertension, sweating, and cardiac arrhythmias (especially atrial fibrillation). Treatment is with carbimazole (30–45mg orally daily for 6–8wk). This inhibits iodination of tyrosyl residues in thyroglobulin. Occasionally in severe cases with a large thyroid, Lugol's iodine is substituted 10d preoperatively to reduce gland vascularity.
- β-blockade (propranolol 30–60mg tds) is also started if there are signs of tremor or palpitations. The non-cardioselective β-blockers such as propranolol are more effective than the selective ones. β_1 adrenergic blockade treats the symptoms of tachycardia, but β_2 adrenergic blockade prevents peripheral conversion of T_4 to T_3.

Preoperative assessment

- Thyroid function: check patient is euthyroid—heart rate of <80bpm and no hand tremor. Delay surgery if possible until this is achieved. Patients with subclinical hypothyroidism usually present no anaesthetic problems and elective surgery can proceed without special preparation.[1]
- Airway: look for tracheal deviation—a large goitre can cause respiratory obstruction. This is a particular problem when the gland extends retrosternally. Ask the patient about positional dyspnoea and dysphagia. Look for evidence of tracheal compression with shortness of breath, dysphagia, or stridor (occurs with 50% compression). Infiltrating carcinomas may make any neck movement difficult and is an independent predictor of difficult intubation.
- Superior vena caval obstruction can occur. Look for distended neck veins that do not change with respiration.
- Check for other autoimmune disorders.

Investigations
- FBC, U&Es, serum calcium, thyroid function tests.
- CXR and thoracic inlet views essential to assess tracheal compression.
- If tracheal compression present, perform CT or MRI scan to reveal site and length of narrowing and also the presence of any calcification.
- Refer to ENT surgeon for indirect laryngoscopy to document any preoperative vocal cord dysfunction.

Conduct of anaesthesia

Hypothyroid patients
- Give all drugs slowly. Susceptible to profound hypotension, which may be relatively resistant to the effects of catecholamine therapy.
- Low metabolic rate predisposes to hypothermia, so actively warm.
- Drug metabolism can be slow. Monitor twitch response and reduce dose of relaxants and opioids.

Hyperthyroid patients
- Continue β-blockade perioperatively to reduce possibility of thyroid storm.

Special considerations

Thyroid storm
- A life-threatening exacerbation of hyperthyroid state with evidence of decompensation in one or more organ systems—mortality 20–30%.
- Usually presents 6–24h post-surgery with fever (>40°C), sweating, sinus tachycardia (>140bpm), coma, nausea, vomiting, and diarrhoea.
- Rehydrate with IV saline and glucose.
- Treat hyperpyrexia with tepid sponging and paracetamol. Do not give NSAIDs or aspirin as this displaces thyroid hormone from serum binding sites.
- Give propranolol (1mg increments up to 10mg) with CVS monitoring to decrease pulse rate to <90bpm. Alternatively give esmolol (loading dose 250–500µg/kg followed by 50–100µg/kg/min).
- Give hydrocortisone (200mg IV qds) to treat adrenal insufficiency and to decrease T_4 release and conversion to T_3 at very high levels.
- Give propylthiouracil (1g loading dose via nasogastric followed by 200–300mg qds). This inhibits thyroid hormone release and also decreases peripheral conversion of T_4 to T_3.
- After blockade by propylthiouracil, give sodium iodide (500mg tds IV), or potassium iodide (5 drops qds via nasogastric) or Lugol's iodine (5–10 drops qds via nasogastric).

Hypothyroid coma
- A rare form of decompensated hypothyroidism—mortality 15–20%.
- Characterised by coma, hypoventilation, bradycardia, hypotension, and a severe dilutional hyponatraemia.

1 Weinberg AD, Brennan MD, Gorman CA, Marsh HM, O'Fallon WM (1983). Outcome of anesthesia and surgery in hypothyroid patients. *Archives of Internal Medicine*, **143**, 893–897.

- Precipitated by infection, trauma, cold, and central nervous system depressants.
- Rehydrate with IV glucose and saline.
- Stabilise cardiac and pulmonary systems as necessary. May require ventilation.
- Sudden warming may lead to extreme peripheral vasodilatation, so use cautious passive external warming.
- IV liothyronine (see p158).
- Hydrocortisone (100mg qds IV) to treat possible adrenal insufficiency, a common result of hypothyroidism.
- Transfer to ICU.

Further reading

Farling PA (2000). Thyroid disease. *British Journal of Anaesthesia*, **85**, 15–28.
http://www.usyd.edu.au/anaes/lectures/thyroid_tmc.html.

Parathyroid disorders

General considerations

The parathyroid glands secrete parathyroid hormone (PTH), which acts on the bones and kidneys to increase serum calcium and decrease serum phosphate. It stimulates osteoclasts to release calcium and phosphate into the extracellular fluid and simultaneously increases phosphate excretion and calcium reabsorption in the kidney. Patients may present for parathyroidectomy (p558) or non-parathyroid related surgery.

Hyperparathyroidism

- Primary hyperthyroidism: usually an adenoma causing a high PTH, high calcium and low phosphate. Associated with familial multiple endocrine neoplasia (MEN) type 1. Tumours rarely palpable and located at surgery. Methylene blue (up to 1mg/kg) is often given preoperatively to localise the parathyroid gland.
- Presentation—50% of cases are asymptomatic and presentation often subtle. May present with anorexia, dyspepsia, nausea, vomiting and constipation, hypertension, shortened QT interval, polydipsia, polyuria, renal calculi, depression, poor memory, and drowsiness.

Hypercalcaemic crisis

- Occurs most commonly in the elderly with undiagnosed hyperparathyroidism and with malignant disease. Dehydration results in anorexia and nausea/vomiting which exacerbates the cycle. Also characterised by weakness, lethargy, mental changes, and coma.
- Serum calcium >4.5mmol/l is life-threatening and can be rapidly but transiently lowered with phosphate (500ml of 0.1M neutral solution over 6–8hr).
- Rehydrate (4–6 litres of fluid often required).
- Pamidronate (60mg in 500ml saline over 4hr) is first-line treatment. Effect is rapid and long lasting.
- Calcitonin (3–4U/kg IV then 4U/kg SC bd). Rapid decrease in skeletal release of calcium and phosphate—results only temporary.
- Second-line treatment, once volume repletion has been achieved, is with forced saline diuresis with furosemide (40mg IV every 4hr). Loop diuretics decrease the proximal tubular resorption of calcium. Consider central pressure monitoring in elderly at risk of left ventricular failure.
- Hydrocortisone (200–400mg IV daily) in patients with malignancy.
- Dialysis is reserved for patients with renal failure.

Secondary hyperparathyroidism

- Complicates chronic renal failure.
- Parathyroid hyperplasia causes a high PTH, normal or low calcium level, and a high phosphate level.
- Usually presents as excessive bone resorption (seen earliest in the radial aspect of the middle phalanx of the second digit) or soft tissue calcification of the vascular and soft tissues including kidneys, heart, lungs, and skin.

- Treat medically with dietary phosphate restriction, calcium, and vitamin D supplements. Medical therapy fails in 5–10% of patients on long-term dialysis and surgery becomes necessary.
- Risks of surgery are bleeding, recurrent hyperparathyroidism, hypoparathyroidism, and injury to the recurrent laryngeal nerves. Patients should undergo dialysis within 1d of surgery and then 48hr postoperatively or as required.
- Watch for postoperative hypocalcaemia and hypomagnesaemia.

Tertiary hyperparathyroidism

- Parathyroid hyperplasia progresses to autonomous secretion, behaving like an adenoma. Excessive secretion of PTH continues, despite correction of renal failure. Only a few require operation.

Perioperative plan

- Restore intravascular volume with 0.9% saline. If the patient has normal cardiovascular and renal systems, a normal ECG, and a total serum calcium <3mmol/l, then proceed with the operation. If the serum calcium is >3mmol/l, the ECG is abnormal or the patient has cardiovascular or renal impairment, then they should be delayed and treated.
- Careful monitoring of neuromuscular blockade should be undertaken if non-depolarising muscle relaxants are used.

Hypoparathyroidism

- Usually caused by parathyroidectomy but post-radiotherapy and idiopathic cases also occur. Patients with a history of extensive neck dissection in the past should have serum calcium measured before further surgery.
- Results in hypocalcaemia—ionised calcium <0.9mmol/l, total calcium (corrected for albumin) <2.2mmol/l. Trough level usually occurs at 20hr following parathyroidectomy and typically normalises by day 2–3.
- Presents with carpopedal spasm, tetany, dysrhythmia, hypotension, and prolonged PR interval on ECG.
- Treat with calcium (calcium gluconate 10ml 10% IV over 10min, followed by 40ml in 1 litre saline over 8hr).
- Low serum magnesium is also common and can be treated with magnesium sulphate (1–5mmol IV slowly).

To adjust calcium concentration for albumin level:
Add 0.1mmol/l to calcium for each 5g/l that albumin is below 40g/l.

Further reading

Edwards R. (1997). Thyroid and parathyroid disease. *International Anesthesiology Clinics*, **35**, 63–83.
Mihai R, Farndon JR (2000). Parathyroid disease and calcium metabolism. *British Journal of Anaesthesia*, **85**, 29–43.

Adrenal insufficiency

Primary (Addison's disease)
- Destruction of adrenal cortex by autoimmune disease (70–80%), infection (TB), septicaemia, AIDS, haemorrhage, metastases, surgery. Associated with glucocorticoid and mineralocorticoid deficiency

Secondary
- Insufficient adrenocorticotrophic hormone (ACTH) to stimulate the adrenal cortex due to pituitary suppression by exogenous steroids or generalised hypopituitarism usually from pituitary or hypothalamic tumours. Associated with glucocorticoid deficiency only

Acute adrenal crisis
- Due to stress in patients with chronic adrenal insufficiency without adequate steroid replacement, acute adrenal haemorrhage or pituitary apoplexy (apoplexy is defined as a sudden neurologic impairment, usually due to a vascular process, i.e. infarction or haemorrhage)

Clinical features of chronic adrenal insufficiency
- Weakness, fatigue (100%), skin hyperpigmentation (90%—primary only), postural hypotension (90%—pronounced in primary), nausea, vomiting, diarrhoea, weight loss (60%), myalgia, joint pain, salt craving (primary only), pale skin (secondary only)

Investigations
- Low serum glucose, low Na^+ (90%), raised K^+ (70%), raised urea and creatinine (primary only), raised Ca^{2+} (primary only)

Biochemical diagnosis of adrenal insufficiency

Test	Normal range	Definite adrenal insufficiency	
		Primary	Secondary
Early morning cortisol	165–680nmol/l	Cortisol <165nmol/l and ACTH >22.0pmol/l	Cortisol <100nmol/l
Early morning ACTH	1.1–11.0pmol/l		Not diagnostic
Standard short Synacthen test[1]	Peak cortisol >500nmol/l	Peak cortisol <500nmol/l	Peak cortisol <500nmol/l
Insulin tolerance test[2]	Peak cortisol >500nmol/l		Peak cortisol <500nmol/l

1 Serum cortisol at 0 and 30min after 250µg Synacthen IV.
2 Serum glucose and cortisol 0, 15, 30, 45, 60, and 90min after insulin (0.1–0.15U/kg IV). Test only valid if symptomatic hypoglycaemia (serum glucose <2.2nmol/l) is achieved. Gold standard test—close supervision mandatory.

Treatment
- Hydrocortisone (20mg in the morning and 10mg at night PO)
- Fludrocortisone (0.1mg PO) to replace aldosterone (primary deficiency only)

Perioperative management of patients with long-standing Addison's disease
- Give all medication up to the morning of surgery. Hydrocortisone (25mg IV) should be given at induction. Small or intermediate cases should be managed as per 'Perioperative steroids' (p166). In major cases, hydrocortisone 200mg/24hr should be used until the patient can be weaned back onto maintenance therapy.
- 4-hourly blood glucose and daily electrolytes.
- Joint care with an endocrinologist is advisable.
- With respect to mineralocorticoid potency, 20mg hydrocortisone is equivalent to 0.05mg fludrocortisone, so with hydrocortisone doses of 50mg or more, mineralocorticoid replacement in primary adrenal insufficiency can be reduced.

Adrenal crisis (Addisonian crisis)
Classically presents as hypotension, hyponatraemia, hyperkalaemia, and hypoglycaemia with abdominal pain. Characteristically resembles hypovolaemic shock, but can also mimic septic shock with fever, peripheral vasodilatation, and a high cardiac output. In patients with type 1 diabetes, deterioration of glycaemic control with recurrent hypoglycaemia can be the presenting sign of adrenal insufficiency.
- 100% oxygen and ventilatory support if necessary. Refer ICU/HDU.
- IV fluids. Colloid to restore blood volume, saline to replace Na^+ deficit initially at 1000ml/hr and glucose for hypoglycaemia.
- Hydrocortisone 200mg stat followed by 100mg qds. Baseline cortisol and ACTH prior to administration of hydrocortisone. Dexamethasone (4mg IV) can be used if the diagnosis has not been confirmed, since this does not interfere with measurement of cortisol and ACTH stimulation testing.
- Inotropes/vasopressors as required. May be resistant in the absence of cortisol replacement.
- Ascertain and treat precipitating cause.

Relative adrenal insufficiency in the critically ill
- Relative hypoadrenalism in ICU patients occurs in ~30–50% of septic patients. Consider in patients who are increasingly vasopressor dependent or require prolonged mechanical ventilation. Treat if suspected—200mg hydrocortisone IV.
- Abnormal response to a short Synacthen test is a poor prognostic indicator.

Further reading
Arlt W, Allolio B (2003). Adrenal insufficiency. Lancet, 361, 1881–1893.
Annane D et al. (2004). Corticosteroids for severe sepsis and septic shock: a systemic review and meta-analysis. British Medical Journal, 329, 480–484.

The patient on steroids

Steroids are used as replacement therapy in adrenocortical insufficiency or to suppress inflammatory and immunological responses. Patients on steroids requiring surgery may develop complications from their underlying disease, or from a potentially impaired stress response due to hypothalamic–pituitary–adrenal (HPA) suppression. Classically these patients were given additional large doses of steroids perioperatively; however, recent research suggests that smaller physiological replacement doses are more than adequate.

HPA suppression

- Endogenous cortisol (hydrocortisone) production is of the order of 25–30mg/24hr (following a circadian pattern). During stress induced by major surgery, it rises to 75–100mg/day and can remain elevated for a variable period of time (up to 72hr following cardiac surgery).
- Prednisolone is a synthetic glucocorticoid with the general properties of the corticosteroids. Prednisolone exceeds hydrocortisone in glucocorticoid and anti-inflammatory activity, being ~3–4 times more potent on a weight basis than the parent hormone, but is considerably less active than hydrocortisone in mineralocorticoid activity.
  Therefore it is often given for chronic conditions to limit water retention, and is found only as an oral preparation. In contrast, the relatively high mineralocorticoid activity of hydrocortisone and the resulting fluid retention make it unsuitable for disease suppression on a long-term basis; however, hydrocortisone can be given as an oral or IV preparation, which is why it is often used perioperatively instead of prednisolone.
- Low-dose steroid treatment, <10mg prednisolone per day, usually carries little danger of HPA suppression. Treatment with >10mg prednisolone (or equivalent) risks HPA suppression. This may occur after treatment via the oral, topical, parenteral, nebulised, or inhaled routes. These patients must be assumed to be suffering from an inability to mount a normal endogenous steroid response to stress and be supplemented accordingly.
- HPA suppression can be measured using various methods. In practice the short Synacthen test is reliable, cheap, and safe. Patients are given Synacthen (synthetic corticotrophin) (250µg IV) and serum cortisol is measured at 0, 30, and 60min. Normal peak cortisol levels range from 420 to 700nmol/l and indicate the ability of the patient to mount a stress response. If the result is equivocal, an insulin tolerance test can be performed under the supervision of an endocrinologist.

Perioperative steroid replacement therapy

<10mg prednisolone/day	Assume normal HPA axis	No additional steroid cover required
>10mg prednisolone/day	Minor surgery, e.g. hernia	Routine preoperative steroid or hydrocortisone 25mg IV at induction
	Intermediate surgery, e.g. hysterectomy	Routine preoperative steroid plus hydrocortisone 25mg IV at induction and then 6-hourly for 24hr
	Major surgery, e.g. cardiac	Routine preoperative steroid plus hydrocortisone 25mg IV at induction then 6-hourly for 48–72hr
High-dose immunosuppression	Should continue usual immunosuppressive dose until able to revert to normal oral intake, e.g. 60mg prednisolone/24hr = 240mg hydrocortisone/24hr	
Patient formerly taking regular steroids	<3 months since stopped steroids—treat as if on steroids	
	>3 months since stopped steroids—no perioperative steroids necessary	

Prednisolone 5mg is equivalent to
- Hydrocortisone 20mg
- Methylprednisolone 4mg
- Betamethasone 750µg
- Dexamethasone 750µg
- Cortisone acetate 25mg
- Deflazacort 6mg
- Triamcinolone 4mg

Fludrocortisone is available only in the oral preparation. It may be withheld on the day of surgery and while the patient is receiving stress doses of hydrocortisone (20mg hydrocortisone has equivalent mineralocorticoid potency of 0.05mg fludrocortisone).

Further reading

British National Formulary (2004). **48**, 356–62.
Nicholson G, Burrin JM, Hall GM (1998). Perioperative steroid replacement. *Anaesthesia*, **53**, 1091–1104.

Cushing's syndrome

A syndrome due to excess plasma cortisol caused by iatrogenic steroid administration (most common), pituitary adenoma (Cushing's disease—80% of remainder), ectopic ACTH (15% of remainder—e.g. oat cell carcinoma of lung), adrenal adenoma (4% of remainder), adrenal carcinoma (rare).

Clinical features
- Moon face, truncal obesity, proximal myopathy, and osteoporosis
- Easy bruising and fragile skin, impaired glucose tolerance, diabetes
- Hypertension, LVH, sleep apnoea
- High Na^+, HCO_3^-, and glucose; low K^+ and Ca^{2+}
- Gastrointestinal reflux.

Diagnosis
- High plasma cortisol and loss of diurnal variation (normal range ~165–680nmol/l; trough level at ~24:00 hr, peak level at ~06:00hr).
- Increased urinary 17-(OH)-steroids
- Loss of suppression with dexamethasone 2mg
- ACTH level:
  - Normal/high—pituitary
  - Low—adrenal, ectopic cortisol administration
  - Very high—ectopic ACTH.

Preoperative assessment
- Many patients have ECG abnormalities (high-voltage QRS and inverted T waves) which may make ischaemic heart disease difficult to exclude but they will revert to normal after curative surgery. These ECG changes seem to be related to the Cushing's disease itself.
- 85% of patients are hypertensive and are often poorly controlled.
- Sleep apnoea and gastro-oesophageal reflux are common.
- 60% of patients have diabetes or impaired glucose tolerance and a sliding scale should be started before major surgery if glucose is >10mmol/l.
- Patients are often obese with difficult veins!

Further reading

Sheeran P, O'Leary E (1997). Adrenocortical disorders. *International Anesthesiology Clinics*, **35**, 85–98.

Smith M, Hirsch NP (2000). Pituitary disease and anaesthesia. *British Journal of Anaesthesia*, **85**, 3–14.

Conn's syndrome

Excess of aldosterone produced from either an adenoma (60%), benign hyperplasia of the adrenal gland (35–40%), or adrenal carcinoma (rare).

General considerations

Aldosterone promotes active reabsorption of sodium and excretion of potassium through the renal tubules. Water is retained with sodium, resulting in an increase in extracellular fluid volume. To a lesser extent, there is also tubular secretion of hydrogen ions and magnesium, resulting in a metabolic alkalosis.

Clinical features

- Refractory hypertension, hypervolaemia, metabolic alkalosis
- Spontaneous hypokalaemia (K^+ <3.5mmol/l); moderately severe hypokalaemia (K^+ <3.0mmol/l) during diuretic therapy despite oral K^+
- Muscle weakness or paralysis especially in ethnic Chinese (secondary to hypokalaemia)
- Nephrogenic diabetes insipidus secondary to renal tubular damage (polyuria)
- Impaired glucose tolerance in ~50% of patients

Preoperative assessment for adrenalectomy

- Spironolactone (competitively inhibits aldosterone production) is usually given to reverse the metabolic and electrolyte effects. It also allows the patient to restore normovolaemia. Doses of up to 400mg/day may be required.
- The patient should have normal serum potassium and bicarbonate, but this may be difficult to achieve.
- Hypertension is usually mild and well controlled on spironolactone, but features of end organ damage, e.g. LVH, should be excluded.
- Calcium channel blockers such as nifedipine are effective antihypertensive agents with aldosterone-secreting adenomas. This is a specific action.

Investigations

- Aldosterone (pg/ml) to renin (ng/ml/h) ratio > 400.
- Secondary hyperaldosteronism has a raised serum aldosterone with a normal ratio.
- Important to distinguish between adenoma and hyperplasia as adenoma is usually treated surgically and hyperplasia medically.
- Adrenal vein sampling, CT, and MRI are all used.

Conduct of anaesthesia for adrenalectomy

Unilateral adrenalectomy can be done laparoscopically or via laparotomy and an appropriate method of analgesia should be discussed. Handling of the adrenal gland during surgery can cause cardiovascular instability but is not as severe as with a phaeochromocytoma (see p560).

- A short-acting α-blocker should be available (phentolamine 1mg boluses IV).
- Check blood glucose perioperatively.
- Chronic hypokalaemia has an antagonistic action upon insulin secretion/release and may result in abnormal glucose tolerance with the stress of surgery.

Postoperative care

- Give hydrocortisone IV postop until the patient can tolerate oral hydrocortisone and fludrocortisone.
- Hypertension may persist after removal of the adenoma, due presumably to permanent changes in vascular resistance.

Management of patients with Conn's syndrome for non-adrenal surgery

Such patients usually have bilateral glomerulosa hyperplasia. Hypertension is usually more severe and may require additional therapy (ACE inhibitors are useful). Try to restore K^+ to normal value preoperatively. Perform cardiovascular assessment as for any hypertensive patient.

Further reading

Winship SM, Winstanley JH, Hunter JM (1999). Anaesthesia for Conn's syndrome. *Anaesthesia*, **54**, 564–574.

Apudomas

Tumours of amine precursor uptake and decarboxylation (APUD) cells which are present in the anterior pituitary gland, thyroid, adrenal medulla, gastro-intestinal tract, pancreatic islet, carotid bodies, and lungs. Apudomas include phaeochromocytoma, carcinoid tumour, gastrinoma, VIPomas, and insulinoma and may occur as part of the multiple endocrine neoplasia (MEN) syndrome.

Phaeochromocytoma (see p560)

Carcinoid tumours

- Carcinoid tumours are derived from argentaffin cells and produce peptides and amines. Most occur in the GI tract (75%), bronchus, pancreas, and gonads. Tumours are mainly benign, and of those that are malignant only about a quarter release vasoactive substances into the systemic circulation, leading to the carcinoid syndrome.
- Mediators are metabolised in the liver; therefore only tumours with hepatic metastases or a primary tumour with non-portal venous drainage lead to the carcinoid syndrome.
- Vasoactive substances include serotonin, bradykinin, histamine, substance P, prostaglandins, and vasoactive intestinal peptide.
- Patients with an *asymptomatic* carcinoid tumour have simple carcinoid disease and do not present particular anaesthetic difficulties. Patients with *carcinoid syndrome* can be extremely difficult to manage perioperatively.

Carcinoid syndrome

Patients may have symptoms related to
- The primary tumour causing intestinal obstruction or pulmonary symptoms, e.g. haemoptysis and respiratory compromise.
- Vasoactive peptides resulting in flushing (90%) especially of the head, neck, and torso, or diarrhoea (78%), which may lead to dehydration and electrolyte disturbances. Other symptoms include bronchospasm (20%), hypotension, hypertension, tachycardia, hyperglycaemia, and right heart failure secondary to endocardial fibrosis affecting the pulmonary and tricuspid valves (mediators are metabolised in the lung before reaching the left heart).

Preoperative assessment

- Treat symptomatically—antidiarrhoeals, bronchodilators, correction of dehydration/electrolyte imbalance, treatment of heart failure.
- Prevent the release of mediators—octreotide (100µg SC tds) for 2wk prior to surgery and octreotide (100µg IV slowly diluted to 10µg/ml) at induction.
- Avoid factors which may trigger carcinoid crises—catecholamines, anxiety, and drugs which release histamine, e.g. morphine.

Investigations

- Crossmatch blood; check LFTs and clotting if metastases present.
- ECG and echocardiography if cardiac involvement is suspected.
- CXR and lung function tests if indicated.

Conduct of anaesthesia

This is best managed by teams/centres familiar with the difficulties. Major complications anticipated in the perioperative period include severe hypotension, severe hypertension, fluid and electrolyte shift, and bronchospasm.

- Premedication: anxiolytic (benzodiazepine) and octreotide (100μg (50–500μg) SC 1hr preoperatively) if not already treated, otherwise continue with preoperative regime.
- Monitoring should include invasive blood pressure monitoring (preinduction as both induction and surgical manipulation of the tumour can cause large swings), CVP monitoring, regular blood sugars, and blood gases. Pulmonary artery flotation catheter if indicated due to cardiac complications.
- Induction: prevent pressor response to intubation (etomidate/propofol and alfentanil/fentanyl). Suxamethonium has been used safely for rapid sequence induction, although fasciculations may theoretically stimulate hormone release by increasing intra-abdominal pressure.
- Maintenance: isoflurane, vecuronium or pancuronium, fentanyl, or low-dose epidural (avoiding hypotension as this may elicit bradykinergic crisis) for analgesia.
- Octreotide (10–20μg boluses IV) to treat severe hypotension.
- Avoid all histamine-releasing drugs and catecholamines (release serotonin and kallikrein, which activates bradykinins).
- Labetalol, esmolol, or ketanserin can be used for hypertension.

Postoperative

- ICU or HDU is required.
- Patients may waken very slowly (thought to be due to serotonin).
- Hypotensive episodes may occur, requiring further IV boluses of octreotide (10–20μg).
- Wean octreotide over 7–10d following tumour resection.

Gastrinoma

Excess production of gastrin by benign adenoma, malignancy, or hyper-plasia of the D cells of the pancreatic islets. Leads to Zollinger–Ellison syndrome, severe peptic ulceration, and diarrhoea. May also have GI bleeds, perforation, electrolyte disturbance, and volume depletion. Treatment includes proton pump inhibitors (e.g. omeprazole), H_2 receptor antagonists, and octreotide. May present for surgery related to gastrinoma, e.g. perforation, or totally unrelated pathology.

- FBC to look for anaemia from bleeding gastric ulceration.
- Check clotting screen and liver function tests, since alterations in fat absorption may influence clotting factors and hepatic function may be affected by liver metastases.
- Antacid prophylaxis preoperatively and rapid sequence induction.
- Invasive pressure monitoring for major surgery.

VIPoma

Rare tumour secreting vasoactive intestinal peptide (VIP) which leads to Verner–Morrison syndrome. Characterised by profuse watery diarrhoea, intestinal ileus, abdominal distension, confusion, drowsiness, hypokalaemia, achlorhydria, hypomagnesaemia, hyperglycaemia, metabolic alkalosis, and tetany.

- VIP inhibits gastrin release; therefore give H_2 receptor blocking drugs preoperatively to prevent rebound gastric acid hypersecretion.
- Replace fluids and electrolytes.
- Treat medically with somatostatin analogues (octreotide). If this fails, try steroids (such as methylprednisolone) and indometacin (a prostaglandin inhibitor).
- Often become malignant (60%) with liver metastases so all warrant resection.
- Use invasive pressure monitoring for major surgery.
- Frequent measurement of arterial blood gases to check acid base status and electrolytes.

Insulinoma

Rare tumour of β cells of pancreas which secrete insulin—diagnosis made by Whipple's triad—symptoms of hypoglycaemia, low plasma glucose, and relief of symptoms when glucose is given.

- Diagnosis also made by a fasting blood glucose <2.2mmol/l, increased insulin, increased C-peptide, and absence of sulphonylurea in the plasma.
- Diazoxide (a non-diuretic benzothiazide which inhibits the release of insulin) has been used where surgery has failed but has unpredictable efficacy.
- Tumours usually non-malignant, but if malignant, hepatic resection may be required.
- Monitor blood glucose closely perioperatively.

Glucagonoma

Tumour of the α cells of the pancreas. Glucagon stimulates hepatic glycogenolysis and gluconeogenesis, resulting in increased blood glucose and diabetes mellitus. Ketoacidosis is rare since insulin is also increased. Characterised by a rash (necrotising migratory erythema which presents in the groin/perineum and migrates to the distal extremities).

- Associated with weight loss, glossitis, stomatitis, anaemia, and diarrhoea.
- Usually have liver metastases at presentation.
- Treatment consists of surgical debulking and somatostatin analogues.
- Increased incidence of venous thromboses so give prophylactic anti-thrombotic therapy.

Further reading

Holdcraft A (2000). Hormones and the gut. *British Journal of Anaesthesia*, **85**, 58–68.
Veall GRQ, Peacock JE, Bax NDS, Reilly CS (1994). Review of the anaesthetic management of 21 patients undergoing laparotomy for carcinoid syndrome. *British Journal of Anaesthesia*, **72**, 335–341.

Hypokalaemia

Defined as plasma potassium <3.5mmol/l.
- Mild   3.0–3.5mmol/l
- Moderate   2.5–3.0mmol/l
- Severe   <2.5mmol/l.

Causes
- Decreased intake.
- Increased potassium loss—vomiting or nasogastric suctioning, diarrhoea, pyloric stenosis, diuretics, renal tubular acidosis, hyper-aldosteronism, magnesium depletion, leukaemia.
- Intercompartmental shift—insulin, alkalosis (0.1 increase in pH decreases K^+ by 0.6mmol/l), β_2-agonists and steroids.

Clinical manifestations
- ECG changes—T wave flattening and inversion, prominent U wave, ST segment depression, prolonged PR interval.
- Dysrhythmias, decreased cardiac contractility.
- Skeletal muscle weakness, tetany, ileus, polyuria, impaired renal concentrating ability, decreased insulin secretion, growth hormone secretion, and aldosterone secretion, negative nitrogen balance.
- Encephalopathy in patients with liver disease.

Management
- Check U&Es, creatinine and Ca^{2+}, phosphate, Mg^{2+}, HCO_3^-, and glucose if other electrolyte disturbances suspected.
- Exclude Cushing's and Conn's syndromes.
- Oral replacement is safest, up to 200mmol per day, e.g. potassium chloride (Sando-K) two tablets four times a day = 96mmol K^+.
- IV replacement—essential for patients with cardiac manifestations, skeletal muscle weakness or where oral replacement not appropriate.
- Aim to increase K^+ to 4.0mmol/l if treating cardiac manifestations.
- Maximum concentration for peripheral administration is 40mmol/l (greater concentrations than this can lead to venous necrosis). 40mmol KCl can be given in 100ml 0.9% saline over 1hr but only via an infusion device, with ECG monitoring, in HDU/ ICU/theatre environment, and via a central vein. Plasma K^+ should be measured at least hourly during rapid replacement. K^+ depletion sufficient to cause 0.3mmol/l drop in serum K^+ requires a loss of ~100mmol of K^+ from total body store.

Anaesthetic considerations
Principal problem is the risk of arrhythmia. The rate of onset is important—chronic, mild hypokalaemia is less significant than that of rapid onset. Patients must be viewed individually and the decision to proceed should be based on the chronicity and level of hypokalaemia, the type of surgery, and any other associated pathologies. Ratio of intracellular to extracellular K^+ is of more importance than isolated plasma levels.

- Classically a K^+ <3.0mmol has led to postponement of elective procedures (some controversy exists about this in the fit, non-digitalised patient who may well tolerate chronically lower K^+ levels, e.g. 2.5mmol/l, without adverse events).
- For emergency surgery, if possible replace K^+ in the 24hr prior to surgery. Aim for levels of 3.5–4.0mmol/l. If this is not possible use an IV replacement regime as documented above intra-/perioperatively.
- If bicarbonate is raised, then loss is probably longstanding with low intracellular potassium and will take days to replace.
- May increase sensitivity to neuromuscular blockade; therefore need to monitor.
- Increased risk of digoxin toxicity at low K^+ levels. Aim for K^+ of 4.0mmol/l in a digitalised patient.

Hyperkalaemia

Defined as plasma potassium >5.5mmol/l.

- Mild   5.5–6.0mmol/l
- Moderate   6.1–7.0mmol/l
- Severe   >7.0mmol/l.

Causes

- Increased intake—IV administration, rapid blood transfusion.
- Decreased urinary excretion—renal failure (acute or chronic), adrenocortical insufficiency, drugs (K^+ sparing diuretics, ACE inhibitors, ciclosporin etc.).
- Intercompartmental shift of potassium—acidosis, rhabdomyolysis, trauma, malignant hyperthermia, suxamethonium (especially with burns or denervation injuries), familial periodic paralysis.

Clinical manifestations

- ECG changes progressing through peaked T waves, widened QRS, prolonged PR interval, loss of P wave, loss of R wave amplitude, ST depression, ventricular fibrillation, asystole. ECG changes potentiated by low calcium, low sodium, and by acidosis.
- Muscle weakness at K^+ >8.0mmol/l.
- Nausea, vomiting, diarrhoea.

Management

Treatment should be initiated if K^+ > 6.5mmol/l or ECG changes present. Unlike hypokalaemia, the incidence of serious cardiac compromise is high and therefore intervention is important. Treat the cause if possible. Ensure IV access and cardiac monitor.

- Insulin (10U in 50ml 50% dextrose IV over 30–60min).
- Calcium (5–10ml 10% calcium gluconate or 3–5ml 10% calcium chloride). Calcium stabilises the myocardium by increasing the threshold potential. Rapid onset, short lived.
- If acidotic, give bicarbonate (50mmol IV).
- β_2-agonist—salbutamol (5mg nebulised—beware tachycardia).
- Ion exchange resin—calcium resonium (15g PO or 30g PR 8-hourly).
- If initial management fails, consider dialysis or haemofiltration.

Anaesthetic considerations

Do not consider elective surgery. If life-threatening surgery, treat hyperkalaemia first.

Avoid Hartmann's solution and suxamethonium if possible. However, if there is a compelling case for rapid intubation conditions without long-term paralysis, suxamethonium has been used safely with a preoperative potassium of >5.5mmol/l.[1] Monitor neuromuscular blockade, since effects may be accentuated.

- Avoid hypothermia and acidosis.
- Control ventilation to prevent respiratory acidosis.
- Monitor K^+ regularly.

Further reading

Gennari FJ (2002). Disorders of potassium homeostasis. Hypokalaemia and hyperkalaemia. *Critical Care Clinics*, **18**, 273–288.

Tetzlaff JE, O'Hara JF Jr, Walsh MI (1993). Potassium and anaesthesia. *Canadian Journal of Anaesthesia*, **40**, 227–246.

Wong KC, Schafer PG, Schultz JR (1993). Hypokalaemia and anaesthetic implications. *Anesthesia and Analgesia*, **77**, 1238–1260.

1 Schow AJ, Lubarsky DA, Olson RP, Gan TJ (2002). Can succinylcholine be used safely in hyperkalaemic patients? *Anesthesia and Analgesia*, **95**, 119–122.

Hyponatraemia

Defined as serum Na^+ <135mmol/l.
- Mild   125–134mmol/l
- Moderate 120–124mmol/l
- Severe   <120mmol/l.

Extracellular fluid volume is directly proportional to total body sodium (Na^+) content. Renal Na^+ excretion ultimately controls extracellular fluid volume and total body Na^+ content. To identify causes of abnormalities of sodium homeostasis it is important to assess plasma and urinary Na^+ levels along with the patient's state of hydration (hypo/eu/hypervolaemic).

Presentation

Important to differentiate between acute and chronic hyponatraemia. Speed of onset is much more important for manifestation of symptoms than the absolute Na^+ level. Rare to get clinical signs if Na^+ >125mmol/l.
- Na^+ 125–130mmol/l causes mostly GI symptoms, i.e. nausea/vomiting.
- Na^+ <125mmol/l—neuropsychiatric symptoms, nausea/vomiting, muscular weakness, headache, lethargy, psychosis, raised intracranial pressure, seizures, coma, and respiratory depression. Mortality high if untreated.

Treatment of symptomatic hyponatraemia

- Acute symptomatic hyponatraemia (develops in <48hr), e.g. TURP syndrome, hysteroscopy-induced hyponatraemia, SIADH. Aim to raise serum Na^+ by 2mmol/l/hr until symptoms resolve. Complete correction is unnecessary, although not unsafe. Infuse hypertonic saline (3% NaCl) at a rate of 1.2–2.4ml/kg/hr through a large vein. In cases of fluid excess give furosemide (20mg IV) to promote diuresis. If there are severe neurological symptoms (seizures, coma) 3% NaCl may be infused at 4–6ml/kg/hr. Electrolytes should be carefully monitored. (See also p571.)
- Chronic symptomatic hyponatraemia (present for more than 48hr or duration unknown). Aim to correct serum Na^+ by 5–10mmol/d. Rapid correction (serum Na^+ rise of >0.5mmol/l/hr) can lead to central pontine myelinosis, subdural haemorrhage and cardiac failure. Give furosemide and replace saline losses with 0.9% saline IV. Monitor electrolytes and urine output carefully. SIADH—fluid restrict and demeclocycline (300–600mg daily).
- Consult with endocrinologist.
- Watch for resolution of symptoms.
- Treat the cause.

Asymptomatic hyponatraemia (often chronic)

- Fluid restrict to 1l/day.
- Treat the cause.

Anaesthetic implications

- No elective surgery if Na^+ <120mmol/l or symptomatic hyponatraemia.
- Emergency surgery: consider risk to benefits. Consult endocrinologist.

Hypernatraemia

Defined as serum Na^+ >145mmol/l.

- Mild   145–150mmol/l
- Moderate 151–160mmol/l
- Severe   >160mmol/l.

Presentation

CNS symptoms likely if serum Na^+ >155mmol/l due to hyperosmolar state and cellular dehydration, e.g. thirst, confusion, seizures, and coma. Features depend on the cause e.g. water deficiency will present with hypotension, tachycardia, and decreased skin turgor.

Management

Correct over at least 48hr to prevent occurrence of cerebral oedema and convulsions. Treat the underlying cause. Oral fluids (water) if possible.

- Hypovolaemic (Na^+ deficiency): 0.9% saline until hypovolaemia corrected, then consider 0.45% saline.
- Euvolaemia (water depletion): estimate the total body water deficit, treat with 5% dextrose.
- Hypervolaemic (Na^+ excess): diuretics, e.g. furosemide (20mg IV) and 5% dextrose, dialysis if required.
- Diabetes insipidus—replace urinary losses and give desmopressin (1–4µg daily SC/IM/IV).

Anaesthetic implications

- No elective surgery if Na^+ >155mmol/l or hypovolaemic.
- Urgent surgery—use central venous pressure monitoring if volume status is uncertain or may change rapidly intra-operatively, and be aware of dangers of rapid normalisation of electrolytes.

Further reading

Kumar S, Beri T (1998). Sodium. *The Lancet*, **352**, 220–228.

Obesity

Obesity is associated with hypertension, ischaemic heart disease, non-insulin-dependent diabetes mellitus, peripheral vascular disease, gallstones, and osteoarthritis.
- Body mass index (BMI) = weight (kg)/height^2 (m^2).
- Obesity is defined by a BMI >28kg/m^2 and morbid obesity by BMI >35kg/m^2.

17% of the UK population are obese and ~1% morbidly obese.

Cardiovascular
- Increase in absolute blood volume, although this is low relative to body mass (occasionally only 45ml/kg).
- Increase in cardiac output and stroke volume in proportion to oxygen consumption and weight gain.
- Systemic hypertension is 10 times more prevalent due to increased cardiac output and blood volume.
- Obesity is a risk factor for ischaemic heart disease.

Respiratory
- Oxygen consumption is increased by metabolically active adipose tissue and the workload of supporting muscles, with concomitant increase in CO_2 production.
- FRC is reduced in the awake obese patient and decreases significantly following induction, which may encroach upon the closing capacity. Pulmonary compliance is decreased by up to 35% (due to heavy chest wall and splinted diaphragm). Increased ventilation/perfusion mismatch.
- Obesity hypoventilation syndrome (OHS) occurs due to loss of central drive. Hypoxaemia, pulmonary hypertension, and polycythaemia can develop.
- Obstructive sleep apnoea (OSA) is also more common in the obese. Occurs due to lack of central drive and peripheral anatomical abnormalities.
- As a result, oxygen desaturation occurs rapidly in the obese apnoeic patient.

Gastrointestinal
- Increased gastric volumes with low pH, raised intra-abdominal pressure, and a higher incidence of hiatus hernia pose a significant risk of aspiration.

Endocrine
- Insulin resistance may cause glucose intolerance and NIDDM.

General
- Potential difficult intubation due to decreased atlanto-axial movement, large tongue, palatal, pharyngeal, and upper thoracic fat pads.
- Technical problems of IV access and nerve blockade.
- Increased risk of skin infections.

Pharmacokinetics/dynamics

- Volume of distribution for drugs is altered due to a smaller proportion of total body water, greater proportion of adipose tissue, increased lean body mass, and increased blood volume and cardiac output.
- Hydrophilic drugs (e.g. neuromuscular blockers) have similar absolute volumes of distribution, clearance, and elimination half-lives. Base dose on lean body mass. Atracurium recovery is similar to the non-obese.
- Lipophilic drugs (e.g. thiopental and benzodiazepines) have increased volumes of distribution, normal clearance, and increased elimination half-lives.
- Increased plasma cholinesterase activity. Give suxamethonium in dose of 1.5mg/kg.

Preoperative assessment

- Calculate the BMI and assess venous access, risk of aspiration, and possibility of a difficult intubation or difficulty with mask ventilation. A BMI of 46 is associated with a 13% risk of difficult intubation. It is useful to assess the airway in both the erect and supine positions.
- Ask about snoring, somnolence, and periodic breathing.
- Evaluate patient for signs of systemic and/or pulmonary hypertension, signs of right and/or left ventricular failure, and ischaemic heart disease.
- Premedication with respiratory depressants should be avoided. An H_2 blocker or proton pump inhibitor plus metoclopramide should be administered on the ward (± 30ml sodium citrate 0.3M in the anaesthetic room).

Preoperative investigations

As per clinical findings and surgical procedure planned, also:
- ECG to look for LVH
- ABGs to identify baseline hypoxaemic and hypercarbic patients

Conduct of anaesthesia

Check that an appropriate operating table and sphygmomanometer cuff are available. Invasive blood pressure monitoring may be required.
- Full preoxygenation is essential. Intubation may be warranted for all but the briefest of procedures due to the risk of aspiration, and IPPV is often necessary because of the increased work of breathing and tendency to hypoventilation. Awake fibreoptic intubation may be indicated, although some use topical anaesthesia and direct laryngoscopy. Traction on the breasts by an assistant or use of a polio blade may help. Reduced FRC can be increased by administering PEEP or large sustained manual inflations. Increasing the I:E ratio may reduce airway pressures.
- Pay particular care to protecting pressure areas.
- Use short-acting agents to ensure rapid recovery. Nitrous oxide is a good choice due to its rapid elimination and analgesic properties, but high oxygen demand may limit its use.

- Aortocaval compression may occur in the supine position and table tilt may help. Avoid head-down positioning, especially in spontaneous ventilation.
- Fluid balance may be difficult to assess clinically and increased blood loss is common due to difficult surgical conditions.
- Local anaesthetic doses for spinals and epidurals should be 75–80% of normal because engorged extradural veins and fat constrict these spaces.

Postoperative care

- Extubate awake, sitting up.
- Thromboembolic events are twice as common and so thromboprophylaxis is important.
- Mobilise as soon as practical—ensure enough staff are available.
- Pulmonary atelectasis is common and lung capacities remain decreased for at least 5d after abdominal surgery. To optimise the FRC/closing capacity ratio the obese patient should be nursed at 30–45° head-up tilt for this period. Humidified oxygen and early, regular physiotherapy should be administered.
- Nocturnal nasal CPAP and continual pulse oximetry may be considered in OSA.
- PCA is more predictable than IM opioids because injections are frequently into SC fat.
- HDU care should be available for higher-risk patients with pre-existing respiratory disease, especially those undergoing thoracic or abdominal surgery.

Further reading

Adams JP, Murphy PG (2000). Obesity in anaesthesia and intensive care. *British Journal of Anaesthesia*, **85**, 91–108.
Ogunnaike BO, Jones SB, Jones DB, Provost D, Whitten CW (2002). Anesthetic considerations for bariatric surgery. *Anesthesia and Analgesia*, **95**, 1793–1805.
Smith HL, Meldrum DJ, Brennan LJ (2002). Childhood obesity: a challenge for the anaesthetist? *Paediatric Anaesthesia*, **12**, 750–761.

Chapter 9

Bone, joint, and connective tissue disorders

Paul Marshall

Rheumatoid arthritis

Rheumatoid arthritis (RA) is a chronic, systemic inflammatory disorder mainly involving joints but with extra-articular effects. Overall prevalence is about 1% but higher in elderly females. Patients are often frail, in chronic pain, and taking medications with adverse effects. Airway problems are common. There is a higher than average mortality due to both the disease itself and the presence of concurrent disorders.

Preoperative assessment

Articular

- Temporomandibular: assess mouth opening as this may be limited.
- Cricoarytenoid: fixation of the cricoarytenoid joints may lead to voice changes, hoarseness, or even rarely to stridor from glottic stenosis. Minimal oedema may lead to airway obstruction postoperatively.
- Atlantoaxial subluxation (AAS) occurs in ~25% of severe rheumatoid patients, but of these only a quarter will have neurological signs or symptoms. Enquire about tingling hands or feet, neck pain, and assess range of neck movement. Excessive movement during anaesthesia can lead to cervical cord compression.
  - Anterior AAS: comprises 80% of all AAS. C1 forward on C2 from destruction of transverse ligament. Significant if there is a gap of >3mm between the odontoid and the arch of the atlas in lateral flexion radiographs. Atlantoaxial flexion is potentially hazardous.
  - Posterior AAS: this is rare. C1 backward on C2 resulting from destruction of the odontoid peg. Can be seen on lateral extension radiographs. Atlantoaxial extension (e.g. from direct laryngoscopy) is potentially hazardous.
  - Vertical AAS: arises from destruction of lateral masses of C1. The odontoid moves upwards through foramen magnum to compress cervicomedullary junction.
  - Lateral AAS: uncommon. Arises from involvement of the C1/C2 facet joints. More than 2mm difference in lateral alignment is significant. Requires a frontal open mouth odontoid view to assess.
- Subaxial subluxation:
  - More than 2mm loss of alignment is significant.
  - Look for this particularly if patient has undergone previous fusion at a higher level.
- Other joints: assess joint deformities with a view to positioning and possible anaesthetic technique (if planning an axillary block can the patient abduct their arm?). Manual dexterity may be important if planning to use standard PCA apparatus after surgery. Special adaptations are available, e.g. trigger by blowing.

Non-articular

- Cardiovascular: association with coronary artery disease. Systemic vasculitis may lead to arterial occlusion in various organs. Myocardial disease due to fibrosis and nodular involvement. Symptomatic pericardial involvement uncommon. Aortic incompetence rare.

- Respiratory: fibrosing alveolitis, frequently asymptomatic. Acute pneumonitis rare. Pleural effusions and/or nodules in pleura may show on X-ray. Association with obliterative bronchiolitis.
- Anaemia: NSAID-associated blood loss. Anaemia of chronic disease. Drug-associated bone marrow depression. Felty's syndrome is combination of splenomegaly and neutropenia and may be associated with anaemia and thrombocytopenia.
- Nervous system: peripheral and compression neuropathies occur. Cord compression may be atlanto-axial or subaxial. Neurological changes may be chronic or acute (trauma).
- Infections: common both from disease itself and drug effects.

Investigations
- All patients should have FBC, U&Es, ECG, and CXR.
- Cervical spine radiographs: the role of preoperative cervical spine flexion/extension views is controversial and interpretation is difficult. The automatic reordering of radiographs in all patients seems unnecessary, particularly if it will not alter management. Flexion/extension views are mandatory in all patients with neurological symptoms or signs, and in those with persistent neck pain. Stabilisation surgery may be necessary before other elective surgery is undertaken. Preoperative cervical spine radiographs may help determine management in some patients with severe disease requiring intubation but only after review of previous radiographs, case notes, and anaesthetic charts. Specialist radiological advice may be required. Unless it is certain that the cervical spine is stable, therefore, all rheumatoid patients should be treated as if they might have an unstable spine. This may involve awake fibre-optic intubation or manual in-line stabilisation when undertaking direct laryngoscopy/LMA insertion/moving patient. MRI and CT may be useful in assessing cord compression.
- Pulmonary function tests should be carried out for patients with unexplained dyspnoea or radiological abnormalities.
- An ENT opinion should be sought and nasendoscopy performed if there is hoarseness or symptoms/signs of respiratory obstruction.
- Echocardiography is needed if there is valvular or pericardial involvement and in symptomatic cardiac disease.

Drugs in the perioperative period
- Steroid supplementation (p167).
- NSAIDs: continue as enables early mobilisation. Stop if postoperative bleeding a potential problem, hypotension, or deterioration in renal function.
- Disease modifying antirheumatoid drugs (DMARDs): these drugs include gold, penicillamine, and immunosuppressant drugs such as methotrexate and azathioprine. Usually continue, as mobilisation important and little evidence that omission reduces postoperative complications (wound infections). If leucopenic consult with rheumatologist.

- TNF-α blockers: etanercept and infliximab belong to new class of drugs blocking effects of tumour necrosis factor α—an inflammatory mediator. Given by injection at twice weekly intervals. Severe infections reported—close monitoring advised.
- DVT prophylaxis (p10): early mobilisation.
- Gastrointestinal agents: continue H_2 antagonists and proton pump inhibitors prior to and after surgery. Consider short-term use in those not receiving treatment.

Anaesthesia

- Take care of the neck and maintain in a neutral position at all times, especially on transfer and turning. Use manual in-line stabilisation during airway manipulation while the patient is unconscious (unless it is certain that spine is stable). If intubation is necessary consider fibreoptic intubation (p948), particularly if there is posterior AAS (rare) and/or predicted difficulty. If direct laryngoscopy is undertaken use manual in-line stabilisation and a gum elastic bougie. If this is difficult have a low threshold for converting to awake fibreoptic intubation.
- Ensure careful positioning and padding/protection of vulnerable areas on the operating table. Note the position before induction, then try to maintain this during surgery.
- Regional techniques may be difficult. Patient discomfort from prolonged immobilisation may favour general anaesthesia, perhaps in combination with regional catheter techniques.
- Normothermia is especially important, as hypothermia may increase the risk of wound infections.
- Strict asepsis with invasive procedures as increased risk of infection.

Postoperative

- Adequate pain control allows early mobilisation. PCA is often impractical due to impaired hand function. A puffer-PCA device has been described.
- Continue NSAIDs unless contraindicated.
- Physiotherapy and mobilisation are important.
- Continue DVT prophylaxis until the patient is fully mobile.
- Maintain fluid intake and monitor renal function.
- Restart DMARDs to avoid exacerbation of joint immobility.

Ankylosing spondylitis

Inflammatory arthritis of the sacroiliac joints and spine, leading to ankylosis and 'bamboo spine'. It is associated with HLA B27 in >90% of cases. The male to female ratio is about 4:1. Important anaesthetic implications are both articular and non-articular.

Articular

- Progressive kyphosis and fixation of the spine may hinder intubation. Conventional intubation and tracheostomy may be impossible. Atlantoaxial subluxation and myelopathy can occur rarely. There may be limited mouth opening from temporomandibular involvement. Use of ILMA described but fibreoptic intubation usually preferred.
- At risk of occult cervical fracture with minimal trauma.
- Cricoarytenoid arthritis may make cords susceptible to trauma.
- Axial skeletal involvement may make neuraxial block difficult or impossible. Spinal anaesthesia using a paramedian approach appears to be the most practical technique for neuraxial block. Reported increased risk of epidural haematoma with epidural block.
- Limited chest expansion may lead to postoperative pulmonary complications. Effective external cardiac massage may be impossible.
- Deformity leads to difficulty with positioning, particularly if a prone position required.

Non-articular

- Fibrosing alveolitis may occur, exacerbating postoperative hypoxia.
- Aortic regurgitation (1%). Mitral valve involvement and conduction defects are rare.
- Amyloid may cause renal involvement.
- Cauda equina syndrome may occur in longstanding cases.
- Associated use of NSAIDs and DMARDs (see p187).

Systemic lupus erythematosus (SLE)

This is a chronic multi-system disease commonest in young females, especially in pregnancy. It is characterised by the presence of numerous antibodies including antinuclear antibody, and immune-mediated tissue damage. Although joints may be affected there is no deformity or bony erosion and no specific airway implications. The main anaesthetic implications are cardiovascular disease, renal disease, coagulation status, and increased risk of infection.

Preoperative assessment

- Skin and joint involvement is common, as are oral and pharyngeal ulceration.
- Cardiovascular: pericarditis in 15%. Myocarditis and endocarditis less common. Raynaud's phenomenon 30%. Coronary artery disease from atherosclerosis and other mechanisms common.
- Respiratory system: infections and pulmonary emboli common. Pleuritis and pleural effusion. Pulmonary fibrosis less common.
- Neurological: cranial and peripheral nerve lesions may occur, secondary to arteritis and ischaemia. Transverse myelitis leading to weakness or paraplegia occurs rarely. Depression, psychosis, and fits.
- Renal: glomerulonephritis is a serious complication and may lead to nephrotic syndrome and renal failure.
- Haematological: clotting disorders or hypercoagulable states can occur. Patients with SLE should have full blood count and clotting status checked. Immune thrombocytopenia or circulating anticoagulants (e.g. antibodies to factor VIII) may be present. Up to a third of patients with SLE may demonstrate features of antiphospholipid syndrome (p227). This is a hypercoagulable state which paradoxically may be associated with the presence of lupus anticoagulant and a prolonged APTT. Since a prolonged APTT may indicate either a clotting disorder or a hypercoagulable state, further haematological advice should be sought.
- Higher risk of stroke with antiphospholipid antibodies.
- Steroids and other immunosuppressant drugs are used.

Anaesthesia

- There may be absolute or relative contraindications to neuraxial blocks in patients taking anticoagulants or in patients with coagulopathy— (p1058). The presence of a peripheral nerve lesion may be a relative contraindication to neuraxial/regional nerve blockade.
- Maintenance of normothermia may reduce the risk of infection as well as lessening the impact of Raynaud's phenomenon if present.
- Laryngeal erythema and oedema are common—try to minimise trauma to the airway.
- Consider hourly urine output and invasive monitoring.
- Steroid supplementation (p167).
- Strict asepsis with invasive procedures as increased risk of infection.

Systemic sclerosis

Limited cutaneous form comprising Calcinosis, Raynaud's, oEsophageal dysfunction, Sclerodactyly, and Telangiectasia (CREST) is more common (60% cases) than the more aggressive diffuse cutaneous form, which has more widespread effects and a high mortality.

The following may be relevant to anaesthesia:

- Cardiovascular: Raynaud's, pericarditis, or myocardial fibrosis. Conduction defects. Pulmonary hypertension common.
- Pulmonary: fibrosing alveolitis in both forms (40% in diffuse form).
- Renal: may develop renal crisis associated with malignant hypertension.
- Gastrointestinal: oesophageal reflux invariable.
- Airway: may have mouth narrowing and tightened skin around neck leading to difficult intubation.

Connective tissue disorders and anaesthesia

	Rheumatoid arthritis	Ankylosing spondylitis	Systemic lupus erythematosus	Systemic sclerosis
Prevalence	1%	0.15%	0.03%	0.001%
Airway and intubation	C Spine instability/ ankylosis Cricoarytenoid arthritis TMJ arthritis	Cervical kyphosis, TMJ arthritis Occult fractures		Limited mouth opening
Respiratory	Fibrosing alveolitis. Pleural effusions Nodules on CXR	Fixed chest wall Apical fibrosis (1%)	Chest infections Pulmonary emboli Pleuritis	Fibrosing. alveolus
Cardiovascular	Ischaemic heart disease (association)	Aortic regurgitation 1%	Raynaud's Hypertension Coronary ischaemia Pericarditis Endocarditis (Libman Sacks)	Raynaud's >90% Hypertension Pulmonary. hypertension Myocardial fibrosis Arrhythmias Pericardial effusions
Neurological	Peripheral neuropathy Radiculopathy Myelopathy	Cauda equina syndrome (rare)	Peripheral neuropathy Psychosis Convulsions	
Renal	Mild renal impairment common		Glomerulo-nephritis	Chronic impairment Hypertensive renal crisis
Gastrointestinal	Drug-related gastritis	Drug-related gastritis	Abdominal pain Nausea Mesenteric vasculitis	Reflux invariable
Haematology	Anaemia—drug-related and disease-related Felty's syndrome (splenomegaly and leucopenia)	Anaemia—drug-related and disease-related	Antiphospholipid syndrome Anaemia Thrombocytopenia	
Neuraxial block	Often difficult ?Infection risk	Difficult Consider lateral approach ?Increased risk epidural haematoma	Check coagulation ?Infection risk	

Scoliosis

Progressive lateral curvature of the spine with added rotation. Scoliosis may be progressive and lead to an increasing restrictive ventilatory defect which in turn leads to hypoxia, hypercarbia, and pulmonary hypertension. Corrective surgery may be carried out in the teens to arrest these changes. Scoliosis may be idiopathic (~75%) or secondary to other conditions with anaesthetic implications:

- Muscular dystrophies
- Poliomyelitis
- Cerebral palsy
- Friedreich's ataxia (See also p296).

Conduct of anaesthesia

- Formal respiratory function tests mandatory in severe cases.
- Check for pulmonary hypertension and right heart failure.
- Some muscular dystrophies may be associated with cardiac abnormalities. Consider echocardiography.
- Avoid sedative premedication in patients with poor respiratory reserve.
- Regional techniques where possible ± GA.
- Plan for high dependency or intensive care in complex cases.

Achondroplasia

The commonest form of dwarfism is caused by premature ossification of bones combined with normal periosteal bone formation, giving a characteristic appearance of short limbs and a relatively normal cranium. The following should be noted:

- The larynx may be small and intubation is occasionally difficult. Have a range of tube sizes and a difficult intubation trolley available.
- Foramen magnum stenosis is common. Avoid hyperextension during intubation.
- Central and peripheral venous access is often difficult. Consider femoral vein cannulation.
- Use an appropriately sized blood pressure cuff.
- Obstructive sleep apnoea is common.
- Restrictive ventilatory defects may occur and can lead to pulmonary hypertension.
- Regional techniques may be difficult.
- The back may be normal. The epidural space is often narrowed.
- The volume of local anaesthetic needed for an epidural is reduced. It is difficult to predict the volume needed for a single injection spinal. Use an incremental spinal or epidural catheter technique.
- The patient is of normal intelligence. Take care to treat on age rather than size.

Further reading

Bandi V, Munnur U, Braman S (2002). Airway problems in patients with rheumatological disorders. *Critical Care Clinics*, **18**, 749–765.

Berkowitz ID, Raja SN, Bender KS, Kopits SE (1990). Dwarfs: pathophysiology and anesthetic implications. *Anesthesiology*, **73**, 739–759.

Dedhia H, DiBartolomeo A (2002). Rheumatoid arthritis. *Critical Care Clinics*, **18**, 841–854.

Park-Kyung W (2004). Antiphospholipid syndrome. *International Anesthesiology Clinics*, **42**, 45–57.

Schelew BL, Vaghadia H (1996) Ankylosing spondylitis and neuraxial anaesthesia—a ten year review. *Canadian Journal of Anaesthesia*, **43**, 65–68.

Haematological disorders

Jonathan Purday

Anaemia

Anaemia—haemoglobin (Hb) below normal for age/sex. Conventionally Hb <13g/dl in an adult male or <12g/dl in an adult female. Common causes of anaemia in the surgical patient are:

- Blood loss: acute or chronic.
- Bone marrow failure: infiltration by tumour or suppression by drugs.
- Megaloblastic anaemias: folate or vitamin B_{12} deficiency.
- Complex anaemias: effects on production and breakdown, e.g. renal failure, rheumatoid arthritis, and hypothyroidism.
- Haemolytic anaemias: either inherited (thalassaemia, sickle cell disease, spherocytosis), acquired (autoimmune, drugs, infections), or physical (mechanical heart valves, DIC, and jogging).

Clinical

- Associated with fatigue, dyspnoea, palpitations, headaches, and angina. Severity often reflects the speed of onset more than the degree of anaemia as there is less time for adaptation.
- Symptoms of the commonest causes should be elicited, including relevant family history; always enquire about aspirin, NSAIDs, and alcohol.
- Respiratory and cardiovascular history may be worsened by the anaemia or make its impact greater.

Investigations

- Measure Hb prior to surgery in appropriate patients (p4) including all those at risk of anaemia undergoing major surgery and anyone with other significant medical problems, especially heart or lung disease.
- Much can be deduced from the Hb and mean corpuscular volume (MCV) alone, but in many instances a blood film gives additional useful information.
- Confirmatory tests such as ferritin, B_{12}/folate levels, reticulocyte count, direct Coombs test, erythrocyte sedimentation rate, liver/renal function, and bone marrow should be requested as appropriate.

Preoperative preparation

- Ideally, patients scheduled for elective surgery should have FBC checked in the weeks approaching the operation so that abnormalities can then be investigated and corrected in time.
- When delay to surgery is possible it is more appropriate and safer to treat the underlying cause and raise the Hb slowly with simple, effective measures, e.g. oral iron, B_{12} injections, etc. Transfusing a patient with pernicious anaemia may precipitate heart failure.

Perioperative blood transfusion (see also p1002)

Recently a more conservative approach has been adopted to blood transfusion. Unfortunately, there are no evidence-based guidelines that set clear target levels. In addition as Hb decreases, cardiac output increases (decrease in blood viscosity) and oxygen delivery may be maintained.

- Hb of 10g/dl (haematocrit of 30%) has traditionally been accepted as the lowest acceptable level, but there is increasing evidence that in fit patients lowering the transfusion trigger to 8g/dl may decrease morbidity.
- Red cell transfusion is indicated if the haemoglobin level is <7g/dl.
- Checking a HemoCue® reading gives comparable results to a Coulter® counter and can help to avoid a transfusion if >8g/dl.
- Each case must be assessed with a view to coexistent disease, expected intra-operative blood loss, and whether acute or chronic.
- For patients with ischaemic heart disease
  - Mild (angina rarely): accept Hb 7–8g/dl.
  - Moderate (angina regularly, but stable): accept Hb 8–9g/dl.
  - Severe (recent MI, unstable angina): accept Hb 10g/dl.
- For patients who may tolerate anaemia poorly, e.g. patients >65yr or those with significant respiratory disease, consider raising transfusion threshold to 9–10g/dl.

Sickle cell disease

Sickle cell disease (SCD) is caused by inheriting sickling haemoglobi-nopathies, either in the homozygous state (HbSS—sickle cell anaemia), heterozygous (HbSA—sickle cell trait) or in combination with another haemoglobin β chain abnormality such as haemoglobin C (HbSC disease), haemoglobin D (HbSD disease) or β-thalassaemia (HbS/β-thal). It is estimated that there are now over 10 000 patients with SCD in Britain. SCD is endemic in parts of Africa, the Mediterranean, the Middle East, and India. The highest incidence is from equatorial Africa; therefore all black patients should have a sickle test preoperatively. The pathology of SCD is primarily a result of vaso-occlusion by sickled red cells leading to haemolysis and tissue infarction. This can be precipitated by hypoxia, hypothermia, pyrexia, acidosis, dehydration, or usually infection. HbC and HbD in association with HbS enhance the sickling process whereas HbF impedes it.

- Susceptibility to sickling is proportional to the concentration of HbS. In the heterozygous state (sickle cell trait) sickling is uncommon—HbS concentration is <50%.
- These patients have a positive sickle test, but normal blood film and Hb level. This can be confirmed by Hb electrophoresis but in an emergency a normal blood film should suffice.
- These patients do not need special treatment, other than avoidance of hypoxia, dehydration, infection, acidosis, hypothermia.

Clinical features

- The manifestations of SCD do not become apparent before 3–4 months of age, when the main switch from fetal to adult haemoglobin occurs.
- There is great variability, not only between patients, but also within individual patients at different periods of life. Many remain well most of the time.
- Vaso-occlusive crises are the most common cause of morbidity and mortality. The presentation may be dramatic with acute abdomen, 'acute chest syndrome' (acute pneumonia-like), stroke, priapism, and painful dactylitis. By the time patients reach adulthood most will have small, fibrotic spleens. A less acute complication is proliferative retinopathy due to retinal vessel occlusion and neovascularisation (more common in HbSC disease).
- Aplastic crises are characterised by temporary shutdown of the marrow manifested by a precipitous fall in Hb and an absence of reticulocytes. Infection with parvovirus B19 and/or folate deficiency are often responsible.
- Sequestration crises occur mainly in children. Sudden massive pooling of red cells in the spleen can cause hypotension and severe exacerbation of anaemia with fatal consequences unless transfusion is given in time.

- Haemolytic crises manifest by a fall in Hb and rise in reticulocytes/bilirubin, and usually accompany vaso-occlusive crises. Chronic haemolysis leads to gallstones in virtually all patients with SCD though many remain asymptomatic.

Laboratory features

- Hb is usually 6–9g/dl (often lower than suggested by clinical picture). Reticulocytes are almost always increased and the film shows sickled cells and target cells. Howell–Jolly bodies are present if the spleen is atrophic. Leucocytosis and thrombocytosis are common reactive features. In sickle cell trait the Hb and film are normal.
- Screening tests for sickling which rely on deoxygenation of HbS are positive in both HbSS and HbAS.
- Hb electrophoresis distinguishes SS, AS, and other haemoglobinopathies. Measurement of the HbS level is important in certain clinical situations (e.g. crises) where a level of <30% is aimed for. It is not necessary to wait for the results of electrophoresis before embarking on emergency surgery; clinical history, Hb level, a positive sickle test, and the blood picture usually allow distinction between SCD and sickle cell trait. A mixed-race patient usually has sickle cell trait.

Management

- As no effective routine treatment exists for SCD, care is directed towards prophylaxis, support, and treatment of complications. Folic acid supplements, pneumococcal/HIB vaccinations, and penicillin prophylaxis (to protect from the susceptibility to infection caused by decreased splenic function) are recommended from an early age, preferably within a comprehensive care programme.
- For crises—rest, rehydration with oral/IV fluids, antibiotics if infection is suspected, maintain PaO_2, keep warm, prompt and effective analgesia (traditionally diamorphine/morphine is used over pethidine; regional anaesthesia very effective).
- Blood transfusions may be life saving, but the indications are limited. Exchange transfusions have a role in some vaso-occlusive crises (acute chest syndrome, stroke). Always discuss with a haematologist. For patients with high perioperative risk, transfusing to achieve an HbS level of <30% may decrease complications but is controversial.

Preoperative preparation

Always seek expert advice from a haematologist well before surgery. A sample for group and antibody screening should be sent well in advance as previously transfused sickle cell patients often have red cell antibodies.

Perioperative and postoperative care

- Special attention must be given to hypoxia, dehydration, infection, acidosis, hypothermia, and pain. These considerations should be continued well into the postoperative period.
- Dehydration: oral fluids as late as possible and pre- and postoperative IV fluids.
- Hypoxia: pulse oximetry and prophylactic oxygen.
- Prophylactic antibiotic cover should always be considered because of increased susceptibility to infection.
- Positive pressure ventilation may be required to achieve normocarbia and avoid acidosis.
- Hypothermia should be avoided by warming the operating room, using a fluid warmer, and the use of a Bair Hugger®. Core temperature should be monitored.
- Regional anaesthesia is not contraindicated and tourniquets can be used if limbs are meticulously exsanguinated prior to inflation.

Haemoglobin SC disease

- Results from double heterozygosity for HbS and HbC.
- Affects 0.1% of American Blacks.
- Intermediate in severity between sickle cell disease and trait.
- Patients develop anaemia, splenomegaly, jaundice, aseptic necrosis of the femoral head, hepatic disease, retinal disease, and bone marrow and splenic infarcts.
- Myocardial necrosis has been described after general anaesthesia.
- Management principles are as for sickle cell disease.

Porphyria

The porphyrias are a group of diseases in which there is an enzyme defect in the synthesis of the haem moiety leading to an accumulation of precursors that are oxidised into porphyrins. There are hepatic and erythropoietic varieties. Only the three acute hepatic forms, inherited in an autosomal dominant manner (although with variable expression), affect the administration of anaesthesia:

- Acute intermittent porphyria (AIP). Common in Sweden—increased urinary porphobilinogen and D-aminolaevulinic acid.
- Variegate porphyria (VP). Common in Afrikaners—increased copro- and protoporphyrin in the stool. Dermal photosensitivity.
- Hereditary coproporphyria (HCP). Very rare, increased urinary porphyrins. Dermal photosensitivity.

Porphyric crises

- Attacks occur most frequently in women in the 3rd–4th decade.
- Acute porphyric crises may be precipitated by drugs, stress, infection, alcohol, menstruation, pregnancy, starvation, or dehydration.
- Symptoms include acute abdominal pain, vomiting, motor and sensory peripheral neuropathy, autonomic dysfunction, cranial nerve palsies, mental disturbances, coma, convulsions, and pyrexia.

General principles

- Patients may never have had an attack, therefore a positive family history must be taken seriously.
- Individuals may have normal biochemical tests between attacks.
- Patients may present with unrelated pathology, e.g. appendicitis.
- Symptoms may mimic surgical pathologies, e.g. acute abdominal pain, acute neurology.
- Any patient giving a strong family history of porphyria must be treated as potentially at risk. Latent carriers may exhibit no signs, be potentially negative to biochemical screening, but still be at risk from acute attacks.

Anaesthetic management

Many commonly used drugs are thought to have the potential to trigger porphyric crises. However, it is difficult to be definitive, as crises can also be triggered by infection or stress, which often occur simultaneously. Drugs which are considered to be definitely unsafe to use, probably safe, and controversial are documented in the table.

Up-to-date information is available from the British National Formulary,[1] the Committee on the Review of Porphyrinogenicity (CORP),[2] the Welsh Medicines Information Centre,[3] or online resources: http://www.leeds.ac.uk/ifcc/SD/porph or http://www.porphyria-europe.com.

Suggested anaesthetic techniques

- Premedication—important to minimise stress: use temazepam/midazolam.
- Minimise preoperative fasting. Use dextrose/saline IV (avoid dextrose alone due to frequency of hyponatraemia).
- Regional anaesthesia—bupivacaine is considered safe for epidural anaesthesia but in the context of any peripheral neuropathy, detailed preoperative examination and documentation is essential. In acute porphyric crises, regional anaesthesia should be avoided as neuropathy may be rapid in onset and progressive.
- General anaesthesia—propofol is the induction agent of choice. Maintenance with nitrous oxide and/or propofol infusion. There are numerous case reports of safe use of halothane and isoflurane.
- Neuromuscular blockade—suxamethonium and vecuronium are considered safe (atracurium controversial). Fentanyl, morphine, and pethidine all considered safe.
- Monitoring—invasive blood pressure during acute crisis as hypovolaemia is common and autonomic neuropathy may cause labile blood pressure. Perform central venous pressure monitoring if clinically indicated.

Problems during anaesthesia

- Hypertension and tachycardia—treat with β-blockers such as atenolol.
- Convulsions—treat with diazepam, propofol, or magnesium sulphate (avoid barbiturates and phenytoin).

Postoperative management

- ICU/HDU if a crisis is suspected.
- Remember that the onset of a porphyric crisis may be delayed for up to 5d.

Treatment of acute porphyric crises

- Withdraw drugs which may have precipitated the crisis.
- Reverse factors which increase ALA synthetase (the initial enzyme responsible for haem production). Give haem arginate 3mg/kg IV once daily for 4d (leads to negative feedback to ALA synthetase). Treat infection, dehydration, electrolyte imbalance, give glucose (20g/hr).
- Treat symptoms with 'safe' drugs.
- Monitor the patient appropriately.

1 http:// www.BNF.org.
2 CORP Secretariat, Lennox Eales Porphyria Laboratories, MRC/UCT Liver Research Centre, University of Cape Town Medical School, Observatory 7925, South Africa. Fax: 010-27-21-448-6815.
3 Welsh Medicines Information Centre, University Hospital of Wales, Cardiff CF14 4XW, UK Telephone +44 029 20742979.

	Definitely unsafe	**Probably safe**	**Controversial**
Induction agents	Barbiturates, etomidate	Propofol	Ketamine
Inhalational agents	Enflurane	Nitrous oxide, ether, cyclopropane	Halothane, isoflurane, sevoflurane,
Neuromuscular blocking agents	Alcuronium	Suxamethonium, tubocurarine, gallamine, vecuronium	Pancuronium, atracurium, rocuronium, mivacurium
Neuromuscular reversal agents		Atropine, glycopyrronium, neostigmine	
Analgesics	Pentazocine	Alfentanil, aspirin, buprenorphine, codeine, fentanyl, paracetamol, pethidine, morphine, naloxone	Diclofenac, ketorolac, sufentanil
Local anaesthetics	Mepivicaine, ropivacaine	Bupivacaine, prilocaine, procainamide, procaine	Cocaine, lidocaine
Sedatives	Chlordiazepoxide, nitrazepam	Lorazepam, midazolam, temazepam, chlorpromazine, chloral hydrate	Diazepam
Antiemetics and H₂ antagonists	Cimetidine, metoclopramide	Droperidol, phenothiazines	Ondansetron, ranitidine
CVS drugs	Hydralazine, nifedipine, phenoxybenzamine	Adrenaline, α-agonists, β-agonists, β-blockers, magnesium, phentolamine, procainamide	Diltiazem, dizopyramide, sodium nitroprusside, verapamil
Others	Aminophylline, oral contraceptive pill, phenytoin, sulphonamides		Steroids

Rare blood disorders

Hereditary spherocytosis

- An autosomal dominant condition in which erythrocytes have a smaller surface to volume ratio and are abnormally permeable to sodium.
- The inflexible red cells are phagocytosed in the spleen, resulting in a microspherocytic anaemia with marked reticulocytosis. The cells' increased osmotic fragility is diagnostic.
- Splenomegaly is common. Splenectomy leads to a 50–70% increase in red cell survival.
- Splenectomy should not be performed in children <10yr of age, and should be followed by pneumococcal, meningococcal, and HIB vaccine and lifelong oral penicillin, to help avoid infection.
- There are no particular anaesthetic considerations.

Glucose-6-phosphate dehydrogenase (G6PD) deficiency

- X-linked trait with variable penetrance in American blacks and people from the Mediterranean.
- The disease may afford some protection against malaria and is prevalent in endemic areas.
- The G6PD enzyme is responsible for the production of NADPH, which is involved in the cell's defence against oxidative stresses such as infections (usually viral, but also septicaemia, malaria, and pneumonia) or oxidative drugs (aspirin, quinolones, chloramphenicol, isoniazid, probenacid, primaquine, quinine, sulphonamides, naphthalene, and vitamin K).
- Additionally, drugs producing methaemoglobinaemia, such as nitro-prusside and prilocaine, are contraindicated as patients are unable to reduce methaemoglobin, thereby diminishing oxygen-carrying capacity.
- Classically, ingestion of broad (fava) beans results in haemolysis (favism).
- Usually the haemolysis of red cells occurs 2–5d after exposure, causing anaemia, haemoglobinaemia, abdominal pain, haemoglobinuria, and jaundice.
- Diagnosis is made by demonstration of Heinz bodies and red cell G6PD assay.
- Treatment includes discontinuation of the offending agent and transfusion may be required.

Thalassaemias

Thalassaemias are due to absent or deficient synthesis of α- or β-globin chains of haemoglobin. The severity of these disorders is related to the degree of impaired globin synthesis.

- The hallmark of the disease is anaemia of variable degree.
- Diagnosis is confirmed by haemoglobin electrophoresis and/or globin chain analysis.

- The disease is prevalent in peoples of Mediterranean (mainly β), African (α and β) and Asian (mainly α) extraction.
- Patients with α-thalassaemia have mild or moderate anaemia.
- Those with severe β-thalassaemia, also called thalassaemia major, are transfusion dependent.
- Since there is no iron excreting mechanism, iron from transfused blood builds up in the reticuloendothelial system, until it is saturated, when iron is deposited in parenchymal tissues, principally the liver, pancreas, and heart.
- Preoperative preparation should include assessment of the degree of major organ impairment (heart, liver, pancreas) secondary to iron overload.
- High-output congestive cardiac failure with intravascular volume overload is common in severe anaemia and should be treated preoperatively by transfusion.
- Previous transfusion exposure may cause antibody production and therefore crossmatching may be prolonged.
- The exceedingly hyperplastic bone marrow of the major thalassaemias may cause overgrowth and deformity of the facial bones leading to airway problems and making intubation difficult.

Coagulation disorders

For regional anaesthesia and coagulation abnormalities see pp1058–1059.

The classical separation of coagulation into extrinsic and intrinsic pathways is overly complicated and is now not thought to occur *in vivo*. Instead there is a common pathway of initiation (see figure 10.1). Tissue factor from damaged vascular beds combines with factor VIIa and activates factors IX and X which leads to the generation of small amounts of thrombin (IIa), followed by amplification. This then activates further factors (V and VIII), leading to massive production of thrombin and generation of fibrin from fibrinogen.

- Congenital disorders of clotting may not present until challenged by trauma or surgery in adult life.
- Acquired disorders are due to lack of synthesis of coagulation factors, increased loss due to consumption (e.g. disseminated intravascular coagulation), massive blood loss, or the production of substances that interfere with their function.
- A family history may be elicited (haemophilia A and B—sex-linked recessives; von Willebrand's disease—autosomal dominant with variable penetrance) but cannot be relied upon (absent in 30% of haemophiliacs).
- Response to previous haemostatic challenges (tonsillectomy, dental extractions) may indicate the severity of the coagulopathy, e.g. in severe haemophilia A (factor VIII <2%) bleeding occurs spontaneously; in mild haemophilia A (factor VIII 5–30%) bleeding occurs only after trauma.
- Concurrent and past medical problems such as liver disease, malabsorption (vitamin K deficiency), infection, malignancy (DIC), autoimmune disease (systemic lupus erythematosus, rheumatoid arthritis) as well as medications (anticoagulants, aspirin, and NSAIDs) may be relevant.
- Abnormalities due to liver disease or vitamin K deficiency—give daily vitamin K (phytomenadione) 10mg slowly IV. FFP (15ml/kg) may be needed in addition if the presenting symptom is bleeding.

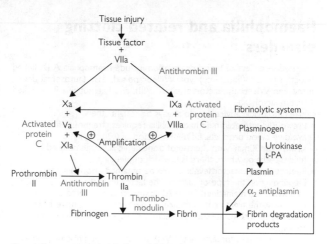

Coagulation cascade (colour indicates inhibitor)

Haemophilia and related clotting disorders

Inherited disorders of blood coagulation include haemophilia A (X-linked defect in factor VIII activity), von Willebrand's disease (autosomal defect in the von Willebrand factor of factor VIII), and haemophilia B (X-linked defect in factor IX).

- Haematological advice should always be sought.
- Previously untreated mild haemophilia requires strenuous efforts at avoiding blood products. DDAVP infusion of 0.3μg/kg in 30ml 0.9% saline over 30min, with the use of tranexamic acid, can be used for mild disease or where there is low risk of bleeding.
- In elective cases factor levels should be obtained prior to surgery. Depending on the type of surgery, the factor level should be 50–100% of normal and maintained for 2–7d postprocedure. If factors are necessary, the treatment of choice is now recombinant material in accordance with established guidelines. Always involve a haemophilia specialist.
- Cryoprecipitate (contains factor VIII) and fresh frozen plasma (contains factor IX) should be used to correct these clotting factors only in an emergency, when concentrate is unavailable, due to their chance of causing factor inhibitor formation and transmission of infection.
- NSAIDs, other anticoagulants, antiplatelet drugs and IM injections should be avoided.
- von Willebrand's disease is divided into three subtypes. After subtyping (type 2B is non-responsive) a therapeutic trial of DDAVP (dose as in haemophilia) with before and after levels of von Willebrand factor is performed. Responders should have DDAVP for bleeding or prophylactively prior to surgery. Non-responders can have factor VIII concentrates with preserved von Willebrand factor or cryoprecipitate.

Disorder	Platelet count	INR	APTT	TT	Fibrinogen	Other
Haemophilia A	Normal	Normal	↑	Normal	Normal	↓VIII
Haemophilia B	Normal	Normal	↑	Normal	Normal	↓IX
von Willebrand's disease	Normal (usually)	Normal	↑	Normal	Normal	↓ VIII, vWF, ↑ bleeding time
Liver disease	Normal or ↓	↑	↑	Normal	Normal or ↓	↓ V
Vitamin K deficiency	Normal	↑	↑	Normal	Normal	↓ II,VII,IX,X
DIC	Normal or ↓	↑	↑	↑	Normal or ↓	↑ FDPs, d-dimers, ↓II,V,VIII
Massive transfusion	↓	↑	↑	Normal or ↑	Normal or ↓	Normal FDPs
Heparin (un-fractionated)	Normal (rarely ↓)	Normal or ↑	↑	↑	Normal	↑ anti-Xa
Heparin (LMWH)	Normal (rarely ↓)	Normal	Normal	Normal	Normal	↑ anti-Xa
Warfarin	Normal	↑	↑	Normal	Normal	↓ II,VII,IX,X
Lupus anti-coagulant	Normal	Normal or ↑	↑	Normal	Normal	DRVVT +ve, cardiolipin antibody

vWF = von Willebrand's factor; FDPs = fibrin degradation products; DRVVT = dilute Russell's viper venom test.

Thrombocytopenia

Defined as a platelet count $<150 \times 10^9/l$.

Spontaneous bleeding is uncommon until the count falls below $10-20 \times 10^9/l$. Thrombocytopenia may be due to:

- Failure of platelet production, either selectively (hereditary, drugs, alcohol, viral infection) or as part of general marrow failure (aplasia, cytotoxics, radiotherapy, infiltration, fibrosis, myelodysplasia, megaloblastic anaemia)
- Increased platelet consumption, with an immune basis (ITP, drugs, viral infections, systemic lupus erythematosus, lymphoproliferative disorders) or without an immune basis (DIC, TTP, cardiopulmonary bypass)
- Dilution, following massive transfusion of stored blood
- Splenic pooling (hypersplenism)
- Platelet function impaired by renal failure and aspirin

Unexpected thrombocytopenia should always be confirmed with a second sample and a blood film.

Preoperative preparation

- Unexplained thrombocytopenia should be investigated before elective surgery, as the appropriate precautions will be determined by the underlying cause.
- Minor procedures such as bone marrow biopsy may be performed without platelet support provided adequate pressure is applied to the wound.
- For procedures such as insertion of central lines, transbronchial biopsy, liver biopsy, or laparotomy, the platelet count should be raised to at least $50 \times 10^9/l$.
- For lumbar puncture, epidural anaesthesia, and operations in critical sites such as the brain or eyes, the platelet count should be raised to $100 \times 10^9/l$ (see also p699 and pp1058–1059).
- In ITP, platelet transfusions should be reserved for major haemorrhage. Preparation for surgery entails the use of steroids or high-dose immunoglobulins initially.

Postoperative management

- If microvascular bleeding continues despite a platelet count of $>50 \times 10^9/l$ suspect DIC. If confirmed by coagulation tests give FFP and cryoprecipitate as appropriate.
- IM injections and analgesics containing aspirin or NSAIDs should be avoided.
- DDAVP 0.3µg/kg in 30ml saline over 30min may improve platelet function in renal failure, haemophilia, and von Willebrand's disease.

Anticoagulants

For anticoagulants and centroneuraxial/regional anaesthesia see p699 (obstetrics) and p1058.

The main indications for anticoagulation are to prevent stroke in atrial fibrillation and patients with mechanical heart valves, and for the treatment and prevention of venous thrombosis and pulmonary emboli.

Warfarin[1]

- Oral anticoagulant that results in the liver synthesising non-functional coagulation factors II, VII, IX, and X as well as proteins C and S, by interfering with vitamin K metabolism. Prolongs the prothrombin time and monitoring is achieved by comparing this with a control—i.e. the international normalised ratio (INR).
- Recommended targets:
  - INR 2–2.5 for prophylaxis of DVT
  - INR 2.5 for treatment of DVT/PE, prophylaxis in AF, cardioversion
  - INR 3.5 for recurrent DVT/PE, or mechanical heart valves
- Reversal of a high INR can be achieved in several ways depending on the circumstances. In the absence of bleeding, with an INR <5, reducing or omitting a dose is usually sufficient, if INR is 5–9 give vitamin K 1–2mg orally in addition. If there is minor bleeding or a grossly raised INR >9, give a small oral or IV dose of vitamin K (2–5mg). Life–threatening bleeding requires slow IV vitamin K (10mg) and either prothrombin complex concentrate or FFP. The last two cases must be discussed with a haematologist.
- Warfarin pharmacokinetics and dynamics can be affected by a multi-tude of other drugs (see BNF[2] for a fuller discussion). The important anaesthetic interactions include:
  - Potentiation (by inhibition of metabolism): alcohol, amiodarone, cimetidine, ciprofloxacin, cotrimoxazole, erythromycin, indometacin, metronidazole, omeprazole, paracetamol.
  - Inhibition (by induction of metabolism): barbiturates, carbamazepine.
  - In addition drugs that affect platelet function can increase the risk of warfarin-associated bleeding, e.g. aspirin and NSAIDs.

Warfarin and surgery/anaesthesia

- Warfarin should be stopped at least 4 days prior to elective surgery to allow the INR to decrease below 1.5—the level usually considered to be safe for surgery (may need to be <1.2 for high-risk surgery).
- The INR should be checked daily and when <2 alternative pre- and postoperative prophylaxis should be considered.
- In patients at high risk of thromboembolism a continuous IV infusion of unfractionated heparin should be started at 1000U/hr and adjusted to keep the APTR between 1.5 and 2.5. This should be stopped 6hr prior to surgery and restarted 12hr afterwards. This should be continued until warfarin therapy is restarted and the INR >2.0.

- For many patients in whom the risk of postoperative thromboembolism is not high enough to warrant IV heparin, the use of SC LMWH is recommended. Again this should be continued until warfarin is restarted and the INR >2.0.
- Alternative methods of embolism prophylaxis should be considered (see p10).
- If the risk of venous thromboembolism is very high (e.g. very recent thromboembolism) and effective anticoagulation cannot be undertaken, the insertion of a caval filter should be considered.
- In emergency surgery there is too little time to withdraw warfarin and specialist haematological advice should be sought. Fresh frozen plasma (10–15ml/kg) and vitamin K (1–2mg IV slowly) can be given, but this may lead to difficulty in regaining anticoagulant control postoperatively.
- Some minor surgery, including skin, dental, and ocular surgery, can be performed without stopping warfarin.
- After warfarin therapy is restarted it takes ~3d for the INR to reach 2.0.

Management of anticoagulation before and after surgery[3]

Indication	Preoperative	Postoperative
Acute venous thromboembolism		
Month 1	IV heparin	IV heparin
Months 2 and 3	Nothing extra	IV heparin
>Month 3	Nothing extra	SC heparin
Recurrent venous thromboembolism	Nothing extra	Nothing extra
Acute arterial thromboembolism		
Month 1	IV heparin	IV heparin[*]
>1 Month	Nothing extra	SC heparin[*]
Mechanical heart valves	Nothing extra	SC heparin
Non-valvular atrial fibrillation	Nothing extra	SC heparin

[*]Only if the risks of bleeding are low.

1 Guidelines on oral anticoagulation: third edition. (1998). *British Journal of Haematology*, **101**, 374–387.
2 http://www.BNF.org.
3 Kearon C, Hirsch J (1997). Management of anticoagulation before and after elective surgery. *New England Journal of Medicine*, **336**, 1506–1511.

Heparin

- A parenterally active anticoagulant that acts by potentiating antithrombin; can be used for both prophylaxis and treatment of thromboembolism.
- Unfractionated heparin is given by IV bolus or infusion. It is monitored by prolongation of the APTT (maintain at 1.5–2.5 times normal laboratory value).
- A validated regime is to give a bolus of 80U/kg followed by an infusion of 18U/kg/hr and check first APTT after 6hr.
- It has a narrow therapeutic window with complex pharmacokinetics and great inter-patient variation in dose requirements.
- Half-life is 1–2hr so stopping it is usually enough to reverse excessive anticoagulation or bleeding. If bleeding is severe protamine can be used.
- Protamine sulphate counteracts heparin. If given within 15min of heparin, 1mg protamine IV neutralises 100U of heparin. After this less protamine is required as heparin is rapidly excreted. It should be given slowly to avoid hypotension to a maximum of 50mg—a higher dose is itself anticoagulant.
- Complications of heparin include heparin-induced thrombocytopenia (HIT), which can cause serious venous and arterial thrombosis. Patients on heparin for 5d or more should have their platelet counts checked. This is less of a problem with SC heparin.
- Low-molecular-weight heparin (LMWH) is replacing unfractionated heparin for both prophylaxis and treatment of thromboembolism and unstable coronary artery disease. Administered once daily by SC injection, it needs no monitoring. Many patients with deep vein thrombosis are now managed as outpatients.
- LMWH is renally excreted so should be used with caution in renal failure.
- The reversal of LMWH is more difficult, although protamine up to 50mg seems to be clinically effective.

Hirudins (lepirudin)

- Lepirudin, a recombinant hirudin, can be for anticoagulation in patients who have Type II (immune) heparin-induced thrombocytopenia (HIT).
- Dose is monitored according to APTT and reduced in renal failure.

Epoprostenol

- Prostaglandin, which inhibits platelet aggregation and is used in renal haemodialysis or haemofiltration and primary pulmonary hypertension
- Given by continuous IV infusion as half-life is ~3min.

New anticoagulants

Direct thrombin inhibitors may soon take over from warfarin, without the need for routine anticoagulant monitoring. Many of these powerful new drugs do not have specific reversal agents (therefore blood products are necessary).

Fondaparinux

- Fondaparinux sodium is a synthetic pentasaccharide that inhibits activated factor X.
- Recently licensed for prophylaxis of venous thromboembolism in major orthopaedic surgery of the lower limbs.
- A recent study has suggested it may be more effective than LMWH.
- The initial dose should not be given until 6hr after surgical closure.

Activated protein C (drotrecogin alfa)

- Recombinant human activated protein C has recently been licensed for the treatment of septic shock with organ failure.
- It must be started within 24–48hr of the onset of sepsis—evidence suggests the earlier the better. It is given as a continuous infusion for 96hr.
- As a natural anticoagulant it inhibits the coagulation pathway at several points.
- It should be stopped at least 2hr prior to invasive procedures or surgery and cannot be started for at least 12hr after surgery.
- Contraindications include any major bleeding risk, other anticoagulants, platelet count <30 × 10^9/l, severe hepatic disease, intracranial pathology, and epidural catheters.
- If serious bleeding occurs, discontinue therapy. There is no specific antidote and supportive therapy with blood and blood products may be required.

Antiplatelet drugs

These decrease platelet aggregation and may inhibit thrombus formation in the arterial circulation, where anticoagulants have little effect.

Aspirin

- Binds irreversibly to platelets and prevents the production of thromboxane. New platelets have to be formed to reverse its effects.
- Should be given immediately in acute myocardial infarction.
- Low-dose aspirin is a mainstay for secondary prevention of thrombotic vascular events in vascular and cardiac disease.
- May also be used in angina, post coronary bypass surgery, intermittent claudication, atrial fibrillation, and primary prevention of ischaemic cardiac disease.
- If aspirin is to be stopped it takes 7–9d for platelet function to return to normal.
- There are few published trials looking at perioperative bleeding.
- In coronary artery bypass grafting aspirin increases perioperative bleeding but increases graft patency.
- In transurethral prostatectomy aspirin considerably increases perioperative bleeding.
- Minor surgery to skin or cataract surgery does not require aspirin to be stopped.
- On balance aspirin should be stopped for at least 7d prior to surgery when the risks of perioperative bleeding are high (major surgery) or where the risks of even minor bleeding are significant (retinal and intracranial surgery). This risk of bleeding must be balanced against the possibility of precipitating a thromboembolic event, particularly in patients with unstable angina.

Dipyridamole

- Used with low-dose aspirin for post coronary artery surgery and valve replacement.
- Also used for secondary prevention of stroke and transient ischaemic attacks.
- Dipyridamole needs to be stopped at least 7d prior to surgery, but probably has less effect than aspirin.

Clopidogrel

- Binds irreversibly with the ADP receptor on platelets.
- Used with aspirin in acute coronary syndrome and for prevention of ischaemic events in symptomatic patients. Also commonly used after stents to maintain patency.
- Can be used in peripheral arterial disease or post ischaemic stroke.
- Needs to be stopped 7d prior to surgery to avoid antiplatelet effect.

- If rapid reversal is necessary for bleeding or emergency surgery, platelet transfusions have been used with some success. However, as it is a prodrug and undergoes biotransfomation these may be ineffective if given just after a dose—therefore try to delay surgery by 24hr. If impossible, case reports have suggested that aprotinin may be useful.

Glycoprotein IIb/IIIa inhibitors

- Prevent platelet aggregation by blocking the binding of fibrinogen to receptors on platelets.
- Abciximab (ReoPro®) is licensed as an adjunct to aspirin and heparin in percutaneous transluminal coronary intervention.
- Eptifibatide (Integrilin®) and Tirofiban (Aggrastat®) are used to prevent early myocardial infarction in unstable angina or non-ST-segment-elevation myocardial infarction.
- These drugs are potent inhibitors of platelet function. Abciximab binds strongly to platelets and has a half-life of several days. Platelet transfusions will be needed to control profound bleeding.
- Eptifibatide and tirofiban are significantly renally eliminated. Therefore if renal function is normal, full reversal will occur within 4–8hr from discontinuation of therapy. For more rapid reversal platelet transfusions are less helpful as free drug is circulating (and the addition of FFP may be beneficial).
- For elective surgery, as the half-life of abciximab is several days it should be discontinued a week prior to surgery. Eptifibatide and tirofiban need only 8hr if renal function is normal.

Fibrinolytics

- Act as thrombolytics by activating plasminogen to plasmin; this degrades fibrin and therefore dissolves thrombi.
- Alteplase (rt-PA, tissue-type plasminogen activator) and streptokinase by continuous infusion.
- Reteplase and tenecteplase by bolus injection (making them ideal for early community injection).
- Used for acute myocardial infarction where benefits outweigh risks.
- Benefit greatest with early injection, ECG changes with ST elevation or new bundle branch block, and anterior infarction.
- Should be used in combination with antithrombin (LMWH) and antiplatelet (aspirin) therapy to reduce early re-infarction.
- Alteplase and streptokinase are also used for life-threatening venous thrombosis and pulmonary embolism.
- Contraindications include any risk of bleeding, especially trauma (including prolonged CPR), recent surgery, GI tract, and intracerebral pathology.
- Streptokinase can cause allergic reactions and should be used only once due to the production of antibodies.
- Serious bleeding calls for the discontinuation of therapy and may require coagulation factors. Cryoprecipitate (high levels of factor VIII and fibrinogen) and FFP (factors V and VIII) as well as platelets may all be required. Antifibrinolytics such as aminocaproic acid, tranexamic acid, and aprotinin may also be useful.
- Bleeding times are prolonged for up to 24hr after these drugs. In emergency surgery reversal will be required.

Antifibrinolytics/haemostatic drug therapy

Tranexamic acid (and aminocaproic acid)

- Both these drugs are synthetic derivatives of the amino acid lysine and reversibly bind to plasminogen, thereby blocking its binding to fibrin.
- Tranexamic acid is 10 times more potent than aminocaproic acid.
- Useful in postoperative bleeding predominantly in prostatectomy and dental extractions (particularly in haemophiliacs).
- Also useful in reversal of thrombolytics.
- Contraindicated in DIC.
- Usual dose of tranexamic acid is 1g tds orally.

Aprotinin

- A proteolytic enzyme inhibitor acting on plasmin, kallikrein, thrombin, and activated protein C.
- Indicated for patients at high risk of major blood loss during open heart surgery.
- Also used for treating life-threatening haemorrhage secondary to hyperplasminaemia (prolonged removal of malignant tumours, promyelocytic leukaemia, thrombolysis) and liver transplantation (unlicensed).
- Usual dose is 50 000U (5ml) over 5min followed by 500 000U (50ml) per hour—but see BNF for different indications.

Desmopressin

- An analogue of arginine vasopressin which induces release of von Willebrand's factor (vWF) from vascular endothelium to increase both vWF and factor VIII.
- Can be used (0.3µg/kg given in 30ml saline over 30min) for haemophilia A and von Willebrand's disease to double or quadruple levels of vWF or factor VIII.
- Platelet function may also be improved in patients in renal failure and aspirin-induced platelet dysfunction.

Factor VIIa

- Recombinant factor VIIa (rFVIIa) acts at the tissue factor–factor VIIa complex at the sight of endothelial damage.
- This effect appears localised to the area where the vessel is damaged, leading to few systemic side effects.
- Numerous case reports have shown rVIIa to have potent haemostatic effects even when other treatments have failed and whatever the cause of bleeding.
- Dosing and mode of delivery (IV bolus or continuous infusion) have still not been established (20–40µg/kg has been used).

Perioperative management of the bleeding patient

- Establish whether the cause of bleeding is surgical or a coagulopathy.
- A coagulopathy is more likely if bleeding is simultaneous from several sites or is slow in onset.
- A single site or sudden massive bleeding suggests a surgical source.
- Coagulation tests may help but often take some time to be obtained.
- Remember blood products also take time to arrive.
- Treatment should be aimed primarily at removal or control of the underlying cause while support is given to maintain tissue perfusion and oxygenation.
- Abnormal coagulation parameters in the presence of bleeding or the need for an invasive procedure are indications for haemostatic support. Transfusion of platelets and FFP (15ml/kg initially or 4U in an average adult) should help restore platelets, coagulation factors, and the natural anticoagulants antithrombin-III and protein C. Cryoprecipitate (10U initially) may also be necessary if the fibrinogen level cannot be raised above 1g/l by FFP alone.
- Indications for heparin, concentrates of antithrombin, and protein C are not established. Antifibrinolytics such as tranexamic acid are generally contraindicated in DIC.
- Massive transfusion of stored blood perioperatively may cause significant coagulation disorders due to the lack of factors V, VIII, and XI. DIC and thrombocytopenia may also be present. Therapy consists of replacement FFP and platelets as guided by coagulation tests.
- Several case reports have shown good results from giving factor VIIa in cases of uncontrollable haemorrhage.

Disseminated intravascular coagulation

- Acute DIC is probably the commonest cause of a significant coagulation abnormality in the surgical setting, especially in the peri- and postoperative phase.
- It is associated with infections (especially Gram-negative bacteraemia), placental abruption, amniotic fluid embolism, major trauma, burns, hypoxia, hypovolaemia, and severe liver disease.
- Haemorrhage, thrombosis, or both may occur.
- Chronic DIC is associated with aneurysms, haemangiomas, and carcinomatosis.
- Laboratory abnormalities are variable, depending on the severity of DIC, and reflect both consumption of platelets and coagulation factors as well as hyperplasminaemia and fibrinolysis.
- Discuss treatment options with a haematologist.

Hypercoagulability syndromes

Polycythaemia

A pattern of red blood cell changes that usually results in a haemoglobin >17.5g/dl in males and >15.5g/dl in females. This is accompanied by a corresponding increase in the red cell count to 6.0 and 5.5 × 10^{12}/l and a haematocrit of 55% and 47%, respectively.

Causes

- Primary: polycythaemia vera
- Secondary: due to compensatory erythropoietin increase (high altitude, cardiorespiratory diseases—especially cyanotic, heavy smoking, methaemoglobinaemia) or inappropriate erythropoietin increase (renal diseases—hydronephrosis, cysts, carcinoma, massive uterine fibromyomata, hepatocellular carcinoma, cerebellar haemangioblastoma)
- Relative: 'stress' or 'spurious' polycythaemia. Dehydration or vomiting
- Plasma loss: burns, enteropathy

Polycythaemia vera

- Presenting features include headaches, dyspnoea, chest pain, vertigo, pruritus, epigastric pain, hypertension, gout, and thrombotic episodes (particularly retinal).
- Splenomegaly.
- Thrombocythaemia in 50% of cases.
- Differential diagnosis is with other causes of polycythaemia. These can be excluded by history, examination, and blood tests including bone marrow aspiration, arterial blood gases, and erythropoetin levels.
- Therapy is aimed at maintaining a normal blood count by venesection and myelosuppression with drugs.
- Thrombosis and haemorrhage are a frequent cause of death and 30% develop myelofibrosis and 15% acute leukaemia.

Essential thrombocythaemia

- Megakaryocyte proliferation and overproduction of platelets are the dominant features with a sustained platelet count >1000 × 10^9/l.
- Closely related to polycythaemia vera with recurrent haemorrhage and thrombosis.
- Recurrent haemorrhage and thrombosis are the principal clinical features.
- Abnormal large platelets or megakaryocyte fragments may be seen on a blood film.
- Differential diagnosis is from other causes of a raised platelet count: e.g. haemorrhage, chronic infection, malignancy, polycythaemia vera, myelosclerosis, or chronic granulocytic leukaemia.
- Platelet function tests are consistently abnormal.
- Radioactive phosphate or alkylating agents are used to keep platelet counts down.

Antiphospholipid syndrome

This is a rare, but increasingly recognised, syndrome resulting in arterial or venous thrombosis or recurrent miscarriage, with a positive laboratory test for antiphospholipid antibody and/or lupus anticoagulant (LA). It may present with another autoimmune disease such as SLE (secondary) or as a primary disease. The main feature of the disease is thrombosis, with a spectrum from subacute migraine and visual disturbances to accelerated cardiac failure and major stroke. Arterial thrombosis helps distinguish this from other hypercoagulable states. Paradoxically the LA leads to a prolongation of coagulation tests such as the APTT but detailed testing is needed before the diagnosis can be confirmed. Patients may present for surgery because of complications (miscarriage, thrombosis) or for incidental procedures. Initially patients are started on aspirin but after a confirmed episode of thrombosis, they usually remain on lifelong warfarin. High risk of thrombosis in these patients means that if warfarin needs to be stopped for surgery, IV heparin should be commenced both pre- and postoperatively.

Anaesthesia and surgery in the hypercoagulable patient

- There are no published guidelines, but it seems prudent that elective patients who are polycythaemic should be venesected to a normal blood count to decrease the risk of perioperative thrombosis.
- Antithrombotic stockings and intermittent compression devices should be used with SC heparin.
- Haematological advice may be required.

Further reading

Association of Anaesthetists of Great Britain and Ireland. *Blood Component Therapy 2005*.

Bombeli T, Spahn DR (2004). Updates in perioperative coagulation: physiology and management of thromboembolism and haemorrhage. *British Journal of Anaesthesia*, **93**, 275–287.

Firth PG, Head CA (2004). Sickle cell disease and anesthesia. *Anesthesiology*, **101**, 766–785.

Guidelines for the clinical use of red cell transfusions (2001). *British Journal of Haematology*, **113**, 24–31.

Guidelines for the use of fresh frozen plasma, cryoprecipitate and cryosupernatant (2004). *British Journal of Haematology*, **126**, 11–28.

Guidelines for the use of platelet transfusions (2003). *British Journal of Haematology*, **122**, 10–23.

James MFM, Hift RJ (2000). Porphyrias. *British Journal of Anaesthesia*, **85**, 143–53.

Kearon C, Hirsch J (1997). Management of anticoagulation before and after elective surgery. *New England Journal of Medicine*, **336**, 1506–1511.

Mahdy AM, Webster NR (2004). Perioperative systemic haemostatic agents. *British Journal of Anaesthesia*, **93**, 842–858.

Spahn DR, Cassutt M (2000). Eliminating blood transfusions. *Anesthesiology*, **93**, 242–255.

Chapter 11

Neurological and muscular disorders

Andrew Teasdale

Jane Halsall

Epilepsy

Epilepsy is a disorder characterised by chaotic brain dysfunction leading to symptoms ranging from behavioural disorder through to life threatening convulsions. Most epileptic patients will be on seizure modifying drug therapy.

General considerations
- Maintain GI function to avoid metabolic disturbance and interference with drug therapy.
- Make provision for therapy if oral antiepileptic medication cannot be given.

Preoperative assessment
- Nature, timing, and frequency of seizures should be recorded.
- Full drug history, including timing of antiepileptic therapy should be noted.
- The effect of the condition on lifestyle and the eligibility to hold a driver's licence should be noted.

Investigations
- Electrolyte and glucose measurement. Disturbance will alter seizure potential.

Conduct of anaesthesia
- Avoid prolonged fasting.
- Sedative premedication, if necessary, may be achieved with benzodi-azepines. Long-acting drugs such as diazepam (10mg PO) or lorazepam (2–4mg PO) are useful.
- Maintain antiepileptic therapy up to the time of surgery.
- All currently used anaesthetic agents are anticonvulsant in conventional doses. Thiopental is powerfully anticonvulsant and may be a preferred induction agent in the poorly controlled epileptic.
- Muscle relaxation is best achieved by drugs without a steroid nucleus (e.g. atracurium, cisatracurium) since enzyme induction by all commonly used anticonvulsant drugs (especially phenytoin, carbamazepine, and the barbiturates) will lead to rapid metabolism (e.g. vecuronium, rocuronium).
- Avoid hyperventilation and consequent hypocarbia since this will lower seizure threshold.
- Regional anaesthesia may assist in preservation of or early return to oral intake. Be aware of maximum local anaesthetic doses.
- Use antiemetic agents unlikely to produce dystonias (e.g. cyclizine 50mg IV/IM, domperidone 30–60mg PR, ondansetron 4mg IV).
- Record any epileptiform activity in the perioperative period carefully. The misdiagnosis of postoperative shivering/dystonic movements on induction as epilepsy may have profound implications.
- Day case anaesthesia is suitable for those with well-controlled epilepsy (seizure free for 1yr or nocturnal seizures only). Patients should be warned of the potential for perioperative convulsions.

Drug issues

The following drugs should be used with caution in epileptics.

Drug	Notes
Methohexitone	Reported to produce seizures in children. Increased EEG evidence of spike activity during administration. No longer marketed in the UK
Ketamine	Avoided because of cerebral excitatory effects although it has been used without incident in many epileptics
Etomidate	Associated with a high incidence of myoclonus (not centrally mediated). May be confused with epileptic activity
Antiemetics: phenothiazines (e.g. prochlorperazine), central dopamine antagonists (e.g. metoclopramide), butyrophenones (e.g. droperidol)	High incidence of dystonic reactions may lead to confusion with epileptic activity
Inhalational agents: enflurane	Associated with abnormal EEG activity after administration—especially in presence of hyperventilation
Neuromuscular blockers: steroid based (e.g. vecuronium, rocuronium)	Pharmacodynamic resistance due to enzyme activation

Propofol

- Propofol is reported to be associated with abnormal movements during both induction and emergence from anaesthesia. This is unlikely to represent true seizure activity (EEG studies fail to demonstrate epileptiform activity during these episodes).
- Epileptic patients may be prone to seizures during the rapid emergence from propofol anaesthesia.
- Profound suppression of abnormal EEG activity is usually noted during propofol infusion.
- Propofol has also been reported to be effective in status epilepticus in ICU.

Caution is advised in the administration of propofol to epileptics (particularly those holding driving licences) unless there is overwhelming clinical need for its administration. Co-induction with benzodiazepine (e.g. midazolam 2–3mg IV) may reduce its potential to produce abnormal movements and reduce the potential for postoperative seizure.

Driving and epilepsy

At present, United Kingdom law mandates the withdrawal of a driving licence from an epileptic until 12 months from the last seizure. The implications of a single convulsion in the postoperative period on a previously well-controlled epileptic cannot be overstated. Up-to-date advice on fitness to drive is available from the DVLA (Driver and Vehicle Licensing Agency: http://www.dvla.gov.uk).

What if oral or nasogastric therapy is not possible?

The following drugs are available in parenteral or rectal formulations. In general, IM administration of antiepileptic medication should be avoided because of unpredictable absorption postoperatively and the irritant nature of the formulations.

Drug levels should be measured during parenteral therapy or after changing the route of administration.

Drug	Notes
Carbamazepine	125mg rectal, equivalent to 100mg oral. Maximum 1g daily in four divided doses
Phenobarbital	200mg IM repeated 6-hourly. Child 15mg/kg. IV administration associated with sedation. Slow infusion of dilute preparation recommended
Phenytoin	Loading dose 15mg/kg IV at rate of no greater than 50mg/min. Maintenance dose (same IV as oral) twice daily. Infusion usually under ECG and BP control
Fosphenytoin	A prodrug of phenytoin. Less irritation and cardiovascular instability on injection. Absorbed very slowly after IM injection although non-irritant. Dose—same dose (in phenytoin equivalents) and frequency as oral phenytoin
Sodium valproate	IV dose same as oral dose, twice daily. Dose to be injected over 3–5min
Clonazepam	IV infusion in high-dependency area only—facilities for airway control available. Child (any age) 500µg. Adult 1mg

Cerebrovascular disease

Stroke is the third leading cause of death in the industrialised world (after heart disease and cancer). Cerebrovascular disease is manifested by either global cerebral dysfunction (multi-infarct dementia) or focal ischaemic disorder ranging from transient ischaemic attack to major stroke.

Transient ischaemic attacks (TIA)

- These are defined as focal neurological deficits that occur suddenly and last for several minutes to hours but never more than 24hr. Residual neurological deficit does not occur.
- They are thought to be related to embolism of platelet and fibrin aggregates released from areas of atherosclerotic plaque. The risk of stroke in untreated patients is said to be ~5% per annum with a mortality of ~30% per episode.
- Patients with a history of TIA should be investigated and assessed by a specialist vascular service if practical. Doppler flow studies, with or without angiography, are indicated in all cases of recurrent TIA or those that have occurred despite aspirin therapy.
- Delay of all but urgent or emergency surgery is warranted until Doppler studies are performed. At present only those with history of TIA with good recovery and a surgically accessible lesion of either >80% stenosis or 'ragged' plaque are routinely referred for carotid surgery. Crescendo TIA is considered by some as an indication for urgent carotid surgery.

General considerations

Cerebrovascular disease is associated with hypertension, diabetes, obesity, and smoking. The incidence rises with age. Medical treatment revolves around the treatment of the underlying disorder, cessation of smoking, and antiplatelet/anticoagulant therapy.

Signs of concurrent cardiac and renal dysfunction should be sought.

When to operate

- Operation within 6wk of a cerebral event is associated with an up to 20-fold increase in the risk of postoperative stroke.
- Hemiplegia of <6–9 months' duration is associated with exaggerated hyperkalaemic response to suxamethonium.

It therefore seems prudent to delay all but life-saving surgery for at least 6wk following a cerebral event and preferably to wait 3–6 months before considering elective surgery.

Preoperative assessment

- Measure blood pressure (both arms) and test blood glucose. The therapeutic aims are for normotension and normoglycaemia.
- Take a full drug history—continue antihypertensive drugs until operation.
- Warfarin should be discontinued and substituted with heparin (unfractionated or LMWH as per local protocol) if necessary.

- Aspirin is discontinued only if the consequences of haemorrhage are great (e.g. tonsillectomy, neurosurgery, etc.).
- Document the nature of any ischaemic events and any residual neurological deficit. These may range from transient blindness (amaurosis fugax) to dense hemiplegia. This will help in differentiating new lesions arising in the perioperative period that may require urgent therapy.
- Ask about precipitating events. Vertebrobasilar insufficiency is most likely to be precipitated by postural changes and neck positioning.

Conduct of anaesthesia

- Ensure that antihypertensive medication (with the possible exception of ACE inhibitors) is continued to the time of operation. ACE inhibitors may predispose to profound, resistant hypotension under anaesthesia.
- Thromboprophylaxis is advisable unless contraindicated (e.g. low-dose LMWH).
- Ensure that pressor and depressor agents are available prior to induction. Use agents with which you are familiar. Maintain blood pressure as close as practical to preoperative levels to maintain cerebral blood flow. Useful pressors are ephedrine/metaraminol; useful depressors are labetalol/esmolol/GTN.
- Blood pressure may 'swing' excessively during surgery. This is due to a rigid vascular system and relative hypovolaemia due to antihypertensive therapy. IV fluid replacement should be proactive rather than reactive, with large-bore IV access and invasive central pressure monitoring if large fluid shifts are expected.
- Ensure that neck positioning is neutral and avoids movements associated with syncope.
- Induction of anaesthesia may result in dangerous hypotension followed by extreme hypertension on intubation. Gentle IV induction is indicated. Cover for intubation may be provided by opioid (e.g. alfentanil 500–1000µg IV) or β-blocker (e.g. labetalol 50mg slow IV).
- Avoid hyperventilation. Hypocapnia is associated with reduced cerebral blood flow and therefore cerebral ischaemia.
- Examine the patient early in the postoperative period to determine any change in neurological status. New neurological signs will require urgent referral to a neurologist/vascular surgeon and urgent treatment if possible.

Parkinson's disease

General considerations

- Parkinsonism is a syndrome characterised by tremor, bradykinesia, rigidity, and postural instability. The aetiology of Parkinson's disease is unknown, but parkinsonism may be precipitated by drugs (especially neuroleptic agents) or be post-traumatic/postencephalitic.
- Parkinsonism is due to an imbalance of the mutually antagonistic dopaminergic and cholinergic systems of the basal ganglia. Pigmented cells in the substantia nigra are lost, leading to reduced dopaminergic activity. There is no reduction in cholinergic activity.
- Drug therapy of parkinsonism is aimed at restoring this balance by either increasing dopamine or dopamine-like activity or reducing cholinergic activity within the brain.
- Drug therapy in parkinsonism is limited by severe side effects (nausea and confusion), especially in the elderly. Up to 20% of patients will remain unresponsive to drug therapy.

Drug therapies

Dopaminergic drugs

- L-dopa is an inactive form of dopamine, which is converted by decarboxylases to dopamine within the brain. It is more useful in patients with bradykinesia and rigidity than tremor and is usually administered with decarboxylase inhibitors (e.g. benserazide, carbidopa) that do not cross into the brain, reducing peripheral conversion into dopamine.
- Monoamine oxidase B inhibitors (MAO-B inhibitors, e.g. selegiline) act by reducing central breakdown of dopamine. Selegiline has fewer drug interactions than the non-specific MAO inhibitors, but may cause a hypertensive response to pethidine and dangerous CNS excitability with SSRI and tricyclic antidepressants (see p274).
- Ergot derivatives such as bromocriptine, cabergoline, lisuride, and pergolide act by direct stimulation of dopamine receptors. They are usually reserved for adjuvant therapy in those already on L-dopa or those intolerant of the side effects of L-dopa.
- Entacapone is an adjuvant agent capable of reducing the dose of L-dopa and increasing the duration of its effect. It is usually reserved for those experiencing 'end of dose' deterioration after long-term dopaminergic therapy.
- Other adjuvant dopaminergic agents are ropinirole, pramipexole, amantadine, apomorphine, and tolcapone.
- There are no parenteral dopaminergic agents currently available for use in parkinsonism.

Anticholinergic (antimuscarinic) drugs

- The most commonly used agents in this group are benzatropine, procyclidine, benzhexol, and orphenadrine.
- These agents are indicated as first-line therapy only when symptoms are mild and tremor predominates. Rigidity and sialorrhoea may be improved by these agents but bradykinesia will not be affected. This class of drugs is useful for drug-induced parkinsonism but not in tardive dyskinesia.
- Parenteral formulations exist for procyclidine and benztropine, making these useful for acute drug-induced dystonias.

Surgical therapies

Surgery for treatment of Parkinson's-induced disability is increasing in popularity. It is normally performed in the awake patient using stereotactic guided probes.

- Thalamotomy is used in those with tremor as the predominant disability, especially if the tremor is unilateral. Anterior thalamotomy is sometimes used for rigidity.
- Pallidotomy is primarily for those with rigidity and bradykinesia, although the tremor (if present) may also be reduced.
- Deep brain stimulation using implantable devices is becoming more commonplace. There is no literature at present relating to incidental anaesthesia in patients with these devices, but it would seem prudent to contact the manufacturer or team responsible for insertion of the device before using diathermy. If diathermy is necessary, bipolar should be used, as far as practical from the device or lead. Device function should be checked after surgery.

Preoperative assessment

Ideally, patients with severe disease should be under the care of a physician with a special interest in Parkinson's disease, who should be involved in the perioperative care.

The following assessment is of particular interest:

- A history of dysphagia or excessive salivation (sialorrhoea) is evidence of increased risk of aspiration and possible failure to maintain an airway in the perioperative period. Gastro-oesophageal reflux is common in this group of patients.
- Postural hypotension may be evidence of both dysautonomia and drug-induced hypovolaemia and should warn of possible hypotension on induction or position changes during surgery.
- Drug-induced arrhythmias, especially ventricular premature beats, are common, although they are usually not clinically significant.
- Respiratory function may be compromised by bradykinesia and muscle rigidity as well as by sputum retention. Chest radiograph, lung function tests, and blood gases may be indicated.
- Difficulty in voiding may necessitate urinary catheterisation. Postoperative urinary retention may be a potent cause of postoperative confusion.
- The severity of the underlying disease should be determined and other likely problems anticipated, e.g. akinesia, muscle rigidity, tremor, confusion, depression, hallucinations, and speech impairment.

Drug interactions

Most patients with severe disease are on several maintenance drugs, many of which have potentially serious interactions.

Drug interactions in parkinsonism

Class of drug	Interaction	Notes
Pethidine	Hypertension and muscle rigidity with selegiline	May resemble malignant hyperpyrexia
Synthetic opioids, e.g. fentanyl, alfentanil	Muscle rigidity	More apparent in high doses
Inhalational agents	Potentiate L-dopa induced arrhythmias	Avoid use of halothane if ventricular arrhythmia present on preop ECG
Antiemetics, e.g. metoclopramide, droperidol, prochlorperazine	May produce extrapyramidal side effects or worsen Parkinson's symptoms	Metoclopramide may increase plasma concentration of L-dopa—use domperidone/ondansetron
Antipsychotics, e.g. phenothiazines, butyrophenones, piperazine, derivatives	May produce extrapyramidal side effects or worsen Parkinson's symptoms	Better to use atypical antipsychotics such as sulpiride, clozapine, risperidone, etc.
Antidepressants: tricyclics (e.g. amitriptyline), serotonin reuptake inhibitors (e.g. fluoxetine)	Potentiate L-dopa induced arrhythmias (tricyclics only) Hypertensive crises and cerebral excitation with selegiline (tricyclics and SSRIs)	
Antihypertensives (all classes)	Marked antihypertensive effect in treated and untreated parkinsonism. Related to postural hypotension and relative hypovolaemia	Most marked with clonidine and reserpine

Conduct of anaesthesia

- Treatment for parkinsonism should be continued up to the start of anaesthesia. Distressing symptoms may develop as little as 3hr after a missed dose.
- Premedication is usually unnecessary unless distressing sialorrhoea is present. Consider glycopyrronium (200–400µg IM) as an antisialogogue.
- The presence of preoperative sialorrhoea or dysphagia is a sign of gastrointestinal dysfunction. Airway control with intubation by rapid sequence induction may be indicated.
- Maintain normothermia to avoid shivering.
- There is no evidence that any anaesthetic technique is superior to any other.
- Analgesia: IV morphine is useful if regional or local analgesia is not possible (PCA may prove difficult for the patient). Oral analgesia may be difficult to administer with coexisting dysphagia (a nasogastric tube may be necessary).

Postoperative care

- In principle, the more disabled the patient preoperatively, the greater the need for postoperative high-dependency and respiratory care.
- Postoperative physiotherapy should be arranged if rigidity is disabling.
- Nasogastric tube insertion may be needed if GI dysfunction is present to allow early return of oral medication.
- Prolonged GI dysfunction postoperatively may lead to severe disability since no parenteral dopaminergic therapy is currently available.

Special considerations

Antiemetic therapy may prove problematic. The following are useful:
- Domperidone (10–20mg 4–6-hourly PO or 30–60mg 4–6-hourly PR). The drug of first choice for PONV in Parkinson's patients. It does not cross the blood–brain barrier to a significant degree and is thus not associated with significant extrapyramidal effects.
- Serotonin antagonists, e.g. ondansetron 4mg IV or granisetron 1mg IV slowly. May be useful rescue agents in PONV if domperidone alone is ineffective.
- Antihistamine derivatives (e.g. cyclizine 50mg IV/IM).

Further reading

Anesthesia and Parkinson's disease (1996). *International Anesthesiology Clinics*, **34**, 133–150.
Nicholson G, Pereira A, Hall G (2002). Review article: Parkinson's disease and anaesthesia. *British Journal of Anaesthesia*, **89**, 904–916.

Anaesthesia in spinal cord lesions

There are ~40 000 patients in the UK with spinal cord injuries. Most are young adults. Fertility in affected females approaches that of the non-injured population and obstetric services are regularly required.

Pathophysiology of spinal cord injury

Spinal injury can be divided into three distinct phases:

- The initial phase: very short (minutes) period of intense neuronal discharge caused by direct cord stimulation. This leads to extreme hypertension and arrhythmias, with risk of LVF, MI, and pulmonary oedema. Steroid usage in acute spinal cord injury remains controversial. If used, they must be given within 8hr of injury, in high dosage (e.g. 30mg/kg methylprednisone).
- Spinal shock follows rapidly and is characterised by hypotension and bradycardia due to loss of sympathetic tone. It is most common after high cord lesions (above T_7). There is associated loss of muscle tone and reflexes below the level of the lesion. Vagal parasympathetic tone continues unopposed, causing profound bradycardia or asystole—especially on tracheal suction/intubation. This phase may last from 3d to 8wk. Paralytic ileus is common.
- Reflex phase: as neuronal 'rewiring' occurs, efferent sympathetic discharge returns, along with muscle tone and reflexes.

Autonomic dysreflexia

Characterised by massive, disordered autonomic response to stimulation below the level of the lesion. It is rare in lesions lower than T_7. Incidence increases with higher lesions. It may occur within 3wk of the original injury but is unlikely to be a problem after 9 months. The dysreflexia and its effects are thought to arise because of a loss of descending inhibitory control on regenerating presynaptic fibres.

Hypertension is the most common feature but is not universal. Other features include headache, flushing, pallor (may be manifest above the level of lesion), nausea, anxiety, sweating, bradycardia, and penile erection. Less commonly pupillary changes or Horner's syndrome occur. Dysreflexia may be complicated by seizures, pulmonary oedema, coma, or death and should be treated as a medical emergency. The stimulus required to precipitate the condition varies but is most commonly:

- Urological: bladder distension, UTI, catheter insertion
- Obstetric: labour, cervical dilation, etc.
- Bowel obstruction/faecal impaction
- Acute abdomen
- Fractures
- Rarely, minor trauma to skin, cutaneous infection (bedsores).

Management of dysreflexia

- Discover the cause if possible and treat.
- If no apparent cause, examine carefully for unrevealed trauma or infection, catheterise, and check for faecal impaction.

- If simple measures fail consider:
  - Phentolamine 2–10mg IV repeated if necessary.
  - Transdermal GTN.
  - Clonidine (150–300µg) if there is hypertension and spasticity.
  - β-blockers are indicated only if there is associated tachycardia—esmolol 10mg IV repeated.

Systemic complications of spinal cord lesions

- Reduced blood volume—may be as little as 60ml/kg, a 20% reduction.
- Abnormal response to the Valsalva manoeuvre with continued drop in blood pressure (no plateau) and no overshoot with release.
- Profound postural hypotension with gradual improvement after initial injury (never to normal). Changes in cerebral autoregulation reduce its effect on CBF and consciousness in the non-anaesthetised patient.
- Lesions above C3—apnoea.
- Lesions at C3/4/5—possible diaphragmatic sparing, some respiratory capacity. Initial lesions may progress in height with shock and oedema, with recovery as the oedema improves, leading to a marked improvement in respiratory capacity.
- Below C5—phrenic sparing, intercostal paralysis. Recruitment of accessory muscles is necessary to improve respiratory capacity (this may take up to 6 months).
- Paralysis of abdominal muscles severely affects the ability to force expiration, reducing the ability to cough.
- The FVC is better in the horizontal or slight head-down position due to increased diaphragmatic excursion.
- Bronchial hypersecretion may occur.
- Poor thermoregulation due to isolation of central regulatory centres from information pathways, inability to use muscle to generate heat and altered peripheral blood flow.
- Muscle spasms and spasticity occur due to intact reflexes below the level of the lesion. They can be caused by minor stimuli. Baclofen and diazepam may be used, the former increasingly via epidural infusion.
- Reduced bone density leading to increased risk of fractures. There is heterotopic calcification around the joints in up to 20% of patients.
- Poor peripheral perfusion—pressure sores and difficult venous access.
- Anaemia, usually mild.
- Tendency to thrombosis and pulmonary embolism. Some centres warfarinise tetraplegics 5d after initial presentation.
- There is delayed gastric emptying in tetraplegics (up to 5 times longer).

Suxamethonium in chronic spinal cord lesions

- After upper motor neuron denervation, the motor endplate effectively extends to cover the entire muscle cell membrane. With administration of suxamethonium, depolarisation occurs over this extended endplate, leading to massive potassium efflux and potential cardiac arrest.
- Recommendations vary as to the period of potential risk. Practically—avoid suxamethonium from 72hr following the initial injury. There are no reports of clinically significant hyperkalaemia with suxamethonium after 9 months.

Conduct of anaesthesia

Spinal shock phase

Surgery usually confined to the management of life-threatening emergencies and coexisting injury. Anaesthesia should reflect this.

- Severe bradycardia or even asystole may complicate intubation—give atropine (300μg IV) or glycopyrronium (200μg IV) prior to intubation.
- Extreme care should be taken if cervical spine injury is suspected.
- Preload with fluid (500–1000ml crystalloid) to reduce hypotension.
- Central line insertion may be necessary to manage fluid balance and guide appropriate inotrope therapy.

Reflex phase

Previous anaesthetic history is vital—many procedures in these patients are multiple and repeated. Pay close attention to the following:

- Is there a sensory level and is it complete? (Risk of autonomic dysreflexia is greater in complete lesions.)
- If complete, is the proposed surgery below the sensory level? (Is anaesthesia necessary?)
- Has there been spinal instrumentation? (Potential problems with spinal/epidural.)
- Is the cervical spine stable/fused/instrumented? (Potential intubation difficulty.)
- Is postural hypotension present? (Likely to be worsened by anaesthesia.)
- Is there a history of autonomic dysreflexia (paroxysmal sweating and/or headache) and, if so, what precipitated it?
- In cervical lesions, what degree of respiratory support is necessary?
- Are there contractures, or pressure sores?

Investigations

- FBC—anaemia
- U&Es—renal impairment
- Liver functions—possible impairment with chronic sepsis
- Lung function tests (FVC)—mandatory with all cervical lesions due to potential respiratory failure.

Is anaesthesia necessary?

In principle, if the planned procedure would require anaesthesia in a normal patient, it will be required for a cord-injured patient.

- Minor peripheral surgery below a complete sensory level is likely to be safe without anaesthesia.
- Even with minor peripheral surgery, minimal stimulation may provoke muscular spasm that may require anaesthesia to resolve. Local anaesthetic infiltration may prevent its occurrence.
- Care should be taken with high lesions (T_5 and above) or patients with a history of autonomic dysreflexia undergoing urological procedures.
- If the decision is made to proceed without anaesthesia, IV access is mandatory and ECG, NIBP, and pulse oximeter should be applied.
- An anaesthetist should be present on 'standby' for such procedures.

General anaesthesia

- Monitoring should be applied prior to induction and blood pressure measured before and after every position change. Invasive monitoring should be performed with the same considerations as normal.
- Despite theoretical risk of gastro-oesophageal reflux there appears to be no increased risk of aspiration. If intubation is necessary for the desired procedure, anticholinergic pre-treatment is recommended.
- Those with cervical cord lesions are likely to require assistance with ventilation under general anaesthesia. If IPPV is performed in tetraplegics, blood pressure may drop precipitously. Fluid preloading and vasopressors (ephedrine) may be required.
- With the exception of paralysis to facilitate intubation, neuromuscular blockade is unlikely to be necessary unless troublesome muscular spasm is present.
- Care should be taken to preserve body temperature (wrapping or forced-air warming blankets). Position with respect to pressure areas.
- Fluid management may be difficult as blood volume is usually low, and with high cord lesions, reflex compensation for blood loss is absent. Fluid preloading coupled with aggressive replacement of blood losses with warmed fluid is recommended.

Centroneuraxial anaesthesia

Advantages
- Prevents autonomic dysreflexia.
- Unlikely to cause cardiovascular instability since sympathetic tone is already low prior to blockade.
- No reported adverse effect of spinal injection of local anaesthetics or opioids on neurological outcome.
- Avoids risks of general anaesthesia.
- Spinal anaesthesia is more common than epidural anaesthesia as it is technically easier and more reliable in preventing autonomic dysreflexia. Use standard doses of local anaesthetic agents (bupivacaine 'heavy' or plain). Intrathecal opioids appear to confer no advantage.

Disadvantages
- May be technically difficult to perform. Spinal anaesthesia is usually possible but epidural techniques are likely to fail in the presence of spinal instrumentation or previous spinal surgery.
- There is difficulty in determining the success or level of blockade in complete lesions. Incomplete lesions are tested as usual.

Postoperative care

- Tetraplegics are best nursed supine or only slightly head up due to improved ventilatory function in this position.
- Temperature should be monitored and hypothermia actively treated.
- Analgesia should be provided by conventional means.
- Dysreflexia may occur and require drug treatment after removal of precipitating causes (such as pain and urinary retention).

Obstetric anaesthesia

Effect of pregnancy on spinal cord injury

- Exaggerated postural hypotension and worsened response to caval occlusion.
- Reduced respiratory reserve with increased risk of respiratory failure and pneumonia. Increased oxygen demand.
- Increased anaemia due to haemodilution.
- Labour is a potent cause of autonomic dysreflexia in those with lesions above T_5 (dysreflexia may be the first sign of labour in such patients).

Effect of spinal injury on pregnancy

- Increased risk of infection (urinary and pressure sores).
- Increased risk of premature labour (increasing risk with higher level injury).
- Increased risk of thromboembolic complications.
- Labour pains will not be felt in complete lesions above T5. Lesion between T_5 and T_{10}—some awareness of some contractions.

Management of labour

- All cord-injured patients should be reviewed early in pregnancy and a plan formulated for the likely need for analgesia. The relative risks and difficulties of epidural catheter insertion should be predicted and discussed with the patient. A plan for anaesthesia in the event of Caesarean section should also be formulated and recorded in the patient notes.
- Epidural analgesia is usually possible in those with high cord lesions without vertebral instrumentation at the level of catheter insertion.
- Spinal anaesthesia is usually possible for elective Caesarean section and may be achievable with both single-shot and microcatheter techniques, irrespective of the presence of spinal instrumentation.
- General anaesthesia may proceed with the precautions outlined above.

Epidural analgesia in labour

- The most effective preventive measure for autonomic dysreflexia is adequate epidural analgesia. Those with high lesions may have an epidural commenced prior to induction of labour.
- Hypotension is not usually a problem after adequate fluid preloading (at least 1 litre of crystalloid or colloid). However, hypotension from any cause should be treated aggressively in those with high lesions due to the lack of compensatory mechanisms and a tendency to progressive hypotension. Aortocaval compression should be avoided by careful positioning for the same reasons.
- Autonomic dysreflexia has been reported up to 48hr after delivery. If successful block is achieved it would appear prudent to leave the epidural in situ for this time.
- Failure to establish adequate epidural blockade may necessitate drug treatment of autonomic dysreflexia (see above).

Further reading

Hambly PR, Martin B (1998). Anaesthesia for chronic spinal cord lesions. *Anaesthesia*, **53**, 273–289.

Myasthenia gravis

Myasthenia gravis is characterised by muscle weakness and fatigability. It is caused by autoimmune disruption of postsynaptic acetylcholine receptors at the neuromuscular junction, with up to 80% of functional receptors lost. The disease may occur at any age but is most common in young adult women. It may be associated with thymus hyperplasia with ~15% of affected patients having thymomas.

- Symptoms range from mild ptosis to life-threatening bulbar palsy and respiratory insufficiency.
- Management is usually with oral anticholinesterase medication with or without steroid therapy.
- Severe disease may require immunosuppressant therapy, plasmapheresis or immunoglobulin infusion.

General considerations

- All patients with myasthenia are sensitive to the effects of non-depolarising muscle relaxants.
- Plasmapheresis depletes plasma esterase levels, prolonging the effect of suxamethonium, mivacurium, ester-linked local anaesthetics, etc.
- Suxamethonium may have an altered effect—patients may be resistant to depolarisation due to reduced receptor activity, requiring increased dose. This, in conjunction with treatment-induced plasma esterase deficiency, leads to an increased risk of non-depolarising (Phase II) block.

Preoperative assessment

- Assess the degree of weakness and the duration of symptoms. Those with isolated ocular symptoms of long standing are unlikely to have progressive disease. Those with poorly controlled symptoms should have their condition optimised.
- Any degree of bulbar palsy is predictive of the need for both intra- and postoperative airway protection.
- Those who have significant respiratory impairment are more likely to require postoperative ventilation.
- Take a full drug history and determine the effect of a missed dose of anticholinesterase. Those with severe disease may be very sensitive to dose omission.

Conduct of anaesthesia

- Maintain anticholinesterase therapy up to the time of induction. Although theoretical inhibition of neuromuscular blockade is possible, this has never been reported.
- Premedication should be minimal.
- Avoid use of neuromuscular blocking drugs if possible. Intubation/ ventilation is often achievable using non-paralysing techniques.
- Non-depolarising drugs should be used sparingly. Monitor the response with a nerve stimulator. Initial doses of ~10–20% of normal are usually adequate.
- Consider topical LA to the airway.
- Short and intermediate duration non-depolarising drugs such as atracurium, mivacurium, or vecuronium are preferable to longer-acting drugs.

- Reversal of neuromuscular blocking drugs should be achievable with standard doses of neostigmine if preoperative symptom control has been good (see below). Avoidance of reversal is preferred since further doses of anticholinesterase may introduce the risk of overdose (cholinergic crisis). Drugs with spontaneous reversal such as atracurium are optimal.
- Consider insertion of nasogastric tube if difficulty with bulbar function is anticipated and early return of oral therapy required.
- Extubation is possible if neuromuscular function is assessed as adequate using nerve stimulation. Beware of preoperative bulbar function abnormality. The best predictor of safe extubation is >5s head lift.
- Regional anaesthesia may reduce the need for postoperative opioids and the risks of respiratory depression.
- Facilities for postoperative ventilation should be available.

Principles of perioperative cholinesterase management

- An easy conversion for oral pyridostigmine to parenteral (IV, IM, or SC) neostigmine is to equate every 30mg of oral pyridostigmine to 1mg of parenteral neostigmine.
- Reversal of neuromuscular blockade is possible with neostigmine if indicated by nerve stimulator—in general, no twitches on train of four means no reversal possible.
- Initial dosage of neostigmine should be used under nerve stimulator control, starting with a 2.5–5mg bolus and increasing if necessary with a 1mg bolus every 2–3min to a maximum equivalent dose to the oral pyridostigmine dose (1:30). For example, if the pyridostigmine dose is 120mg 3–4-hourly, then the maximum neostigmine dose should be 4mg (to be repeated after 2–4hr if necessary).

Rapid sequence induction

- Suxamethonium may be used if indicated—doses of 1.5mg/kg are usually effective.
- If doubt exists as to the ease of intubation consider awake techniques.
- If suxamethonium is used, do not use any other neuromuscular blocker until muscle function has returned and no fade is present.

Postoperative care

- Rapid return of drug therapy is mandatory. Use NG tube if necessary.
- In the event of gastrointestinal failure, parenteral therapy is indicated.

Preoperative predictors of need for postop ventilation

- Major body cavity surgery.
- Duration of disease >6yr.
- A history of coexisting chronic respiratory disease.
- Dose requirements of pyridostigmine >750mg/d.
- A preoperative vital capacity of <2.9l.

The best monitors of postoperative respiratory capacity are:
- Repeated peak flow measurements.
- Vital capacity should be at least twice tidal volume to allow for cough.
- Blood gases and pulse oximetry may be normal up to the point of respiratory failure.

Specific drugs of interest in myasthenia gravis

Drug	Interaction	Notes
Non-depolarising neuromuscular blockers	Marked sensitivity	Avoid use if possible. Start with 10% normal dosage. Always monitor neuromuscular function. Use short- and intermediate-acting agents only
Suxamethonium	Resistance to depolarisation and delayed onset of action	No reported clinical ill effects using 1.5mg/kg. Delayed recovery in patients with induced esterase deficiency (plasmapheresis, anticholinesterase treatment). Follow with non-depolarising agents only when full recovery of neuromuscular function noted
Inhalational anaesthetics	All inhalational agents reduce neuromuscular transmission by up to 50%	Avoiding need for neuromuscular blocking agents
IV anaesthetics	No discernible clinical effect on neuromuscular transmission	Total IV anaesthesia with propofol may be useful if neuromuscular function is precarious
Local anaesthetics	Prolonged action and increased toxicity in ester-linked agents with anticholinesterase therapy and plasmapheresis. Exacerbation of myasthenia reported	Use minimum dosage required for adequate block. Monitor respiratory function as with general anaesthesia
Drugs dependent on esterases for elimination	Prolonged effect and increased toxicity if patient on plasmapheresis or (theoretically) anticholinesterase therapy	Suxamethonium, remifentanil, mivacurium, ester-linked local anaesthetics, esmolol etc.
Antibiotics	Neuromuscular blocking effects may become clinically important	Avoid aminoglycosides (e.g. gentamicin). Similar effects reported with erythromycin and ciprofloxacin
Miscellaneous	All the following agents have a reported effect on neuromuscular transmission: procainamide, β-blockers (especially propranolol), phenytoin	

Table contd.

Drug	Interaction	Notes
Pyridostigmine	Adult: 30–120mg at suitable intervals (usually 4–6-hourly). Do not exceed total daily dose of 720mg Child: <6yr initial dose 30mg; 6–12yr initial dose 60mg. Total daily dose 30–360mg Neonate: 5–10mg every 4hr, 30–60min before feeds	Useful duration of action. No parenteral preparation available. Less potent and slower onset than neostigmine
Neostigmine (oral)	Adult: 15–30mg PO at suitable intervals (up to 2-hourly). Total daily dose 75–300mg Child: <6yr initial dose 7.5mg PO; 6–12yr initial dose 15mg PO. Total daily dose 15–90mg Neonate: 1–5mg PO 4-hourly, 30min before feeds	More marked GI effects than pyridostigmine. Useful if parenteral therapy indicated but more likely to require antimuscarinic (atropine or glycopyrronium) cover if used by this route
Neostigmine (SC/IM)	Adult: 1–2.5mg at suitable intervals (usually 2–4-hourly). Total daily dose 5–20mg Child: 200–500µg 4-hourly Neonate: 50–250µg 4-hourly	IV usage increases side effects and has reduced duration of action. If IV usage is necessary, anticholinergic agents (atropine/ glycopyrronium) should be administered
Edrophonium	Adult: 2mg by IV injection followed after 30s by 8mg if no adverse reaction Child: 20µg/kg IV followed by 80µg/kg after 30s if no adverse reaction	Use limited to diagnosis of myasthenia and differentiation of myasthenic and cholinergic crises
Distigmine	Adult: 5mg daily half an hour before breakfast. Maximum 20mg daily	Very long acting with risk of cholinergic crisis due to dosage accumulation. Not recommended in small children or neonates

Special considerations

Thymectomy

- Consensus now favours thymectomy in all adults with generalised myasthenia gravis. Remission rates are high and improvement of symptoms is almost universally attainable (96% gain benefit regardless of preoperative characteristics).
- Best results are achieved in those with normal or hyperplastic thymus.
- The approach most used is trans-sternal. Transcervical approaches provide less satisfactory access for surgery.
- Thoracoscopic thymectomy is gaining acceptance, although its reputed benefit of reduced complications and need for postoperative ventilation is yet to be proven.
- Anaesthetic management follows the same general principles outlined above, although all patients need postoperative care in HDU or require ventilation for a short period in the early postoperative period.
- Fewer than 8% of patients requiring sternotomy for thymectomy need ventilation for >3hr postoperatively.
- Almost all patients will require a degree of muscle relaxation if preoperative preparation has been optimal. Postoperative analgesia can be achieved satisfactorily with epidural or PCA.

Eaton–Lambert syndrome

Eaton–Lambert syndrome (myasthenic syndrome) is a proximal muscle weakness associated with cancer (most often small cell carcinoma of the lung).

- The condition is thought to be due to a reduction in the release of acetylcholine (prejunctional failure).
- It is not reversed by anticholinesterase therapy and muscle weakness is improved by exercise.
- Associated dysautonomia may manifest as dry mouth, impaired accommodation, urinary hesitance, and constipation.
- Unlike myasthenia gravis, patients with myasthenic syndrome are sensitive to both depolarising and non-depolarising neuromuscular blockers.
- Reduced doses should be used if the disease is suspected. Maintain a high index of suspicion in those undergoing procedures related to diagnosis and management of carcinoma of the lung.

Further reading

Baraka A (1992). Anaesthesia and myasthenia gravis. *Canadian Journal of Anaesthesia*, **39**, 476–486.

Krucylak PE, Naunheim KS (1999). Preoperative preparation and anesthetic management of patients with myasthenia gravis. *Seminars in Thoracic and Cardiovascular Surgery*, **11**, 47–53.

Wainwright AP, Brodrick PM (1987). Suxamethonium in myasthenia gravis. *Anaesthesia*, **42**, 950–957.

Multiple sclerosis

An acquired disease of the central nervous system characterised by demyelinated plaques within the brain and spinal cord. The onset of symptoms usually occurs in early adulthood with 20–30% following a benign course and 5% a rapid deterioration. It is most common in geographical clusters within Europe, North America, and New Zealand.

General considerations

Incurable disease, but steroids and interferon have been associated with improved symptom-free intervals. Most patients suffer from associated depression. Baclofen and dantrolene are useful for painful muscle spasm.

- Symptoms range from isolated visual disturbance and nystagmus to limb weakness and paralysis.
- Respiratory failure due to both respiratory muscle failure and bulbar palsy may be a feature in end-stage disease.
- Symptoms are characterised by symptomatic episodes of variable severity with periods of remission for several years.
- Permanent weakness and symptoms develop in some patients, leading to increasingly severe disability.
- Demyelinated nerve fibres are sensitive to heat. A temperature rise of 0.5°C may cause a marked deterioration in symptoms.

Preoperative assessment and investigation

- Preoperative evaluation must include a history of the type of symptoms suffered and a detailed neurological examination. This will allow comparison with postoperative state to elucidate any new lesions.
- Respiratory function may be affected. Bulbar palsy causes increased risk of aspiration and reduced airway reflexes in the postop period.

Conduct of anaesthesia

- General anaesthesia does not affect the course of multiple sclerosis.
- Regional anaesthesia does not affect neurological symptoms, but it may be medicolegally prudent to avoid nerve blockade.
- Centroneuraxial blockade has been associated with recurrence of symptoms. However, this is reduced by use of minimal concentrations of local anaesthetic/opioid in combination. Epidural analgesia for labour is not contraindicated—keep LA concentration to a minimum.
- Suxamethonium is associated with a large efflux of potassium in debilitated patients and should be avoided.
- Response to non-depolarising drugs is normal, although caution and reduced dosages are indicated in those with severe disability.
- Careful cardiovascular monitoring is essential since autonomic instability leads to marked hypotensive responses to drugs and sensitivity to hypovolaemia.
- Temperature is important and should be monitored in all patients. Pyrexia must be avoided and should be treated aggressively with antipyretics (paracetamol 1g PR/PO), tepid sponging, and forced-air blowers. Hypothermia may delay recovery from anaesthesia.

Guillain Barré syndrome

Guillain Barré syndrome is an immune-mediated progressive demyelinating disorder characterised by acute or subacute proximal skeletal muscle paralysis. The syndrome is often preceded by limb paraesthesia/back pain and in more than half of affected patients by a viral illness. No single viral agent has been implicated.

More than 85% of patients achieve a full recovery, although this may take several months. The use of steroids in the management of this condition remains controversial.

- One-third of patients will require ventilatory support.
- The more rapid the onset of symptoms, the more likely the progression to respiratory failure. Impending respiratory failure may be evidenced by difficulty in swallowing and phonation due to pharyngeal muscle weakness.
- Inability to cough is a marker of severe respiratory impairment and usually indicates the need for intubation and ventilation.
- Autonomic dysfunction is common.

Conduct of anaesthesia

- Respiratory support is likely to be necessary, both during surgery and in the postoperative period.
- Autonomic dysfunction leads to potential severe hypotension during induction of anaesthesia, initiation of positive pressure ventilation, and postural changes under anaesthesia or recovery.
- Hydration should be maintained with wide-bore IV access and pressor agents (ephedrine 3–6mg bolus IV) prepared prior to induction.
- Tachycardia due to surgical stimulus may be extreme and atropine may elicit a paradoxical bradycardia.
- Suxamethonium should be avoided due to potential catastrophic potassium efflux. The risk of hyperkalaemia may persist for several months after clinical recovery.
- Non-depolarising muscle relaxants may not be needed and should be used cautiously.
- Epidural analgesia is useful and may avoid the need for systemic opioid analgesia. Epidural opioids have been used to manage distressing paraesthesia in these patients.

Motor neuron disease (amyotrophic lateral sclerosis)

This is a degenerative disorder of upper and lower motor neurons in the spinal cord. It manifests initially with weakness, atrophy, and fasciculation of peripheral muscles (usually those of the hand) and progresses to axial and bulbar weakness.

- Progression is relentless, with death from respiratory failure usually occurring within 3yrs of diagnosis.
- Patients remain mentally competent up to the point of terminal respiratory failure, leading to ethical and moral difficulty in the provision of long-term ventilation.

Conduct of anaesthesia

- Bulbar palsy increases the risk of sputum retention and aspiration. Intubation may be necessary. Many patients with advanced disease will have a long-term tracheostomy for airway protection and episodes of mechanical ventilation.
- Respiratory support is likely to be necessary, both during surgery and in the postoperative period.
- Autonomic dysfunction leads to potentially severe hypotension during induction of anaesthesia, initiation of positive pressure ventilation, and postural changes under anaesthesia or recovery.
- Hydration should be maintained with wide-bore IV access if necessary and pressor agents (ephedrine/metaraminol) prepared prior to induction.
- Suxamethonium should be avoided due to potential catastrophic potassium efflux.
- Non-depolarising agents should be used in reduced dosage if necessary and their action monitored with a nerve stimulator.

Dystrophia myotonica

Dystrophia myotonica (myotonic dystrophy, myotonia atrophica) is the most common of the dystonias (1:20 000), the others being myotonia congenita and paramyotonia. It is an autosomal dominant disease, presenting in the second or third decade of life.

General considerations

- Persistent contraction of skeletal muscle follows stimulation. Characterised by prefrontal balding and cataracts.
- The main clinical features are related to muscular atrophy, especially of facial, sternomastoid, and peripheral muscles.
- Progressive deterioration/atrophy of skeletal, cardiac, and smooth muscle over time leads to a deterioration in cardiorespiratory function and a (possibly severe) cardiomyopathy.
- Further respiratory deterioration occurs due to degeneration of the central nervous system, leading to central respiratory drive depression.
- Progressive bulbar palsy causes difficulty in swallowing/clearing secretions and an increased risk of aspiration.
- Degeneration of the cardiac conduction system causes dysrhythmia and atrioventricular block.
- Mitral valve prolapse occurs in ~20% of patients.
- Mental deterioration after the second decade.
- Endocrine dysfunction may lead to diabetes mellitus, hypothyroidism, adrenal insufficiency, and gonadal atrophy.
- Death usually occurs in the fifth or sixth decade.
- Pregnancy may aggravate the disease and Caesarean section is more common due to uterine muscle dysfunction.
- Therapy is supportive using antimyotonic medications such as procainamide, phenytoin, quinine, and mexiletine.

Preoperative assessment

- Assess respiratory reserve, including signs of bulbar palsy (difficulty with cough or swallowing).
- Seek signs of cardiac failure and dysrhythmia.
- Gastric emptying may be delayed. Premedication with an antacid (ranitidine 150–300mg PO) or a prokinetic (metoclopramide 10mg PO) may be indicated.

Investigations

- CXR, spirometry, and arterial blood gases if indicated by respiratory symptoms.
- ECG to exclude conduction defects and echocardiography for myocardial dysfunction.
- U&Es and glucose to exclude endocrine dysfunction.

- s...
  tion, ve...
- Non-depolarisin... relaxation. Use of a ne... leading to misdiagnosis of teta... muscle contraction (and potas-
- Reversal with neostigmine may also p... action may make intuba- depolarising agents with short action and spo... always cause muscle curium, mivacurium) are preferred. ...uscle contraction,
- Intubation and maintenance of anaesthesia can often be achie... without the use of any muscle relaxant.
- Invasive arterial monitoring is indicated for significant cardiovascular impairment.
- Even small doses of induction agents can produce profound cardio-respiratory depression.
- Bulbar palsy increases the need for intubation under general anaesthesia.
- Regional anaesthesia does not prevent muscle contraction. Trouble-some spasm may be helped by infiltration of local anaesthetic directly into the affected muscle. Quinine (600mg IV) or phenytoin (3–5mg/kg IV slowly) have been effective in some cases.
- High concentrations of inhaled anaesthetics should be avoided because of their effect on myocardial contraction and conduction.
- Patient warmth must be maintained. Postoperative shivering may pro-voke myotonia.

Postoperative care

- High-dependency care is indicated after anything but minor peripheral surgery. Discharge to low-dependency areas should be considered only if the patient is able to cough adequately and maintain oxygenation on air or simple supplemental oxygen.
- Analgesia is best provided, if possible, by regional or local block to avoid the systemic depressant effects of opioids.

Myotonia congenita

This develops in infancy and early childhood and is characterised by pharyngeal muscle spasm leading to difficulty in swallowing. It improves with age and patients have a normal life expectancy.

Paramyotonia

This is extremely rare. It is characterised by cold-induced contraction, only relieved by warming the affected muscle. Anaesthetic management is the same as for myotonic dystrophy. Patient warmth is paramount.

Further reading

Imison AR (2001). Anaesthesia and myotonia—an Australian experience. *Anaesthesia and Intensive Care*, **29**, 34–37.

Muscular dy...

The muscular dys... of congenital muscular disor-
ders characteri... ...kness of affected muscle groups.
They can be ... ...o inheritance:
- X-linked... ...ker's
- Autos... ...limb-girdle, childhood, congenital
- A...e's muscular dystrophy ...nant: facioscapulohumeral, oculopharyngeal.

...ost common and most severe form.

General considerations

- Sex-linked recessive trait, clinically apparent in males.
- Onset of symptoms of muscle weakness at 2–5yr.
- The patient is usually confined to a wheelchair by 12yr.
- Death usually by 25yr due to progressive cardiac failure or pneumonia.
- Cardiac: myocardial degeneration leading to heart failure and possible mitral valve prolapse. Evidence of heart failure is often apparent by 6yr (reduced R wave amplitude and wall motion abnormalities). Isolated degeneration of the left ventricle may lead to right outflow obstruction and right heart failure.
- Respiratory: progressive respiratory muscle weakness, leading to a restrictive ventilation pattern, inadequate cough, and eventual respiratory infection and failure.
- Possible vascular smooth muscle dysfunction, leading to increased bleeding during surgery
- Associated progressive and severe kyphoscoliosis.
- Disease progression may be tracked by serum creatinine kinase levels. These are elevated early in the disease but reduce to below normal as muscles atrophy.

Other muscular dystrophies (Becker's, facioscapulohumeral, and limb-girdle dystrophy) are less severe than Duchenne's dystrophy, with onset at a later age and slower progression of the disease. Isolated ocular dystrophy is associated with a normal lifespan.

Preoperative assessment and investigations

- Patients are usually under the care of specialist paediatricians.
- CXR, spirometry, and blood gases may be indicated by respiratory symptoms.
- Echocardiography is mandatory if the patient is wheelchair bound—myocardial and valve function can be assessed.
- Reduced gut muscle tone leads to delayed gastric emptying and increased risk of aspiration.

Conduct of anaesthesia
- Antacid premedication (H_2 receptor blocker or proton pump inhibitor) with a prokinetic such as metoclopramide may be useful to reduce risk of aspiration.
- An antisialogogue such as glycopyrronium may be needed if secretions are a problem.
- Careful IV induction of anaesthesia with balanced opioid/induction agent.
- Potent inhalational anaesthetics should be used cautiously in these patients because of the risk of myocardial depression.
- Suxamethonium should be avoided because of potassium efflux and potential cardiac arrest.
- Non-depolarising neuromuscular blockers are safe, although reduced doses are required. Nerve stimulator monitoring should be used.
- Respiratory depressant effects of all anaesthetic drugs are enhanced and postoperative respiratory function should be monitored carefully. Those with pre-existing sputum retention and inadequate cough are at high risk of postoperative respiratory failure and may need prolonged ventilatory support.
- Regional analgesia is useful to avoid opioid use and potential respiratory depression after painful surgery. Caudal epidural may be technically easier to perform than lumbar epidural in those with kyphoscoliosis.

Malignant hyperthermia

Aetiology

- Malignant hyperthermia (MH) is a pharmacogenetic disease of skeletal muscle induced by exposure to certain anaesthetic agents such as, suxamethonium, and all the anaesthetic volatile agents.
- It is inherited as an autosomal dominant condition and caused by loss of normal Ca^{2+} homeostasis at some point along the excitation–contraction coupling process on exposure to triggering agents. Any defect along this complex process could result in the clinical features of MH and may explain why differing chemical agents trigger MH and the heterogeneity seen in DNA studies.
- Most likely site is the triadic junction between T tubule, involving the voltage sensor of the dihydropyridine receptor (DHPR), and sarcoplasmic reticulum (SR), involving the Ca^{2+} efflux channel of the ryanodine receptor (RYR1).
- About 60% of MH families are linked to the RYR1 gene located on chromosome 19q. Over 100 mutations have been identified in RYR1 but only 22 have evidence of causality. Other loci have been identified (e.g. chromosomes 1, 3, and 7) but only for small numbers of families.

Epidemiology

- Incidence is about 1:10 000–15 000 but difficult to estimate. All races are affected.
- Mortality rates have fallen dramatically from 70–80% to 2–3% due to increased awareness, improved monitoring standards, and the availability of dantrolene.
- Commonly seen in young adults, males > females, but this may be a lifestyle, rather than a true sex difference.
- More frequent in minor operations e.g. dental/ENT due to anaesthetic technique, i.e. suxamethonium and vapour commonly used.
- Previous uneventful anaesthesia with triggering agents does not preclude MH. 75% of MH probands (index cases) have had previous anaesthesia prior to their MH crisis.
- Annual U.K. incidence of confirmed MH cases is falling (currently ~10–15/yr) due to changes in anaesthetic techniques, e.g. decreased use of suxamethonium, increased use of TIVA and local anaesthesia. However, there is an increased referral rate due to increased index of suspicion.

Clinical presentation

- The clinical diagnosis can be difficult as the presentation of MH varies considerably and no one sign is unique to MH. It can be a florid dramatic life-threatening event or have an insidious onset. Rarely can develop 2–3d postoperatively with massive myoglobinuria and/or renal failure due to severe rhabdomyolysis.

Clinical signs

- Signs of increased metabolism: tachycardia, dysrhythmias, increased CO_2 production, metabolic acidosis, pyrexia, DIC. Often called a 'metabolic storm'. Pyrexia develops as a consequence of metabolic stimulation, so occurs after other signs. A pyrexia developing after recovery from normal anaesthesia is not indicative of MH.
- Muscle signs: masseter spasm after suxamethonium, generalised muscle rigidity, hyperkalaemia, high CK, myoglobinuria, renal failure.

Masseter muscle spasm

- Masseter muscle spasm after suxamethonium (MMS), defined as impeding intubation and persisting for ~2min. 30% of patients presenting with MMS alone, even when anaesthesia has proceeded uneventfully, prove to be MH susceptible.
- If possible abandon surgery; if not convert to 'MH safe' technique (volatile free); allow approximately 15min to ensure that the patient is stabilised. Monitor $ETCO_2$, temperature, and consider an arterial line.
- Additional MH signs increase the likelihood of MH significantly: 50–60% if metabolic signs present, 70–80% if muscle signs present.
- Investigations that are particularly useful are the initial and 24hr creatine kinase (CK) and examination of the first voided specimen for myoglobinuria, indicating evidence of muscle damage.
- Prolonged severe muscle stiffness greatly in excess of the 'normal scoline pains' may occur.
- MMS maybe the first indication of a previously unsuspected muscle disease, particularly the myotonic conditions. Perform resting CK and EMG. Consider neurological opinion.

Treatment of a crisis

See p894.
- A poster 'Guidelines for the treatment of an MH crisis' is available from the AAGBI for display in theatres.

After treating a suspected MH crisis

- If MH was suspected clinically refer the patient to an MH unit with all the relevant clinical details/anaesthetic chart/laboratory results. The timing of various events is important.
- In the meantime warn the patient and/or family of the potential implications of MH.
- MH is not a diagnosis to be made lightly without adequate follow-up.
- Unless MH can be clearly excluded on clinical grounds the patient/family will be offered screening to confirm of refute the clinical diagnosis.
- The proband is always screened even if the clinical reaction is undoubted. If the proband cannot be screened (e.g. died or too young) the most appropriate relative is screened (e.g. parents of a young child).

Diagnosis of MH susceptibility

• Muscle biopsy using the *in vitro* contracture test (IVCT) remains the gold standard of MH diagnosis. This is an open invasive procedure usually performed under a femoral nerve block to remove 8–10 muscle specimens ~3–4cm long from the vastus medialis muscle. As living samples are used, the patient has to travel to the MH centre.

• The IVCT follows a European MH Group (EMHG) protocol exposing muscle tissue to halothane and separately to caffeine under preset conditions in a dedicated laboratory.

• The diagnosis is considered positive if the muscle contracts in response to halothane and/or caffeine.

• There is a potential for 'false positive' MH diagnoses in order to ensure the accuracy of the MH negative diagnosis. The combined EMHG data indicate a specificity of 93.6% and sensitivity of 99%.

• If the proband is confirmed as MH susceptible by IVCT, they are screened for the 22 RYR1 mutations currently used for diagnostic purposes by the EMHG for DNA testing of MH.

• If a mutation is identified in the proband, family members can be offered an initial DNA blood test for the familial mutation; if a muta-tion carrier they are classified as MH susceptible without a muscle biopsy; if mutation negative a confirmatory biopsy is required for reasons of safety because MH is heterogeneous and there is a small incidence of discordant results within families.

• If a mutation is not identified in the proband, family members are offered IVCT only.

• Family screening is organised on the basis of the autosomal dominant pattern of inheritance, so relatives with a 50% risk are screened first, i.e. parents, siblings, and children; the latter are not screened until aged 10–12yr.

• The purpose of family screening is to identify the small number of indi-viduals in a family who are susceptible to MH rather than labelling the whole family. Screening will involve only a small proportion of the family.

• Once identified as MH susceptible the MH unit can provide written information about MH, warning cards/discs, and information about the British MH Association (BMHA), a patient support charity.

• MH centres should co-ordinate family screening to ensure the appro-priate method of testing is offered.

Anaesthesia for known or suspected MH susceptible patients

• MH patients should not be denied necessary surgery solely because of MH.

• Preoperative questioning about personal and family anaesthetic history is essential to identify potential MH patients.

• It is not absolutely essential to screen suspected cases prior to surgery, providing careful individual assessment has been made of the risks involved.

• An MH 'safe' technique, i.e. avoiding suxamethonium and all anaes-thetic volatile agents, may not pose any additional risk in many circumstances, but will do so in certain situations, e.g. when the preferred technique would have necessitated use of these agents.

- All local anaesthetic agents are safe.
- Dantrolene is not required prophylactically because of its side effects, but should be readily available.
- Standard monitoring is adequate, i.e. ECG, NIBP, SaO$_2$, ETCO$_2$. A baseline core temperature should be established before the procedure and monitored ~4hr postoperatively.
- If no volatile-free machine is available, remove all vaporisers and circuitry from the machine and ventilator and purge with oxygen for 20–30min. Use new circuits/LMAs/ETT, etc.
- The MH unit can be contacted for further advice if required.

Anaesthesia for a patient with a known or suspected family history of MH

- Establish the family history and the relationship of your patient to the named proband or other tested family members. The MH centre will then be able to advise about the risk to your patient and need for further investigation.
- If anaesthesia is urgent and more details unavailable, proceed as for an MH susceptible patient.

Suspicious previous anaesthetic history

- Unexplained/unexpected cardiac arrest/death during anaesthesia carries a 50% risk of MH.
- History of postoperative myoglobinuria (red/black urine).
- Renal failure in otherwise healthy patient.
- Postoperative pyrexia. Establish timing of the pyrexia in relation to surgery. If intra-operative/immediate recovery period was uneventful with the pyrexia developing later on the ward, MH is not implicated. If timing unclear, the likelihood of MH is low but cannot be excluded.
- Take a thorough history of the event. If possible obtain old records and seek further advice from the MH centre. If surgery is urgent proceed as if MH susceptible and resolve problem later.

Obstetric patients

- Baby of susceptible parent:
  - Has 50% chance of being affected if one parent is MH susceptible, so should be treated as potentially MH.
- Mother MH susceptible:
  - Plans for any emergency situation should be prepared with obstetric anaesthetist prior to EDD.
  - It is essential to anticipate airway problems and consider other options, e.g. awake intubation.
  - Regional techniques preferred.
  - For general anaesthesia use an MH safe technique substituting suxamethonium with a rapid onset non-depolarising muscle relaxant, e.g. rocuronium and maintaining anaesthesia with a propofol infusion.
  - Ephedrine, syntocinon, ergometrine can be used.

- Father MH susceptible (fetus at risk)
  - Avoid MH triggering agents which cross the placenta, i.e. inhalational agents, until after delivery of the baby.
  - Suxamethonium, being highly charged, can be used as it does not cross the placenta to any great extent.

Associated conditions

- Central core disease (CCD) is a non-progressive inherited condition causing peripheral muscle weakness and occasionally musculoskeletal and cardiac problems. It is the only condition known to be associated with MH, but this is not invariable. CCD patients should be treated as potentially MH susceptible but offered screening because of the discordant association. Other muscle diseases are not thought to be related to MH but clearly cause anaesthetic problems in their own right.
- Heat stroke and King–Denborough syndrome remain controversial.
- Neuroleptic malignant syndrome and sudden infant death syndrome are not associated with MH (see p276).

Anaesthesia for the MH susceptible patient	
MH 'triggering' agents	Avoid suxamethonium and all anaesthetic vapours/volatiles
MH 'safe' agents	All induction agents including ketamine, all analgesics, all non-depolarising agents, all local anaesthetics (preferably plain solutions)
	Atropine/glycopyrronium/neostigmine
	Ephedrine and other vasopressors
	Metoclopramide/droperidol Nitrous oxide, benzodiazepines
Monitoring	ECG, NIBP, ETCO$_2$, core temperature. Check temp 2hr preop to establish baseline and 4–6hr postop
Anaesthetic equipment	If no vapour-free machine is available, remove the vaporisers and blow both the anaesthetic machine and the ventilator with oxygen for 20–30min. Use fresh clean tubing/masks/ET tubes, etc. If possible select a ventilator with little inner tubing, e.g. Nuffield Penlon
Dantrolene	This is not required prophylactically, as no reaction should occur. It is unpleasant for the patient and markedly prolongs the action of non-depolarising muscle relaxants. However, it should be readily available

MH centres and the British MH Association (BMHA)

- There is only one MH centre in the United Kingdom: Dr P. J. Halsall, MH Investigation Unit, Clinical Sciences Building, St James's University Hospital, Leeds LS9 7TF. Tel: 0113 2065274; Fax: 0113 2064140; Hotline: 07947 609601 (usually available for medical emergencies only).
- The British MH Association (BMHA) is a charitable patient support group which provides the 'hotline', warning cards/discs, and translations for travel abroad, newsletters, as well as fundraising for research. Secretary: Mrs A. Winks, 11 Gorse Close, Newthorpe, Nottingham NG16 2BZ. Tel: 01773 717901.
- There are 22 MH centres in Europe. Contact the European MH Group Secretary Dr P. J. Halsall (address above) for further details or see the EMHG website: http://www.emhg.org
- For the USA and Canada contact MHAUS, 39 East State St, PO Box 1069, Sherburne, NY 13460, USA. Tel: in North America, 1–800-MH-Hyper; outside North America, 1–315–464–7079; http://www.mhaus.org. Hotline: 1–800–98-MHAUS.
- For Australia contact Dr Neil Street, Anaesthetic Dept, The New Children's Hospital, Westmead, NSW, PO Box 3515, Parramatta 2124. Tel: (02) 9845 0000; Fax: (02) 9845 3489.
- For New Zealand contact Dr Neil Pollock, Anaesthetic Dept, Palmerston North Hospital, Mid Central Health, Palmerston North Tel: (06) 3569169; Fax: (06) 3508566.

Further reading

Ellis FR, Halsall PJ, Christian AS (1990). Clinical presentation of suspected malignant hyperthermia during anaesthesia in 402 probands. *Anaesthesia*, **45**, 838–841.

Guidelines for the treatment of an MH crisis. A poster published by the Association of Anaesthetists of Great Britain and Ireland. Bedford Square, London.

Halsall PJ, Hopkins PM (2003). Inherited disease and anaesthesia. In: *A Practice of Anaesthesia, 7th ed.* Eds. Healy TEJ and Knight PR, 363–376.

MacLennan DH, Phillips MS (1992). Malignant hyperthermia. *Science*, **256**, 789–794.

Urwyler A, Deufel T, McCarthy TV, West SP for the European MH Group (2001). Guidelines for the molecular genetic testing of susceptibility to malignant hyperthermia. *British Journal of Anaesthesia*, **86**, 283–287.

Chapter 12

Psychiatric disorders and drugs

Aidan O'Donnell

Colin Berry

Aidan O'Donnell

See also:

Psychiatric disorders

- Psychiatric illness is present in about 10% of UK population.
- 1% of population have a major psychiatric disorder.
- Anaesthetic implications are usually due either to the psychiatric comorbidity itself or the interactions between psychiatric drugs and anaesthetic techniques.
- Many patients are on long-term drug therapy which should be continued perioperatively where possible.
- Alcohol and drug misuse is common among the psychiatric population
- Most patients can give consent normally (see p16) but some may be held for treatment under the Mental Health Act. (In Scotland the Adults with Incapacity Act (2000) clarifies capacity and consent issues.)
- Stress of hospitalisation for surgery may exacerbate coexisting psychiatric problems.

Schizophrenia

- Lifetime risk ~1%, M = F. Peak incidence in late teens.
- Schneider's first-rank symptoms suggest diagnosis. These include thought echo, withdrawal, insertion or broadcast, auditory hallucinations, somatic passivity, and delusional perceptions. Patients may have poverty of thought, flat or incongruous affect, and amotivation. 10% die by suicide.
- Acute schizophrenics may be very agitated and delusional and unable to give informed consent.
- Chronic schizophrenics may be withdrawn and uncommunicative.
- Schizophrenia is often treated with antipsychotic drugs (p276), which should be continued perioperatively.

Bipolar affective disorder

- Lifetime risk ~1%, slight female preponderance. Peak incidence in early twenties.
- Recurrent episodes of altered mood and activity with both mania and depression.
- Manic patients lack insight and may be detained under the Mental Health Act.
- Patients may be treated with antipsychotic drugs, lithium (p276), or anticonvulsant drugs (which have mood-stabilising properties), e.g. carbamazepine and valproate. Abrupt withdrawal of any of these is dangerous.

Depression

- Lifetime risk 10–20%, F:M ratio 2:1, peak incidence in late twenties.
- Persistent low mood, sometimes associated with cognitive and functional impairment (disturbances of appetite, sleep, or libido).
- Antidepressant medication includes TCAs, SSRIs, MAOIs, and occasionally lithium (p272–276).
- Severe depression with strong risk of suicide may be treated with ECT (see p280).

Anxiety

- Anxiety in the anaesthetic room is extremely common and usually managed with explanation, reassurance, premedication (p6), or IV sedation (e.g. midazolam 2mg IV) titrated to effect.
- Anxiety disorder may be acute or chronic (symptoms are similar) or occur as part of other disorders (e.g. depression).
- Extreme agitation may make cannulation difficult. Patients may hyperventilate and have high levels of circulating catecholamines.

Dementia

- Irreversible global deterioration in higher mental functioning. 50% of cases due to Alzheimer's disease.
- Prevalence: 1% aged 65–74 rising to 10% aged >75, and 25% aged >85yr.
- Mean life expectancy is 7yr from diagnosis.
- Patients are unable to give informed consent: an incapacity form should be completed by the consultant responsible.
- Patients are usually confused, and may be agitated (occasionally violent) or profoundly withdrawn.
- Patients may be on anticholinesterases such as donepezil which may prolong the action of suxamethonium and partially antagonise the effects of non-depolarising neuromuscular blocking drugs.
- Regional anaesthesia may still be desirable if significant comorbidity: ketamine (eg 5–20mg IV) may facilitate this and preserves airway reflexes and BP (titrate to effect). (Midazolam may cause disinhibition, which may paradoxically worsen agitation.)

Anorexia nervosa[1]

- Anorexia nervosa is a chronic, severe, multi-system disorder which carries the highest morbidity and mortality rate of any psychiatric disorder.
- Anorexia (fear of fatness with deliberate weight loss) is present in 1–2% of females aged 13–20. Bulimia (uncontrolled binge eating and purging) is commoner (1–3%). F:M ratio for both is about 50:1.
- Typically anorexics are 25% below their ideal weight (bulimics may be normal or overweight).
- Many sufferers experience major depressive illness.
- IV drug misuse is common (p278).
- Clinical features are those of malnutrition and starvation: cachexia, hair loss, amenorrhoea, and osteoporosis. Patients may require nasogastric feeding. Immunocompetence is usually preserved until >50% of normal body weight is lost. Endocrine changes may mimic panhypopituitarism.
- CVS: significant bradycardia and hypotension are common (e.g. systolic BP <100mmHg). ECG changes may be present in up to 80% of patients (AV block; ST depression; T wave inversion and prolonged QT (associated with significant risk of sudden death)). Arrhythmias are common. Myocardial impairment may occur. Patients are at risk of cardiac failure if overfilled intra-operatively.

1 Seller CA, Ravalia A (2003). Anaesthetic implications of anorexia nervosa. *Anaesthesia*, **58**, 437–443.

- RS: prolonged starvation causes loss of lung elasticity. Airway pressures may be high.
- Renal: GFR is reduced. Two-thirds of patients are proteinuric. Excessive losses of Na^+, K^+, Cl^-, and H^+ from the stomach result in hypochloraemic metabolic alkalosis and hypokalaemia. Severe hypokalaemia is uncommon but should be corrected with caution preoperatively. Hypocalcaemia may accompany hypokalaemia.
- GI: anorexics and bulimics may have paradoxically delayed gastric emptying. Fasting is not a reliable way of ensuring an empty stomach.
- Anaesthetic management: patients need more laboratory tests than their age alone would suggest. Check FBC, U&Es, LFTs, glucose, Ca^{2+}, Mg^{2+}, phosphate, ECG. Rehydrate patient preoperatively and correct any abnormal electrolyte levels. Rapid sequence induction is advisable. Hypokalaemia and hypocalcaemia may potentiate neuromuscular blockade. Patients are prone to hypothermia. Position patient carefully as prone to pressure necrosis and nerve palsies.
- Hypoalbuminaemia may cause elevated levels of unbound drugs in the plasma; and drug metabolism and elimination may be slowed. Avoid hyperventilation (exacerbates hypokalaemia). Avoid large infusions, which may precipitate pulmonary oedema.

Chronic alcohol abuse

- Alcoholic liver disease: earliest form is reversible fatty liver progressing to alcoholic hepatitis (abdo pain, weight loss, jaundice, fever) and later cirrhosis (jaundice, ascites, portal hypertension and hepatic failure).
- Alcoholic cardiomyopathy is characterized by a dilated, hypokinetic LV and decreased EF. Patients may present with congestive cardiac failure and oedema, exacerbated by low serum albumin. Consider echo.
- Hypoglycaemia may complicate acute alcohol intoxication, alcoholic liver disease and pancreatic disease. More common in adolescents.
- Ketoacidosis may present after binge drinking in association with vomiting and fasting. Blood alcohol levels may already have normalised.
- Patients with acute alcohol ingestion are partially anaesthetised and reduced concentrations of volatile agents are required. Chronic exposure to alcohol induces tolerance to some anaesthetic agents.
- Avoid non-emergency surgery if there is acute alcohol toxicity.
- If emergency surgery is unavoidable, ensure adequate rehydration with careful attention to electrolyte and glucose disturbances. Give IV vitamins (e.g. Pabrinex slow IV bd for 7 days).
- Correct clotting abnormalities. Transfuse appropriately if required.
- Patients with liver failure require intensive care if surgery is planned (see also p138).
- Anticipate alcohol withdrawal symptoms. Most patients can tolerate 24–48h abstinence perioperatively. Do not complicate management by attempting alcohol withdrawal perioperatively.
- Seizures are most commonly seen 7–48h after cessation of drinking, typically tonic-clonic. Several fits over a period of a few days are common. Low K^+ and Mg^{2+} predispose. Seizures may be preceded by disorientation and agitation (*delirium tremens*).

Tricyclic antidepressants (TCA)

- Formerly the mainstay of treatment of depressive illness, they have largely been superseded by SSRIs (fewer side effects and safer in overdose).
- May be used in treatment of other problems, e.g. chronic pain.
- Block reuptake of amines from the synaptic cleft by competing for transport protein. Need to be given for 2–4wk before effective.
- Most have atropine-like side effects: dry mouth, blurred vision, urinary retention, and constipation. Other common side effects are sedation and postural hypotension.
- Strongly bound to plasma proteins, and their effects may be enhanced by competing drugs (e.g. aspirin, warfarin, digoxin).
- In overdose, TCAs are extremely toxic, producing agitation, delirium, respiratory depression, and coma. Cardiac arrhythmias with prolongation of the QT interval are frequent. There is no specific antidote and treatment is supportive, although intensive care may be required. Alkalinisation of plasma reduces the amount of free drug.

Anaesthesia for patient on TCA

- It is not necessary (and may be harmful) to withdraw TCAs preoperatively.
- Increased sensitivity to catecholamines may result in hypertension and arrhythmias following administration of sympathomimetic drugs (adrenaline, noradrenaline). Indirect sympathomimetics (e.g. ephedrine, metaraminol) should be avoided (see p274).
- Ventricular arrhythmias may occur with high concentrations of volatile agents, especially halothane.
- TCAs may delay gastric emptying.
- Anticholinergic drugs (e.g. atropine) which cross the blood–brain barrier may precipitate postoperative confusion.
- Tramadol increases risk of CNS toxicity.

St John's Wort (*Hypericum perforatum*)

- Extract of the plant contains several alkaloids which are similar in structure to tricyclic antidepressant drugs.
- Useful and safe as monotherapy in mild depressive illness.
- May induce certain cytochrome 'p450' enzymes, thereby enhancing the metabolism of many drugs, including warfarin, digoxin, theophylline, ciclosporin, tacrolimus, HIV protease inhibitors, and oral contraceptive drugs.
- May interact with other drugs, e.g. SSRIs, to cause serotonin syndrome (see p273).

Selective serotonin reuptake inhibitors (SSRIs)

- Most commonly prescribed antidepressants, and are increasingly being prescribed for other conditions (e.g. panic disorder, obsessive-compulsive disorder).
- Highly specific inhibitors of presynaptic reuptake of serotonin from the synaptic cleft and are much less toxic than TCAs.
- Common side effects affect the GI tract (nausea, vomiting, diarrhoea) and the CNS (insomnia, agitation, tremor, headache, sexual dysfunction). Cardiovascular side effects are rare (occasional reports of bradycardia).
- In patients with pre-existing ischaemic heart disease, SSRIs may precipitate coronary vasoconstriction.
- SIADH has been described with the use of SSRIs, especially in the elderly, and may present with hyponatraemia (p180).
- High doses of SSRIs may impair platelet aggregation, and cause prolonged bleeding times.
- Serotonin **syndrome**[1] is a toxic crisis resulting from increased synaptic levels of serotonin in the brainstem and spinal cord due to overdose of SSRIs, or combination of SSRIs with other drugs affecting serotonin (especially TCAs, MAOIs, pethidine, tramadol, and dextromethorphan). It presents as alteration in behaviour (agitation, confusion), motor activity (rigidity, myoclonus, hyperreflexia), and autonomic instability (pyrexia, tachycardia, diarrhoea, unstable BP). It may progress to seizures, oculogyric crises, DIC, rhabdomyolysis, myoglobinuria, acute renal failure, arrhythmia, coma, and death. It may mimic the neuroleptic malignant syndrome (p276). The patient is likely to require intensive care. Treatment is mainly supportive, and the episode usually lasts <24hr.
- SSRIs inhibit cytochrome p450 enzymes, which may prolong or enhance the activity of other drugs, notably warfarin, theophylline, phenytoin, carbamazepine, tolbutamide, benzodiazepines (diazepam, midazolam), Type 1c antiarrhythmics (e.g. flecainide), tricyclic antidepressants, and some NSAIDs.

Anaesthesia for patient on SSRI

- Abrupt withdrawal of SSRIs can precipitate withdrawal syndrome.
- Check urea and electrolytes to exclude hyponatraemia, especially in the elderly.
- A coagulation screen should be assessed and corrected if necessary.
- Benzodiazepines should be used cautiously as their effects may be prolonged.
- Pethidine, pentazocine, tramadol, and dextromethorphan should be avoided (see above).

---

1 Jones D, Story OA (2005). Serotonin syndrome and the anaesthetist. *Anaesthesia and Intensive Care*, **33**, 181–187.

Monoamine oxidase inhibitors (MAOIs)[1]

- MAOIs are third-line antidepressants, used in refractory cases.
- The enzyme monoamine oxidase is present on mitochondrial membranes, where it deaminates (thereby inactivating) monoamine neurotransmitters in the cytoplasm. It has two isoenzymes, A and B.
- MAOA preferentially metabolises serotonin, noradrenaline and adrenaline, and predominates in the CNS.
- MAOB preferentially metabolises non-polar aromatic amines such as phenylethylamine and methylhistamine. It predominates in the liver, lungs, and non-neural cells. 75% of all MAO activity is due to MAOB.
- Tyramine (a noradrenaline precursor found in cheese and other foods) and dopamine are substrates for both A and B.
- Indirect sympathomimetics, which are metabolised by MAO, may have greatly exaggerated effects. They may displace noradrenaline from neurotransmitter vesicles in such high amounts that a fatal hypertensive crisis may be precipitated.
- Older drugs (**tranylcypromine, phenelzine, isocarboxazid**) bind covalently to the MAO enzyme and are non-selective for A or B. Regeneration of new enzyme takes 2–3wk.
- Newer drugs are reversible, and selective for MAOA: known as reversible inhibitors of monoamine oxidase A (**RIMA**). **Moclobemide** is the only RIMA available in the UK, and its use may be rising.
- **Linezolid** (antibacterial used in MRSA) is a non-selective but reversible MAOI: equal caution should be observed.
- **Selegiline** is an MAOB inhibitor used in Parkinson's disease.

Preoperative withdrawal

- If the patient is taking **moclobemide**, it can safely be omitted for 24hr preoperatively.
- If the patient is taking **tranylcypromine, phenelzine,** or **isocarboxazid**, ideally it must be stopped at least 2wk prior to surgery to be of benefit. This may provoke drastic relapses in symptoms and should not be done without consultation with a senior psychiatrist. If stopped for <2wk patients should be considered as still on MAOI.
- It is not necessary to stop **selegiline** if taken in doses of <10mg/d. At this dose there is no reaction with sympathomimetics. Pethidine, however, should still be avoided.

Anaesthesia for a patient on MAOI

- General anaesthesia can be undertaken with caution in patients who are taking an MAOI.
- The most dangerous interactions are with indirect sympathomimetics and some opioids (especially pethidine, which is absolutely contraindicated with any MAOI).
- Indirect sympathomimetics (ephedrine, metaraminol, amphetamine, cocaine, tyramine), which release stored noradrenaline from vesicles, may precipitate potentially fatal hypertensive crises and are absolutely contraindicated with any MAOI.

- **Direct sympathomimetics** (e.g. noradrenaline, adrenaline, phenylephrine, methoxamine, dopamine, dobutamine, isoprenaline) may have an exaggerated effect and should be used with caution.
- Treat hypotension initially with IV fluid, then cautious doses of phenylephrine (e.g. 10–20µg).
- There are two types of opioid interaction:
  - Type I ('excitatory'): drugs which inhibit serotonin re-uptake (including pethidine and dextromethorphan) may precipitate serotonin syndrome (see p273).
  - Type II ('depressive'): MAOIs can inhibit hepatic microsomal enzymes, prolonging the action of all opioids and enhancing their effect. This can be treated with naloxone.
- **Phenelzine** decreases plasma cholinesterase levels and prolongs the action of suxamethonium. This is specific to phenelzine and is not typical of MAOIs.
- Pancuronium releases stored noradrenaline and should be avoided.
- Safe drugs: induction agents propofol, thiopental, and etomidate; nondepolarising neuromuscular blocking drugs (except pancuronium); volatile agents and nitrous oxide; NSAIDs; benzodiazepines.
- Local anaesthetic drugs (except cocaine) are safe (caution if contain adrenaline). Axial and regional blocks are ideal; however, hypotension should be treated cautiously. Felypressin is a satisfactory alternative to adrenaline if a vasoconstrictor is required.
- Anticholinergic drugs (atropine, glycopyrronium) are considered to be safe.
- Morphine is the opioid of choice and should be titrated cautiously to effect. There is no direct evidence of problems with fentanyl, alfentanil, remifentanil, or sufentanil.

Drug interactions with MAOIs

Drugs to be avoided	Reason	Suitable alternative treatment
Pethidine, tramadol	Hyperpyrexia, hypotension/ hypertension, also risk of serotonin syndrome	Morphine, fentanyl
Ephedrine, metaraminol, cocaine	Severe hypertension	Phenylephrine, noradrenaline
Pancuronium	Releases stored noradrenaline	Vecuronium, atracurium
Suxamethonium	Phenelzine only (decreased cholinesterase activity)	Mivacurium, rocuronium

1 Luck JF, Wildsmith JAW, Christmas DMB (2003). Monoamine oxidase inhibitors and anaesthesia. *Royal College of Anaesthetists Bulletin*, **21**, 1029–1034.

Antipsychotic drugs and lithium

Antipsychotic drugs

- Formerly known as major tranquillisers or neuroleptics.
- Main action is antagonism at CNS dopamine (D_2) receptors.
- Most antagonise other receptors, including histamine (H_1), serotonin ($5HT_2$), acetylcholine (muscarinic), and α-adrenergic receptors.
- Main side effects include sedation, extrapyramidal motor disturbances, and the development of tardive dyskinesia with chronic use. Other side effects include gynaecomastia, weight gain, postural hypotension, antimuscarinic effects, obstructive jaundice (uncommon), and agranulocytosis (rare but severe).
- Many drugs prolong the QT interval, especially when combined with other drugs which may do the same (e.g. antidepressants).
- **Neuroleptic malignant syndrome** is a rare idiosyncratic reaction to antipsychotic drugs which resembles malignant hyperthermia (p260). Typical patients are young males. Features include hyperthermia, tachycardia, extrapyramidal dysfunction (rigidity, dystonia), and autonomic dysfunction (sweating, labile BP, salivation, urinary incontinence). CK and WCC are raised. Patients should be treated in ICU. Mortality is ~20%.
- Anaesthesia for a patient on antipsychotic medication:
  - Abrupt withdrawal of antipsychotic medication is dangerous.
  - Antipsychotic drugs potentiate sedative and hypotensive effects of anaesthetic agents (including opioids)—marked antiemetic action.

Lithium

- Inorganic ion used in treatment of bipolar affective disorder.
- Low therapeutic ratio, with optimal plasma concentration 0.4–1.0mmol/l.
- Mimics sodium in excitable tissues, being able to permeate voltage-gated ion channels, and accumulates inside cells, causing slight loss of intracellular potassium and partial depolarisation.
- Chronic use causes weight gain, renal impairment, and hypothyroidism.
- Lithium toxicity occurs at >1.5mmol/l. Toxicity is exacerbated by hyponatraemia, diuretic therapy, and renal disease. Features include lethargy/restlessness, nausea/vomiting, thirst, tremor, polyuria, renal failure, ataxia, convulsions, coma, and death. Haemodialysis is effective.
- Lithium potentiates both depolarising and nondepolarising neuromuscular blockade: nerve stimulator monitoring should be used (p992).
- Lithium may cause T wave flattening or inversion, but clinically important cardiovascular effects are rare.
- NSAIDs should be used with caution (risk of exacerbating renal impairment and causing toxicity).

Sedation of agitated patients on the ward

Anaesthetists may be asked to help with sedation of agitated patients on general wards, and are more likely to be familiar with effects of sedation than other junior medical or surgical staff.

- Patients are likely to be in an acute confusional state: exacerbated by pain, unfamiliar/threatening surroundings, and strangers. They may be disoriented, agitated, disinhibited, or violent, and may experience visual or auditory hallucinations.
- When presentation is acute in a previously lucid patient, the cause is usually organic. Establishing and treating the cause may remove the need for sedation.
- Exclude hypoglycaemia, hypoxia, pain, alcohol withdrawal, full bladder.
- Differential diagnosis includes infection (chest, urine, lines), drugs (cocaine, LSD, sedatives, analgesics), metabolic derangement (e.g. hyponatraemia). Less frequently: head injury, stroke, acute psychiatric disorder (e.g. mania), acute porphyria.

Approach to the patient

- Ensure the safety of yourself and other staff. A calm and reassuring approach will help the patient and any onlookers.
- If physical restraint is necessary, ensure plenty of help is available (hospital security, porters, or even police) and discuss with psychiatrist.
- Establish venous access if possible and bandage the cannula.
- Aim to render patient calm and cooperative rather than unconscious.

Drug therapy

- Haloperidol 5mg IV initially (reduce dose in elderly e.g. 1mg). Repeat after 5min if no effect. Titrate to effect. Maximum dose: 18mg/24hr according to BNF but higher doses are occasionally warranted.
- Midazolam 1–2mg IV may also be useful (titrate to effect). May cause paradoxical disinhibition, especially in the elderly.
- Alcohol withdrawal: give diazepam 5–10mg IV (or chlordiazepoxide 50mg PO) and repeat as required. Avoidance is better than treatment. A *small* amount of alcohol daily may prevent acute withdrawal. Clomethiazole and IV alcohol are no longer advised.
- Ketamine is useful in emergencies if patient is extremely violent or dangerous. Give 0.5–1mg/kg IV (or 5–10mg/kg IM).
- Do not use propofol (too short acting), opioids (respiratory depression), or drugs you may be unfamiliar with.
- In A&E, or where the history is unknown, further investigation (e.g. CT scan) may be appropriate. In this circumstance, rapid sequence induction of anaesthesia with full monitoring may be required.

Anaesthesia for drug-misusing patients

General considerations

- In the UK around 1 in 3 of the population aged over 16 have taken illegal drugs.
- Misuse of street drugs is common in all socio-economic groups.
- Consider drug misuse in all patients requiring emergency surgery and anaesthesia. An accurate drug history is unlikely to be forthcoming.
- Drug misuse may contribute to a reduced conscious level even if other causes are present (especially trauma).
- IV drug misuse is associated with IV infective complications. HIV and viral hepatitis are commonest. Bacterial endocarditis is rare but serious, and associated with pulmonary abscesses, embolic phenomena from vegetations, and vasculitis.
- Drugs in common use fall into four groups (see table). Combinations of drugs are common, often with alcohol.

Street drugs in common use

Drug	Clinical signs
Cannabis	Tachycardia, abnormal affect (e.g. euphoria, anxiety, panic, or psychosis), poor memory, fatigue
Stimulants: cocaine, amphetamines, ecstasy	Tachycardia, labile blood pressure, excitement, delirium, hallucinations, hyperreflexia, tremors, convulsions, mydriasis, sweating, hyperthermia, exhaustion, coma
Hallucinogens: LSD, phencyclidine, ketamine	Sympathomimetic, weakly analgesic, altered judgement and perceptions, toxic psychosis, dissociative anaesthesia
Opioids: morphine, heroin, opium	Euphoria, respiratory depression, hypotension, bradycardia, constipation pinpoint pupils, coma

Anaesthesia

- High index of suspicion—especially in trauma.
- Difficult venous access—IV drug users may be able to direct you to a patent vein. May need central venous cannulation or cut-down for relatively minor procedures. Consider gas induction.
- Take full precautions against infection risk.
- Plan postoperative analgesia with patient preoperatively (see below) .

Opioid-misusing patient

- Patients who are misusing opioids should expect the same quality of analgesia as other patients. Combinations of regional nerve blocks and NSAIDs may avoid the need for opioids.

- If opioids are the only method of providing analgesia they should be administered in the same way as for normal patients, with doses titrated to effect (large doses may be required—see p1044 for a suitable dosing regime).
- A small group of 'ex-addicts' will have fears about being prescribed opioids after addiction treatment. This should not become an obstacle to treating postoperative pain, but opioids should not be given without first obtaining consent.
- Opioid-addicted surgical patients should be supported by specialist addiction services during the perioperative period (usually contactable via the local psychiatric services).

Cocaine and crack cocaine

- Cocaine toxicity is mediated by central and peripheral adrenergic stimulation. Presenting symptoms include tachycardia, hypertension, aortic dissection, arrhythmias, accelerated coronary artery disease, coronary spasm, infarction, and sudden death. Intracerebral vasospasm can lead to stroke, rigidity, hyperreflexia, and hyperthermia. Inhalation of cocaine can cause alveolar haemorrhage or pulmonary oedema.
- Psychiatric symptoms range from elation and enhanced physical strength to full toxic paranoid psychosis.
- Patients needing surgery following ingestion of cocaine may need intensive care while they are stabilised. Most of the life-threatening side effects of cocaine are due to vasospasm and can be reversed using combinations of vasodilators, antiarrhythmic agents, and α/β-blockers titrated against effect using full invasive monitoring.
- Combination local anaesthetic/vasoconstrictors (or any vasopressor) should be avoided. Tachycardia or hypertensive crisis may result. If vasopressors are required in theatre use very small doses and titrate against response.
- Intra-arterial injections of cocaine have lead to critical limb and organ ischaemia. Successful treatment has included regional plexus blockade, IV heparin, stellate ganglion block, intra-arterial vasodilators or urokinase, and early fasciotomy.

Ecstasy (3,4-methylenedioxymethamphetamine (MDMA))

- Approximately 20 people die from taking ecstasy annually in the United Kingdom.
- Hyperthermia (>39°C), disseminated intravascular coagulation, and dehydration are common features.
- Excessive ADH release may also cause hyponatraemia leading to coma.
- Carefully monitor fluid and electrolyte replacement.

Anaesthesia for electroconvulsive therapy (ECT)

Procedure	Electrically-induced seizure
Time	5–10 min
Pain	+
Position	Supine
Blood loss	Nil
Practical technique	Short IV GA, FM only, bite block

General considerations
ECT is commonly carried out an isolated site: ensure skilled assistance and adequate resuscitation facilities. Anaesthetic equipment may be old or unfamiliar.

Physiological effects of ECT
- Immediately parasympathetic stimulation: bradycardia and hypotension, lasting about 15s, followed by a more prolonged (5min) sympathetic stimulation: tachycardia, hypertension, dysrhythmias, increased myocardial oxygen requirement.
- CNS: increased ICP, increased CBF, increased cerebral oxygen requirement.
- Other: hypersalivation, increased intragastric pressure, increased intraocular pressure.

Preoperative
- A careful preoperative assessment (including investigations) should be undertaken.
- Consent is normally arranged by the psychiatrist responsible.
- ECT is usually given several times weekly for several weeks: read the notes for documentation of previous problems.
- Absolute contraindications: recent MI or CVA, phaeochromocytoma, intracranial mass lesions, intracranial or aortic aneurysm.
- Relative contraindications: uncontrolled angina, congestive cardiac failure, severe osteoporosis, major bone fractures, glaucoma, retinal detachment.
- Avoid sedative premedication.
- Glycopyrronium (0.1–0.3mg IV) may be used to reduce secretions and to counteract bradycardia.

Perioperative
- Efficacy of ECT is dependent on the duration of seizure activity (ideally 25–50s).
- Good technique provides short GA, muscle relaxation to lessen risk of trauma, attenuation of physiological effects, and rapid recovery.

- Propofol is widely used for induction as it provides quick onset and offset with some attenuation of sympathetic response. (Thiopental, etomidate and ketamine have all been used with success). Inhalational sevoflurane is effective but takes longer. All general anaesthetics shorten the seizure in a dose-related fashion.
- Suxamethonium (0.5–1 mg/kg) is given to 'modify' the seizure (reduce muscle power to prevent injury during seizure). Mivacurium (0.2mg/kg) may be used instead, although it will probably require reversal.
- Insert a bite-block to prevent damage to the mouth and teeth.
- Maintain the airway with a facemask and oral airway. Hand-ventilate the patient with oxygen until breathing resumes.
- The psychiatrist may titrate the magnitude of the stimulus to the length of seizure: be prepared to maintain anaesthetic with further boluses of induction agent if a second shock is required.
- Sympathetic response may be attenuated with alfentanil (10µg/kg) or esmolol (e.g. 0.25mg/kg). Labetalol, sodium nitroprusside and hydralazine have also been used.
- Seizure augmentation: both caffeine and theophylline lower the seizure threshold and prolong seizures. Etomidate gives slightly longer seizures. Hyperventilation with bag and mask before the seizure is also effective.
- If the seizure lasts longer than 150–180s it should be terminated e.g. with diazepam 10mg IV.

Postoperative

- Post-ictal agitation, confusion, or aggression may occur in up to 10% of patients. They should be nursed in a calm environment and may require sedation (e.g. midazolam 1mg).
- Headache is commonly reported and usually responds to simple analgesics.
- Memory loss and cognitive impairment are very common but usually reversible.
- Other complications include nausea, exacerbation of ischaemic heart disease, fractures and dislocations, dental and oral injury, and laryngospasm.
- ECT does not increase risk of other types of seizure.
- Overall mortality is quoted as 0.02–0.04%.

Further Reading

Folk JW, Kellner CH, Beale MD, et al. (2000). Anesthesia for electroconvulsive therapy: A Review Journal of ECT 16, 157–170.

Tecoult E, Nathan N (2001). Morbidity in electroconvulsive therapy. European Journal of Anaesthesiology 18, 514–518.

Uncommon conditions

Graham Hocking

Aarskog–Scott syndrome

Cervical spine hypermobility/odontoid anomaly, mild/moderate short stature, cleft lip/palate, skin and skeletal anomalies/laxity, interstitial pulmonary disease, pectus excavatum, difficult intubation.[1]

Achalasia of the cardia

Motor disorder of the distal two-thirds of the oesophagus, failure of relaxation, dysphagia and regurgitation, risk of malignant change, increased risk of gastric reflux.[2]

Achondroplasia

Dwarfism, normal size trunk, short limbs, disproportionately large head, flat face, possible small larynx, bulging skull vault and kyphoscoliosis, spinal stenoses in the canal/foramen magnum can occur, difficult intubation, care on neck flexion (cord compression), central neural blocks may have unpredictable spread (use smaller amounts), increased risk of obstructive sleep apnoea.[3,4] (See also p195.)

Acromegaly

Enlarged jaw/tongue/larynx, nerve entrapment syndromes, respiratory obstruction including sleep apnoea, diabetes mellitus, hypertension, cardiac failure, thyroid, and renal impairment, difficult intubation and airway maintenance, possible narrow cricoid ring, associated organ dysfunction, perioperative glucose intolerance.[5] (See also p156.)

Alagille's syndrome (syndromic bile duct paucity)

Paucity of interlobular bile ducts, chronic cholestasis, cardiac/musculo-skeletal/ocular/facial abnormalities, coagulopathy, pathological fractures, neuropathies (vitamin deficiencies), retinopathy, pretreat with vitamin K, splenomegaly may cause thrombocytopenia, CVS assessment (stenosis/hypoplasia common), sagittal spinal cleft, cerebellar ataxia, document pre-existing peripheral neuropathy, gastric reflux risk (abdominal distension).[6]

Albers–Schönberg disease (marble bones), see osteopetrosis

Albright's osteodystrophy (pseudohypoparathyroidism type 1a)

Resistance of target tissues to parathyroid hormone, short stature, round face, short neck, diabetes mellitus, hypocalcaemia, neuromuscular irritability, convulsions.

Albright's syndrome (McCune-Albright syndrome)

Defective regulation of cAMP, multiple unilateral bone lesions, skin pigmentation, sexual precocity in females, bony deformity (including skull) and fractures, spinal cord compression, acromegaly, thyrotoxicosis, Cushing's syndrome may coexist, identify endocrine abnormalities, may need larger than expected ETT, cardiac arrhythmias may occur, bony deformity may complicate regional blocks.[7]

Alport syndrome

Hereditary nephropathy, predominantly affecting males, characterised by nephritis progressing to renal failure, sensorineural deafness, myopia, and thrombocytopenia with giant forms of platelets, check renal function and clotting, hypertension.[8]

Alstrom syndrome

Obesity from infancy, nystagmus, sensitivity to light, progressive visual impairment with blindness by age 7, sensorineural hearing loss, diabetes mellitus and renal failure in early adult life, cardiac disease, problems associated with obesity/organ dysfunction.[9]

Alveolar hypoventilation

Central hypoventilation due to midbrain lesion or severance of the spinal tracts from the midbrain (Ondine's curse), periods of prolonged apnoea, hypoxia, hypercarbia, abnormal respiratory drive, care with O_2 supplements if relying on hypoxic drive, re-establishing spontaneous ventilation may be difficult, consider regional techniques, postoperative respiratory failure, cor pulmonale, polycythaemia, autonomic dysfunction.[10,11]

Amyloidosis

Abnormal deposition of hyaline material in tissues, macroglossia, beware laryngeal amyloid, unexpected cardiac or renal failure can occur, associated with other pathologies, assess to detect systems affected, risk of postoperative organ failure.[12]

Amyotonia congenita, see spinal muscular atrophy

Amyotrophic lateral sclerosis

Progressive degeneration of lower motor neurons, motor nuclei of the brainstem, descending pathway of the upper motor neurons, atrophy and weakness involving most of the skeletal muscles including tongue, pharynx, larynx, and chest wall muscles, fasciculation occurs, sensation normal, impaired ventilation, altered response to muscle relaxants, aspiration risk (laryngeal incompetence), sensitive to respiratory depressants.[13,14]

1 Teebi AS et al. (1993). Am J Med Genet, **46**, 501–509.
2 Hay H (2001). Eur J Anaesthesiol, **17**, 398–400.
3 Krishnan BS et al. (2003). Paediatr Anaesth, **13**, 547–549.
4 Wardall GJ, Frame WT (1990). Br J Anaes, **64**, 367–370.
5 Seidman PA et al. (2000). Br J Anaes, **84**, 179–182.
6 Choudhry DK et al. (1998). Paed Anaesth, **8**, 79–82.
7 Langer RA et al. (1995). Anesth Analg, **80**, 1236–1239.
8 Kashtan CE et al. (1999). Medicine, **78**, 338–360.
9 Russell-Eggitt LM et al. (1998). Ophthalmology, **105**, 1274–1280.
10 Wiesel S, Fox GS (1990). Can J Anaesth, **37**, 122–126.
11 Strauser LM et al. (1999). J Clin Anesth, **11**, 431–437.
12 Noguchi T et al. (1999). J Clin Anesth, **11**, 339–341.
13 Rowland LP, Schneider NA (2001). N Engl J Med, **344**, 1688–1700.
14 Mishima Y et al. (2002). Masui, **51**, 762–764.

Analbuminaemia
Deficiency of albumin. Sensitivity to all protein-bound drugs, titrate drugs carefully.[1]

Andersen's disease, see glycogenoses, type IV

Andersen's syndrome
Triad of potassium-sensitive periodic paralysis/ventricular arrhythmias/dysmorphic features, long QT, spontaneous attacks of paralysis with acute K^+ changes, baseline level may be hypokalaemia/ normokalaemia/ hyperkalaemia.[2]

Anhidrotic/hypohidrotic ectodermal dysplasia (Christ–Siemens–Touraine syndrome)
Characterised by hypodontia, hypotrichosis, and hypohidrosis, difficult intubation, heat intolerance, recurrent chest infections (poor mucus formation).[3]

Ankylosing spondylitis
Asymmetric oligoarthropathy, total vertebral involvement, cardiomegaly, aortic regurgitation, cardiac conduction abnormalities, pulmonary fibrosis, bamboo spine, difficult airway, and central neural blockade.[4,5] (See also p190.)

Antley–Bixler syndrome
Autosomal recessive disorder, multiple bone and cartilaginous abnormalities, significant craniosynostosis, midface hypoplasia, choanal stenosis/atresia, femoral bowing, radiohumeral synostosis, multiple joint contractures, CVS/Renal/GI malformations, potential difficult airway, extremity deformities may complicate vascular access and positioning.[6]

Apert's syndrome
Craniosynostosis, high forehead, maxillary hypoplasia, relative mandibular prognathism, cervical synostosis, visceral malformations, congenital heart anomalies, airway difficulties, perioperative respiratory problems (especially wheezing), assess for other organ involvement and raised ICP.[7]

Arnold–Chiari malformation
Group of congenital hindbrain anomalies causing downward displacement of pons and medulla with variable neurological sequelae, preoperative assessment of CNS function and response to neck movement and ICP, careful neuroanaesthetic (usual potential problems).[8]

Arthrogryposis (congenital contractures)
Skin and SC tissue abnormalities, contracture deformities, micrognathia, cervical spine and jaw stiffness, congenital heart disease (10%), difficult airway and venous access, sensitive to thiopental, hypermetabolic response is probably not MH.[9,10]

Asplenia syndrome

Complex congenital heart defects, asplenia, visceral anomalies, cardiac failure, hiatus hernia/reflux, recurrent pneumonias.[11]

Ataxia-telangiectasia

Progressive cerebellar ataxia, conjunctival telangiectasia, progressive neurological degeneration, recurrent chest and sinus infections, bronchiectasis, malignancies (leukaemias), sensitive to X-rays/radiotherapy (cellular damage), premature ageing.[12]

Axenfeld–Rieger syndrome

Ocular and dental defects, maxillary hypoplasia, heart defects, short stature, mental deficiency, airway problems.[13]

Bardet–Biedl syndrome, see also Laurence–Moon syndrome

Obesity, retinitis pigmentosa, polydactyly, mental retardation, hypogonadism, renal failure.[14]

Bartter syndrome

Growth retardation, hypertrophy and hyperplasia of the juxtaglomerular apparatus, ADH antagonism by protaglandins, hyperaldosteronism, hypokalaemic alkalosis, normal BP, diminished response to vasopressors, platelet abnormalities, maintain CVS stability, control serum K^+, meticulous fluid balance, caution with renally excreted drugs, central neural anaesthesia may be hazardous (stature, clotting, pressor response).[15]

Beckwith–Wiedemann syndrome (infantile gigantism)

Macroglossia, microcephaly, omphalocele, perinatal/postnatal gigantism, neonatal hypoglycaemia (hyperinsulinism), possible congenital heart disease (ASD/VSD/PDA/hypoplastic LV), abnormal airway anatomy, congenital heart disease, and severe hypoglycaemia, extubate awake.[16,17]

1 Koot BG (2004). *Eur J Pediatr*, **163**, 664–670.
2 Sansone V *et al.* (1997). *Ann Neurol*, **42**, 305–312.
3 Sugi Y *et al.* (2001). *Can J Anaesth*, **43**, 105–1019.
4 Schelew BL, Vaghadia H (1996). *Can J Anaesth*, **43**, 65–68.
5 Lu PP *et al.* (2001). *Can J Anaesth*, **48**, 1015–1019.
6 LeBard SE, Thiemann LJ (1998). *Paed Anaesth*, **8**, 89–91.
7 Elwood T *et al.* (2001). *Paed Anaesth*, **11**, 701–703.
8 Semple DA, McClure JH (1996). *Anaesthesia*, **51**, 580–582.
9 Hopkins PM *et al.* (1991). *Anaesthesia*, **46**, 374–375.
10 Nguyen NH *et al.* (2000). *J Clin Anesth*, **12**, 227–230.
11 Uchida K *et al.* (1992). *Masui*, **41**, 1793–1797.
12 Gatti RA *et al.* (1991). *Medicine*, **70**, 99–117.
13 Asai T *et al.* (1998). *Paediatr Anaesth*, **8**, 444.
14 Puebla G *et al.* (2001). Rev Esp Anestesiol Reanim, **48**, 99–100.
15 Abston PA, Priano LL (1981). *Anesth Analg*, **60**, 764–766.
16 Suan C *et al.* (1996). *Paediatr Anaesth*, **6**, 231–233.
17 Gurkowski MA *et al.* (1989). *Anesthesiology*, **70**, 711–712.

Behçet's syndrome

Chronic multisystem vasculitis of unknown aetiology, triad of recurring iritis/mouth ulceration/genital ulceration, vasculitis may involve other organ systems, possible altered fibrinolysis, previous oral ulceration/ scarring may complicate airway management, fully assess other organ function, minimise needle punctures (diffuse inflammatory skin reaction), autonomic hyper-reflexia may occur with spinal cord involvement.[1]

Bernard–Soulier syndrome (giant platelet syndrome)

Congenital lack of membrane glycoprotein GP1b, reduced number of huge platelets, prolonged bleeding time, severe bleeding tendency, possibly improves with age, platelet infusions may be needed.

Blackfan–Diamond syndrome (congenital red-cell aplasia)

Congenital hypoplastic anaemia, growth retardation, congestive cardiac failure, hepatosplenomegaly (may reduce FRC), hypersplenism, thrombocytopenia.[2]

Bland–White–Garland syndrome

Anomalous origin of left coronary artery from pulmonary trunk, chronic myocardial ischaemia/subendocardial fibrosis/LV dilation/valvular insufficiency (papillary muscle damage), congestive cardiac failure, perioperative myocardial failure, often difficult to wean ventilation.[3]

Bloom's syndrome

Rare autosomal recessive disorder, chromosome breakage/ recombination, short stature, photosensitive, facial telangiectasic erythema, predisposition to malignant diseases, potential difficulties with mask fit and laryngoscopy, limit X-rays (may damage cells).[4]

Brugada syndrome

Abnormal human cardiac sodium channel, right bundle branch block/ST elevation in leads V1–3/sudden death from VF (up to 1 in 1000 young SE Asian males), normal cardiac anatomy, tachyarrhythmias not responsive to medical therapy—may have implantable cardioverter defibrillator if pre-existing syncope (requires usual care during surgery), treat intra-operative tachyarrhythmias by cardioversion, avoid neostigmine (worsens ST elevation—risk of VT/VF), safety of techniques needing high doses of local anaesthetics not yet tested, spinal anaesthesia appears safe.[5]

Buerger's disease (thromboangiitis obliterans)

Peripheral vascular disease with ulceration, Raynaud's phenomenon, hyperhidrosis, bronchitis and emphysema, non-invasive BP may over-read.

Bullous cystic lung disease

Non-communicating lung cysts may be more compliant than normal lung, risk of pneumothorax with IPPV, avoid N_2O, high-frequency jet ventilation used successfully.[6]

Burkitt's lymphoma

Undifferentiated lymphoblastic lymphoma most commonly affecting the jaw (also abdominal organs/breasts/testes), difficult intubation.[7]

Cantrell's pentalogy

Defect of supraumbilical abdominal wall, agenesis of lower part of sternum/anterior portion of diaphragm, absence of diaphragmatic part of pericardium, cardiac malformation (VSD/ASD), check for right-to-left shunting, avoid pressure to lower thorax/abdomen, hypoplastic lungs.[8]

Carpenter's syndrome

Cranial synostosis, small mandible, congenital heart disease (PDA/VSD), obesity, umbilical hernia and mental retardation, cerebrospinal malformations (narrowed foramen magnum, hypoplastic posterior fossa, kinked spinal cord), difficult intubation, system anomalies.[9]

Central core disease, see congenital myopathy

Cerebrocostomandibular syndrome

Micrognathia, cleft palate, rib defects/microthorax, mental deficiency, early death from respiratory complications, difficult intubation, tracheal anomalies.[10]

Chagas' disease (American trypanosomiasis)

Many asymptomatic, malaise, anorexia, fever, unilateral oedema, hepatomegaly, cardiac failure, chronic myocarditis, mega-colon/mega-oesophagus, gastric reflux risk, and associated organ dysfunction.[11]

Charcot–Marie–Tooth disease (peroneal muscular atrophy)

Chronic peripheral neuromuscular denervation/atrophy, spinal/lower limb deformities, hyperkalaemia, may affect respiratory muscles (restrictive pattern), evidence suggests low MH risk, avoid suxamethonium, pulmonary complications.[12]

CHARGE association

Coloboma/Heart anomaly/choanal Atresia/Retardation/Genital/Ear anomalies, difficult intubation (micrognathia).[13]

Chediak–Higashi syndrome (immunodeficiency, with some albinism)

Albinism, photophobia, nystagmus, weakness, tremor, thrombocytopenia, susceptible to infection.[14]

1 Turkoz A et al. (2001). J Cardiothorac Vasc Anesth, **16**, 468–470.
2 Willig TN et al. (2000). Curr Opin Hematol, **7**, 85–94.
3 Kleinschmidt S et al. (1996). Paediatr Anaesth, **6**, 65–68.
4 Aono J et al. (1992). Masui, **41**, 255–257.
5 Kim JS et al. (2004). Acta Anaesthesiol Scand, **48**, 1058–1061.
6 Normandale JP et al. (1985). Anaesthesia, **40**, 1182–1185.
7 Palmer CD et al. (1998). Paediatr Anaesth, **8**, 506–509.
8 Laloyaux P et al. (1998). Paediatr Anaesth, **8**, 163–166.
9 Islek I et al. (1998). Clin Dysmorphol, **7**, 185–189.
10 Smith KG, Sekar KC (1985). Clin Pediatr (Phila), **24**, 223–225.
11 Saraiva RA et al. (1980). Trop Doct, **10**, 62–65.
12 Antognini JF (1992). Can J Anaesth, **39**, 398–400.
13 Davenport SLH et al. (1986). Clin Genet, **29**, 298–310.
14 Ulsoy H et al. (1995). Middle East J Anesthesiol, **13**, 101–105.

Cherubism

Tumourous mandibular and maxillary lesions, intraoral masses, difficult intubation, profuse bleeding, may develop acute respiratory distress, tracheostomy may be needed.[1]

Chronic granulomatous disease

Rare genetically transmitted disorder, recurrent life-threatening infections with catalase-positive micro-organisms, excessive inflammatory reactions, granuloma formation, multiple organ system involvement including pulmonary granulomata, regurgitation/aspiration risk (GI granulomata), long-term prophylactic antibiotics.[2]

Cockayne's syndrome

Rare autosomal recessive condition, failure of DNA repair, dysmorphic dwarf, mentally retarded infant/child, airway management problems, increased risk of gastric aspiration, hypertension, hepatic deficiencies, osteoporosis, deafness, blindness, other effects of premature ageing (see progeria).[3]

Congenital adrenal hyperplasia (adrenogenital syndrome)

Congenital disorders leading to defects in cortisol biosynthesis, increased ACTH, disordered androgens, may mimic pyloric stenosis in neonate, electrolyte abnormalities, adequate perioperative fluid/steroid therapy.

Congenital analgesia

Rare hereditary disorder leading to self-mutilation, defective thermoregulation, careful positioning, vasomotor control and possible sensitivity to anaesthetic drugs.[4]

Congenital myopathy (central core disease) (see also p260)

Non-progressive extremity weakness (lower > upper), difficulty rising from sitting, increased lumbar lordosis, ptosis, most test positive for MH *in vitro*, avoid trigger factors, ventilatory weakness, sensitive to muscle relaxants.[5,6]

Conradi–Hunermann syndrome (chondrodysplasia punctata)

Epiphyseal calcifications, short stature, hypertelorism, saddle nose, short neck, tracheal stenosis and scoliosis, renal and congenital heart disease, ventilatory failure due to airway and thoracic deformities, renal impairment, skin protection (use patient's creams/padding), attention to thermoregulation (lose heat quicker).[7]

Cornelia de Lange syndrome

Duplication/partial trisomy chromosome 3, psychomotor retardation, skeletal craniofacial deformities, VSD, GI anomalies, assess cardiorespiratory function, possible difficult airway, gastric reflux risk, susceptible to infections.[8]

Costello syndrome

Mental and growth retardation, potential airway difficulties (short neck, macroglossia, hypertrophied tonsillar/supraglottic tissues, laryngeal papillomata, choanal atresia), cardiac arrhythmias, hypertrophic cardiomyopathy, talipes, scoliosis, gastric reflux, arrhythmias.[9]

CREST syndrome

Form of scleroderma, widespread necrotising angiitis with granulomata, Calcinosis/Raynaud's phenomenon/oEsophageal dysfunction/Sclerodactyly/Telangiectasia, multiple organ involvement, airway difficulties, gastric reflux risk, arrhythmias, nerve compression syndromes, contractures, pulmonary fibrosis.

Cretinism

Congenital hypothyroidism, neurological and intellectual damage, muscle weakness, cardiomyopathy, intubation problems (macroglossia), sensitive to anaesthetic drugs, respiratory complications, steroid cover, glucose and electrolyte abnormalities.

Creutzfeldt–Jacob disease (CJD)

One of the transmissible spongiform encephalopathies, progressive fatal encephalopathy, responsible for recent changes in surgery/anaesthesia relating to re-use/sterilisation of equipment, four types: *sporadic CJD* (85–90% cases, older patients, rapidly progressive over few months); *familial CJD* (5–10%, due to gene mutation); *iatrogenic CJD* (<5%, transmission from surgical instruments/implants/growth hormone); *variant CJD* (young patients, slowly progressive 1–2yr); caused by prions (small proteinaceous infectious particles resistant to inactivation—contain abnormal isoform of a cellular protein), highest concentration in CNS/eye/lymphoid tissue, progressive neurological signs—psychiatric symptoms/altered sensation/visual loss/ ataxia/weakness/involuntary movements/cognitive impairment/aphasia, involve staff from communicable diseases, follow protocols for handling fluids/waste, remove unnecessary equipment/staff from theatre, universal precautions, consider antisialogue to reduce secretions, portable suction to stay with patient throughout entire theatre visit/recovery, consider recovering in theatre—send directly back to ward, quarantine all used equipment (ventilator etc.), use disposable equipment where possible, bipolar diathermy plume may contain inhalable prions (monopolar better), warn laboratory staff.[10]

1 Maydew RP et al. (1985). Anesthesiology, **62**, 810–812.
2 Wall RT et al. (1990). J Clin Anesth, **2**, 306–311.
3 Wooldridge WJ et al. (1996). Anaesthesia, **51**, 478–481.
4 Nagasako EM et al. (2003). Pain, **101**, 213–219.
5 Johi RR et al. (2003). Br J Anaesth, **91**, 744–747.
6 Farbu E et al. (2003). Acta Anaesthesiol Scand, **47**, 630–634.
7 Pandit JJ, Evans FE (1996). Anaesthesia, **51**, 992–993.
8 Corsini LM et al. (1998). Paediatr Anaesth, **8**, 159–161.
9 Katcher K et al. (2003). Paediatr Anaesth, **13**, 257–262.
10 Farling P et al. (2003). Anaesthesia, **58**, 627–629.

Cri-du-chat syndrome

Inherited disease resulting in mental retardation, abnormal cry (due to abnormal larynx), laryngomalacia, microcephaly, micrognathia, macroglossia, spasticity, congenital heart disease (30%), potential airway problems, long curved epiglottis, narrow diamond-shaped epiglottis, hypotonia (possible airway obstruction by soft tissues), temperature instability.[1]

Crouzon's disease

Craniosynostosis, hydrocephalus, raised ICP, maxillary hypoplasia, mandibular prognathism, prominent nose, coarctation, airway difficulty, postoperative respiratory obstruction, assess other organ involvement/ICP, correction procedures can bleed profusely.[2]

Cutis laxa (elastic degeneration)

Defective elastin cross-linking probably related to copper deficiency, extreme laxity of facial and trunk skin, no retraction after stretching, fragile skin and blood vessels, pendulous pharyngeal/laryngeal mucosa may obstruct airway, respiratory infections and emphysema common, careful positioning.

Cystic hygroma

Benign multilocular lymphatic tumour of neck/oral cavity/tongue causing local pressure symptoms, including airway compromise, potential airway problems, partially obstructed airway in awake patient may totally obstruct on induction, oral intubation often impossible (enlarged tongue), tracheostomy complicated with sub-mandibular involvement.[3]

Dandy–Walker syndrome

Congenital obstruction to foramina of Luschka/Magendi, progressive head enlargement, hydrocephalus, craniofacial abnormalities, cardiac/renal/skeletal malformations, altered medullary respiratory control, usually require CSF shunt, control ICP, risk of respiratory failure, postoperatively consider ICU (recurrent apnoea).[4]

Delleman syndrome (oculocerebrocutaneous syndrome)

Somatic mutation of autosomal dominant gene only compatible with life in mosaic form, multiple brain/skin/eye/bony abnormalities, seizures can occur under general anaesthesia (seen as unexplained autonomic changes), aspiration pneumonitis, hydrocephalus, vertebral anomalies, difficult intubation, postoperative apnoea monitoring.[5]

Dermatomyositis (polymyositis)

Inflammatory myopathy, skeletal muscle weakness may result in dysphagia/recurrent pneumonia/aspiration, myocarditis, occult cancer, restricted mouth opening, enhanced/delayed effect of muscle relaxant, cardiomyopathy (arrhythmias and cardiac failure), anaemia, steroid supplementation.[6]

DiGeorge syndrome (velocardiofacial syndrome 'CATCH 22' syndrome)

Cardiac abnormalities/Abnormal facies/Thymic hypoplasia/Cleft palate/Hypocalcaemia/chromosome 22 affected, immune deficiency, recurrent chest infections, upper airway problems/stridor, obstructive apnoea, hyperventilation-induced seizures (low calcium), gastro-oesophageal reflux, hypotonia.[7]

Down's syndrome

Commonest congenital abnormality (1.6 per 1000), higher morbidity and mortality, characteristic dysmorphic features, impaired global development, congenital cardiac defects (40%—predominantly endocardial cushion defects/VSD), Eisenmenger's syndrome (especially if there is associated obstructive sleep apnoea), recurrent respiratory tract infection (relative immune deficiency and a degree of upper airway obstruction from tonsillar/adenoidal hypertrophy), atlantoaxial instability (30% but frequently asymptomatic—routine X-ray not indicated), epilepsy (10%), obesity and potentially difficult venous access, hypothyroidism (40%), careful airway assessment (relatively large tongue, crowding of midfacial structures, high arched narrow palate, micrognathia, short broad neck), careful cardiorespiratory assessment (including investigation) as indicated—beware asymptomatic disease, optimise where possible, reduced threshold for postoperative HDU/ICU, often uncooperative (sedative premed often helpful—caution if airway obstruction), drying agents useful if hypersalivation (caution—?exaggerated sensitivity to mydriatic/cardiac effects of atropine), high incidence gastro-oesophageal reflux, avoid excessive neck movement, prone to hypoventilation—consider IPPV, postoperative pain management may be problematic (consider regional blocks/LA, PCA possible in selected patients), parents/carers often indispensable in managing postoperative agitation, hypotonia (up to 75%) may compromise airway maintenance, prone to atelectasis/respiratory tract infections—consider humidified oxygen/physiotherapy.[8]

Dubowitz syndrome

Retarded growth, microcephaly, craniofacial deformations, difficult intubation, dysmorphia of the extremities, psychomotor development varies between normal and retarded, thin hair, cryptorchism, hyperactivity, thorough assessment required since the condition may involve the cutaneous, ocular, dental, digestive, musculoskeletal, urogenital, cardiovascular, neurological, haematological, and immune systems.[9]

1 Brislin RP et al. (1995). Paediatr Anaesth, **5**, 139–141.
2 Payne JF, Cranston AJ (1995). Paediatr Anaesth, **5**, 331–333.
3 Sharma S et al. (1994). Singapore Med J, **35**, 529–531.
4 Ewart MC, Oh TE (1990). Anaesthesia, **45**, 646–648.
5 Sadhasivam S, Subramaniam R (1998). Anesth Analg, **87**, 553–555.
6 Ganta R et al. (1988). Br J Anaesth, **60**, 854–858.
7 Flashburg MH et al. (1983). Anesthesiology, **58**, 479–481.
8 Borland LM et al. (2004). Paediatr Anaesth, **14**, 733–738.
9 Tsukahara M, Opitz JM (1996). Am J Med Genet, **63**, 277–289.

Dwarfism

Manifestation of over 55 syndromes, disproportionate short stature (cf. 'midgets'—proportionate), atlantoaxial instability, spinal stenosis and/or compression, difficult airway management, thoracic dystrophy (ventilatory problem/frequent pneumonia), scoliosis/kyphoscoliosis, congenital cardiac disease, evaluate and protect the cervical spine, document pre-existing neurological deficit if central blockade considered.

Dyggve–Melchior–Clausen syndrome

Autosomal recessive, mental retardation, small stature (short vertebral column) thoracic kyphosis, protruding sternum, reduced articular mobility, microcephaly, difficult intubation.[1]

Dysautonomia (Riley–Day syndrome)

Inherited disease, abnormally active parasympathetic nervous system/sporadic sympathetic storms, highly emotional, unexplained BP fluctuations, autonomic instability, salivation, poor thermoregulation, bouts of sweating, regurgitation, sensitivity to respiratory depressants with reduced hypercapnic drive (need IPPV), reduced pain sensitivity, volatile agents can cause hypotension and bradycardia.[2,3]

Eaton–Lambert syndrome, see myasthenic syndrome (also p248).

Ebstein's abnormality (tricuspid valve disease)

Congenital heart defect, downward displacement of deformed tricuspid valve, atrialisation of RV, may be no obvious clinical signs, risk of SVT during induction.[4]

Edward's syndrome (trisomy 18)

Craniofacial anomalies, congenital heart disease, mental/physical delays, pain assessment difficult, only less severe cases survive.[5]

Ehlers–Danlos syndrome

Group of conditions with defective collagen cross-linking, variable features depending upon the tissue distribution of different collagens, extensible fragile skin, joint laxity/hypermobility, recurrent dislocations, prolonged/spontaneous bleeding, rupture of cerebral/other vessels, bowel perforation, ocular abnormalities, kyphoscoliosis, spontaneous pneumothorax, careful positioning/padding, beware undiagnosed pneumothorax, intubation may cause severe tracheal bruising.[6]

Eisenmenger's syndrome (pulmonary hypertension, VSD, right ventricular failure) (see also p72)

Cyanotic congenital heart disease, usually uncorrectable, pulmonary hypertension/VSD/RV failure, medical therapy may prolong life (thirties), high mortality in pregnant patients due to reductions in SVR and increased shunt (termination has been advocated), prevent increases in right-to-left shunt (caused by e.g. increased PVR/reduced SVR from volatiles/histamine release, etc.), avoid dehydration, consider pancuronium (sympathetic stimulation beneficial), air from infusions/syringes can cross VSD, risk of asystole under GA, slow equilibration of inhaled gases.[7]

Ellis–Van Creveld disease (chondroectodermal dysplasia)
Dwarfism, pulmonary/cardiac abnormalities (ASD/VSD/single atrium), polydactyly, underlying anomalies, respiratory failure.[8]

Epidermolysis bullosa
Rare autosomal recessive, extreme bullae formation of skin and mucosa, typical dystrophic nails, flexion contractures/deformities, carious teeth/ small mouth caused by scarred lip contractures are characteristic, avoid skin/mucous membrane trauma (e.g. care with positioning, electrodes, tape, padding below BP cuff, longest acceptable inflation interval), shearing force worse than direct pressure, lubricate everything well, keep upper airway manipulations to a minimum, consider postoperative ICU.[9]

Erythema multiforme
Acute self-limiting condition of skin and mucous membranes, concentric rings of erythematous papules/bullae (epidermal necrosis), severe cases can be fatal (Stevens–Johnson syndrome), beware postintubation laryngeal oedema, consider drug-related cause.

Fabry syndrome
α-Galactosidase deficiency, deposition of glycosphingolipid in many organs, ischaemic heart disease, neurological disorder, renal failure, hypohidrosis, assess CVS/CNS/renal, document any neurological deficit prior to regional techniques, monitor/control core temperature.[10]

Factor V Leiden mutation
Resistance to anticoagulant effect of protein C, high risk of PE, careful control of anticoagulation.

Familial dysautonomia, see dysautonomia

Familial periodic paralysis, see also hypokalaemic familial periodic paralysis.
Muscular weakness related to K^+ changes (absolute K^+ value is not important).

Fanconi's anaemia
Congenital aplastic anaemia, defective DNA regeneration, limit exposure to X-rays (sensitive).

1 Eguchi M et al. (2001). *Masui*, **50**, 116–117.
2 Axelrod FB et al. (1988). *Anaesthesiology*, **68**, 631–635.
3 Challands JF, Facer EK (1998). *Paediatr Anaesth*, **8**, 83–88.
4 Takahashi K et al. (1992). *Masui*, **41**, 1163–1167.
5 Courreges P et al. (2003). *Paediatr Anaesth*, **13**, 267–269.
6 Campbell N, Rosaeg OP (2002). *Can J Anaesth*, **49**, 493–496.
7 Lovell AT (2004). *Br J Anaesth*, **93**, 129–139.
8 Wu CL, Litman RS (1994). *Paediatr Anaesth*, **4**, 335–337.
9 Herod J et al. (2002). *Paediatr Anaesth*, **12**, 388–397.
10 Watanabe H (1995). *Masui*, **44**, 1258–1260.

Fanconi syndrome (renal tubular acidosis)

Generalised defect in proximal tubular function, phosphate wasting, glycosuria, aminoaciduria, bicarbonate wasting, excess potassium loss, polydipsia, polyuria, muscle weakness, acidosis, dwarfing, osteomalacia, usually secondary to other disease, correct/maintain careful fluid/electrolyte balance.[1]

Farber's disease (lipogranulomatosis)

Ceramidase deficiency, hoarse cry, painful swollen joints, periarticular nodules, pulmonary infiltrates, mental handicap, thickened heart valves, cardiomyopathy, renal/hepatic failure, usually die by 2yr (airway problems), difficult intubation, laryngeal granulomata may complicate intubation, postextubation laryngeal oedema/bleeding, risk of postoperative renal/hepatic failure, anatomical neck deformity may complicate urgent tracheostomy.[2]

Felty's syndrome

Hypersplenism in rheumatoid arthritis, pancytopenia, haemolysis due to red cell sequestration, increased plasma volume. (See also p186.)

Fibrodysplasia ossificans

Progressive bony infiltration of tendons/muscles/fascia/aponeuroses leading to joint ankylosis throughout the body, permanent ankylosis of the jaw may follow minimal soft tissue trauma, intubation difficulties, atlantoaxial subluxation possible, restrictive pulmonary disease, cardiac conduction abnormalities.[3]

Fibromatosis (including juvenile and hyaline forms)

Large cutaneous nodules (especially head/neck/lips), joint contractures, gingival hypertrophy, osteolytic lesions, potential airway problems.[4]

Fraser syndrome (cryptophthalmos—'hidden eye')

Cryptophthalmos, laryngeal atresia/hypoplasia, fixed posterior arytenoids, cleft lip/palate, airway problems, genitourinary abnormalities, possible congenital heart disease/neurological abnormalities.[5]

Freeman–Sheldon (craniocarpotarsal dysplasia or 'whistling face') syndrome

Progressive congenital myopathy, multiple deformities of face/hands/feet, microstomia with pursed lips, difficult intubation (micrognathia/neck rigidity/anterior larynx), postoperative respiratory complications, difficult venous access, possible MH risk.[6]

Friedreich's ataxia

Autosomal recessive progressive ataxia with additional myopathy, myocardial degeneration with failure/arrhythmias, respiratory failure, diabetes, peripheral neuropathy, ?suxamethonium sensitivity—not supported by the evidence.[7]

Gaisbock's syndrome

Relative polycythaemia due to decreased plasma volume in middle-aged obese smoking hypertensive men, arterial thrombotic risk, myocardial/cerebral ischaemia, consider venesection to normal haematocrit.

Gardner's syndrome (familial polyposis coli)

Multiple colonic polyps (risk of malignant change), soft tissue tumours, osseous neoplasms, possible laryngeal polyps.

Gaucher's disease

Autosomal recessive disorder of lipid catabolism, end-organ dysfunction from glycosphingolipid accumulation, three variants differ in onset/CNS involvement, seizures, gastro-oesophageal reflux, chronic aspiration, possible upper airway obstruction (bulbar involvement/infiltration of upper airway), hypersplenism, thrombocytopenia, anaemia.[8,9]

Gilbert's disease

Asymptomatic familial unconjugated non-haemolytic hyperbilirubinaemia, perioperative jaundice may be precipitated by stress/surgery/starvation.[10]

Glanzmann's disease (thrombasthenia)

Lack of membrane protein GPIIb and GPIIIa, normal number/sized platelets, no clot retraction, defective aggregation, moderately severe bleeding diathesis, platelet transfusions sometimes ineffective due to antiplatelet antibodies.[11]

Glomus jugulare tumours

Highly vascular benign tumour of glomus body, invades locally, may affect cranial nerves (progressive deafness/tinnitus), sudden severe haemorrhage during excision (?hypotensive technique), may need to sacrifice local structures (carotid etc.), consider cerebral protection measures.[12,13]

Glucagonoma

Rare tumour of pancreatic islet α cells, marked increases in blood glucagons/glucose levels, potential significant metabolic/myocardial dysfunction, control blood glucose—large amounts of glucagon can be released during tumour handling, careful evaluation of nutrition/fluid/electrolytes, thromboembolic prophylaxis.[14] (See also p172.)

1 Joel M, Rosales JK (1981). *Anesthesiology*, **55**, 455–456.
2 Asada A et al. (1994). *Anesthesiology*, **80**, 206–209.
3 Singh A et al. (2003). *J Clin Anesth*, **15**, 211–213.
4 Norman B et al. (1996).*Br J Anaesth*, **76**, 163–166.
5 Jagtap SR et al. (1995). *Anaesthesia*, **50**, 39–41.
6 Munro HM et al. (1997). *Paediatr Anaesth*, **7**, 345–348.
7 Bell CF et al. (1986). *Anaesthesia*, **41**, 296–301.
8 Kita T et al. (1998). *Masui*, **47**, 69–73.
9 Tobias JD et al. (1993). *J Clin Anesth*, **5**, 150–153.
10 Taylor S (1984). *Anaesthesia*, **39**, 1222–1224.
11 Monte S, Lyons G (2002). *Br J Anaesth*, **88**, 734–738.
12 Braude BM et al. (1986). *Anaesthesia*, **41**, 861–865.
13 Mather SP, Webster NR (1986). *Anaesthesia*, **41**, 856–860.
14 Sanders WC, Wolpert LA (1991). *J Clin Anesth*, **3**, 48–52.

Glucose-6-phosphate-dehydrogenase deficiency (see also p208)
Predominantly male, attacks of haemolytic anaemia precipitated by infections/some drugs (including aspirin, vitamin K, chloramphenicol), chronic anaemia (increased 2,3-DPG) of 5–10g/dl, may benefit from splenectomy.

Glycogenoses (glycogen storage diseases)

Type I (Von Gierke's disease)
Mental retardation, hepatosplenomegaly, renal enlargement, hypoglycaemic convulsions, stomatitis, bleeding diathesis, leucopenia, tendency to hypoglycaemia during fasting, lactic acidosis, cautious attention to metabolic/homeostatic derangements, abdominal distension may affect ventilation.[1]

Type II (Pompe's disease)
Wide spectrum of severity, neonatal acyanotic cardiac death to normal life, cardiomegaly/cardiomyopathy, progressive cardiac failure, outflow obstruction, generalised hypotonia, neurological deficits, macroglossia, normal glucose tolerance, postoperative respiratory insufficiency, potential exaggerated hyperkalaemic response to suxamethonium, consider local anaesthetic alternatives.[2]

Type III (Forbes' disease)
Perioperative hypoglycaemia.

Type IV (Andersen's disease)
Hepatosplenomegaly, cirrhosis, hepatic dysfunction, severe growth retardation, death before 3yr, muscular hypotonia, muscle relaxants generally unnecessary, reduced doses of IV drugs, prone to perioperative hypoglycaemia/heat loss.

Type V (McArdle's disease)
Muscle weakness, cardiac failure.

Goldenhar syndrome (oculoauriculovertebral syndrome, hemifacial microsomia)
Eye/ear abnormalities, difficult intubation, micrognathia, maxillary hypoplasia, cleft/high arched palate, cervical synostosis, congenital heart anomalies (Fallot/VSD), craniovertebral anomalies, atropine-resistant bradycardia.[3]

Goltz–Gorlin syndrome (focal dermal hypoplasia)
Dental/facial asymmetry, stiff neck, difficult airway, hypertension.[4,5]

Goodpasture's syndrome
Severe repeated intrapulmonary haemorrhages with fibrosis, restrictive lung defect, hypertension, anaemia, renal failure.

Gorham syndrome ('disappearing bone disease')

Massive osteolysis—replacement of bone by fibrovascular tissue (most common in second/third decade), pathological fractures, lymphangiomatosis, respiratory and neurological deficits, relapsing pleural effusions, chylothorax/pericardium, assess respiratory function, check cervical spine (often involved), avoid suxamethonium (may cause/worsen pathological fractures), consider postoperative ICU respiratory support, poor prognosis.[6]

Gronblad–Strandberg disease, see pseudoxanthoma elasticum.

Haemochromatosis (bronze diabetes and haemosiderosis)

Iron deposits in liver/pancreas/joints/skin/heart, cirrhosis, diabetes, arthritis, late cardiac failure, may be having weekly venesections.

Haemolytic uraemic syndrome

Triad of renal failure/haemolytic anaemia/thrombocytopenia, multisystem disorder may also involve CVS/respiratory/CNS/hepatic systems.[7]

Haemorrhagic telangiectasia (Osler–Weber–Rendu syndrome)

Familial telangiectasia of mucous membranes (nose/oropharynx/viscera/skin), avoid trauma, repeated haemorrhages, bleeding difficult to control, GI bleeding, may have pulmonary AV fistulae, invasive procedures complicated (poor tissues).[8]

Hallermann–Streiff syndrome

Oculomandibulodyscephaly, dwarfism, direct laryngoscopy may be hazardous/difficult (brittle teeth, temporomandibular joint dislocation).

Hallervorden–Spatz disease

Rare progressive disorder of basal ganglia, myotonia/dystonic posturing, scoliosis, dementia, trismus, difficult intubation, volatile agents relieve the posturing (returns after discontinuation).[9,10]

Hand–Schuller–Christian disease (histiocytic granulomata)

Diabetes insipidus, hepatic failure, respiratory failure, difficult intubation (small larynx), pancytopenia, electrolyte problems.

Hartnup disease

Defective tubular/jejunal reabsorption of most neutral amino acids leading to tryptophan malabsorption/nicotinamide deficiency, pellagra, psychiatric disorders, cerebellar ataxia

1 Shenkman Z et al. (1996). Can J Anaesth, **43**, 467–470.
2 Ing RJ et al. (2004). Paediatr Anaesth, **14**, 514–519.
3 Madan R et al. (1990). Anaesthesia, **45**, 49–52.
4 Ezri T et al. (1994). Anaesthesia, **49**, 833.
5 Holzman RS (1991). J Clin Anesth, **3**, 422–425.
6 Szabo C, Habre W (2000). Anaesthesia, **55**, 157–159.
7 Johnson GD, Rosales JK (1987). Can J Anaesth, **34**, 196–199.
8 Waring PH et al. (1990). Anesth Analg, **71**, 96–99.
9 Roy C et al. (1983). Anesthesiology, **58**, 382–384.
10 Keegan MT et al. (2000). J Neurosurg Anesthesiol, **12**, 107–111.

Hay–Wells syndrome
Difficult intubation (maxillary hypoplasia).

Hecht–Beals syndrome (trismus pseudocamptodactyly/Dutch–Kennedy syndrome)
Arachnodactyly, kyphoscoliosis, difficult intubation (restricted mandible—LMA beneficial), multiple joint contractures, crumpled ears, ventilatory defect, mitral valve prolapse, aortic root dilatation.[1,2]

Henoch–Schönlein purpura
Abnormal vascular reaction, normal platelets, nephritis (30%), haemorrhagic risk, renal failure.

Hepatolenticular degeneration (Kinnier–Wilson disease)
Defective copper metabolism, hepatic failure, epilepsy, trismus, weakness, sensitive to muscle relaxants.

Holt–Oram syndrome (hand–heart syndrome)
Rare disorder combining congenital cardiac anomalies (ASD/VSD/occasionally others) and upper limbs (hypoplastic thumbs/clavicles), hypoplastic vasculature, arrhythmias frequent even with normal anatomy, risk of sudden death, potentially difficult venous access (especially central), often previous cardiac surgery.[3]

Homocystinuria
Homocystine excreted in urine, mental handicap, Marfan-like syndrome, venous/arterial thrombotic episodes, pulmonary embolisms (requiring heparinisation), renal failure, hypoglycaemia.[4]

Hunter syndrome (mucopolysaccharidosis II), see mucopolysaccharidoses

Huntington's chorea/juvenile Huntington's disease
Similar conditions, progressive degenerative involuntary choreoathetoid movement, dysphagia/regurgitation/pulmonary aspiration, poor respiratory function, possible associated autonomic neuropathy, avoid precipitating convulsions/clonic spasms, depression/apathy lead to cachexia and malnourishment, exaggerated response to thiopental and suxamethonium.[5,6]

Hurler syndrome (gargoylism, mucopolysaccharidosis I)
Most severe mucopolysaccharidosis, death at early age. See mucopolysaccharidoses.

Hutchinson–Gilford syndrome (premature ageing syndrome), see progeria

Hyperviscosity syndrome (Waldenstom's macroglobulinaemia, multiple myeloma)
Thrombotic risk, preoperative plasmapheresis may be needed.

Hypokalaemic familial periodic paralysis

Attacks of severe muscle weakness/flaccid muscle paralysis with low serum K^+, perioperative attack may compromise spontaneous ventilation, avoid drugs known to cause K^+ shifts (e.g. β-agonists), arrhythmias, sensitive to muscle relaxants.[7,8]

Hypoplastic left heart syndrome

Hypoplasia of LV/mitral valve/ascending aorta, aortic valve atresia, previously 100% mortality, survival depends upon PDA, balance of PVR and SVR (both circulations in parallel supplied by single ventricle), control of pulmonary blood flow, VF may occur with surgical manipulation.[9]

Ichthyosis

Hyperkeratotic plates of flaky/fissured skin, difficulty placing and securing catheters/cannulae/electrodes (consider bandaging), perioperative temperature control.[10]

Idiopathic thrombocytopenic purpura (see also p214)

Thrombocytopenia <50 000 cells/mm³, petechiae, avoid heparin/aspirin, consider platelet infusions, beware rebound thrombosis after splenectomy, minimise airway trauma, avoid regional blocks.

Isaacs' syndrome (continuous muscle fibre activity syndrome, neuromyotonia, quantal squander)

Autoimmune condition, continuous involuntary muscle fibre activity, fasciculation, delayed relaxation, ataxia, incoordination, anticonvulsants effective, regional blocks acceptable, probable exaggerated response to muscle relaxants.[11]

Ivemark syndrome

Asplenia, complex cardiac pathology (needs full assessment), abnormal abdominal viscera.

Jervell–Lange–Nielsen syndrome

Congenital prolonged QT interval/enlarged T wave, deafness, prone to ventricular arrhythmias/cardiac arrest, consider pacemaker insertion/β-block (for CVS stability), select drugs/technique known to minimise catecholamine levels.[12]

1 Nagata O et al. (1999). *Paediatr Anaesth*, **9**, 444–447.
2 Vaghadia H, Blackstocki D (1988). *Can J Anaesth*, **35**, 80–85.
3 Shono S et al. (1998). *Br J Anaesth*, **80**, 856–857.
4 Teng YH et al. (2002). *Acta Anaesthesiol Sin*, **40**, 153–156.
5 Cangemi CF, Miller RJ (1998). *Anesth Prog*, **45**, 150–153.
6 Gupta K, Leng CP (2000). *Paediatr Anaesth*, **10**, 107–109.
7 Ahlawat SK, Sachdev A (1999). *Postgrad Med J*, **75**, 193–197.
8 Viscomi CM et al. (1999). *Anesth Analg*, **88**, 1081–1082.
9 Testa L et al. (1994). *J Clin Anesth*, **65**, 127–132.
10 Kubota R et al. (2003). *Masui*, **52**, 1332–1334.
11 Shyr MH et al. (1997). *Acta Anaesthesiol Sin*, **35**, 241–245.
12 Ryan (1988). *Can J Anaesth*, **35**, 422–424.

Jeune's syndrome (asphyxiating thoracic dystrophy)
Pulmonary hypoplasia, severe thoracic defect preventing normal intercostal function, minimise ventilator pressures, renal dysfunction, myocardial dysfunction in older patients.[1]

Joubert syndrome
Abnormal respiratory control (brainstem/cerebellar hypoplasia), hypotonia, ataxia, mental retardation, sensitive to respiratory depressant effects of anaesthetic agents (including. N_2O), spontaneously breathing general anaesthetic problematic, care with opioids, close postoperative observation.[2,3]

Kartagener's syndrome
Sinusitis/brochiectasis/situs inversus (50%), (abnormal cilia), immunoincompetence, dextrocardia (reverse ECG lead position/defibrillator paddles, etc.), right lateral displacement (obstetrics), chronic/recurrent chest infections, fully assess CVS/RS function, preoperative physiotherapy, humidify gases, local/regional block preferred.[4]

Kawasaki disease (mucocutaneous lymph node syndrome)
Acute childhood (<5yr) febrile illness, coronary arteritis, aneurysms/thrombotic occlusions/IHD/sudden death, degree of CVS dysfunction determines technique, invasive lines have higher complication risk, accelerated atherosclerosis.[5]

Kearns–Sayer syndrome
Extremely rare mitochondrial myopathy, cardiac conduction abnormalities common (range from bundle branch block to third degree AV block), risk of complete heart block, generalised CNS degeneration (see progressive external ophthalmoplegia), sensitive to induction agents/muscle relaxants, consider inhalation induction with deep anaesthesia intubation, ophthalmic complications, depressed respiratory drive (care with opioids etc.).[6]

Kelly–Paterson syndrome, see Plummer–Vinson syndrome.

Kenny–Caffey syndrome
Proportional dwarfism, macrocephaly, eye anomalies, dysmorphic facies, mandibular hypoplasia, difficult airway, episodic hypocalcaemic tetany, may be associated with Mournier–Kuhn syndrome, hypocalcaemia, anaemia, thoracic/skeletal abnormalities.[7]

King Denborough syndrome
Slowly progressive myopathy, short stature, kyphoscoliosis, pectus carinatum, cryptorchidism, characteristic facial appearance, MH risk.[8]

Klinefelter syndrome
Chromosomal abnormality 47XXY, poor sexual development, tall stature, reduced intelligence, vertebral collapse from osteoporosis, may have reduced muscle bulk/power, care during positioning.[9]

Klippel–Feil syndrome

Three main types—differ in severity, congenital fusion of cervical and/or thoracic vertebrae, short neck, limited range of motion, possible cervical cord compression, syncope on sudden rotation of head, kyphoscoliosis, cardiac/respiratory/renal anomalies, difficult intubation, keep neck in neutral axis (basilar insufficiency).[10]

Klippel–Trenaunay syndrome (angio-osteohypertrophy)

Generalised haemangiomas, soft tissue hypertrophy, bone overgrowth and/or arteriovenous malformations, possible airway/respiratory problems, high output cardiac failure, consumptive coagulopathy, pulse oximeter may under-read if placed on limb with large A-V fistula (pulsatile venous flow) (see also Proteus syndrome).[11,12]

Kniest syndrome

Difficult intubation (stiff neck).[13]

Kugelberg Welander syndrome (spinal muscular atrophy type III), see spinal muscular atrophy

Larsen's syndrome

Multiple congenital dislocations, difficult intubation (subglottic stenosis), unstable cervical spine, prominent forehead, flattened face, chronic respiratory disease from kyphoscoliosis.[14]

Laurence–Moon syndrome, see also Bardet–Biedl syndrome

Mental retardation, spastic paraplegia, retinitis pigmentosa, hypogonadism.

Leber's disease, see also alveolar hypoventilation

Idiopathic hypoventilation, sensitive to sedatives/analgesics.[15]

Leigh's syndrome

Necrotising encephalomyelopathy in children, hypotonia, seizures, aspiration.[16]

1 Borland LM (1987). *Anesthesiology*, **66**, 86–88.
2 Habre W et al. (1997). *Paediatr Anaesth*, **7**, 251–253.
3 Matthews NC (1989). *Anaesthesia*, **44**, 920–921.
4 Reidy J et al. (2000). *Br J Anaesth*, **85**, 919–921.
5 Waldron RJ et al. (1993). *Anaesth Intensive Care*, **21**, 213–217.
6 Lauwers MH et al. (1994). *Anaesthesia*, **49**, 876–878.
7 Janke EL et al. (1996). *Paediatr Anaesth*, **6**, 235–238.
8 Watsubo T et al. (2001). *Masui*, **50**, 390–393.
9 Lanfranco F et al. (2004). *Lancet*, **364**, 273–283.
10 Farid IS et al. (2003). *J Cardiothorac Vasc Anesth*, **17**, 502–505.
11 Christie IW et al. (1998). *Anaesth Intensive Care*, **26**, 319–321.
12 Ezri T et al. (1996). *Paediatr Anaesth*, **6**, 81.
13 Felius GM et al. (1985). *Rev Esp Anestesiol Reanim*, **32**, 127–129.
14 Lauder GR, Sumner E (1995). *Paediatr Anaesth*, **5**, 133–138.
15 Hunter AR (1984). *Anaesthesia*, **39**, 781–783.
16 Ward DS (1981). *Anesthesiology*, **55**, 80–81.

LEOPARD syndrome
Rare inherited progressive disorder, similar to Noonan syndrome, Lentigines/ECG abnormalities/Ocular hypertelorism and obstructive cardiomyopathy/Pulmonary valve stenosis/Abnormal male genitalia/Retarded growth/Deafness, CVS assessment will determine technique, cardiomyopathy may be occult.[1]

Leprechaunism
'Gnome' facies, cutis laxa, adipose tissue atrophy, dwarfism, extreme wasting, dysphagia requiring parenteral feeding, abnormal endocrine state, mentally defective (see cutis laxa; dwarfism), maintain blood sugar during fasting (hyperinsulinism).[2]

Lesch–Nyhan syndrome (hyperuricaemia)
Disorder of purine metabolism, hyperuricaemia, spasticity, choreoathetosis, dystonia, self-injurious behaviour, aggression, normal cognitive function, possible atlantoaxial instability, sudden unexplained death, seizures, abnormalities in respiration, apnoea, absent adrenergic pressor response—severe bradycardia, caution with exogenous catecholamines, increased incidence of vomiting/regurgitation, chronic pulmonary aspiration.[3]

Letterer–Siwe disease (histiocytosis-X)
Histiocytic granulomata in viscera/bones, similar clinical course to acute leukaemia, pancytopenia, anaemia, purpura, haemorrhage, pulmonary infiltration, hepatic involvement, tooth loss.

Lipodystrophy (total lipoatrophy)
Generalised loss of body fat, fatty fibrotic liver, hepatic failure, portal hypertension, splenomegaly, hypersplenism, anaemia, thrombocytopenia, nephropathy, renal failure, diabetes mellitus.[4]

Long QT syndrome
Mutations in cardiac ion channels, prolonged ventricular repolarisation, genetic/drug induced, 60% are symptomatic (syncope, seizure-like episodes, cardiac arrest), high risk of perioperative malignant ventricular arrhythmias (may be refractory), preoperative β-blockade, normalise all electrolytes, prevent sympathetic activation (pain, laryngoscopy, extubation, normocapnia, etc), invasive monitoring advisable, maintain temperature (hypothermia prolongs QT), adequate analgesia essential, torsades de points may be self-limiting/require cardioversion/magnesium/pacing, consider postoperative ICU.[5]

Lowe syndrome (oculocerebrorenal syndrome)
Metabolic acidosis due to renal-tubular dysfunction, renal failure, convulsions, mental retardation, abnormal skull shape, bone fragility, hypotonia, hypocalcaemia, glaucoma/cataracts.[6]

Maffucci syndrome

Progressive condition, enchondromatosis and multiple soft tissue haemangiomata (including airway/cervical spine), increased risk of malignancy, intracranial lesions, anaemia, coagulopathy, increased risk of epidural haematoma (spinal lesions), assess for raised ICP, pathological fractures, GI bleeding, may be sensitive to vasodilating drugs.[7]

Mandibulofacial dysostosis (Treacher–Collins syndrome)

Mandibulofacial dysostosis, deafness, hypoplasia of facial bones (mandible/maxilla/cheek), characteristic facies, cardiovascular malformations, postoperative laryngeal/pharyngeal oedema may develop, difficult airway, sleep apnoea, respiratory distress, sudden death all reported.[8]

Maple syrup urine disease

Branched chain ketoacid decarboxylase deficiency, failure to thrive, fits, cerebral degeneration, neonatal acidosis.

Marchiafava–Micheli syndrome

Autoimmune haemolytic anaemia, venous thromboembolism, paroxysmal nocturnal dyspnoea.

Marfan's syndrome

Autosomal dominant disorder of connective tissue metabolism, tall with long/thin fingers, dilation of ascending aorta, dissecting aneurysms, aortic/mitral regurgitation, coronary thrombosis, cataracts/retinal detachment/lens dislocation, emphysema, spontaneous pneumothorax, pectus excavatum, beware possible tracheomalacia, obstructive sleep apnoea, easy joint dislocation, cervical spine bony/ligamentous abnormality (routine X-ray not indicated), high arched palate, crowded teeth, kyphoscoliosis, perioperative β-blockade if not already treated, minimise sympathetic response, control BP, consider invasive monitoring, central blocks are acceptable.[9]

Maroteaux–Lamy syndrome (mucopolysaccharidosis IV)

see mucopolysaccharidoses

1 Torres J et al. (2004). Paediatr Anaesth, 14, 352–356.
2 Cantani A (1987). Ann Genet, 30, 221–227.
3 Larson LO, Wilkins RG (1985). Anesthesiology, 63, 197–199.
4 Koga Y et al. (1987). J Anesth, 1, 112–114.
5 Booker PD et al. (2003). Br J Anaesth, 90, 349–366.
6 Watoh Y (1992). Masui, 41, 1004–1007.
7 Chan SK et al. (1998). Anaesth Intensive Care, 26, 586–589.
8 Takita K et al. (2003). Can J Anaesth, 50, 969–970.
9 Gordon CF, Johnson MD (1993). J Clin Anesth, 5, 248–251.

Marshall–Smith syndrome

Accelerated bone maturation, dysmorphic facial features, airway abnormalities, death in early infancy from respiratory complications, generally die in infancy, airway difficulties including possible atlantoaxial instability/laryngomalacia/tracheomalacia, facemask ventilation may be impossible, maintain spontaneous breathing if possible, consider elective use of nasopharyngeal airway during induction/emergence.[1,2]

Meckel's syndrome (Meckel–Gruber syndrome)

Microcephaly, micrognathia, difficult intubation, cleft epiglottis/palate, congenital CVS disease, polycystic kidneys, renal failure, encephalocele.

Meig's syndrome

Large ovarian cyst in peritoneal space (space/pressure effects), respiratory distress, pleural effusion drainage, poor nutrition, intravascular volume correction.[3]

Menkes' disease

Suppression of copper-dependent enzymes resulting from copper deficiency, kinky hair, convulsions, mental retardation, bone/connective tissue lesions, hypothermia, seizures, gastro-oesophageal reflux, airway complications (poor pharyngeal motor tone).[4]

MERRF syndrome

Mitochondrial encephalomyopathy, mixed seizures, myoclonus, progressive ataxia, spasticity, mild myopathy, growth retardation, deafness, dementia.

Mikulicz's syndrome

Salivary/lacrimal gland enlargement, glandular tissue may complicate airway management, anticholinergics probably best avoided.

Miller–Fisher syndrome Variant of Guillain Barre syndrome (p253).

Miller's syndrome

Rare congenital disorder, facies similar to Treacher–Collins syndrome, congenital heart disease (ASD/VSD/PDA), limb abnormalities, consider early tracheostomy for airway maintenance (especially if repeated procedures planned), difficult venous access, gastric reflux.[5]

Moebius syndrome

Multiple cranial nerve palsies, difficult/failed intubation, orofacial malformations, limb anomalies, high incidence of other anomalies (congenital cardiac/spinal/corneal abrasions/peripheral neuropathies), potential aspiration of oral secretions due to salivary drooling (consider antisialogogue premedication).[6]

Morquio syndrome (mucopolysaccharidosis IV)

Short stature, short neck, hypoplastic odontoid/atlantoaxial instability (compression of long tracts/paraplegia can occur), difficult airway, potential narrowed lumen (infiltration), sleep apnoea, loss of muscle tone, hypermobility/loose skin, aortic incompetence, prominent sternum, respiratory and cardiac failure in early adult life, end organ dysfunction.[7]

Moschcowitz disease (thrombotic thrombocytopenic purpura)

Triad of haemolytic anaemia/consumptive thrombocytopenia/CNS dysfunction, renal disease, bleeding risk (padding/positioning important), often need splenectomy (rebound thrombocytosis).[8]

Mounier–Kuhn syndrome

Diffuse tracheobronchomegaly, communicating paratracheal cysts, intubate trachea/pack pharynx if ventilation needed.[9]

Moya–moya disease (in the German literature 'Nishimoto–Takeuchi–Kudo–Suzuki's disease')

Severe internal carotid artery stenosis, fine network of vessels around basal ganglia, CNS deterioration can follow general anaesthesia, optimise cerebral perfusion (BP/CO_2, etc).[10]

Mucopolysaccharidoses (Hunter, Hurler, Morquio, Maroteaux–Lamy, Scheie)

Abnormal mucopolysaccharide metabolism (lack of lysosomal enzyme), anatomical abnormalities/organ dysfunction from progressive deposition in tissues, upper airway obstruction (infiltration of lips/tongue/epiglottis/tonsils/adenoids) and lower airway, obstructive/restrictive ventilatory defects (abnormal laryngeal/tracheal cartilage, copious airway secretions, vertebrae/thoracic deformities), recurrent infection, cardiovascular abnormalities (coronary infiltration/ valvular disease/myocardial insufficiency), difficult intubation (craniofacial abnormalities—short neck/stiffened temporomandibular joints/large tongue/anterior larynx), difficulty increases with age, protruberant abdomen, increased muscle tone, generally die from pneumonia/cardiac complications. (see also Further reading).[11]

Multiple myeloma

Neoplastic proliferation of plasma cells characterised by immunoglobulin disorders, renal failure, haemorrhagic tendency, hyperviscosity syndrome, anaemia, increased susceptibility to infections, pathological fractures (care positioning), hypercalcaemia.[12]

1 Antila H et al. (1998). Paediatr Anaesth, **8**, 429–432.
2 Dernedde G (1998). Can J Anaesth, **45**, 660–663.
3 Hirota M et al. (1995). Masui, **44**, 874–879.
4 Tobias JD (1992). Can J Anaesth, **39**, 712–715.
5 Stevenson GW (1991). Can J Anaesth, **38**, 1046–1049.
6 Ferguson S (1996). Paediatr Anaesth, **6**, 51–56.
7 Morgan KA et al. (2002). Paediatr Anaesth, **12**, 641–644.
8 Pivalizza EG (1994). Anesth Analg, **79**, 1203–1205.
9 Sane AC et al. (1992). Chest, **102**, 618–619.
10 Bingham RM, Wilkinson DJ (1985). Anaesthesia, **40**, 1198–1202.
11 Walker RWM et al. (2003). Paediatr Anaesth, **13**, 441–447.
12 Wake M (1995). Masui, **44**, 1282–1284.

Myasthenic syndrome (Eaton–Lambert syndrome) (see also p246)

Paraneoplastic condition, defective acetylcholine release at neuromuscular junctions, proximal muscle weakness in ocular/bulbar muscles, post-tetanic facilitation, muscle weakness, sensitive to muscle relaxants, respiratory complications, autonomic dysfunction, impaired oesophageal motility.[1,2]

Myositis ossificans

Bony infiltration of tendons/fascia/muscle/aponeuroses, airway problems if neck involved, thoracic involvement reduces compliance, asphyxia, aspiration.

Myotonia congenita (Thomsen's disease) (see also p256)

Defective skeletal muscle chloride channel (failure of muscle relaxation), widespread dystrophy and/or hypertrophy, unresponsive to non-depolarising muscle relaxants, palatopharyngeal dysfunction, aspiration risk, cardiomyopathy, no apparent association with MH, can be precipitated by cold/surgery/diathermy/anticholinesterases, suxamethonium may cause myotonia with difficult intubation/ventilation.[3]

Nager syndrome

Oromandibular hypogenesis (like Treacher–Collins syndrome), mandibular/midface manifestations may complicate perioperative/postoperative airway management, vertebral malformations (cervical spine involvement), congenital cardiac defects.[4]

Nance Insley syndrome (otospondylomegaepiphyseal dysplasia 'OSMED')

Disrupted cartilaginous growth leading to midface hypoplasia/micrognathia/cleft palate, difficult airway, disproportionate short stature/short limbs, progressive sensorineural deafness, joint contractures, vertebral abnormalities.[5]

Nemaline myopathy

Congenital myopathy, non-progressive hypotonia/symmetrical muscle weakness (including skeletal/diaphragm, sparing cardiac/smooth), skeletal deformities, facial dysmorphism, airway difficulties, poor respiratory function (restrictive), chronic aspiration, abnormal drug responses (including relaxants), rarely cardiomyopathy, MH not described.[6,7]

Nesidioblastosis

Autonomous insulin secretion unaffected by blood glucose, neonatal/infantile apnoea, hypoglycaemia, hypotonia, seizures, total pancreatectomy needed, monitor perioperative blood glucose.[8]

Neurofibromatosis

Café au lait spots, astrocytomas, seizures, kyphoscoliosis, potential difficult airway and positioning, avoid proconvulsants, occult phaeochromocytoma (5%) (see Further reading).

Niemann–Pick disease

Sphingomyelin accumulation in organs (liver/spleen/bone marrow), progressive central/peripheral nervous system degeneration, mental retardation, anaemia, hepatosplenomegaly, thrombocytopenia, difficult intubation/ventilation, respiratory failure.[7]

Noonan's syndrome

Short stature, cardiac defects (pulmonary stenosis/hypertrophic cardio-myopathy/VSD), mental retardation, micrognathia, short webbed neck, difficult intubation, pectus excavatum, vertebral anomalies, lymphoedema, platelet/coagulation defects, renal failure.[10]

Ondine's curse/Ondine–Hirschsprung disease, see alveolar hypoventilation

Opitz–Frais syndrome (hypospadias dysphagia syndrome)

Recurrent pulmonary aspiration of intestinal contents, achalasia of the oesophagus, subglottic stenosis, hypertelorism, micrognathia, high arched palate.[11]

Osler–Weber–Rendu syndrome, see haemorrhagic telangiectasia

Osteogenesis imperfecta (fragilitas ossium)

Inherited connective tissue disorder, four types ranging in severity, bone fragility, frequent fractures and/or deformities, blue sclera (not all types), teeth easily damaged, excessive bleeding, tendency to hyperthermia—probably not MH.[12]

Osteopetrosis (Albers–Schönberg disease)

Group of disorders, increased bone density, changes in modelling with over-growth, range of severity, brittle bones, nerve compression syndromes, mental retardation, hearing loss, leucoerythroblastic anaemia (bone marrow involvement), airway/ventilation problems, head/mandibular involvement may affect intubation, cervicomedullary stenosis (cord trauma during intubation), thrombocytopenia, hepatosplenomegaly (reduced FRC), reduced myocardial contractility (hypocalcaemia), careful moving and positioning—risk of fractures.[13]

1 Seneviratne U, deSilva R (1999). Postgrad Med J, 75, 516–520.
2 Telford RJ, Holloway TE (1990). Br J Anaesth, 64, 363.
3 Farbu E et al. (2003). Acta Anaesthesiol Scand, 47, 630–634.
4 Groeper K et al. (2002). Paediatr Anaesth, 12, 365–368.
5 Denton R (1996). Anaesthesia, 51, 100–101.
6 Asai T et al. (1992). Anaesthesia, 47, 405–408.
7 Stackhouse R (1994). Anesth Analg, 79, 1195–1197.
8 Bellwoar C et al. (1996). Paediatr Anaesth, 6, 61–63.
9 Bujok LS et al. (2002). Paediatr Anaesth, 12, 806–808.
10 Grange CS (1998). Can J Anaesth, 45, 332–336.
11 Bolsin SN, Gillbe C (1985). Anaesthesia, 40, 1189–1193.
12 Karabiyik L et al. (2004). Paediatr Anaesth, 14, 524–525.
13 Burt N et al. (1999). Anesth Analg, 88, 1292–1297.

Paramyotonia congenita (Eulenberg's disease)

Variant of hyperkalaemic periodic paralysis, cold-induced myotonia, flaccid paralysis, worsened by exercise, assess sensitivity to cold/frequency of myotonic episodes, warm theatre/fluids/patient, normal response to non-depolarising muscle relaxants, avoid suxamethonium, central neural blocks safe, no MH tendency.[1]

Patau's syndrome (trisomy 13)

Multiple craniofacial/cardiac/neurological/renal anomalies, 'rockerbottom feet', difficult airway, thoracic kyphoscoliosis, ineffective cough, postoperative respiratory problems, apnoeic episodes, full cardiac assessment (severe malformations in 80%), impaired renal function, polycythaemia, platelet dysfunction.[2,3]

Pemphigus vulgaris

Autoimmune disease, impaired cell adhesion within epidermis, bullous eruptions of skin/mucous membrane, avoid friction (airway manipulation/monitors/positioning lines, etc.), possible ulceration/bullae/oedema of glottis after intubation (lubricate everything well), careful fluid/electrolyte balance (include losses from bullae), perioperative steroids to reduce exacerbation, regional/general anaesthetic acceptable.[4]

Pendred's syndrome

Genetic defect in thyroid hormone synthesis, hypothyroidism, goitre, deafness, treat as hypothyroidism.[5]

Pfeiffer's syndrome (acrocephalosyndactyly type V)

Growth/developmental retardation, sagittal craniosynostosis, hypertelorism, low set ears, micrognathia with mandibular ankylosis, congenital heart defects, genital anomalies, solid cartilaginous trachea lacking rings may be present.[6]

Pharyngeal pouch

Epithelial-lined diverticulum above the upper oesophageal sphincter, often asymptomatic, dysphagia, tracheal soiling not prevented by cricoid pressure, empty pouch manually (by patient) prior to induction or with large bore nasopharyngeal tube, consider intubation in head-down position or under local anaesthetic.

Phenylketonuria

Defective phenylalanine-4-hydroxylase, mental retardation, cerebral damage, epilepsy, sensitive to opioids/barbiturates, consider inhalation induction, monitor blood glucose, B12 deficiency—avoid nitrous oxide.[7]

Pickwickian syndrome

Morbid obesity, episodic somnolence, hypoventilation, hypoxaemia, polycythaemia, pulmonary hypertension, cardiac failure, difficult access/positioning, prone to wound infection, DVT/PE risk, sensitive to respiratory depressants, regional anaesthesia ideal for peripheral surgery, alert ICU following major surgery, CPAP beneficial.[8]

Pierre–Robin syndrome

Difficult airway, cleft palate, micrognathia, mandibular hypoplasia, receding mandible fails to hold tongue forward—falls against posterior pharyngeal wall, congenital heart disease.[9]

Plott's syndrome

Laryngeal-abductor paralysis, psychomotor retardation, sixth nerve palsy, stridor at rest, cyanosis during crying/exertion, postoperative upper airway control.[10]

Plummer–Vinson syndrome (Patterson–Brown–Kelly syndrome)

Upper oesophageal web, dysphagia, regurgitation risk, iron-deficiency anaemia, glossitis, angular stomatitis, increased risk of postcricoid carcinoma.[11]

Pneumatosis cystoides intestinalis

Multiple intramural gas-filled cysts in gut, disturbed bowel function, avoid N_2O, systemic sclerosis association.[12]

Pompe's disease, see Glycogenoses, type II

Post-poliomyelitis syndrome

New neuromuscular symptoms occurring >15yr after clinical stability attained in patients with prior history of symptomatic poliomyelitis, limb atrophy, slow progression with periods of stabilisation, respiratory muscle involvement, bulbar dysfunction.

Potter's syndrome (bilateral renal agenesis)

Incompatible with life, bilateral renal agenesis, pulmonary hypoplasia, characteristic facial features, ventilation may be impossible despite intubation.[13]

Prader–Willi syndrome

Mental retardation, severe obesity, polyphagia, dental caries, congenital muscle hypotonia, short stature, hypogonadism, cardiovascular anomalies, difficult venous access, arrhythmias, altered thermoregulation, convulsions, blood glucose should be maintained IV during fasting, perioperative respiratory problems may occur.[14]

1 Grace RF et al. (1999). Anaesth Intensive Care, **27**, 534–537.
2 Martlew RA et al. (1995). Anaesthesia, **50**, 980–982.
3 Pollard RC et al. (1996). Paediatr Anaesth, **6**, 151–153.
4 Mahalingam TG et al. (2000). Anaesthesia, **55**, 160–162.
5 Reardon W (1999). J Med Genet, **36**, 595–598.
6 Moore MH et al. (1995). Cleft Palate Craniofac J, **32**, 62–70.
7 Lee P et al. (1999). Lancet, **353**, 554.
8 Neuman GG et al. (1986). Anesth Analg, **65**, 985–987.
9 Rasch DK et al. (1986). Can Anaesth Soc J, **33**, 364–370.
10 McDonald D (1998). Paediatr Anaesth, **8**, 155–157.
11 Hoffman RM et al. (1995). Arch Intern Med, **155**, 2008–2011.
12 Sutton DN et al. (1984). Anaesthesia, **39**, 776–780.
13 Van der Weyden (1982). Anaesth Intensive Care, **10**, 90.
14 Dearlove OR et al. (1998). Paediatr Anaesth, **8**, 267–271.

Progeria (premature ageing)

Feature of numerous syndromes, IHD/hypertension/cardiomyopathy at young chronological age, plan technique around 'physiological age'.[1]

Progressive external ophthalmoplegia (PEO)

Progressive mitochondrial myopathy, ptosis, diabetes mellitus, hypothyroidism, hyperparathyroidism, short stature, sensitive to all induction agents, increased MH risk.[2]

Proteus syndrome

Congenital progressive hamartomatous disorder, partial bilateral gigantism, hemihypertrophy (often one whole side of the body), macrocephaly, scoliosis, cystic lung changes (probably explains 'the Elephant Man'), difficult airway (see also Bullous cystic lung disease; Klippel–Trenaunay syndrome.[3]

Prune-belly syndrome (Eagle–Barrett syndrome)

Almost exclusively male, absent abdominal muscles, genitourinary malformations/bilateral undescended testes, pulmonary hypoplasia, poor cough (muscle weakness), beware postoperative respiratory distress, difficult airway (micrognathia), congenital heart disease, skeletal anomalies, imperforate anus, careful fluid balance, renal failure may coexist.[4]

Pseudoxanthoma elasticum (Gronbald–Strandberg disease)

Hereditary disorder of elastic tissue, four types—variable features, fragile connective tissue, vascular complications (slow progressive occlusive arterial disease), retinal changes with early blindness/myopia, blue sclera, high arched palate, lungs not affected, fragile tissue—haemorrhage with minor trauma (including airway), valvular disease/hypertension/IHD/arrhythmias, care in fixing IV lines.[5]

Pulmonary cysts

Can increase in size and rupture during anaesthesia (especially with N_2O).

Refsum's disease

Defective metabolism of phytanic acid, sensorimotor polyneuropathy, ataxia, retinal damage, deafness, document any neurology before performing regional blocks.

Rett syndrome

Devastating disabling female neurological disease, second commonest cause of mental retardation in females after Down's, abnormal respiratory control when awake (hyperventilation/apnoea), respiratory pattern normal under general anaesthesia, long QT, sudden death, full respiratory assessment ideal but may be technically difficult, prolonged weaning, high pain threshold (abnormal processing), scoliosis, may be sensitive to sedative drugs/resistant to muscle relaxants, consider depth of anaesthesia monitoring.[6]

Rigid spine syndrome

Very limited spinal flexion, generalised proximal limb weakness, limb contractures, progressive scoliosis, restrictive ventilatory defect, cardiomyopathy, conduction defects, pulmonary hypertension, RV failure, difficult intubation, flexible ETT provides better fit in hyperextended trachea, avoid suxamethonium (K^+), low MH risk, care with muscle relaxants, careful positioning/padding, consider postoperative HDU/ICU.[7]

Riley–Day syndrome, see Familial dysautonomia

Romano–Ward syndrome

Congenital delay of cardiac depolarisation, prolonged QT interval, risk of sudden death during induction of anaesthesia, consider preoperative pacing.[8]

Rubinstein–Taybi syndrome

Microcephaly, craniofacial abnormalities, difficult airway, mental retardation, broad thumbs/toes, recurrent respiratory infections/chronic lung disease, congenital heart disease (33%), arrhythmias.[9]

Russell–Silver syndrome

Short stature, facial/limb asymmetry, mandibular hypoplasia, micrognathia, macroglossia, difficult airway (including mask fit), sweating, fasting hypoglycaemia (intra-operative glucose monitoring), mental retardation, congenital heart disease, temperature control (minimal body fat), monitor neuromuscular block (normal doses may underdose).[10]

Saethre–Chotzen syndrome

Craniosynostosis, micrognathia, difficult intubation, renal failure.

Scheie syndrome (mucopolysaccharidosis V), see mucopolysaccharidoses

Scimitar syndrome

Anomalous venous drainage of right lung into IVC, right lung hypoplasia, scimitar-shaped radiographic shadow of the anomalous vein gives syndrome its name.

Seckel syndrome

Chromosome aberration, bird-headed dwarfism, microcephaly, minor deformities, preop laryngeal/renal assessment.[11]

1 Nguyen NH et al. (2001). Paediatr Anaesth, 11, 370–371.
2 Guasch E et al. (2003). Anaesthesia, 58, 607–608.
3 Cekman N et al. (2004). Paediatr Anaesth, 14, 689–692.
4 Baris S et al. (2001). Paediatr Anaesth, 11, 501–504.
5 Krechel SL et al. (1981). Anesth Analg, 60, 344–347.
6 Khalil SN et al. (2002). Paediatr Anaesth, 12, 375.
7 Jorgensen BG et al. (1999). Paediatr Anaesth, 9, 352–355.
8 Ponte J et al. (1981). Br J Anaesth, 53, 1347–1350.
9 Twigg SJ et al. (2002). Br J Anaesth, 89, 786–787.
10 Dinner M et al. (1994). Anesth Analg, 78, 1197–1199.
11 Shiraishi N et al. (1995). Masui, 44, 735–738.

314 CHAPTER 13 **Uncommon conditions**

Shprintzen syndrome (velocardiofacial syndrome)

Facial dysmorphism, cleft palate, cardiovascular malformations, mild/moderate mental retardation/learning difficulties.[1]

Shy–Drager syndrome (central nervous and autonomic degeneration)

Progressive neurovegetative disorder with primary autonomic failure, severe orthostatic hypotension/syncope, anhidrosis, disordered thermoregulation, impotence/urinary incontinence, respiratory obstruction/sleep apnoea, increased aspiration risk (gut motility disorder plus laryngeal weakness), IPPV may cause CVS instability (reduced venous return), ensure normovolaemia, regional blocks used successfully, consider fludrocortisone to sustain plasma volume.[2]

Simmond's syndrome and Sheehan's syndrome (postpartum pituitary necrosis)

Pituitary infarction following postpartum haemorrhage, variable degree of pituitary insufficiency, assess endocrine derangement.

Sipple syndrome (multiple endocrine neoplasia type IIa) (see also p172)

Phaeochromocytoma, medullary carcinoma of thyroid with or without parathyroid hyperplasia, assess degree of endocrine dysfunction, treat as for phaeochromocytoma.[3]

Sjogren's syndrome (keratoconjunctivitis sicca)

Dry eyes without rheumatoid arthritis, may also have other autoimmune disease, dysphagia/abnormal oesophageal motility, renal defects, pulmonary hypertension, peripheral neuropathy, vasculitis, assess for other systemic conditions, worsened by anticholinergic drugs, improved by humidification.[4]

Smith–Lemli–Opitz syndrome

Abnormal cholesterol biosynthesis, severe growth failure, congenital anomalies affecting most organ systems, early death, developmental delay, self-injurious/ritualistic behaviour, typical dysmorphic facial features (micrognathia/cleft palate/small and abnormally hard tongue), thymic hypoplasia, intrinsic lung disease, possibly susceptible to infection.[5]

Spinal muscular atrophy (see also p256)

Peripheral motor neurons affected, upper motor neurons spared, increase in rate of progression through types I–IV, muscular wasting (see also amyotrophic lateral sclerosis), proximal/respiratory muscle weakness (IPPV advisable), kyphoscoliosis, restrictive chest defects, bulbar dysfunction, regional blocks may be technically difficult, beware altered distribution of local anaesthetics, difficult intubation (spinal deformity/aspiration risk), avoid suxamethonium (chronic denervation/K^+), abnormal reaction to muscle relaxants (if essential, monitor blockade and ensure full reversal), postoperative respiratory support may be indicated.[6]

Strumpell's disease

Progressive spastic paresis predominantly lower extremities, avoid suxamethonium, sensitive to non-depolarising muscle relaxants, regional anaesthesia probably OK, poor respiratory function/reserve.[7]

Sturge–Weber syndrome

Unilateral angiomatous lesions of the leptomeninges/upper face, contralateral hemiparesis, seizures, mental retardation, evaluate for associated abnormalities, careful intubation/extubation (angiomas of mouth/upper airway), prevent rise in ICP/IOP.[8]

Takayasu's disease (pulseless disease, occlusive thromboaortopathy, or aortic arch syndrome)

Chronic autoimmune inflammatory disease, elastic tissue replaced by fibrous tissue leading to blood vessel narrowing/occlusion/aneurysms (preferentially large arteries—aorta and branches), often self-limiting, hypertension (usually renovascular), IHD, cerebrovascular disease, maintain organ perfusion (BP, CO_2, etc.), non-invasive blood pressure measurements may be inaccurate, many have postoperative CVS complications from poorly controlled hypertension, consider regional blocks (care—cardiovascular effect of spinal).[9]

Tangier disease (familial α-lipoprotein deficiency)

Deficient HDL apoprotein, accumulation of cholesterol in reticuloendothelial tissue, enlarged orange tonsils, hepatosplenomegaly, corneal opacities, polyneuropathy, sensitivity to muscle relaxants, IHD, anaemia, thrombocytopenia.[10]

TAR syndrome (thrombocytopenia, absent radius)

May also have Fallot's tetralogy.

Tay–Sachs disease (familial amaurotic idiocy)

Accumulation of GM2 gangliosides in CNS/peripheral nerves, progressive cerebral degeneration/seizures/dementia/blindness, usually die in <2yr, characteristic macular cherry spot appearance, progressive neurology leads to respiratory complications.

1 Meinecke P et al. (1986). Eur J Pediatr, **145**, 539–544.
2 Niquille M et al. (1998). Anesth Analg, **87**, 396–399.
3 Luo A et al. (2003). Chin Med J (Engl), **116**, 208–211.
4 Takahashi S et al. (1990). Masui, **39**, 1393–1396.
5 Quezado ZM et al. (2000). Anesthesiology, **97**, 1015–1019.
6 Kitson R et al. (2004). Anaesthesia, **59**, 94–95.
7 McTiernan C et al. (1999). Can J Anaesth, **46**, 679–682.
8 Batra RK et al. (1994). Can J Anaesth, **41**, 133–136.
9 Kathirvel S et al. (2001). Anesth Analg, **93**, 60–65.
10 Mentis SW (1996). Anesth Analg, **83**, 427–429.

Thrombotic thrombocytopenic purpura
Rare severe disease triad of haemolytic anaemia/consumptive thrombocytopenia/CNS dysfunction, often have therapeutic splenectomy, preferably postpone elective surgery until remission, check coagulation/renal/liver function, consider prophylactic antiplatelet drugs/corticosteroids, platelet transfusion contraindicated (may worsen disease), use packed cells/FFP, strict asepsis (often immunocompromised), avoid IM route/nasal intubation, control BP (renal/cerebral perfusion), care with positioning.[1]

Tourette syndrome
Profane vocalisations, repetitious speech, muscle jerking, do not confuse tic like behaviour with seizure activity on induction/emergence, sedating premedication beneficial, continue normal medication, pimozide may cause prolonged QT, beware interaction of psychotropic drugs and sympathomimetics.[2]

Toxic epidermal necrolysis ('scalded skin syndrome')
Split at level of stratum granulosum, epidermal erythema/blistering/necrosis, made worse by lateral shearing forces, can be drug related, prevent friction (monitors/lines/airway manipulation/positioning, etc.), consider fluid losses from blisters/exposed areas of dermis, manage like severe second-degree burn.[3]

Treacher–Collins syndrome, see mandibulofacial dysostosis

Trisomy 13, see Patau's syndrome

Trisomy 18, see Edward's syndrome

Trisomy 21, see Down's syndrome

Tuberous sclerosis (Bourneville's disease)
Neurocutaneous syndrome, facial angiofibromas, seizures, mental retardation, CVS/CNS/renal hamartomas, may affect airway/lungs/CVS—spontaneous rupture/bleeding, spontaneous pneumothoraces, careful positioning/padding, avoid pro-convulsants, consider full preoperative CVS assessment (cardiac rhabdomyoma 30–50%).[4]

Turner's syndrome
XO chromosome, micrognathia, short webbed neck, possible difficult intubation, coarctation/dissecting aortic aneuryms/pulmonary stenosis, renal anomaly (50%).

Urbach–Wiethe disease
Type of histiocytosis (see Hand–Schuller–Christian disease), hyaline deposits in larynx and pharynx—hoarseness/aphonia, cautious intubation, laryngeal opening may be small.

Von Recklinghausen's disease, see Neurofibromatosis

Von Willebrand's disease (pseudohaemophilia), see p212

WAGR syndrome

Wilms tumour/Aniridia/Genitourinary abnormalities/Retardation.

Weaver's syndrome

Unusual craniofacial appearance, micrognathia, airway/intubation problems, may have large stature in adulthood.

Weber–Christian disease

Global fat necrosis (including retroperitoneal/pericardial/peritoneal/meningeal), associated organ dysfunction (e.g. adrenals, constrictive pericarditis), avoid trauma to superficial fat during movement/positioning during surgery (cold, heat, pressure).

Wegener's granulomatosis

Necrotising granulomata in inflamed vessels of multiple organ systems (CNS/CVS/renal/RS), consider laryngeal stenosis, pneumonia, bronchial destruction, valvular dysfunction, abnormal cardiac conduction, arteritis (cerebral aneurysms, arterial line difficulty), IHD, renal failure, peripheral neuropathy.

Welander's muscular atrophy

Peripheral muscular atrophy, sensitive to thiopental/muscle relaxants/opioids, good prognosis.

Werdnig–Hoffman disease (spinal muscular atrophy type I acute, and type II chronic), see Spinal muscular atrophy

Wermer syndrome (multiple endocrine neoplasia types MEN1)

Parathyroid/pituitary/adrenal/thyroid adenomas, pancreas islet cell tumours, assess endocrine dysfunction.

Werner syndrome (premature aging syndrome), see progeria

Wiedemann–Rautenstrauch syndrome (premature aging syndrome), see progeria

William's syndrome

Characteristic elfin facies, congenital heart disease (aortic/pulmonary stenosis), hypercalcaemia, feeding problems, severe gag reflex, dental abnormalities, stellate blue eyes, retardation but social personality, hyperacusis.[5]

Wilson's disease

Inborn error of copper metabolism, basal ganglia degeneration, neurological symptoms, hepatic and renal failure. Respiratory complications, difficulty reversing muscle relaxants.[6,7]

1 Pivalizza EG (1994). *Anesth Analg*, **79**, 1203–1205.
2 Morrison JE et al. (1986). *Anesth Analg*, **65**, 200–202.
3 Rabito SF et al. (2001). *J Clin Anesth*, **13**, 133–137.
4 Shenkman Z et al. (2002). *Paediatr Anaesth*, **12**, 700–704.
5 http://www.williams-syndrome.org/fordoctors/anesthesia.html
6 el Dawlatly AA et al. (1992). *Middle East J Anesthesiol*, **11**, 391–397.
7 http://www.wilsonsdisease.org

Wiskott–Aldrich disease
Faulty presentation of antigen to macrophages, thrombocytopenia, coagulopathy, anaemia, immunodeficiency, recurrent infections.

Wolf–Hirschhorn syndrome
Rare chromosomal abnormality, severe psychomotor retardation, seizures, VSD/ASD, characteristic facies, midline fusion abnormalities, many die by age 2 (cardiac failure/bronchopneumonia), assess for system dysfunction, MH risk unproven.[1]

Wolfram syndrome
Diabetes insipidus, diabetes mellitus, optic atrophy, deafness, fluid/electrolyte problems.

Wolman's syndrome
Familial xanthomatosis, adrenal calcification, hepatosplenomegaly, hypersplenism, anaemia, thrombocytopenia, platelet transfusion may only be successful after splenectomy.

Zellweger syndrome (cerebrohepatorenal syndrome)
Reduced/absent peroxisomes in brain/liver/kidney, flat/round face, micrognathia, cleft palate, polycystic kidneys, apnoeas, congenital heart defects, hypotonia, areflexia, seizures, hepatomegaly/biliary dysgenesis, difficult intubation, care with muscle relaxants.[2]

Further reading
Benumof JL (1998). *Anesthesia and Uncommon Diseases, 4th ed.* Philadelphia: WB Saunders.

Diaz JH (2000). Perioperative management of children with congenital phakomatoses. *Paediatr Anaesth*, **10**, 121–8.

Merlin GB et al. (2000). Specific genetic diseases at risk for sedation/anesthesia complications. *Anesth Analg*, **91**, 837–55. [good review]

Russell SH, Hirsch NP (1994). Anaesthesia and myotonia. *Br J Anaesth*, **72**, 210–16.

For online information about rare conditions try:

http://www.diseasesdatabase.com.

http://www.rarediseases.org/.

MedlinePlus has extensive information from the National Institutes of Health and other trusted sources on over 650 diseases and conditions. http://www.nlm.nih.gov/medlineplus/healthtopics.html.

Online Mendelian Inheritance in Man, OMIM (TM). McKusick-Nathans Institute for Genetic Medicine, Johns Hopkins University (Baltimore, MD) and National Center for Biotechnology Information, National Library of Medicine (Bethesda, MD), 2000. http://www.ncbi.nlm.nih.gov/omim/. [Click on 'Search the OMIM Database' and enter the name of the condition in the search field.]

---

1 Ginsburg R et al. (1988). *Anaesthesia*, **43**, 386–388.
2 Govaerts L et al. (1982). *Eur J Pediatr*, **139**, 125–128.

Chapter 14

Cardiac surgery

Michael Sinclair and Rhys Evans

Determinants of myocardial oxygen supply and demand

Coronary blood flow to the left ventricle occurs only during diastole. Increased heart rate decreases the diastolic interval, with little change in the length of systole.

Myocardial oxygen **supply** depends upon:
- O_2 content of arterial blood (Hb and SaO_2).
- Myocardial (coronary) blood flow; this is further determined by
  - Diastolic blood pressure (dependent upon systolic pressure and heart rate)
  - Diastolic interval (length of diastole, again dependent upon heart rate)
  - Blood viscosity (decreased on cardiopulmonary bypass)
  - Coronary vascular resistance (variable coronary vascular tone and fixed atheromatous lesions)
  - LVEDP (higher pressures decrease flow)

Myocardial oxygen **demand** depends upon:
- Myocardial wall tension (systolic blood pressure).
- Number of contractions per minute (i.e. heart rate).
- 'Physiological' heart rates and systemic arterial pressures provide optimal coronary flow.
- Bradycardia provides long diastolic intervals and hence more time for coronary blood flow, together with few contractions demanding oxygen, but falling diastolic pressure during prolonged diastole decreases coronary perfusion pressure and hence CBF becomes limited in late diastole.
- Tachycardia increases mean diastolic pressure and hence coronary perfusion pressure but allows relatively little time for the flow to occur; increased numbers of contractions also increase myocardial O_2 consumption.
- High blood pressure provides higher diastolic pressures for improved coronary perfusion and hence O_2 supply, but generation of increased systolic pressures increases O_2 consumption.
- Low blood pressures are generated by low myocardial wall tension, and hence low systolic pressures and O_2 demand, but the associated low diastolic pressure limits coronary blood flow and hence O_2 supply.

Risk scoring

Parsonnet risk stratification scheme

Risk factor		Score
Female gender		1
Age	70–74yr	7
	>75yr	12
Ejection fraction	Good	0
	Fair (30–49%)	2
	Poor (<30%)	4
Obesity	>1.5 times ideal weight	3
Diabetes		3
Hypertension	Systolic >140mmHg	3
Re-operation	First re-operation	5
	Second or subsequent re-operation	10
Preop intra-aortic balloon pump	Present for surgery	2
LV aneurysm		5
Valve surgery		5
Aortic	Gradient <120mmHg	5
	Gradient >120mmHg	7
Mitral	PA pressure <60mmHg	5
	PA pressure >60mmHg	8
Valve and CABG		2
Emergency surgery following cardiac catheter		10
Dialysis dependent		10
Catastrophic states		10–50
Other circumstances (asthma etc.)		2–10

Score	Risk	Predicted mortality
0–4	Good	1%
5–9	Fair	5%
10–14	Poor	9%
15–19	High	17%
>20	Very high	31%

Cardiopulmonary bypass

- Cardiopulmonary bypass (CPB) replaces the function of heart and lungs while the heart is arrested, allowing for a bloodless and stable surgical field.
- Membrane oxygenators are most commonly used. These contain minute hollow fibres, giving a large surface area for gas exchange ($2–2.5m^2$). Gas exchange occurs down concentration gradients; increasing the gas flow removes more CO_2 and increasing FiO_2 increases oxygenation.
- Prior to CPB, full anticoagulation of the patient is required with an activated clotting time (ACT) recorded at >400s.
- The bypass circuit is primed with crystalloid (e.g. Hartmann's solution), heparin, and occasionally mannitol. The bypass machine normally delivers non-pulsatile flow of $2.4l/min/m^2$ (to correspond to a typical cardiac index).
- Mean arterial pressure (MAP) is normally maintained between 50 and 70mmHg by altering SVR.
- Volume, as crystalloid/colloid/blood, can be added to or removed by ultrafiltration, to maintain a haematocrit of 20–30%.
- Cardiopulmonary bypass causes haemolysis, platelet damage, and consumption of coagulation factors. This is usually minimal for the first 2hr.
- Other problems include poor venous drainage, aortic dissection, and gas embolisation.
- Risk of a cerebrovascular episode (CVE) ranges from 1% to 5% and is associated with increasing age, hypertension, aortic atheroma, previous CVE, diabetes, and type of surgery (aortic arch replacement > valve replacement > coronary artery surgery).
- Hypoperfusion and emboli are main aetiological factors. Strategies to reduce cerebral injury (thiopental, steroids, mannitol, use of arterial filters in the bypass circuit) lack evidence base. Maintaining optimum perfusion pressures, normoglycaemia, and careful temperature control may decrease the incidence of neurological sequelae.

Instituting cardiopulmonary bypass

- Prior to instituting bypass, the patient should be anticoagulated with heparin 300IU/kg (use central rather than peripheral line for administration to minimise risk of delivery failure). ACT must be confirmed at >400s prior to aortic cannulation.
- Before cannulation, systolic blood pressure should be decreased (to 80–100mmHg) to reduce the risk of aortic dissection.
- Prepare and pressurise cardioplegia to 300mmHg, ensuring a bubble-free circuit if cold crystalloid cardioplegia is to be used.
- Once on bypass the ventilator is turned off and an IV anaesthetic (e.g. propofol 6mg/kg/h) started. A bolus of midazolam or a volatile agent administered by vaporiser mounted on the bypass machine are alternatives.

- The perfusionist maintains a perfusion pressure of 50–70mmHg by the use of vasoconstrictors (metaraminol) and vasodilators (GTN, phentolamine).
- Blood gases and ACT are checked every 30min.
- Note: aprotinin, if used during CPB (see p346), affects ACT measured with celite (prolongation) but not with kaolin.
- The patient's temperature is actively lowered, or allowed to drift, to 28–34°C, depending on the type of surgery and surgical preference.

Coming off bypass

- This is a team effort between surgeon, anaesthetist, and perfusionist. The aim is to wean the patient from the bypass machine, allowing the heart and lungs to re-establish normal physiological function.
- Before coming off bypass:
  - The temperature should have returned to 37°C.
  - Potassium should be 4.5–5mmol/l.
  - Haematocrit should be >20%.
  - Acid/base should be in the normal range.
- Heart rate should be 70–100bpm and sinus rhythm (if possible). Defibrillate and use atropine/isoprenaline/adrenaline as necessary.
- Ventilate with 100% oxygen and ensure the lung bases are expanded.
- The venous line is progressively clamped and the heart gradually allowed to fill/eject. It is usual practice to come off bypass with the patient relatively 'underfilled'. This avoids over-distension of the ventricles, which may not yet function normally.
- The perfusionist will transfuse 100ml boluses as required. Be vigilant, watch the heart performance and filling carefully. If the ventricle is performing poorly, commence inotropic support (e.g. adrenaline).
- Do not draw up protamine (1mg/100 IU heparin—usually 3mg/kg) until off CPB. When the surgeon requests protamine, clearly inform the perfusionist to turn off the suction, and administer slowly IV. Protamine may cause systemic hypotension and pulmonary hypertension. Rapid volume administration may be required.

Following bypass

- Ensure adequate anaesthesia and analgesia with a volatile agent (e.g. isoflurane) and an opioid.
- Systolic blood pressure should be controlled at 80–140mmHg by careful filling and adjustments of vasodilator/inotrope infusions, as necessary.
- Maintain serum potassium levels at 4–5mmol/litre. Hypokalaemia should be treated with aliquots of 20mmol KCl (in 100ml over 30min).

Cardioplegia

- Based on Ringer's solution containing potassium (20mmol/litre), magnesium (16mmol/litre), and procaine.
- When rapidly infused renders the heart asystolic.
- Cold (4°C) cardioplegia affords myocardial protection against ischaemia. Further doses are repeated every 20min or when electrical activity returns.

- Can be blood or crystalloid based. The advantages of blood cardioplegia are largely theoretical and based on the assumption that haemoglobin will carry oxygen and thus help reduce myocardial damage. Reperfusion (warm blood) cardioplegia is sometimes used towards the end of bypass to wash out products of metabolism.
- Cardioplegia is usually administered anterograde (via the coronary arteries), but retrograde cardioplegia may be delivered via the coronary sinus.

Temperature management

- During bypass, the patient's temperature may be allowed to 'drift' down to 34°C, or the patient can be actively cooled to a lower temperature (28–34°C).
- Generally, a cooler temperature allows better cerebral protection.
- Different centres vary in approach, but marked hypothermia is usually reserved for more complex cases.

Intermittent cross-clamping and fibrillation

- Coronary arterial grafts can be undertaken using either cardioplegia or intermittent cross-clamping with fibrillation.
- Intermittent cross-clamping—the aorta is clamped and a fibrillator pad placed underneath the heart. The lower end of a graft can then be sutured. After each graft the cross-clamp is removed and the heart cardioverted into sinus rhythm.
- Advantages are that no cardioplegia is used (hence a lower incidence of complete heart block) and after each graft is attached, the ECG can be inspected for ischaemia.
- As the heart is not protected by cardioplegia, surgical time needs to be kept to a minimum to avoid myocardial damage.

Volatile agents and CPB

- All volatile agents cause vasodilatation, cardiac depression, and brady-cardia in a dose-dependent manner.
- Isoflurane has been shown in the animal model to cause a 'steal' phenomenon, but this has not been convincingly demonstrated in man.
- A large study compared all different anaesthetic techniques then in use for cardiac surgery and concluded that there was no difference between the anaesthetic used in terms of either morbidity or mortality[1].
- Halothane is the volatile agent that has been used the longest and the more recently introduced volatile agents (enflurane, isoflurane, sevoflurane) would not appear to offer any major advantages.
- For repeated anaesthetics isoflurane is probably the agent of choice.

1 Slogoff S, Keats AS (1989). Randomised trial of primary anaesthetic agents on outcome of coronary artery bypass operations. *Anesthesiology*, **70**, 179– 188.

Coronary arterial bypass grafting

Procedure	Bypassing a coronary artery stenosis with an arterial or venous graft
Time	3hr
Pain	+++/++++
Position	Supine ± crucifix
Blood loss	Moderate (X-match 2U)
Practical techniques	ETT, IPPV, arterial/CVP, urinary catheter, temperature monitoring, usually on CPB. Consider PA flotation catheter and/or TOE

Preoperative

- Commonly associated medical problems include hypertension, COPD, diabetes, cerebrovascular disease, and renal dysfunction.
- History of angina, recent MI, or CVE.
- Investigations: recent FBC, U&Es, clotting screen, chest radiograph, ECG. Respiratory function tests and arterial blood gases may be appropriate.
- Careful assessment of left ventricular function:
    - Orthopnoea and paroxysmal dyspnoea are important symptoms of LV failure.
    - Exercise ECG.
    - Coronary angiography within past 12 months.
    - Echocardiography assessment (transthoracic or transoesophageal).
    - Most useful assessment of left ventricular function is exercise tolerance.
- Parsonnet's scoring system (see p321).
- Premedication with IM opioid and anticholinergic (e.g. papaveretum/hyoscine 15.4mg/0.4mg for an adult male, very amnesic, soporific, and analgesic; alternatively an oral anxiolytic but this lacks analgesia for awake line placement). Prescribe oxygen supplementation from time of premedication.
- Continue all cardiac medication preoperatively (some centres stop aspirin/anti-platelet drugs/ACE inhibitors).

Echocardiography

40–50% ejection fraction	mild LV impairment
30–40% ejection fraction	moderate LV impairment
<30% ejection fraction	severe LV impairment

Perioperative

- Peripheral venous and arterial lines pre-induction, preoxygenate and induce with fentanyl 10–15µg/kg and a cardiostable induction agent. Paralyse with non-depolarising muscle relaxant, intubate, and maintain anaesthesia with a volatile agent in an oxygen and air mixture. Insert internal jugular lines and urinary catheter.
- Five-lead ECG with ST segment monitoring is advised (lead II for rhythm and V5 for ischaemia).
- Use a nasopharyngeal temperature probe.
- Indications for a pulmonary artery flotation catheter include:
  - All ventricles with an ejection fraction <30%.
  - All mitral valves, as filling and PA pressures are important post-operatively.
  - All patients with raised preoperative creatinine.
  - A peroperative alternative is to insert a left atrial line, or use transoesophageal echo to assess filling and ventricular function.
- Avoid hypertension and tachycardia. Aim for cardiovascular stability with volume, GTN infusion, and careful boluses of vasoconstrictor (e.g. metaraminol 0.5–1mg).
- Prophylactic antibiotics timed to coincide with skin incision:
  - Flucloxacillin 25mg/kg (vancomycin 1g IV with premed if penicillin allergy or MRSA risk)
  - Gentamicin 1.5mg/kg
- Anticipate blood pressure surge during sternotomy, cover with fentanyl/volatile supplements and/or GTN.
- Give heparin 300IU/kg and ensure ACT >400s pre-bypass.
- Maintain systolic blood pressure in range 80–100mmHg for aortic cannulation.
- Continue as for 'Bypass' (p322).
- Once the chest is closed and the patient stable, transfer intubated to recovery.
- Patients require optimum filling postoperatively, particularly if bleeding, diuresing well, and vasodilating as they warm up. If cardioplegia has been used, temporary pacing wires will be inserted and temporary pacing may be needed.

Postoperative

- Check FBC, clotting, ABGs, and ensure blood loss is <200ml/hr.
- Once warm, awake, weaned, and not bleeding (i.e. a stable patient) extubate. Administer morphine (0.02mg/kg/hr) with GTN to keep systolic BP <140mmHg—to protect the graft 'top-ends' and reduce bleeding.

Special considerations

- For severe left main stem disease, adequate myocardial perfusion must be preserved by maintaining diastolic pressure and diastolic interval (i.e. heart rate) at preoperative values.
- Unstable angina with poor ventricles: consider PAFC and insertion of an intra-aortic balloon pump (IABP) in the anaesthetic room.

- Thoracic epidurals are used in some centres, claiming improved haemodynamic stability and excellent postoperative pain relief, but this is controversial due to the perceived risk of epidural haematoma and tetraplegia following anticoagulation for CPB.
- Arterial grafts (internal mammary/radial artery) are prone to spasm; therefore maintain GTN infusion postoperatively. Avoid noradrenaline if possible.

Off-pump coronary artery bypass grafting (OPCAB)

Management is as for CABG but without bypass and using a 'stabiliser' to keep the heart as still as possible.

- Keep patient well filled with crystalloid.
- Keep patient warm (blood/fluid warmer, warming mattress/blanket, HME, etc).
- May need vasoconstrictor when surgeon manipulates heart to maintain adequate BP.
- Consider TOE or oesophageal Doppler probe.
- Patient may still require full or half-dose heparin (surgical preference).
- If patient unstable, may need to go on bypass (1–10%).
- For right/posterior descending coronary artery grafts, patient is placed in Trendelenberg position to increase venous return.
- Postoperatively: as for CABGs on bypass.

Emergency coronary arterial bypass graft (failed angioplasty)

Preoperative
- The patient will be collapsed in peri-arrest with the need for urgent surgery to correct ischaemia.
- Should have good arterial access from the 'cath lab'.
- Patient will probably need inotropes, if not already started. Ideally attain some degree of stability or cardiac arrest may follow induction.
- An IABP can help poor coronary perfusion by increasing diastolic pressure, plus improve left ventricular function by off-loading the heart.
- Consider placement of central venous access under local anaesthetic before induction (administration of cardioactive drugs in case of cardiac arrest during induction).
- Patient may have had abciximab or other anti-platelet drug and may require platelets post-bypass.

Perioperative
- May need a pulmonary artery flotation catheter, but do not waste time if speed is important. It can be done later during the case.
- Cautious induction with a reduced dose of fentanyl (250–500µg) and etomidate (4–6mg). Cardiovascular stability is essential.
- Adrenaline should be prepared to be given as a bolus, 10 or 100µg/ml as appropriate.
- Do not forget to give heparin (300IU/kg) before aortic cannulation.
- Institute CPB as soon as possible.

Postoperative
- Inotropes should be maintained post-CPB; restart IABP if placed pre-operatively and consider insertion of IABP if not.
- There is no urgency to extubate the patient. A period of stability is required.
- There is a high risk of renal failure.

Aortic valve replacement: stenosis

(See also p56)

Procedure	Replacement of aortic valve
Time	3hr
Pain	+++/++++
Position	Supine
Blood loss	Moderate (X-match 2U)
Practical techniques	As for CABG

The anatomical problems and consequences of particular valve lesions should be understood to appreciate the physiological requirements necessary for forward flow of blood before and after valve replacement.

Mechanical valves tend to be used in younger patients, as they are longer lasting; however, anticoagulation (warfarin) is needed to prevent clot formation around the valve. In elderly patients, biological tissue (homograft) valves can be used, as long-term anticoagulation is not needed. These valves probably only last for ~15yr.

Preoperative
- A sudden change in heart rhythm (e.g. atrial fibrillation) can precipitate LV failure.
- Perform echocardiography and angiography to assess LV function and coronary blood flow.
- Aortic stenosis causes LV hypertrophy, with no increase in LV volume and a stiff non-compliant ventricle with poor diastolic function (relaxation). This increases oxygen demand, and requires higher filling pressures. If long-standing, the LV fails, LVEDP increases (causing mitral regurgitation and a high PAP) and ultimately RV failure.

- An LV–aorta gradient exceeding 40mmHg or aortic orifice of <0.8cm represents significant obstruction to LV outflow.
- Surgery indicated if gradient >70mmHg with good LV (>50mmHg with poor LV).
- If a known gradient is decreasing, this is a sign of LV failure.

Perioperative
- Heart rate: 'aortic stenosis—always slow'. Tachycardia is not well tolerated as it shortens diastole, hence time for coronary blood flow, and increases oxygen demand. The atrial kick of sinus rhythm improves filling of a stiff LV.
- Preload: should be increased to aid filling of stiff LV; beware vasodilators reducing preload and cardiac output.
- SVR: afterload must be meticulously maintained with α_1 agonists (e.g. metaraminol, noradrenaline). A reduction in diastolic pressure may critically reduce coronary blood flow to a hypertrophied LV; again, extreme caution with vasodilators.
- Contraction: the stiff and thickened LV may require adrenaline.

Post-bypass

- Preload: volume is still very important for adequate filling and perfusion of a stiff LV; consider sequential A-V pacing to stimulate atrial contraction and augment ventricular filling.
- SVR: an infusion of noradrenaline may be required once well filled.
- Contraction: inotropic support (e.g. adrenaline) may be required to improve LV performance.

Special considerations

- Consider a pulmonary artery flotation catheter as filling is crucial, particularly in the postoperative period. Pre-bypass, the high pulmonary arterial pressure in long-standing aortic stenosis may underestimate LV filling.
- Good myocardial protection for a hypertrophied ventricle by meticulous cardioplegic technique during CPB is the key to a good outcome.

Aortic valve replacement: regurgitation

(See also p58)

Procedure	Replacement of aortic valve
Time	3hr
Pain	+++/++++
Position	Supine
Blood loss	moderate (X-match 2U)
Practical techniques	As for CABG

Preoperative

- Aortic regurgitation (AR) may be associated with aortic root dilation or dissection.
- In AR the LV is volume overloaded with LV dilation. There is increased sympathetic drive, causing tachycardia, increased contractility, peripheral vasodilatation, and fluid retention to increase preload.
- Surgery is indicated once symptomatic; angina is a late symptom indicating end-stage disease.

Perioperative

- 'Full, fast, and forward for a regurgitant lesion.'
- Heart rate: cardiac output is rate dependent, increasing the rate reduces diastole and forward flow is encouraged (regurgitation occurs during diastole). Avoid bradycardia and aim for a rate of 90bpm. Collapsing diastolic pressure due to AR also decreases coronary perfusion, so again keep HR up to maintain mean diastolic pressure and hence coronary blood flow.
- Preload: LV is stiff with increased volume; therefore maintain adequate filling. Sinus rhythm is of benefit but patients are often in atrial fibrillation. Consider A-V sequential pacing.
- SVR: anaesthesia causes a reduction in SVR, reducing the regurgitant fraction and encouraging forward flow. Vasodilators have similar effects, but may also reduce venous return/preload. Pre-bypass, beware excessive systemic vasodilatation decreasing diastolic pressure and hence coronary perfusion.
- Contraction: if LV function is poor, inotropic support/inodilators may be required.

Severity of AR is assessed by echocardiography with colour flow Doppler: dimensions of jet into LV cavity on apical five-chamber view indicates severity. Jet width >60% at cusp level indicates severe AR (fifth chamber is aortic root).

Post-bypass
- Preload: because of LV dilatation, adequate filling is essential and must be maintained.
- SVR: a reduction will encourage forward flow, particularly if the LV is impaired.
- Contraction: inotropic support may be required. An inodilator (e.g. milrinone, enoximone) will both reduce the SVR and improve LV function.

Special considerations
- An intra-aortic balloon pump is contraindicated in aortic regurgitation, but may be useful post-bypass when the aortic valve is competent to offload the LV/optimise cardiac output, and to augment diastolic pressure and hence coronary blood flow.
- Careful control of blood pressure is needed pre-bypass in patients with aortic root dilatation or dissection. Aim to keep systolic blood pressure <120mmHg with vasodilators/volatile agents.

With mixed regurgitant/stenotic lesions manage the dominant lesion.

Mitral valve replacement: stenosis

(See also p60)

Procedure	Replacement of mitral valve
Time	3–4hr
Pain	+++/++++
Position	Supine
Blood loss	Moderate (X-match 2U)
Practical techniques	As for CABG; PAFC and TOE likely to be indicated.

Prosthetic mitral valves are usually mechanical—tissue mitral valve prostheses are uncommon, and most patients are anticoagulated anyway because of chronic AF.

Preoperative
- Frail, flushed, in atrial fibrillation and often on warfarin, with a fixed cardiac output and possible pulmonary hypertension.
- Almost always due to rheumatic heart disease, normally asymptomatic for 20yr.
- Surgery required if dyspnoea on mild exertion/at rest.
- Continue antiarrhythmic therapy and convert those on warfarin to heparin preoperatively.
- Echocardiography and angiography to assess pulmonary arterial pressure, ventricular function, and coronary arteries.
- Opioid/anticholinergic premedication with oxygen supplementation.

Normal valve surface area	4–6cm^2
Symptom-free until	1.5–2.5cm^2
Moderate stenosis	1–1.5cm^2
Critical stenosis	<1cm^2

Perioperative
- Heart rate: mitral flow is relatively fixed, keep <100bpm and sinus rhythm if possible to maximise time for diastole and coronary blood flow.
- Preload: does not normally need augmenting pre-bypass.
- SVR: because of fixed cardiac output the SVR is often raised—avoid reducing it as the diastolic pressure will fall and with it coronary blood flow. Venodilation will also reduce cardiac return and cardiac output for which the heart cannot compensate.

- PVR: pulmonary hypertension secondary to raised PVR and PA pressures may be at least partially reversible. Avoid pulmonary vasoconstriction, and consider techniques to improve pulmonary vasodilatation:
  - Maintain filling pressures.
  - Avoid hypoxia/hypercapnia even at the expense of raised mean intrathoracic pressures
  - Check ABGs regularly—avoid acidosis.
  - Pulmonary vasodilators if PA pressure >two thirds systemic pressure: nitric oxide = first-line choice, alternatively inhaled prostacyclin, and consider inodilators (milrinone, sildenafil) depending on availability.
- Contraction: severe mitral stenosis leads to pulmonary hypertension and with it right ventricular failure. The left ventricle is normally unaffected until end-stage disease. Inotropic support (e.g. adrenaline) may be required if the right ventricle is very dilated and failing.
- Heart rate: disruption of conducting pathways from surgery can cause heart block and arrhythmias requiring pacing and/or chronotropic agents (e.g. atropine, isoprenaline).

Post-bypass

- Preload: keep well filled as obstruction to flow has been removed (PAWP 13–16mmHg).
- SVR: a reduction will now encourage forward flow.
- PVR: maintain pulmonary vasodilatation to optimise pulmonary blood flow and left-sided filling.
- Contraction: inotropic support (e.g. adrenaline) may be required if the right ventricle is failing in order to optimise cardiac output.

Special considerations

- Use a pulmonary arterial flotation catheter to assess filling, PVR, and requirement for inotropes.
- Pulmonary arterial pressures take several days/weeks to decrease. Nitric oxide/pulmonary vasodilators may help.
- Catastrophic atrioventricular disruption (rupture) in the early postoperative period is rare and usually fatal.

Mitral valve replacement: regurgitation

(See also p62)

Procedure	Replacement or repair of mitral valve
Time	3hr
Pain	+++/++++
Position	Supine
Blood loss	Moderate (X-match 2U)
Practical techniques	As for CABG plus PAFC and TOE

Preoperative

- May result from papillary muscle rupture due to MI; therefore ischaemic heart disease may co-exist. If acute may cause pulmonary oedema.
- 75% have atrial fibrillation. Continue anti-arrhythmic therapy and change warfarin to heparin.
- The LV is volume overloaded; mitral regurgitation (MR) increases pulmonary arterial pressure and may cause RV failure.

Perioperative

- 'Full, fast, and forward for a regurgitant lesion.'
- Heart rate: avoid bradycardia, maintain HR >70/min (increases forward flow but also increases regurgitation).
- Preload: keep the patient well filled, again to encourage forward flow.
- SVR: an increase in SVR increases the regurgitant fraction. Vasoconstrictors should be avoided if there is a drop in blood pressure—fluids should be given to supplement circulating blood volume. Avoid bradycardia.
- PVR: avoid pulmonary vasoconstriction and attempt to decrease PVR (see mitral stenosis above). PA pressure monitoring is useful.
- Contraction: inotropes are rarely needed pre-bypass; however, with acute MR an intra-aortic balloon pump decreases afterload and improves cardiac output.

Severity of MR relates to regurgitant fraction and PVR.
- Echocardiography with colour flow Doppler:
  - If regurgitant jet fills area of LA >8cm^2 = severe MR
  - If regurgitant jet fills area of LA <4cm^2 = mild MR
- Raised PA pressure = chronic significant MR (pulmonary hypertension).

Post-bypass

- LV function is often overestimated in mitral regurgitation, as the pulmonary circulation provides a low-pressure release system for a poor ventricle. On replacing the valve the LV has to work harder, which may precipitate failure and the need for inotropes/inodilators.
- Preload: adequate filling is still essential.
- SVR: afterload reduction will benefit forward flow and cardiac output.
- PVR: the pulmonary vasculature is often highly reactive and prone to vasoconstrictive spells. Avoid factors causing pulmonary vasoconstriction and consider pulmonary vasodilators. Although IPPV raises mean intrathoracic pressure and hence PVR, this is more than offset by the pulmonary vasodilatation resulting from optimised ABGs (see also p337).
- Contraction: inotropic support may be required for a failing LV.

Special considerations

- A pulmonary arterial flotation catheter is indicated in MR as PA pressure monitoring and correct ventricular filling are essential.
- An IABP may also be of use in the short term for a failing LV.

Thoracic aortic surgery

Procedure	Replacement of ascending aorta/aortic arch with a tubular graft
Time	3–4hr
Pain	+++/++++
Position	Supine
Blood loss	Moderate/severe (X-match 4U)
Practical techniques	As for CABG ± deep hypothermic circulatory arrest

- Thoracic aortic aneurysms and dissection are usually due to atherosclerosis. They can be divided into two groups, those with hypertension and those with hereditary conditions such as Marfan's syndrome.
- More than 66% have co-existing ischaemic heart disease, and dilatation of the aortic root with aortic regurgitation is common.
- They are classified as type A, involving the ascending aorta to the brachiocephalic artery, and type B, the arch/descending aorta.
- Type A and those involving the arch are treated surgically; the remainder of type B (descending lesions) are treated medically.
- Arch involvement, although rare, is treated surgically, under deep hypothermic circulatory arrest.
- They may present as elective or emergency procedures.

Preoperative

- For emergency dissections, control of blood pressure, bleeding, and fluid resuscitation are the main priorities. Wide-bore venous access is essential; consider inserting a PA catheter sheath (for rapid transfusion through the side-arm and later placement of PAFC). An arterial line should be inserted under LA pre-induction.
- Blood (6U) needs urgent crossmatching; warn the laboratory regarding the need for clotting factors, platelets, and more blood later.
- Vasodilators (e.g. GTN, labetalol) may be required to keep the systolic pressure <120mmHg.

Managing hospital transfer of patient for emergency thoracic aortic surgery

- Adequate analgesia
- Oxygen
- Wide-bore IV access
- Monitoring: invasive BP plus non-invasive BP monitoring on contralateral arm, pulse oximeter, ECG
- BP control/antihypertensive therapy (e.g. labetalol infusion)

Perioperative

- It is essential to avoid hypertension during induction as this can rupture the thoracic aorta.
- Once stable they should be treated as patients with aortic regurgitation (see p334)—avoid bradycardia, reduced afterload, and keep well filled.
- Inotropes/vasoconstrictors should be avoided as any dissection can extend or rupture.
- Be aware that a dissection, and surgical clamps, may interfere with invasive arterial monitoring.
- Aprotinin (2 million units) is administered to the patient, 2 million units added to the bypass prime, and then continued IV at 500 000U/hr per-operatively to reduce clot breakdown.
- Femoral artery cannulation is usually required as the ascending aorta is to be resected; administer heparin (300IU/kg) and ensure adequate anticoagulation (ACT >400s) before femoral cannulation.
- If the aortic root is involved the aortic valve may need replacement and coronary arteries re-implanting.
- Regular ABGs and monitoring of acid–base for indices of organ perfusion.
- Inotropic support (e.g. adrenaline) may be required before coming off bypass.

Post-bypass

- Bleeding and control of the arterial pressure are major problems.
- Continue aprotinin infusion (500 000U/hr). Following administration of protamine check coagulation; if indicated administer FFP and platelets.
- Meticulous control of systolic pressure at <120mmHg.
- Aortic dissection may involve renal and mesenteric vessels—monitor indices of kidney/gut perfusion.

Special considerations

Circulatory arrest

- Protection of the central nervous system by deep hypothermia during prolonged periods of circulatory arrest is necessary if the arch of the aorta is to be operated on (during this procedure it is not possible to perfuse the cerebral vessels easily on bypass).
- Hypothermia depresses the metabolic rate and oxygen consumption in the brain and also seems to protect cerebral integrity during reperfusion. The maximum safe duration of deep hypothermic circulatory arrest (DHCA) is thought to be ~45min at 18°C. In neonates, this can be extended to 60min.
- Most centres do not rely solely on hypothermia to protect the brain; the head can be packed in ice, and consider adding thiopental (7mg/kg), steroid (e.g. methyl prednisolone (15mg/kg), and mannitol (0.5g/kg)) to the pump prime in an effort to decrease cerebral metabolic demand further and protect against ischaemic damage.
- The shorter the period of DHCA the better. Incidence of postoperative neurological problems is directly proportional to the time of DHCA.

- To aid rapid cooling, and to ensure that the brain is cooled, a vasodilator (e.g. GTN) is given. This prevents localised vasoconstriction due to hypothermia.
- Once the circulation has been arrested, all infusions and pumps are stopped.
- It is essential to measure both core and skin temperature and to make sure the core temperature reaches <20°C.
- On rewarming, switch on warming blankets but do not set to >10°C above patient temperature in order to avoid burns. Start propofol infusion (3–6mg/kg/hr as tolerated), check coagulation and if necessary order FFP (4U) and platelets (1 pooled donor pack), as these patients frequently encounter bleeding problems. A vasodilator (e.g. GTN), if tolerated, may be used to maintain vasodilatation and help rewarming.
- Mannitol (0.5g/kg) may also be given to encourage a diuresis.
- When core temperature reaches 35°C start inotrope (e.g. adrenaline) to improve cardiac function.
- A steep head-down tilt is used to allow air out of the aortic graft. Keeping the patient warm is difficult as it takes a considerable time to warm thoroughly. Skin temperature must be >33°C with a core temperature of ≥37°C, before attempting to come off bypass. Do not be rushed as rebound cooling occurs in recovery, which will exacerbate poor myocardial function and any coagulopathy.

Pulmonary thromboembolectomy

Procedure	Removal of clot/tumour from pulmonary artery
Time	2–3hr
Pain	++/+++
Position	Supine
Blood loss	Moderate (X-match 4U)
Practical techniques	As for CABG

Preoperative

- The patient is often collapsed—resuscitation may be in progress.
- Presentation with tachycardia, tachypnoea, hypoxia, cyanosis with distended neck veins, and signs of RV failure.
- A healthy heart requires 50–80% of the pulmonary trunk to be obstructed before RV failure.
- The patient may have recently received thrombolytic therapy
- Urgent cardiopulmonary bypass to re-establish oxygenation is the priority, so rapid decision-making is essential.

Diagnosis of PE

- Chest pain, dyspnoea, tachypnoea, haemoptysis, cyanosis, tachycardia, dysrhythmia, raised JVP, hypotension, oliguria, collapse, arrest
- ABGs: hypoxia, hypo/hypercapnia, metabolic acidosis
- CXR: oligaemic lung fields, prominent PA
- ECG: S1Q3T3, RV strain, normal in 50%
- Te/Xe lung scan, pulmonary angiography, spiral CT

Assessment of severity

- Minor (<30% pulmonary obstruction, no RV dysfunction):
  - Non-specific symptoms, pleuritic chest pain, dyspnoea, tiredness
  - Specific treatment = anticoagulation (heparin, then warfarin)
- Moderate (30–50% pulmonary obstruction, some RV dysfunction but normotensive):
  - Haemoptysis, tachypnoea → respiratory alkalosis, raised JVP, tachycardia
  - Specific treatment = thrombolysis
- Massive (>50% pulmonary obstruction, severe RV failure and haemodynamic impairment/collapse):
  - Severe chest pain, dyspnoea, hypotension, hypoxia, syncope, shock, arrest
  - Specific treatment = embolectomy

General treatment

- Oxygen, IV access, fluid resuscitation, analgesia, inotropic support, ventilatory support, as required. Specific treatment (above) according to severity

Perioperative
- Once the decision is taken to operate speed is the key—allow no delays. Heparin (300IU/kg) is easily forgotten.
- Intubate and ventilate with 100% oxygen, maintaining perfusion with inotropes as necessary and institute CPB as soon as possible.
- There may be substantial airway haemorrhage from pulmonary infarction. Ventilation may be difficult and the ETT may require frequent suctioning. A double lumen ETT may be helpful to control pulmonary bleeding and aid ventilation.
- The surgeons should consider placing an IVC filter post-embolectomy.

Post-bypass
- Inotropic support is likely to be needed; keep well filled and reduce SVR with vasodilators if tolerated.
- Nitric oxide, inhaled prostacyclin, or an inodilator (e.g. milrinone, sildenafil (IV administration if available)) may help reduce a raised pulmonary arterial pressure. Delay heparinisation (following CPB) for 24hr to reduce surgical bleeding.

Special considerations
- Very high right-sided pressures may open the foramen ovale and cause right-to-left shunting. This will worsen hypoxia and may allow paradoxical emboli, causing a CVE.
- With significant pulmonary emboli the capnograph will detect very little or no expired CO_2. Following embolectomy, if successful, this should show dramatic improvement, as the pulmonary circulation is re-established.

Redo cardiac surgery

Preoperative

- There is often poor LV function.
- Venous/arterial access as for CABG but often more difficult.
- Crossmatch 6U.

Perioperative

- Place external defibrillator pads on the patient, as VF is a risk at sternotomy and during dissection of adhesions. This can be a problem with extensive use of diathermy as it obscures the ECG and with VF all you may notice is a flat arterial trace (be vigilant)!
- There is a risk of torrential bleeding as the right ventricle may be stuck by adhesions to the underside of the sternum. Ensure adequate wide-bore venous access (e.g. PAFC sheath) and have blood checked and available in theatre.
- Consider using aprotinin during the procedure. Test dose of 1ml, then 2 million units (200ml) loading dose, 2 million units into the pump prime, and then 500 000U/hr (50ml) peroperatively.

Postoperative

- There is increased risk of postoperative bleeding. After administering protamine, check coagulation and administer clotting factors if indicated.
- There may be problems related to poor LV function.

Cardioversion

Procedure	DC shock to convert an arrhythmia back to sinus rhythm
Time	5–10min
Pain	—
Position	Supine
Blood loss	Nil
Practical techniques	Monitor ECG/SpO$_2$/NIBP; propofol ± LMA; COETT if full stomach

Preoperative
- Atrial fibrillation is the commonest arrhythmia—acute or chronic.
- Often a remote site, with patients who are cardiovascularly unstable.
- If possible transfer to an anaesthetic room in theatre with help nearby.
- Treat as for any surgical procedure, and have a physician ready to cardiovert the patient.
- Potassium should be in the normal range as the myocardium may become unstable.
- If in AF >24hr and not anticoagulated the left atrium should be checked for clot with a transoesophageal echo before cardioversion. This can be done under propofol sedation. If clot is present anticoagulation for 4wk is required and then check again. If clear, continue with propofol and secure the airway as appropriate.

Perioperative
- Attach monitoring, with ECG leads connected through the defibrillator and synchronised to R wave.
- Any GA suitable for day-case surgery, including sevoflurane by inhalation, is appropriate.
- Preoxygenate, induce slowly with e.g. a minimal dose of propofol. Maintain the airway using a facemask. RSI/COETT if risk of aspiration.
- Consider etomidate if haemodynamically unstable.
- Opioids/muscle relaxants are not usually necessary.
- Obese patients and those who are likely to have an awkward airway can be defibrillated in the lateral position.
- Safety during defibrillation—follow the ALS protocol. Remove oxygen during shock.
- AF—start at 150J biphasic defibrillator, 200J standard defibrillator.
- Atrial flutter—start with 50J, and increase by increments of 50J.

Postoperative
- Turn the patient into the recovery position with supplemental oxygen and recover with full monitoring as for any anaesthetic.

Special considerations
- Digoxin increases the risk of arrhythmia—omit on the day.
- Amiodarone improves the success of cardioversion to sinus rhythm.

Anaesthesia for implantable defibrillators

Procedure	Implanting pacemaker/defibrillator
Time	1–3hr
Pain	+
Position	Supine
Blood loss	Nil
Practical techniques	LA + sedation; GA: ETT/IPPV or LMA/SV ± invasive arterial monitoring

- Implantable defibrillators are placed in patients who are at risk of sudden death due to malignant cardiac arrhythmias. Patients range from young and otherwise fit adults with normal cardiac contractility to extremely compromised cardiac patients.
- The procedure may be straightforward, when two venous wires (sensing and shocking) are positioned transvenously, or complex when pacemakers are replaced or the coronary sinus is catheterised to gain access to the LV myocardium.
- In some units cardiologists provide their own sedation service.
- During the procedure VF is induced on a number of occasions to test the device. The patient needs to be sedated during this phase.
- Invasive monitoring (arterial line) is advisable for any patients with impaired contractility.
- The cardiologist usually gains access via the left cephalic vein and uses fluoroscopy to guide the position of the leads.
- Careful asepsis is important to avoid infection of the prosthesis. IV antibiotics are usually given.
- Monitor the total doses of local anaesthetic used by the cardiologist.

Preoperative

- Careful assessment is required to assess the functional cardiac reserve. Use local anaesthesia and sedation for anyone who is compromised.
- Ensure resuscitation drugs and equipment are available, as well as an external defibrillator (applied via stick-on pads).
- Draw up vasopressors and vagolytic drugs ready for use (ephedrine/ metaraminol/glycopyrronium). Have dedicated, skilled assistance.
- Give a good explanation to the patient of what will happen.

Perioperative

- If sedation is planned, give small doses of a short-acting sedative (e.g. midazolam) and an opioid (e.g. fentanyl) until comfortable, co-operative, but sleepy. Administer oxygen. Deepen the sedation immediately before defibrillator testing—propofol TCI is ideal at minimal doses.
- If the defibrillator is to be placed under the muscle, it is often difficult to get fully effective regional anaesthesia, and a short period of deeper sedation/anaesthesia may be required.

- If GA is planned ensure recovery is organised preoperatively. Use light anaesthesia with careful induction as many of these patients have limited cardiac reserve. An X-ray table may not tip and induction may be safer on a tilting trolley.
- ECG is recorded by the cardiologist.
- Antibiotics will be required according to local protocols.

Special considerations

- During VF testing, if the device does not work, do not allow the heart to be stopped for long! Repeated shocks may be required.
- After VF and defibrillation the BP may remain low for a short period. Vasopressors may be required.
- If the patient has an existing pacemaker which is to be changed and the cardiologist is using diathermy, complete loss of pacemaker function can occur.
- Cardiac catheter laboratories are difficult places to work in—space may be at a premium. Do not allow yourself to be distracted by the range of other activities taking place.
- A large plastic sheet (similar to an awake carotid set-up) allows the anaesthetist access to the patient's airway without compromising sterility. Infection is a disaster.

Further reading

Belisle S, Hardy JF (1996). Hemorrhage and the use of blood products after adult cardiac operations: myths and realities. *Annals of Thoracic Surgery*, **62**, 1908–1917.
Berton C, Cholley B (2002). Equipment review: new techniques for cardiac output measurement—oesophageal Doppler, Fick principle using carbon dioxide, and pulse contour analysis. *Critical Care*, **6**, 216–221.
Gothard J, Kelleher A, Haxby E (2003). *Cardiovascular and Thoracic Anaesthesia.* London: Butterworth Heinemann.
Hwang NC, Sinclair M (ed.) (1997). *Cardiac Anaesthesia: A practical Handbook.* Oxford: Oxford University Press.
Kaplan J (ed.) (1998). *Cardiac Anesthesia.* New York: Grune & Stratton.
Mets B (2000). The pharmacokinetics of anesthetic drugs and adjuvants during cardiopulmonary bypass. *Acta Anaesthesiologica Scandinavica*, **44**, 261–273.
Myles PS, Daly DJ, Djaiani G, Lee A, Cheng DC (2003). A systematic review of the safety and effectiveness of fast-track cardiac anesthesia. *Anesthesiology*, **99**, 982–987.
Patel RL, Turtle MRJ, Chambers DJ, *et al.* (1993). Hyperfusion and cerebral dysfunction: effect of differing acid-base management during cardiopulmonary bypass. *European Journal of Cardio-thoracic Surgery*, **7**, 457–464.
Reeves JG (1999). Towards the goal of optimal cardiac anesthesia. *Journal of Thoracic and Cardiovascular Anesthesia*, **13**, 1–2.
Ridley S (2003). Cardiac scoring systems—what is their value? *Anaesthesia*, **58**, 985–991.
Singh S, Hutton P (2003). Cerebral effects of cardiopulmonary bypass in adults. *British Journal of Anaesthesia CEPD Reviews*, **3**, 115–119.
Slogoff S, Keats AS (1989). Randomised trial of primary anesthetic agents on outcome of coronary artery bypass operations. *Anesthesiology*, **70**, 179–188.
Stone KR, McPherson CA (2004). Assessment and management of patients with pacemakers and implantable cardioverter defibrillators. *Critical Care Medicine*, **32**, S155–S165.
Troncy E, Francoeur M, Blaise G (1997). Inhaled nitric oxide: clinical applications, indications, and toxicology. *Canadian Journal of Anaesthesia*, **44**, 973–98.
Tuman KJ, McCarthy RJ, Spiess BD, *et al.* (1989). Does choice of anesthetic agent significantly affect outcome after coronary artery surgery. *Anesthesiology*, **70**, 189–198.
van Dijk D, Keizer AM, Diephuis JC, Durand C, Vos LJ, Hijman R (2000). Neurocognitive dysfunction after coronary artery bypass surgery: a systematic review. *Journal of Thoracic and Cardiovascular Surgery*, **120**, 632–639.

Thoracic surgery

David Sanders

General principles

Successful thoracic anaesthesia requires the ability to control ventilation of the patient's two lungs independently, skilful management of the shared lung and airway, and a clear understanding of planned surgery. Good communication between surgeon and anaesthetist is essential.

Patients undergoing thoracic surgery are commonly older and less fit than other patients (30% > 70yr, 50% > ASA 3). Long-term smoking, bronchial carcinoma, pleural effusion, empyema, oesophageal obstruction, and cachexia are all common and can significantly reduce cardiorespiratory physiological reserve.

General considerations

• Discuss planned procedure and any potential problems with the surgeon.
• Optimise lung function before elective surgery—try to stop patients smoking, arrange preoperative physiotherapy and incentive spirometry.
• The lateral decubitus position with operating table 'broken' to separate ribs is used for many operations.
• Postoperative mechanical ventilation stresses pulmonary suture lines and increases air leaks and the risk of chest infection, so avoid if possible.
• Minimise postoperative respiratory dysfunction by providing good analgesia and physiotherapy.
• Prescribe postoperative oxygen therapy routinely to compensate for increased V/Q mismatch. Warmed humidified 40% oxygen via a facemask is recommended after pulmonary surgery. Nasal cannulae delivering oxygen at 3litres/min are better tolerated and satisfactory for most other patients.

Important clinical scenarios which may be encountered by the thoracic anaesthetist include:

• Sub-glottic obstruction of the trachea/carina from extrinsic compression (retrosternal thyroid, lymph node masses, etc.) or invasion of the lumen, usually by a bronchial or oesophageal carcinoma.
• Dynamic hyperinflation of the lungs following positive pressure ventilation in patients with severe emphysema, bullae, lung cysts, or in the presence of an airway obstruction which acts as a 'flap valve' and results in gas trapping. Progressive lung distension creates the mechanical equivalent of a tension pneumothorax. This increase in intrathoracic pressure and pulmonary vascular resistance compromises venous return and right ventricular function and dramatically reduces cardiac output. If undiagnosed the situation can rapidly degenerate into a 'PEA arrest'. Emergency treatment is to disconnect the patient from the ventilator, open the tracheal tube to atmosphere, relieve any airway obstruction, and support right ventricular function. Remember—'if in doubt let it [the trapped gas] out!'[1]
• Mediastinal shifts can occur due to large pleural effusions, tension pneumothorax, and lateral positioning. Significant shifts cause lung compression and a severe reduction in cardiac output. Prompt recognition and correction of the underlying cause is vital.

- Sudden falls in cardiac output presenting as acute severe hypotension and caused by surgical manipulation within the chest obstructing venous return or cardiac filling. The effects can be reduced by volume loading the patient, but the surgeon or assistant should be advised and requested to 'stop squashing the heart!'

Preoperative assessment

- Patients require a standard assessment with particular emphasis on cardiorespiratory reserve.
- Examine most recent CXR and CT scans. Check for airway obstruction and tracheal or carinal distortion/compression which can cause difficulties with double lumen tube placement.
- Patients with significant cardiac disease are clearly a high-risk group.

Lung resection[2]

Based on history, examination, and simple pulmonary function tests (PFTs), patients may be classified as:

- Clinically fit with good exercise tolerance and normal spirometry—accept for surgery
- Major medical problems, minimal exercise capacity, and grossly impaired PFTs—high risk for surgery, consider alternative treatment
- Reduced exercise capacity (short of breath on climbing two flights of stairs) and abnormal spirometry with or without moderate co-existing disease—require careful evaluation of risks/benefits of surgery

Pulmonary function (see p98) tests are often used to determine suitability for lung resection surgery by estimating postoperative lung function. Always consider the results in context of patient's general health and proposed resection.

- Spirometry reflects the 'bellows' function of the respiratory system while tests of diffusion capacity (e.g. carbon monoxide transfer factor, DLCO) assess the ability to transfer oxygen to the circulation. It is important to realise that patients with diffuse alveolar lung disease can have severely impaired gas transfer with relatively normal spirometry.
- Generally accepted minimum preoperative values of FEV_1 for the following procedures are pneumonectomy >55%, lobectomy >40%, wedge resection >35% of patient's predicted value.
- Predicted postop value of PFTs is preop value × (5 − number of lobes resected)/5. Goal is for estimated postoperative FEV_1 and DLCO >40% of predicted normal (FEV_1 0.8–1.0 litre for average male).
- If preoperative DLCO <40% predicted normal, estimated postop FEV_1 <800ml, or estimated postop FVC <15ml/kg it is likely that postoperative ventilation will be needed (poor cough with an FVC <1 litre).
- Exercise testing or exercise pulse oximetry should be used to refine clinical assessment in borderline cases. Failure to cover at least 200m or a fall in SpO_2 of more than 4% in a '6 min walk test' indicates a very high risk.[3]

1 Conacher I (1998). Dynamic hyperinflation—the anaesthetist applying a tourniquet to the right heart. *British Journal of Anaesthesia*, **81**, 116–117.
2 British Thoracic Society and Society of Cardiothoracic Surgeons Working Party (2001). Guidelines on the selection of patients with lung cancer for surgery. *Thorax*, **56**, 89–108.
3 Burke JR, Duarte IG, Thourani VH, Miller JI (2003). Preoperative risk assessment for marginal patients requiring pulmonary resection. *Annals of Thoracic Surgery*, **76**, 1767–1773.

Analgesia

Thoracotomy incisions are extremely painful. Inadequate pain relief increases the neurohumoral stress response, impairs mobilisation/respiration, leading to an increase in respiratory complications and a post-thoracotomy chronic pain syndrome. Good analgesia is crucial and a technique combining NSAIDs, a regional block, intra-operative opioids, and regular postoperative oral analgesia is recommended.

Perioperative intercostal nerve blocks or percutaneous paravertebral blocks are useful for thoracoscopic procedures and can be combined with postoperative patient-controlled opioid analgesia. Unless specifically contraindicated, patients undergoing thoracotomy or thoracoabdominal incisions should receive continuous thoracic epidural or paravertebral regional analgesia. Match the level of block to that of the incision—usually T5/6 or T6/7. Perioperative epidural blockade should be established cautiously (3–4ml of 0.25% bupivacaine) as an extensive thoracic sympathetic block can cause a major reduction in cardiac output and severe hypotension. Pre-incision percutaneous paravertebral injection of 0.5% bupivacaine (0.3ml/kg) followed by a continuous postoperative infusion of bupivacaine (0.5% for 24hr, then 0.25% for 3–4d) at 0.1ml/kg/hr via a surgically placed paravertebral catheter provides excellent post-thoracotomy analgesia.[1]

1 Richardson J, Lönnqvist PA (1998). Thoracic paravertebral block. *British Journal of Anaesthesia*, **81**, 230–238.

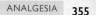

Isolation of the lungs

- Achieving independent ventilation of the two lungs is not always straightforward.
- One lung ventilation (OLV) is associated with a number of complications and should be used only when benefits outweigh the risks.

Advantages of OLV

- Protects dependent lung from blood and secretions.
- Allows independent control of ventilation to each lung.
- Improves surgical access and reduces lung trauma.

Disadvantages of OLV

- One lung ventilation inevitably creates a shunt and may cause hypoxia.
- Correct choice and positioning of endobronchial tubes is crucial.
- Increases technical and physiological challenge.

Indications for isolation and separation of the two lungs

- To avoid contamination of a lung in cases of infection, massive pulmonary haemorrhage, or bronchopulmonary lavage.
- Control the distribution of ventilation in massive air leaks or severe unilateral lung disease (e.g. giant bullae or lung cysts).
- Improving access for surgery is a *relative* indication for one lung ventilation. If isolation of the lung proves difficult the need to pursue OLV should be discussed with the surgeon since satisfactory access can often be achieved by careful lung retraction.

Techniques

- Double lumen endobronchial tubes (DLTs). Commonest and most versatile approach.
- Bronchial blockers (Univent tube or Arndt endobronchial blocker). Occasionally useful, especially in patients who are difficult to intubate or have distorted tracheobronchial anatomy/tracheostomy.
- Single lumen endobronchial tubes are rarely used.

Double lumen endobronchial tubes

- Traditional reusable red rubber DLTs are still used in some specialist centres but disposable plastic (polyvinyl chloride—PVC) tubes are probably in wider general use.
- Described as 'right' or 'left' according to main bronchus they are designed to intubate.
- Right-sided tubes have a hole or slit in the wall of the endobronchial section to facilitate ventilation of the right upper lobe.
- Sizes of plastic DLTs are given in Charriere (Ch) gauge (equivalent to French gauge), which is the external circumference of the tube in mm. Thus a 39Ch tube has an external diameter of about 13mm.
- The lumens of DLTs are small compared with standard single lumen tubes used in adults. The internal diameters of the lumens of the 39 and 35Ch 'Broncho-Cath' DLTs are only 6.0 and 4.5mm, respectively.

- Bronchoscopic placement and checking requires a narrow scope (<4mm diameter) ideally with an integral battery light source for ease of manipulation.
- A major contraindication to use of a DLT is very distorted tracheo-bronchial anatomy or an intraluminal lesion—placement likely to be difficult and possibly dangerous.

Types of DLT

- Carlens (left-sided): has a carinal 'hook' to aid correct placement
- Whites (right-sided): has a carinal hook and slit in the tube wall for right upper lobe
- Robertshaw (right- and left-sided): D-shaped lumens; traditionally a red rubber reusable tube, now available as a single use version in small, medium, and large sizes
- Single-use PVC (right- and left-sided): high-volume, low-pressure cuffs; bronchial cuff and pilot tube coloured blue; radiopaque marker stripe running to tip of bronchial lumen; available in sizes 28–41Ch, e.g. 'Broncho-Cath' (Mallinckrodt) or 'Sheribronch' (Sheridan)

Selection of DLT

- Use the largest DLT that will pass easily through the glottis. 41Ch or 39Ch gauge PVC tube (large or medium Robertshaw) for males, 37Ch gauge PVC tube (medium Robertshaw) for females. Small individuals may need a 35Ch gauge or small Robertshaw tube.
- Use a left-sided tube unless the surgery involves a left pulmonary resection or abnormal bronchial anatomy is likely to obstruct intubation of the left main bronchus. A left-sided tube is less likely to block a lobar bronchus and gives a greater tolerance to shifts in tube position, which inevitably occur when the patient is moved.

Placement of DLT

- Assess the risks/benefits of using a DLT. Examine the X-Rays, CT scans and any previous bronchoscopy reports for tracheobronchial anatomy and lung pathology—is there distortion or narrowing which will interfere with bronchial intubation?
- Check the Y connector and ensure that 15mm connectors are inserted into proximal ends of the DLT ('Broncho-Caths' come with these connectors separately wrapped).
- Most plastic DLTs are supplied with a malleable stylet which can be used to adjust the curve of the tube to facilitate intubation.
- Commence intubation with the concavity of the endobronchial section of the DLT facing anteriorly—once the tip is past the glottis, partially withdraw the stylet and rotate the tube 90° to bring the oropharyngeal curve into the sagittal plane. Turn the patient's head to the side opposite to the bronchus to be intubated (i.e. to the right for a left-sided DLT) and gently slide the tube down the trachea until resistance is felt to further advancement.
- At this stage treat DLT as an ordinary ETT—inflate only the tracheal cuff to achieve a seal and confirm ventilation of both lungs.

- It is easy to push plastic DLTs in too far. The patient's height is the main determinant of correct insertion depth—the usual insertion depth to the corner of the mouth in a patient 170cm (5' 7") tall is 29cm (depth changes by 1cm for every 10cm (4") change in the patient's height).[1]

Clinical confirmation of DLT position

- Next check the tube position and establish isolation of lungs. Beware of pathology affecting clinical signs—compare with preop clinical examination findings and radiology. Be systematic—it is easy to get confused!
- Start by checking ventilation through the bronchial lumen. Clamp off the gas flow to the tracheal lumen at the Y connector and open the sealing cap on the tracheal lumen to air.
- Look for chest movement—is there appropriate unilateral expansion?
- Listen—auscultate both lungs and listen at proximal end of open lumen for leaks around bronchial cuff. Inflate bronchial cuff 1ml at a time (use a 5ml syringe) until leak stops. If a reasonable seal cannot be obtained with <4 ml of air, the tube is either incorrectly placed or too small for the patient. Check specifically that all lobes are ventilated, especially the right upper if using a right-sided DLT.
- Feel—assess compliance by 'bagging' right, left, and both lungs. Very poor compliance (high inflation pressures) which is not explained by the patient's pathology suggests malposition—peak pressure on OLV should be <35cmH$_2$O.
- Close the sealing cap, remove the Y connector clamp and then confirm it is possible to isolate and achieve OLV of the opposite lung via the tracheal lumen.
- Endobronchial tubes often move when the patient is placed in the lateral position. Recheck isolation and OLV once the patient is in position and before surgery starts.

Fibre-optic bronchoscope

- Ideally the position of every DLT should be checked bronchoscopically. At the very least a suitable bronchoscope must be immediately available to assess DLT placement if there are clinical problems with the tube or with OLV.
- This is invaluable where bronchial intubation is difficult and can be used to 'railroad' the tube into the correct main bronchus. Insert the bronchoscope via the bronchial lumen, partially withdraw the DLT so its tip lies in the trachea, locate the carina with the scope and advance into the appropriate main bronchus, then slide the tube into position.
- Several bronchoscopic studies have shown that up to 80% of DLTs are mal-positioned to some extent even when clinical signs are satisfactory. The upper surface of the bronchial cuff (blue) should lie just below the carina when visualised via the tracheal lumen.
- Always confirm positioning of right-sided tube by bronchoscopy. Lateral 'slit' in the wall of the distal bronchial lumen should be aligned with the right upper lobe bronchus.

Bronchial blocker technique

- A balloon-tipped catheter ('blocker') is manipulated through a single lumen tracheal tube into the appropriate main (or lobar) bronchus with the aid of a narrow fibre-optic bronchoscope.
- Good lubrication of both bronchoscope and blocker is essential.
- The position of the blocker should be rechecked after the patient has been positioned for surgery.
- The lung or lobe is isolated from ventilation by inflating the balloon within the bronchus. The isolated lung slowly collapses as the trapped gas is absorbed or escapes via blocker's narrow central lumen.
- Collapse can be accelerated by ventilating with 100% oxygen for a few minutes and then inflating the blocker at end expiration when lung volume is at its minimum.
- Re-inflation of the collapsed lung requires deflation of the blocker and consequently loss of isolation of the lungs. (A correctly positioned DLT will maintain separation of the airways to each lung until extubation.)
- During pneumonectomy or sleeve resection (bronchial reanastomosis) the blocker has to be withdrawn to allow surgical access to the bronchus.

There are two modern forms of bronchial blocker:

- Univent tube: a single lumen tube with an internal channel in its wall containing an adjustable blocker bearing a high-volume, low-pressure cuff.
- Arndt wire-guided endobronchial blocker (COOK™): a stiff catheter with a cylindrical cuff and an adjustable 'wire' loop at its tip which guides the blocker along the outside of a fibre-optic bronchoscope into the required bronchus. Supplied with a special adapter which allows it to be deployed through a conventional single lumen or cuffed tracheostomy tube.

Indications for using a bronchial blocker[2]

- On the rare occasions when isolation of a lobar bronchus is required (localised bronchiectasis or haemorrhage, lung abscess, or bronchopleural fistula)
- In patients who are difficult to intubate or have a permanent tracheostomy
- To avoid the reintubation required to change to or from a DLT in patients receiving pre- or postoperative IPPV

1 Brodsky JB, Benumof JL, Ehrenwerth J, Ozaki GT (1991). Depth of placement of left double-lumen endobronchial tubes. *Anesthesia and Analgesia*, **73**, 570–572.
2 Campos JH (2003). An update on bronchial blockers during lung separation techniques in adults. *Anesthesia and Analgesia*, **97**, 1266–1274.

Management of one lung ventilation

The physiology is complex and some aspects remain controversial.[1] One lung ventilation inevitably creates a shunt through the unventilated lung and the crucial factor in managing OLV is to minimise the effects of this shunt. Hypoxic pulmonary vasoconstriction, and the influence of anaesthetic agents, have little relevance to the routine clinical management of thoracic anaesthesia.

Initiating OLV

- Start with typical ventilator settings during two lung ventilation (FiO_2 0.33, V_T 9–10ml/kg, and P_{AW} ≤25cmH$_2$O).
- Increase FiO_2 to 0.5 and decrease V_T to 6–8ml/kg before initiating OLV.
- Clamp Y connection to non-dependent lung and open sealing cap on that lumen of the DLT to allow the gas to escape.
- Observe the airway pressure closely. It will normally increase, often by 30–40%.
- If P_{AW} is excessive (>35cmH$_2$O) or rises abruptly with each inspiration exclude mechanical causes (e.g. kinked connector, clamp incorrectly placed) and DLT malposition or obstruction (e.g. ventilating lobe rather than lung, sputum plugs, opening of tracheal lumen against wall of trachea).
- Adjust V_T and ventilation profile to limit P_{AW}, ideally to ≤30cmH$_2$O.
- Observe SaO_2 and $ETCO_2$ closely. If necessary increase ventilatory rate to maintain acceptable minute volume and carbon dioxide clearance.
- Check with surgeon that lung is collapsing (may take a few minutes in patients with obstructive airways disease) and that mediastinum has not 'sunk' into dependent hemithorax.

Hypoxia on OLV

- Hypoxia is a frequent complication of OLV, and is more common when right lung is collapsed.
- It usually occurs after a few minutes of OLV (as oxygen in non-ventilated lung is absorbed).
- SaO_2 dips but then often rises again a few minutes later as non-ventilated lung collapses more completely and blood flow through it decreases.
- Increase FiO_2 and try to ensure an adequate cardiac output.
- Confirm correct positioning of DLT—are all lobes ventilated? Check with fibre-optic bronchoscope if unsure.
- If partial collapse of the ventilated (dependent) lung is suspected ('sinking' mediastinum) try 5–10cmH$_2$O PEEP on that lung—this may help, but the effect is unpredictable.
- If still hypoxic, warn surgeon, partially re-inflate non-dependent lung, and then apply 5–10cmH$_2$O CPAP via a simple reservoir bag/APL valve arrangement (CPAP System, Mallinckrodt™) supplied with 100% oxygen from an auxiliary oxygen flowmeter or cylinder. This will reliably improve saturations—simply insufflating oxygen into the collapsed non-dependent lung will not.

- If hypoxia persists use intermittent inflation of non-dependent lung with oxygen breaths from the CPAP circuit—needs to be co-ordinated with surgical activity.
- If these manoeuvres are not successful return to two lung ventilation.
- Persisting with OLV in the face of continuing hypoxia (SaO_2 <92%) is dangerous and can rarely be justified.

Returning to two lung ventilation

- Gently suction the non-ventilated lung to clear any blood or pus—use the long suction catheters supplied with the DLT.
- Close sealing cap on lumen to non-ventilated lung and remove clamp on the Y connector.
- Switch to manual ventilation and re-inflate the collapsed lung under direct vision using sustained inflations. Inflation pressures up to 35–40cmH$_2$O are often required to fully re-expand all areas of the lung.
- Return patient to mechanical ventilation and, unless significant volumes of lung have been resected, return to original two lung ventilator settings and FiO$_2$.
- Adjust respiratory rate to maintain normocapnia.
- Always be prepared to return to OLV immediately should problems occur, e.g. large air leak from operated lung.

1 Wilson WC, Benumof JL (2005). Physiology of one lung ventilation. In: Miller RD, ed. *Miller's Anesthesia*, 6th ed, Chapter 49, 1890–1894. Philadelphia: Elsevier, Churchill Livingstone.

Rigid bronchoscopy and stent insertion

Procedure	Endoscopic inspection of tracheobronchial tree—± biopsy, stents, removal of foreign body
Time	5–20min
Pain	+
Position	Supine with head and neck extended
Blood loss	Usually minimal
Practical techniques	TIVA with propofol boluses/infusion, alfentanil/remifentanil, intermittent suxamethonium. IPPV through bronchoscope with oxygen via Venturi needle and Sanders injector

Preoperative

- Check for airway obstruction—stridor, tracheal tumour on CT scan, or foreign body.
- Suitable as day-case procedure in appropriate patients.
- Warn about postoperative coughing, haemoptysis, and suxamethonium myalgia.
- Often combined with mediastinoscopy to assess suitability for lung resection.

Perioperative

- Give full pre-oxygenation.
- Confirm surgeon is in the theatre before inducing the patient.
- Boluses of midazolam (2–3mg) and alfentanil (500–1000μg) facilitate induction and may reduce risk of awareness.
- A preinduction 'taming' dose of non-depolarising relaxant (e.g. vecuronium 0.5mg) can reduce suxamethonium pains.
- Normally induce in the anaesthetic room, transfer to theatre with a face mask, and give suxamethonium just prior to bronchoscopy.
- If there is potential airway obstruction (foreign body or tracheal compression) inhalation induction in theatre with sevoflurane in oxygen is recommended until airway is secure.
- Co-ordinate ventilation with surgical activity.
- Observe or palpate abdomen to detect recovery of muscle tone.
- Suction upper airway and confirm adequate muscle power before removing the scope.

Postoperative

- Turn patient biopsied side down to avoid bleeding into normal lung.
- Sit fully upright as soon as awake.
- Blood clot can cause severe lower airway obstruction requiring immediate intubation, suction, and repeat bronchoscopy.

Special considerations

- The airway is unprotected so patients at risk of regurgitation should be pretreated to reduce the volume and acidity of gastric secretions (omeprazole 40mg PO the night before and 40mg 2–6hr before procedure).
- The procedure is very stimulating and can generate a marked hypertensive response.
- Extreme cardiovascular responses need to be obtunded and profound relaxation provided, but with prompt return of laryngeal reflexes and spontaneous respiration.
- Vocal cords can be sprayed with local anaesthetic (4% topical lidocaine) but this will not prevent carinal reflexes and may impair postoperative coughing.
- Rarely, biopsy can precipitate a life-threatening airway bleed.
- Stent insertion can be technically difficult and may involve periodic loss of airway control.
- A short acting non-depolarising muscle relaxant can be employed but it is difficult to achieve the profound paralysis required using mivacurium.
- Bradycardias caused by repeat doses of suxamethonium are rarely seen during rigid bronchoscopy in adults. Atropine should be drawn up but routine administration is not recommended since this will exacerbate any tachycardia.

Mediastinoscopy/mediastinotomy

Procedure	Inspection and biopsy of tumours and lymph nodes in superior and anterior mediastinum via small suprasternal or anterior intercostal incision
Time	20–30min
Pain	+
Position	Supine or slightly head up, arms by sides and head ring with bolster under shoulders
Blood loss	Usually minimal but potential for massive haemorrhage, G&S
Practical techniques	IPPV via single lumen tube

Preoperative
- Suitable as day-case procedure in appropriate patients.
- Check for superior vena cava obstruction and tracheal deviation or compression due to large mediastinal masses.
- Often preceded by rigid bronchoscopy ('Bronch & Med').

Perioperative
- Tape eyes and check tracheal tube connectors—head will be obscured by drapes.
- Boluses of IV fentanyl during surgery.
- Insert 16G cannula in lower leg vein after induction (see below).
- Watch for surgical compression of trachea—monitor tidal volume and airway pressures.
- Monitor BP in left arm and put pulse oximeter on right hand (see below).

Postoperative
- Paracetamol and NSAID with PRN codeine phosphate.

Special considerations
- There is the potential for massive haemorrhage from the great vessels—risk increased in patients with SVC obstruction (hence cannula in leg)—may require immediate median sternotomy.
- The brachiocephalic artery can be compressed by mediastinoscope, restricting blood flow to right arm and carotid artery creating a risk of cerebral ischaemia. Place pulse oximeter on right hand to monitor perfusion.
- Mediastinotomy can cause a pneumothorax.

Lung surgery: wedge resection, lobectomy, and pneumonectomy

Procedure	Excision of pulmonary tissue either selectively (wedge resection or lobectomy) or a whole lung (pneumonectomy)
Time	2–4hr
Pain	+++++
Position	Lateral decubitus with table 'broken', elbows flexed to bring forearms parallel to face with upper arm in gutter support
Blood loss	200–800ml—occasionally significantly more; G&S, X-match 2U for lobectomy/ pneumonectomy
Practical techniques	IPPV via DLT using OLV during resection phase. Epidural or paravertebral regional anaesthesia with catheter for postoperative analgesia, art line for pneumonectomy and less fit patients

Preoperative

- Cancer is the commonest indication for lung resection—others include benign tumours, bronchiectasis, and TB.
- Assess cardiorespiratory reserve and estimate post-resection lung function (see p353).
- Assess airway with respect to placement of DLT.
- Plan postoperative analgesia regime.

Perioperative

- Select appropriate DLT and check lung isolation carefully after intubation.
- Use a left-sided tube unless the surgery involves a left lobectomy or pneumonectomy or abnormal bronchial anatomy is likely to obstruct intubation of the left main bronchus.
- IV infusion in upper arm—14–16G cannula.
- Radial arterial lines function better in the dependent arm as that wrist is usually extended.
- CVP monitoring is unreliable in lateral position with open chest. Central lines are not recommended for routine use but may be indicated for access purposes or postoperative monitoring.
- One lung ventilation facilitates surgery and prevents soiling of dependent lung.
- Continuous display of the airway pressure/volume loop is a valuable adjunct to monitoring and managing OLV.
- Surgical manipulation often causes cardiac and venous compression, which reduces cardiac output/blood pressure and may cause arrhythmias.
- Suction the airway to the collapsed lung prior to re-inflation.

- The bronchial suture line is 'leak tested' under saline by manual inflation to $40cmH_2O$.
- Titrate IV fluids to losses and duration of surgery. Avoid excessive fluid replacement especially in pneumonectomy.
- Preoperative epidural or paravertebral block with surgically inserted catheter. Epidural can be used preoperatively but cautious incremental boluses are recommended (3ml of 0.25% bupivacaine ± opioid).

Postoperative

- Aim to extubate patient awake at end of procedure and sit upright in theatre.
- Prescribe continuous supplementary oxygen—humidified is preferable but nasal cannulae are more likely to stay on the patient in the ward.
- Ensure good analgesia is achieved.
- A CXR is usually required in recovery room.

Special considerations

- Occasionally patients with bronchial carcinoma may have 'non-metastatic' manifestations (Eaton–Lambert myasthenic syndrome or ectopic hormone production). See pp248, 308.
- Perioperative mortality from pneumonectomy is 5%. Acute lung injury occurs in 4–5% of resections, is three times more common after pneumonectomy, and is responsible for 43% of deaths. Additional risk factors include chronic alcohol abuse, intra-operative plateau pressures $>15cmH_2O$ and >4000ml of IV fluid in first 24hr.[1]
- Arrhythmias, especially atrial fibrillation, are quite common after pneumonectomy and many advocate prophylactic digitalisation (digoxin 500µg IV over 30min given during surgery followed by 250µg/d orally for 4–5d).

1 Licker M, de Perrot M, Spiliopoulos A, Robert J, Diaper J, Chevalley C, Tschopp JM (2003). Risk factors for acute lung injury after thoracic surgery for lung cancer. *Anesthesia and Analgesia*, **97**, 1558–1565.

Thoracoscopy and video-assisted thoracoscopic surgery (VATS) procedures

Procedure	Inspection of thoracic cavity via scope passed through intercostal incision. Used for drainage of effusions, lung and pleural biopsy, pleurectomy/pleurodesis, pericardial biopsy/window
Time	30–120min
Pain	++/+++
Position	Lateral decubitus with table 'broken', elbows flexed to bring forearms parallel to face with upper arm in gutter support
Blood loss	minimal–200ml, G&S
Practical techniques	IPPV and OLV via left-sided DLT. Percutaneous paravertebral block/catheter or intercostal blocks, ± art line

Preoperative
- Assess as for a thoracotomy.
- Much less invasive than thoracotomy with less postoperative deterioration of lung function.
- Discuss regional analgesia and where appropriate PCA.

Perioperative
- Consider invasive arterial pressure monitoring for high-risk or compromised patients.
- IV infusion in upper arm; arterial line in radial artery of dependent arm.
- Boluses of fentanyl (50–100µg) for intra-operative analgesia.
- Commence OLV (using left-sided DLT) before insertion of trocar.
- Good collapse of the lung in operative hemithorax is required for surgical access.
- Intercostal or paravertebral blocks. A paravertebral catheter can be inserted under thoracoscopic guidance for more extensive procedures.

Postoperative
- Extubate, sit up, and start supplementary oxygen in theatre before transfer to recovery.
- CXR in recovery is required to confirm full lung re-expansion.
- Although a thoracotomy is avoided, patients still need balanced analgesia as for lung resection. PCA morphine may be required for 24–48hr for more painful procedures such as pleurectomy, pleurodesis or wedge resections.
- Encourage early mobilisation.

Special considerations
- Not a minor procedure—there is always the possibility of conversion to an open thoracotomy.
- Epidural not necessary but worth considering if bilateral.

Lung volume reduction surgery and bullectomy

Procedure	Non-anatomical resection of regions of hyperinflated and poorly functioning pulmonary tissue
Time	2–5hr
Pain	+++/+++++
Position	Median sternotomy (bilateral surgery)—supine with arms to sides. Thoracotomy—lateral decubitus (as for lung resection)
Blood loss	200–800ml, X-match 2U
Practical techniques	Thoracic epidural pre-induction. GA with TIVA, relaxant, DLT—extreme care with IPPV and OLV

Lung volume reduction surgery is a surgical treatment for selected patients with severe respiratory failure secondary to emphysema. The aim is to reduce total lung volume to more physiological levels by resecting most diseased areas, thereby improving respiratory function. Most of these patients belong to a group in which general anaesthesia would normally be avoided at all costs.

Preoperative
- Patients require intensive assessment, careful selection/optimisation prior to surgery.
- Cardiac assessment for lung volume reduction surgery often includes coronary angiography and right heart catheterisation to evaluate IHD, ventricular function, and pulmonary artery pressures.
- Patients are often on corticosteroids—perioperative supplementation is required.
- A clear understanding of pathophysiology and adequate thoracic experience is essential to safe anaesthetic management.[1]

Perioperative
- Surgery may be performed via sternotomy, thoracotomy, or by video-assisted thoracoscopic surgery.
- There is a serious risk of rupturing emphysematous bullae with IPPV, causing leaks and tension pneumothorax.
- Nitrous oxide is contraindicated and, since an increased alveolar–arterial gradient may exist for volatile agents, total IV anaesthesia with remifentanil and propofol may be preferable.
- Continuous spirometry, invasive arterial and CVP monitoring are essential.
- Clinical assessment of DLT placement is difficult—verify position bronchoscopically.
- Limit risk of 'gas trapping' and dynamic pulmonary hyperinflation (see p352) by deliberate hypoventilation and permissive hypercapnia ($PaCO_2$ up to 8.5kPa). Recommend V_T 6–7ml/kg, 10–12bpm, I:E ratio 1:4, and peak airway pressure <30cmH$_2$O.

- Disconnect from ventilator intermittently to allow lungs to 'empty'.
- Bronchospasm and sputum retention with mucus plugging can be a problem.
- Use colloids for fluid replacement to minimise risk of pulmonary oedema.

Postoperative

- HDU or ICU care will be required—extubate as soon as possible.
- Anticipate and accept raised $PaCO_2$ (7–9kPa) and adjust FiO_2 to maintain SaO_2 in range 90–92%.
- Watch closely for air leaks—use a maximum of 10cmH_2O suction on intercostal drains.
- Requires excellent pain relief, skilled physiotherapy, and a pulmonary rehabilitation programme.

Special considerations

- Commonest complication is prolonged air leak—>7d in 50% of patients.
- Mortality from recent series is 5–10%.
- The National Emphysema Treatment Trial demonstrated that lung volume reduction surgery benefits patients with predominantly upper lobe disease and a low baseline exercise capacity.
- Patients with an isolated congenital bulla or 'lung cyst' require same careful intra-operative anaesthetic management but are usually much fitter and do not normally require invasive cardiological assessment.

1 Hillier J, Gillbe C (2003). Anaesthesia for lung volume reduction surgery. *Anaesthesia*, **58**, 1210–1219.

Drainage of empyema and decortication

Procedure	Surgical removal of pus (empyema) and organised thick fibrinous pleural membrane (decortication)
Time	Drainage 20–40min; decortication 2–3hr
Pain	+++/+++++
Position	Lateral decubitus for thoracotomy
Blood loss	Simple drainage: minimal Decortication: 500–2 000ml, X-match 2U
Practical techniques	GA with IV induction, relaxant, intubation, IPPV DLT advised for decortication (risk of air leaks); single lumen tube adequate for drainage procedures; art line/CVP

Preoperative

- Intrapleural infection usually secondary to pneumonia, intercostal drains, or chest surgery.
- Patients are often debilitated by infection and may be frankly septic.
- Respiratory function often already compromised by pneumonia or prior lung resection.
- Check for bronchopleural fistula created by erosion into the lung.

Perioperative

- Empyema usually drained by rib resection and insertion of a large-bore intercostal drain.
- Thoracoscopy may be used to break down a loculated effusion or empyema and free pleural adhesions.
- Decortication requires 'thoracotomy' anaesthetic with epidural analgesia since pleural changes preclude a paravertebral catheter.
- Decortication frequently causes significant haemorrhage.
- Art line/CVP monitoring are advisable for all but fittest patients.

Postoperative

- Balanced analgesia with regular paracetamol, NSAID, regional block (intercostal blocks useful for drainage procedures), and opioids.
- High-dependency care is recommended for debilitated patients undergoing decortication.

Special considerations

- The surgical principle is to remove infected tissue including pleural 'peel', fully re-expand the lung, and obliterate the infected pleural space.
- Air leaks are common following decortication of the visceral pleura and lobectomy is occasionally required if a massive air leak or severe parenchymal lung damage occurs.
- Decortication is a major procedure which requires careful evaluation of risks and benefits in elderly, frail, and sick patients.

Repair of broncho–pleural fistula

Procedure	Closure of communication between pleural cavity and trachea or bronchi
Time	2–3hr (for thoracotomy approach)
Pain	++++/+++++
Position	Keep sitting upright with affected side tilted down until good lung isolated, then lateral decubitus for thoracotomy
Blood loss	300–800ml, G&S, X-match 2U if anaemic
Practical techniques	Rapid IV induction and fibre-optic guided endobronchial intubation with DLT Awake fibre-optic guided intubation with DLT Intubation with DLT under deep inhalation anaesthesia with spontaneous ventilation

Preoperative

• Features are productive cough, haemoptysis, fever, dyspnoea, SC emphysema, and falling fluid level in post-pneumonectomy space on the chest radiograph.
• The severity of symptoms is proportional to the size of the fistula—big fistulae with large air leaks cause severe dyspnoea and may necessitate urgent respiratory support.
• Patients are often debilitated with respiratory function compromised by infection and prior lung resection.
• Check previous anaesthetic charts for ease of intubation and type of DLT used.
• Check the anatomy of the lower airway carefully on chest radiograph—it is often distorted by previous surgery.
• Require supplementary oxygen, a functioning chest drain, IV antibiotics, and fluids.

Perioperative

• Key principles are to protect 'good' lung from contamination and to control the distribution of ventilation. Failure to adequately isolate lungs after induction will put the patient at grave risk.
• Small or moderate fistulae are usually assessed by bronchoscopy and may be amenable to sealing with tissue glue.
• Commence invasive arterial pressure monitoring before induction.
• Traditionally, awake intubation under local anaesthesia has been recommended as the safest option but ultimately the technique should be selected to give the best balance of risks and benefits for each patient. Many thoracic anaesthetists use a modified rapid sequence induction and advance the DLT under direct vision with a fibre-optic bronchoscope to ensure correct placement in the bronchus contralateral to fistula. The potential exists to enlarge the fistula by inappropriate placement of the DLT.

- IPPV increases gas leakage, causing loss of tidal volume and the risk of tension pneumothorax.
- TIVA is recommended—delivery of volatile agents may be unreliable with large gas leaks. Ketamine may be useful in high-risk patients.

Postoperative
- Plan HDU/ICU care for all but most straightforward cases.
- Minimise airway pressures during ventilation and extubate as soon as possible.
- Use standard post-thoracotomy analgesic regimen but watch renal function with NSAIDs.

Special considerations
- Most fistulae are postoperative complications of pneumonectomy or lobectomy but some are secondary to pneumonia, lung abscesses, or empyema.
- Anaesthesia for repair of bronchopleural fistula is challenging and not recommended for an 'occasional' thoracic anaesthetist!

Tips for controlling a massive air leak
(i.e. unable to ventilate effectively)

If a DLT cannot be positioned satisfactorily these are worth attempting:
- Intubate with an uncut cuffed 6mm diameter single lumen tube—pass fibre-optic bronchoscope through tube into intact main bronchus and 'railroad' the tube into the bronchus to isolate and ventilate good lung.
- Ask the surgeon to pass a rigid bronchoscope into the intact main bronchus and slide a long flexible bougie or COOK™ airway exchange catheter (which allows jet ventilation) into bronchus—remove bronchoscope and railroad single lumen tube.
- If all else fails an Arndt endobronchial blocker or a large Fogarty embolectomy catheter passed into the fistula via a rigid bronchoscope may control the leak temporarily.

Pleurectomy/pleurodesis

Procedure	Stripping of parietal pleura from inside of chest wall (pleurectomy). Production of adhesions between parietal and visceral pleura either chemically (talc, tetracycline) or by physical abrasion (pleurodesis)
Time	Pleurectomy 1–2hr; pleurodesis 20–40min
Pain	+++/++++
Position	Lateral decubitus for open thoracotomy or VATS. May be supine for pleurodesis
Blood loss	Minimal if thoracoscopic; up to 500ml for thoracotomy, G&S
Practical techniques	IPPV, DLT and OLV advised for open/VATS procedures. A single lumen tube is usually adequate for talc pleurodesis

Preoperative
- Patients fall into two groups: the relatively young and fit with recurrent pneumothoraces (check for asthma) and older patients compromised by COPD or recurrent pleural effusions (check respiratory reserve).
- Even very large unilateral effusions rarely cause orthopnoea in previously healthy patients. Symptomatic orthopnoea should alert the anaesthetist to possible additional pathology such as heart failure.
- Check a recent CXR for pneumothorax and/or effusion.
- A preoperative intercostal drain is advised if pneumothorax present.
- Check the planned surgical approach.
- Discuss postoperative analgesia and regional technique.

Perioperative
- Keep airway pressures as low as possible in patients with history of pneumothorax.
- Be alert for pneumothoraces—they can tension rapidly on IPPV even with drain in situ and can be on the 'healthy' side—avoid nitrous oxide.
- Collapse the lung during instillation of irritant to facilitate pleural coating—if using a single lumen tube pre-oxygenate and then briefly disconnect lungs from ventilator.
- Aim for full expansion of lung at end of procedure to appose parietal and visceral pleura.

Postoperative
- Extubate and sit the patient upright before transfer to recovery room.
- A CXR is needed to check full lung expansion—suction on intercostal drains is often prescribed to assist expansion.
- Pleural inflammation can cause severe pain.
- A balanced analgesic regime with regular paracetamol, NSAID, and either a thoracic epidural (bilateral procedures), sited and used as for a thoracotomy, or combination of morphine PCA with intercostal blocks or, if feasible, a paravertebral catheter.

Special considerations

- Pleurectomy usually performed for recurrent pneumothorax—combined with stapling of lung tissue responsible for recurrent air leaks (usually apical 'blebs' or small bullae).
- Pleurodesis often used to manage malignant pleural effusions (mesothelioma, metastatic carcinoma)—there can be large volumes of fluid causing significant respiratory compromise.
- Patients with massive pleural effusions (more than two-thirds of the hemithorax on chest radiograph or >2 000 ml) should have these 'tapped' and partially drained at least 12hr before surgery because rapid intra-operative re inflation of the collapsed lung can precipitate unilateral postoperative 're-expansion' pulmonary oedema.
- Patients with extensive effusions are also at risk of circulatory collapse when turned 'effusion side up' for surgery. The mechanism is probably a combination of mediastinal shift and high intrathoracic pressure on IPPV reducing venous return and cardiac output. If this occurs return the patient to the supine position and drain the effusion before proceeding.

Oesophagectomy

Procedure	Total or partial excision of oesophagus with mobilisation of stomach (occasionally colon) into chest
Time	3–6hr
Pain	+++++
Position	Supine with arms by sides and/or lateral decubitus for thoracotomy
Blood loss	500–1 500ml; X-match 2U
Practical techniques	IPPV, DLT useful if thoracotomy. Art/CVP lines, urinary catheter, thoracic epidural or paravertebral catheter for thoracoabdominal incision

Preoperative

- Establish indication for surgery—usually oesophageal cancer but occasionally for non-malignant disease (benign stricture, achalasia).
- The anaesthetic plan requires understanding of surgical approach:
  - Transhiatal: laparotomy and cervical anastomosis
  - Ivor–Lewis: laparotomy and right thoracotomy
  - Thoracoabdominal: left thoracotomy crossing costal margin and diaphragm
  - McKewan 3 stage: laparotomy, right thoracotomy, and cervical anastomosis
  - Minimally invasive: thoracoscopic oesophageal mobilisation, laparoscopic gastric mobilisation, and cervical anastomosis
- Preoperative malnutrition or cachexia is common and associated with higher risk of postoperative morbidity and mortality. Requires careful cardiorespiratory assessment.
- Plan for duration of surgery and need to reposition patient during procedure.
- Preoperative adjuvant chemotherapy may leave residual immunosuppression but can dramatically improve dysphagia.
- Book HDU or ICU according to patient's fitness and local protocols.

Perioperative

- Consider all patients with oesophageal disease to be at risk of regurgitation, so rapid sequence induction with cricoid pressure advised.
- If thoracotomy is planned use a DLT and OLV to facilitate surgical access and reduce trauma to the lung.
- Plan regional anaesthesia according to surgical approach— paravertebral LA infusion with morphine PCA for thoracoabdominal approach. For laparotomy/thoracotomy a mid-thoracic epidural (using 3ml boluses of 0.25% bupivacaine perioperatively and postoperative infusion of 5mg diamorphine in 50ml 0.167% bupivacaine at 2–8ml/hr).
- A nasogastric tube will be required initially. It is removed for resection and re-inserted under surgical guidance following anastomosis.

- Do not put internal jugular line on side required for cervical anastomosis.
- Monitor core temperature and be obsessional about keeping patient warm (efficient fluid warmer and forced-air warming blanket).
- Stay ahead with fluid replacement—for open procedures aim for 10ml/kg/hr of crystalloid plus colloid or red cells to replace blood loss.
- Check Hb (HemoCue® ideal) and blood gases intra-operatively— watch for metabolic acidosis suggesting inadequate tissue perfusion.
- Arrhythmias and reduced cardiac output causing hypotension may occur during intra-thoracic oesophageal mobilisation.
- Change DLT to a single lumen tube to improve surgical access prior to cervical anastomosis (if performed).

Postoperative

- Require intensive and experienced postoperative nursing care in a specialist ward, high-dependency unit, or intensive care.
- If cold (<35.5°C) or haemodynamically unstable ventilate until condition improves.
- Aim for minimum urine output of 1ml/kg/hr.
- Use a jejunostomy or nasoduodenal tube for early enteral feeding.

Special considerations

- Oesophagectomy has one of the highest perioperative mortality rates of all elective procedures (up to 5% even in specialist centres).
- 66% of deaths are from systemic sepsis secondary to respiratory complications or anastomotic breakdown.
- Over 30% of patients suffer a major complication.
- In some centres minimally invasive (endoscopic) oesophagectomy is replacing the traditional open approaches.
- Occasional practice in anaesthesia (or surgery) for oesophagectomy is not recommended.

Chest injury

The emergency diagnosis and initial treatment of major thoracic trauma is described on pp828–830. This section deals with the anaesthetic management for definitive repair of ruptures of the diaphragm, oesophagus, and tracheobronchial tree.

General considerations

- Serious chest injuries are frequently associated with major head, abdominal, or skeletal injuries and appropriate attention and priority must be given to their management (cervical spine immobilisation, laparotomy to arrest bleeding, splintage of limb fractures).
- Fewer than 30% of patients with thoracic trauma require a thoracotomy but persistent bleeding from intercostal drains exceeding 200ml/hr is an indication for urgent surgery.
- Most deaths from thoracic trauma are due to exsanguination. Good IV access with two large-bore cannulae will allow rapid infusion.
- Emergency thoracotomy in the resuscitation room is seldom indicated and rarely associated with a favourable outcome.
- Standard principles of emergency anaesthesia should be applied.
- Maintain a high index of suspicion for tension pneumothorax during IPPV—an intercostal drain does not guarantee protection.
- Massive air leaks usually indicate significant tracheobronchial injury (see below).
- Patients with major thoracic trauma are at high risk of multiple organ failure and require postoperative management in an intensive care unit.

Repair of ruptured diaphragm

- Clinical features and diagnosis are described on p829.
- May present as a chronic condition or as intestinal obstruction of herniated bowel—check preoperative fluid and electrolyte status.
- Defect should be closed promptly but seldom needs to be done as an emergency.
- The surgical approach is via standard lateral thoracotomy or thoracoabdominal incision.
- Intra-operative management is as for a fundoplication (p383).
- Avoid nitrous oxide—it distends bowel and may make reduction of the hernia more difficult.
- DLT and OLV facilitate surgical access for repair.
- A nasogastric tube should be used to decompress the stomach.

Repair of ruptured oesophagus

- Clinical features and diagnosis are described on p830—surgical emphysema and pleural effusions frequently present.
- Other causes of oesophageal rupture include excessive abdominal straining and unco-ordinated vomiting (Boerhaave's syndrome). Oesophageal perforation can be caused by foreign bodies but is often iatrogenic (during endoscopic procedures).
- Mediastinitis is followed rapidly by sepsis and a systemic inflammatory response syndrome with associated problems of circulatory shock, renal failure, and ARDS.

- The principles of surgical management are initially drainage and prevention of further contamination.
- A careful endoscopic assessment will determine extent of oesophageal disruption.
- Small tears in unfit frail patients may be managed conservatively with chest drainage and nasogastric suction, but normally urgent surgery is required.
- Patients should be stabilised preoperatively in ICU with chest drainage, IV fluid replacement, analgesia, invasive monitoring, and inotropic support.
- Intra-operative management is as for oesophagectomy (see p378).
- Upper and lower oesophageal injuries require right and left thoracotomy, respectively.
- Primary closure may be possible if the oesophagus is healthy; if not oesophagectomy will be required.
- Arrhythmias common, particularly atrial fibrillation, due to mediastinitis.
- Change the DLT for a single lumen tube before transfer to intensive care for postoperative ventilation.
- Even patients who are stable at the end of the repair procedure remain at high risk of major complications for several days.
- Early postoperative feeding—feeding jejunostomy or parenterally.
- There is a significant incidence of dehiscence resulting in oesophagopleurocutaneous fistula with high mortality.

Repair of tracheobronchial injury

- Most patients with significant tracheal/bronchial disruption do not reach hospital alive.
- Clinical features of laryngeal and tracheobronchial injuries are described on p830.
- The priority is 100% oxygen and relief of tension pneumothorax, which may require two large-bore intercostal drains with independent underwater seals.
- If ventilation and oxygenation are acceptable call for thoracic surgical assistance and try to assess and identify site of airway injury by fibre-optic bronchoscopy before intubation.
- Airway management and anaesthetic principles apply as for a large bronchopleural fistula (p374).
- Adequate positive pressure ventilation may be impossible with single lumen tube.
- A torn bronchus can be isolated by fibre-optic guided intubation of the contralateral intact main bronchus with an appropriate DLT.
- An uncut single lumen tube can be guided past an upper tracheal tear with a bronchoscope so its cuff lies distal to the injury.
- Once the airway is secure and ventilation is stabilised proceed to urgent thoracotomy for repair.
- Carinal disruption may require cardiopulmonary bypass to maintain oxygenation during repair.
- Inappropriate management can lead to later stenosis and long-term airway problems.

Further reading

Ghosh S, Latimer RD (1999). *Thoracic Anaesthesia Principles and Practice*. Butterworth Heinemann.
Wilson WC, Benumof JL (2005). Anesthesia for thoracic surgery. In: Miller RD, ed. *Miller's Anesthesia*, 6th ed, Chapter 49. Philadelphia: Elsevier Churchill Livingstone.

Operation	Description	Time	Pain	Position/approach	Blood loss/X-Match	Notes
Fibre-optic bron-choscopy	Visual inspection of tracheo-bronchial tree ± biopsy and bronchial brushings/lavage	5–10min	+	Supine	None	GA rarely used. Single lumen tube (SLT) (8–9mm) with bronchoscopy diaphragm on angle piece. IPPV with relaxant appropriate to duration. Expect high airway pressures while scope in ETT. Suction can empty breathing system
Lung biopsy	Diagnostic sampling of lung tissue for localised or diffuse abnormality	30–60min	+++/++++	Lateral/VATS or minithoracotomy	Minor/G&S: X-match if anaemic	DLT and OLV facilitates VATS procedures. Patients with diffuse disease can have very poor lung function—risk of ventilator dependence and significant mortality
Oesophagoscopy and dilatation (O&D)	Visual inspection of oesophagus via rigid or fibre-optic scope ± dilatation of stricture with flexible bougies or balloon	5–20min	–/+	Supine	None	Regurgitation risk so rapid sequence induction advised. SLT on left side of mouth—watch for airway obstruction and ETT displacement during procedure. Flexible oesophagoscopy often done under IV sedation
Oesophageal stent insertion	Endoscopic placement of tubular stent through oesophageal stricture	10–30min	+/++	Supine	None	Often emaciated, may be anaemic. Preop IV fluids to correct dehydration. Rapid sequence induction, SLT, and awake extubation in lateral position. Small risk of oesophageal rupture

Procedure	Description			Position/incision		Notes
Fundoplication/ hiatus hernia repair	'Anti-reflux' procedure—fundus of stomach wrapped round lower oesophagus, may require a gastroplasty to lengthen oesophagus	2–3min	++++/ +++++	Supine/laparotomy Lateral/left thoracotomy. Now often done laparoscopically	Moderate/ G&S; if Hb <12 X-match 2U	Often obese—check respiratory function Rapid sequence induction or awake fibre-optic intubation mandatory. Nasogastric tube required. DLT helpful for thoracic approach. Epidural or paravertebral catheter and PCA recommended
Pectus excavatum/ carinatum repair	Correction of 'funnel chest'/'pigeon chest' deformity of sternum	3–5hr	++/+++	Supine—arms to sides/midline sternal incision	Moderate to severe/ X-match 2U	Primarily cosmetic unless deformity severe. Usually young fit adults. GA, IPPV via SLT, and mid-thoracic epidural recommended. Risk of pneumothoraces
Thymectomy	Excision of residual thymic tissue and/or thymoma from superior and anterior mediastinum	2–3hr	++/+++	Supine—arms to sides/median sternotomy	Moderate/ X-match 2U	Usually for myasthenia gravis. Check for airway compression, other autoimmune diseases, thyroid function, and steroid, immunosuppressive, and anticholinesterase therapy (see p246). GA, IPPV via SLT, minimal or no relaxant, and monitoring of neuromuscular transmission. May need postop ventilatory support

Neurosurgery

Tracey Clayton and Alex Manara

Steve Townley

General principles

Intracranial pressure (ICP)

Normal ICP is 5–12mmHg. Changes in ICP reflect changes in the volume of intracranial contents held within the confines of the skull (brain substance 1200–1600ml, blood 100–150ml, CSF 100–150ml, ECF <75ml). Compensatory mechanisms initially reduce the effect of an intracranial space-occupying lesion on ICP. These mechanisms involve displacement of CSF into the spinal subarachnoid space, increased absorption of CSF, and a reduction in intracranial blood volume. Eventually these mechanisms are overwhelmed and further small increases in intracranial volume result in a steep rise in intracranial pressure. If a lesion develops slowly it may reach a relatively large volume before causing a significant rise in ICP. A lesion that appears relatively small on a CT scan may have developed quickly, allowing little time for compensation.

Causes of raised ICP

- Increased brain substance: tumour, abscess, and haematoma
- Increased CSF volume: hydrocephalus, benign intracranial hypertension, blocked shunt
- Increased blood volume:
  - Increased cerebral blood flow: hypoxia, hypercarbia, volatile anaesthetic agents
  - Increased cerebral venous volume: increased thoracic pressure, venous obstruction in the neck, head-down tilt, coughing
- Increased extracellular fluid: cerebral oedema

Cerebral perfusion pressure (CPP)

CPP is the effective pressure that results in blood flow to the brain.

$$CPP = MAP - (ICP + VP)$$

Venous pressure (VP) at the jugular bulb is usually zero or less, and therefore CPP is related to ICP and mean arterial pressure (MAP) alone. The ICP is normally 5–12mmHg. The CPP therefore varies with the individual patient's MAP but cerebral blood flow is maintained constant by autoregulation.

Cerebral blood flow (CBF)

CBF is autoregulated to maintain blood flow between a MAP of 50 and 140mmHg. Outside these limits CBF varies passively with perfusion pressure. In patients with chronic hypertension the lower and upper limits of autoregulation are higher than normal, so that a blood pressure that may be adequate in a normal patient may lead to cerebral ischaemia in the hypertensive patient. Autoregulation is also impaired or abolished acutely in the presence of a brain tissue acidosis, i.e. with hypoxia, hypercarbia, acute intracranial disease, and following head injury.

CBF varies with:
- Metabolism: CBF is primarily determined by the metabolic demands of the brain. It increases during epileptic seizures and with pain/anxiety. It is reduced in coma, hypothermia, and following the administration of anaesthetic agents.
- Carbon dioxide tension: hypocapnia results in cerebral vasoconstriction and a reduction in CBF. The greatest effect is at normal $PaCO_2$, where a change of 1kPa results in a 30% change in blood flow. Arterial pressure modifies the response of CBF to hyperventilation. High perfusion pressures increase the responsiveness to hyperventilation, whereas hypotension of 50mmHg abolishes the effect of $PaCO_2$ on CBF.
- Oxygen tension: PaO_2 is not an important determinant of CBF, a value of <7kPa being required before cerebral vasodilatation occurs.
- Temperature: hypothermia reduces cerebral metabolism by ~5% for every degree centigrade, thereby reducing CBF.
- Viscosity: there is no effect on CBF when the haematocrit is between 30 and 50%. CBF will increase with reduced viscosity outside this range.
- Anaesthetic agents: see below.

Measuring intracranial pressure
- Ventricular: a catheter inserted into a lateral ventricle via a burr hole is the gold standard for measuring ICP. This also allows drainage of CSF as a treatment option. Risks of the technique include haemorrhage at insertion and ventriculitis with prolonged use. Insertion may be difficult in patients with cerebral oedema and small ventricles.
- Subdural: a hollow bolt is inserted into the skull via a burr hole. The dura is incised and a pressure transducer or fibre-optic device is passed into the subdural space. Haemorrhage and infection are possible. Subdural ICP monitoring tends to underestimate ICP.
- Intra-parenchymal: Micro-miniature silicone strain gauge monitors can be inserted into the brain parenchyma to monitor ICP. They are accurate and relatively easy to insert even by non-neurosurgical staff.
- Extradural: catheters in the extradural space are not a reliable method of monitoring ICP and are rarely used.

General principles of anaesthesia in the presence of raised ICP
Symptoms and signs to identify patients with a raised ICP preoperatively:
- Early: headache, vomiting, seizures, focal neurology, papilloedema.
- Late: increasing blood pressure and bradycardia. Agitation, drowsiness, coma, Cheyne Stokes breathing, apnoea. Ipsilateral then bilateral pupillary dilatation, decorticate then decerebrate posturing.
- Investigations: evaluate CT/MRI scans for the presence of generalised oedema, midline shift, acute hydrocephalus and site/size of any lesion.

Management aims
Do not increase ICP further.
- Avoid increasing cerebral blood flow by avoiding hypercarbia, hypoxia, hypertension, and hyperthermia. Use IPPV to control $PaCO_2$ and ensure good oxygenation, adequate analgesia, and anaesthetic depth.

- Avoid increasing venous pressure. Avoid coughing and straining, the head-down position, and obstructing neck veins with ET tube ties.
- Prevent further cerebral oedema. While patients are generally fluid restricted, it is important to maintain intravascular volume and CPP. Do not use hypotonic solutions—fluid flux across the blood–brain barrier is determined mainly by plasma osmolality not oncotic pressure. Maintenance of a high normal plasma osmolality is essential.
- Maintain CPP: hypotension will result in a decreased CPP in the presence of a raised ICP. Control blood pressure using fluids and vasopressors as necessary. Aim for a CPP >70mmHg.
- Avoid anaesthetic agents that increase ICP (see below).

Specific measures to decrease ICP:

- Reduce cerebral oedema using osmotic or loop diuretics, or both. Give mannitol 0.25–1g/kg over 15min or furosemide 0.25–1mg/kg. Insert a urinary catheter in patients receiving diuretics.
- Modest hyperventilation to $PaCO_2$ of 4.0–4.5kPa has a transient effect in reducing ICP for 24hr. Excessive hyperventilation will result in cerebral ischaemia and a loss of autoregulation. Note: $ETCO_2$ is lower than $PaCO_2$.
- Corticosteroids reduce oedema surrounding tumours and abscesses but have no role in head injury. They take several hours to work. Dexamethasone 4mg 6-hourly is often given electively preoperatively.
- Cerebrospinal fluid may be drained via a ventricular or lumbar drain.
- Position the patient with a head-up tilt of 30° to reduce central venous pressure. Ensure that MAP is not significantly reduced as the overall result could be a reduction in CPP.

Anaesthetic agents and ICP

- Volatile agents uncouple metabolism and flow, reducing cerebral metabolism while increasing CBF and ICP. They abolish autoregulation in sufficient doses. Halothane causes the greatest increase in ICP and isoflurane the least. ICP is unaffected by concentrations of <1 MAC of isoflurane, sevoflurane, and desflurane. Enflurane may cause seizures, particularly with hypocapnia, and has no place in neuroanaesthesia. Nitrous oxide is a weak cerebral vasodilator causing an increase in CBF and therefore ICP. It has also been shown to increase cerebral metabolic rate.
- IV anaesthetic agents all decrease cerebral metabolism, CBF and ICP with the exception of ketamine (increases ICP and should be avoided). CO_2 reactivity and autoregulation of the cerebral circulation are well maintained during propofol/thiopental anaesthesia.
- Other drugs:
  - Suxamethonium causes a rise in ICP through muscle fasciculation increasing venous pressure. This effect is moderate and of little clinical relevance. Suxamethonium should still be used when rapid intubation is required in the presence of a potentially full stomach (e.g. head injury).
  - Opioid analgesics have little effect on CBF and ICP if an increase in $PaCO_2$ is avoided. CO_2 reactivity is maintained.

Craniotomy

Procedure	Excision or debulking of tumour, brain biopsy, drainage of cerebral abscess
Time	1–12hr
Pain	+/+++
Position	Supine, head-up tilt or lateral decubitus
Blood loss	0–2000ml, G&S or X-match 2U
Practical techniques	ETT, IPPV, arterial line, CVP

Preoperative

- Assess the patient for symptoms and signs of raised intracranial pressure. Document any neurological deficits. Assess the gag reflex.
- Intracranial tumours may be metastatic: primary sites include the lung, breast, thyroid, and bowel.
- Check CT/MRI scans—the duration and complexity of the procedure are determined by the size, site, and vascularity of lesions being excised.
- Patients receiving diuretic therapy or who have been vomiting may have disordered electrolytes. Patients receiving preoperative dexamethasone may be hyperglycaemic.
- Restrict IV fluids to 30ml/kg/d if cerebral oedema present. Avoid glucose-containing solutions. They may cause hyperglycaemia, which is associated with a worse outcome after brain injury. They also reduce osmolality, resulting in increased cerebral oedema.
- Avoid sedative premedication in patients with raised ICP.
- Ensure graduated compression stockings are fitted to prevent DVT.
- Prophylactic or therapeutic phenytoin may be required (a loading dose of 15mg/kg followed by a single daily dose of 3–4mg/kg).
- Discuss with the surgeon the anticipated duration of procedure since this is very variable (multiply the estimate by two!).

Perioperative

- Patients undergoing burr hole biopsy require standard monitoring. Those scheduled for craniotomy also need art line/CVP, neuromuscular monitoring, and core temperature. Insert a urinary catheter for long procedures and in patients who receive diuretics.
- Induce with thiopental 3–5mg/kg or propofol 2–3mg/kg combined with remifentanil (0.2–0.5µg/kg/min). Give IV induction agents slowly to avoid reducing BP and CPP. A non-depolarising relaxant (vecuronium 0.15mg/kg) is used to facilitate intubation. Remifentanil usually attenuates the hypertensive response to intubation—if not use additional agents such as lidocaine 1.5mg/kg or a β-blocker (labetalol 5mg increments). Use an armoured ETT to prevent kinking and secure in place with tapes as ties may cause venous obstruction. Cover and protect the eyes.

- Avoid N_2O. Maintain anaesthesia using either volatile agent (sevoflurane/isoflurane <1 MAC) or TCI propofol (3–6µg/ml). Remifentanil infusion is continued at a lower rate (0.15–0.25µg/kg/min) titrated to response. Requirement for further top-up doses of muscle relaxants is virtually eliminated with remifentanil. In the absence of remifentanil use fentanyl 5µg/kg at induction followed by top-up doses as required or an alfentanil infusion (25–50µg/kg/hr). In this case maintain neuromuscular relaxation throughout.
- Patients may be placed in the supine or lateral position. Avoid extreme neck flexion or rotation, which may impair cerebral venous return, and maintain a head-up tilt. If the head is turned for surgery, support the shoulder to reduce the effect on neck veins.
- Application of the Mayfield 3 point fixator to secure the head can cause a marked hypertensive response. Pin sites should be infiltrated with local anaesthetic and if necessary give a further dose of remifentanil (0.5–1µg/kg) or propofol (0.5–1mg/kg).
- Aim for normotension during most procedures. Modest hypotension may infrequently be required to improve surgical field. Mild hypocapnia is used in tumour surgery. Aim for $PaCO_2$ of 4.0–4.5kPa. Use 0.9% saline as maintenance fluid, replacing blood loss with colloid or blood.
- Maintain normothermia. Hypothermia is rarely indicated.
- Use intermittent pneumatic compression device to the calves or feet.
- Closure of the dura, bone flap, and scalp takes at least half an hour. Administer IV morphine at this stage to provide analgesia when the remifentanil is stopped. Sudden hypertension on awakening may be treated with small boluses of labetalol. Avoid coughing if possible.

Postoperative

- Further incremental doses of IV morphine may be required in the immediate postoperative period in the recovery area.
- Many routine craniotomies can be managed postoperatively on an adequately staffed neurosurgical ward. Continued monitoring of the patient's conscious level and neurological state is essential. Consider postoperative sedation and ventilation if there is continuing cerebral oedema or if the patient was severely obtunded preoperatively.
- On return to the ward the majority of patients will experience pain in the mild to moderate range after craniotomy. At this stage codeine phosphate (60–90mg) combined with regular paracetamol is usually sufficient in >90% of patients. If not PCA with morphine may be used.

Special considerations

- NSAIDs should be used only for postoperative analgesia after careful consideration. While they reduce opioid requirements and enhance opioid analgesia, they also increase bleeding time—a postoperative intracranial haematoma is potentially disastrous. Many patients will have also received diuretics and are potentially hypovolaemic.
- A central line is indicated for the majority of craniotomies to allow measurement of CVP, infusion of vasoactive drugs, and aspiration of air in the case of venous air embolism. This is most commonly inserted in the antecubital fossa using a long line. However, in experienced hands, the insertion of an internal jugular line does not worsen raised ICP.

Ventriculo-peritoneal shunt

Procedure	CSF drainage for hydrocephalus
Time	45–120min
Pain	++
Position	Supine, head-up tilt
Blood loss	Nil
Practical techniques	ETT, IPPV

Shunts are inserted for hydrocephalus. CSF is diverted from the cerebral ventricles to other body cavities, from where it is absorbed. Most commonly a ventriculo-peritoneal shunt is created. On rare occasions ventriculo-atrial or ventriculo-pleural shunts are inserted. An occipital burr hole enables a tube to be placed into the lateral ventricle. This is then tunnelled subcutaneously down the neck and trunk and inserted into the peritoneal cavity through a small abdominal incision. A flushing device can be placed in the burr hole to keep the system clear, and a valve system is incorporated to prevent CSF draining too rapidly with changes in posture.

Preoperative
- As for craniotomy (p390).
- Many patients requiring shunts are children and the usual paediatric considerations apply.
- Patients often have raised intracranial pressure.
- Emergency cases may have a full stomach, requiring a rapid sequence induction.

Perioperative
- Shunt procedures are shorter and simpler than craniotomies. Use routine monitoring. Arterial and central venous lines are not required.
- Antibiotic treatment or prophylaxis is required and strict antisepsis protocols are normally followed to reduce the incidence of shunt infection.
- Advancing the trocar to allow tunnelling of the shunt is particularly stimulating. Additional analgesia and/or muscle relaxation is often required at this stage.

Postoperative
- Any deterioration in the patient's conscious level is an indication for CT scan to exclude shunt malfunction or subdural haematoma.

Special considerations
- Patients are at risk of intracranial haemorrhage if CSF is drained too rapidly.
- Shunts often block or become infected, requiring revision.
- Watch for signs of pneumothorax as the trocar is placed subcutaneously.

Evacuation of traumatic intracranial haematoma

Procedure	Evacuation of extradural or subdural haematoma
Time	1.5–3hr
Pain	+/+++
Position	Supine, head-up
Blood loss	200–2000ml, X-match 2U
Practical techniques	ETT, IPPV, art line, CVP

Intracranial haematoma may be extradural, subdural or intracerebral.
- Extradural: urgent evacuation is required and certainly within an hour of pupillary dilation. The haematoma is usually the result of a tear in the middle meningeal artery. It is virtually always associated with a skull fracture, except in children, when the fracture may be absent.
- Subdural haematoma results from bleeding from the bridging veins between the cortex and dura. Early evacuation of acute subdural haematoma improves outcome. Chronic subdural haematomas occur in the elderly, often after trivial injury. They present insidiously with headaches and confusion and can be evacuated via burr hole under local anaesthesia.
- Intracerebral haematoma occurs in hypertensive individuals, as a complication of treatment with warfarin, or as a result of bleeding from an intracranial aneurysm.

Preoperative
- As for head injury (p824).
- Most patients will have a reduced or deteriorating GCS.
- Intracranial pressure is usually raised.
- Patients may have associated injuries to chest, pelvis, or abdomen requiring resuscitation and treatment in their own right—see p818. Protect C-spine if necessary.
- Patients may have a full stomach, requiring rapid sequence induction. Insert an orogastric tube after intubation.
- Check blood clotting profile and the availability of blood products prior to surgery.

Perioperative

- As for craniotomy (p390).
- Patients require standard monitoring, including invasive blood pressure monitoring. CVP monitoring should be instituted.
- Ensure smooth induction and normotension. Maintain CPP using fluids and vasopressors if necessary. Assume that the ICP is 20mmHg—the minimum acceptable MAP is therefore 90mmHg to achieve a CPP of 70mmHg.
- Ensure head-up tilt; avoid nitrous oxide, ventilate to an $ETCO_2$ of 4.0kPa and give mannitol (0.5–1g/kg) or 5% saline (100ml) and furosemide (0.25–1mg/kg) as required.
- Once decompression has occurred there may be a decrease in systemic blood pressure, which can usually be treated with volume replacement.

Postoperative

- Most patients should be transferred to ITU. Further management should be guided by a protocol to maintain CPP and prevent secondary insults to the brain (see below).

Special considerations

- It is essential for the various teams to communicate and set priorities in the management of patients with multiple injuries. Priorities will vary from patient to patient—see p845.
- Hypotension in a head-injured patient is a medical emergency and must be treated promptly and aggressively.

Postoperative and ICU management of the head-injured patient

- Management of head injured patients is similar for postoperative patients and those not requiring surgery. Patients are best managed using a protocol designed primarily to maintain an adequate CPP/cerebral oxygenation and control ICP. It involves identifying and treating causes of secondary brain insults.[1]
- Causes of secondary insult are:
  - Intracranial—haematoma, oedema, convulsions, hydrocephalus, abscess, hyperaemia
  - Systemic—hypotension, hypoxia, hyponatraemia, pyrexia, anaemia, sepsis, hypercarbia
- On current evidence, steroids should not be administered to patients following severe head injury.

1 Clayton TJ, Nelson RJ, Manara AR (2004). Reduction in mortality from severe head injury following introduction of a protocol for intensive care management. *British Journal of Anaesthesia*, **93**, 761–767.

Guidelines for managing adults with severe head injuries in ICU

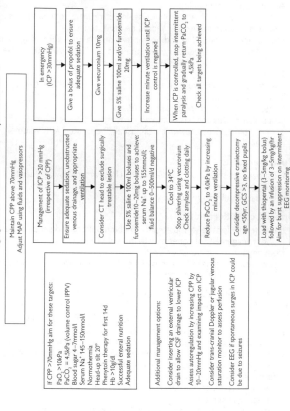

Maintain CPP above 70mmHg
Adjust MAP using fluids and vasopressors

If CPP >70mmHg aim for these targets:

PaO$_2$ >10kPa
PaCO$_2$ = 4.5kPa (volume control IPPV)
Blood sugar 4–7mmol/l
Serum Na$^+$ 145–150mmol/l
Normothermia
Head-up tilt 20°
Phenytoin therapy for first 14d
Hb >10g/dl
Successful enteral nutrition
Adequate sedation

Additional management options:

Consider inserting an external ventricular drain to allow CSF drainage to lower ICP

Assess autoregulation by increasing CPP by 10–20mmHg and examining impact on ICP

Consider trans-cranial Doppler or jugular venous saturation monitor to assess perfusion

Consider EEG if spontaneous surges in ICP could be due to seizures

Management of ICP >20 mmHg
(irrespective of CPP)

Ensure adequate sedation, unobstructed venous drainage, and appropriate ventilation

Consider CT head to exclude surgically treatable lesion

Use 5% saline 100ml boluses and furosemide 10–20mg boluses to achieve: serum Na$^+$ up to 155mmol/l; fluid balance 0–500ml/d negative

Cool to 34°C
Stop shivering using vecuronium
Check amylase and clotting daily

Reduce PaCO$_2$ to 4.0kPa by increasing minute ventilation

Consider decompressive craniectomy age <50yr, GCS >3, no fixed pupils

Load with thiopental (3–5mg/kg bolus) followed by an infusion of 3–5mg/kg/hr
Aim for burst suppression on intermittent EEG monitoring

In emergency
(ICP >30mmHg)

Give a bolus of propofol to ensure adequate sedation

Give vecuronium 10mg

Give 5% saline 100ml and/or furosemide 20mg
Check all targets being achieved

Increase minute ventilation until ICP control is regained

When ICP is controlled, stop intermittent paralysis and gradually return PaCO$_2$ to 4.5kPa

Pituitary surgery

Procedure	Trans-sphenoidal hypophysectomy
Time	90–180min
Pain	++
Position	Supine, head-up tilt
Blood loss	Nil usually, but large if venous sinus disrupted, G&S
Practical techniques	ETT, IPPV, art line

Pituitary tumours account for 15% of all intracranial tumours. They present with either hypersecretion of hormones (acromegaly/Cushing's syndrome), or mass effects (headaches, visual field defects, hydrocephalus, hypopituitarism). Hypophysectomy is undertaken urgently if the patient's sight is deteriorating rapidly.

Preoperative

Special considerations for acromegalic patients (see also p156):
- Possible airway compromise due to macroglossia, prognathism, and hypertrophy of epiglottis/vocal cords
- Hypertension and left ventricular hypertrophy
- Sleep apnoea, diabetes mellitus

Special considerations for Cushing's patients (see also p168):
- Hypertension, truncal obesity
- Electrolyte abnormalities (hypokalaemia, hyperglycaemia)
- Steroid cover necessary pre- and postoperatively

Perioperative

- As for craniotomy (p390).
- A throat pack should be inserted following intubation. Moffett's solution (p606) may be instilled into each nostril to improve surgical conditions.
- Surgical access is via the sphenoidal air sinuses.
- If there is suprasellar extension a lumbar drain is inserted into the CSF. The anaesthetist may be required to instil a volume of sterile saline to advance the tumour into the operative field.
- Major haemorrhage may occur if there is disruption of the cavernous sinus/carotid arteries which lie lateral to the pituitary gland.

Postoperative

- Codeine phosphate is the analgesic of choice.
- Diabetes insipidus may occur in up to 50% of patients. It is managed initially with IV DDAVP (0.25–1µg).
- Cerebrospinal rhinorrhoea may occur. It is usually self-limiting but, if persistent, intermittent drainage via a lumbar drain may be required.

Special considerations

Patients with preoperative pan-hypopituitarism or who develop postoperative endocrine disturbances should be referred to an endocrinologist for advice on hormone replacement.

Posterior fossa surgery

Procedure	Excision or debulking of tumour, vascular procedures, foramen magnum decompression
Time	3–14hr
Pain	+/+++
Position	See below
Blood loss	100–2000ml, G&S
Practical techniques	ETT, IPPV, art line, CVP, ?monitoring for venous air embolism

The posterior fossa lies below the tentorium cerebelli and contains the pons, medulla, and cerebellum. Within the brain stem lie the main motor and sensory pathways, the lower cranial nerve nuclei, and the centres that control respiration and cardiovascular function. An increase in pressure in this area results in decreased consciousness, hypertension, bradycardia, respiratory depression and loss of protective airway reflexes. The exit pathways for CSF from the ventricular system are also located here and obstruction results in hydrocephalus. Space-occupying lesions and surgical disturbance in this area can therefore have a profound physiological impact.

Preoperative

- Patients with posterior fossa lesions may have a reduced level of consciousness and impaired airway reflexes. Bulbar palsy may lead to silent aspiration. Pulmonary function must be assessed.
- Assess intracranial pressure—may be raised. If hydrocephalus is present, ventricular drainage may be required before the definitive procedure.
- Assess fluid status—may be dehydrated if vomiting. A reduced intravascular volume will result in hypotension on induction or if placed in the sitting position.
- Check electrolytes and glucose, particularly if taking diuretics or steroids.
- Assess cardiovascular function, particularly the presence of untreated hypertension, postural hypotension, and septal defects.

Perioperative

- As for craniotomy (p390).
- Insert an NG tube if the patient has, or is at risk of, postoperative bulbar dysfunction.
- Further specialised monitoring is required for posterior fossa surgery, including monitoring for venous air embolism (p414) and nerve tract injury. The appropriate electrophysiological monitor used to detect nerve tract injury depends upon the neural pathway at risk during the procedure. Spontaneous or evoked electromyographic activity, somatosensory evoked potentials, or brainstem auditory evoked potentials are frequently monitored.

- Lumbar CSF drainage is occasionally requested to improve surgical conditions and to reduce the incidence of postoperative CSF leaks.
- Avoid N_2O—it increases cerebral metabolic rate and CBF and may worsen the outcome of air embolism. Finally, there is a risk that any residual intracranial air will increase in volume and cause postoperative pneumocephalus.
- While some still recommend spontaneous respiration for posterior fossa surgery, the consensus is to use muscle relaxation and IPPV.
- Surgical interference with vital centres may result in sudden and dramatic cardiovascular changes. Inform the surgeon—more gentle retraction or dissection usually resolves the problem. Use drugs such as atropine and β-blockers only if absolutely necessary as they make the interpretation of further changes difficult.

Patient positioning

Surgical access to the posterior fossa requires the patient to be sitting, prone or lateral. Careful attention is required in positioning the patient as procedures are often prolonged.

- Sitting position: use of this position is declining. It provides optimum access to midline lesions, improves cerebral venous drainage, and lowers intracranial pressure. However, complications include haemodynamic instability, venous air embolism, and the possibility of paradoxical air embolism, pneumocephalus, and quadriplegia. Absolute contraindications include cerebral ischaemia when upright and awake, and the presence of a patent ventriculo-atrial shunt or patent foramen ovale (should be screened preoperatively). Relative contraindications are uncontrolled hypertension, extremes of age, and COPD. To achieve this position the head and shoulders are gradually elevated with the neck partially flexed and the forehead resting on a horseshoe ring mounted on a frame. Avoid excessive head flexion since this can cause jugular compression, swelling of the tongue and face, and cervical cord ischaemia.
- Prone position: allows good surgical access without the risks specifically associated with the sitting position. Abdominal compression should be avoided as it results in increased cerebral venous pressure. This is achieved by adequately supporting the chest and pelvis.
- Lateral position: the lateral or 'park bench' position is particularly suitable for lateral lesions such as acoustic neuroma or operations on a cerebellar hemisphere. The neck is flexed and the head rotated towards the floor ensuring that the jugular veins are not obstructed. Pressure points over the shoulder, greater trochanter, and peroneal nerves should be protected.

Postoperative

- Most patients can be safely extubated and managed on a properly staffed neurosurgical ward postoperatively.
- Airway obstruction can occur after posterior fossa surgery due to macroglossia, partial damage to the vagus, or excessive flexion of the cervical spine.

- Surgery on medulla or high cervical lesions carries a significant risk of postoperative impairment of respiratory drive.
- The patient should be admitted to ICU for ventilation if the preoperative state was poor, the surgical resection was extensive, there is significant cerebral oedema, or there are intra-operative complications.

Special considerations

- **Acoustic neuroma:** the facial nerve is particularly vulnerable and is monitored using electromyographic needles placed over the face. This allows the surgeon to identify when the nerve is at risk. Neuromuscular blockade should be used only at induction to allow intubation. Often 8th nerve function is also monitored to preserve any residual hearing. This requires a constant level of anaesthesia so that neurophysiological changes can be attributed to surgery rather than variations in anaesthetic depth. These requirements are best met using a remifentanil infusion combined with a constant level of anaesthesia using a low concentration of an inhalation agent or a propofol infusion.
- **Venous air embolism** (see p414).
- Postoperative analgesia is managed as for craniotomy. Posterior fossa surgery is reputed to cause more postoperative pain than supratentorial surgery, although this is questionable.

Posterior fossa lesions

Tumour	Notes
Gliomas	Cerebellar astrocytomas, ependymomas, particularly arising from the fourth ventricle
Medulloblastoma	Often arising from the vermis of the cerebellum, usually in children
Acoustic neuroma	Arising from the 8th nerve in the cerebello-pontine angle, usually benign
Haemangioblastoma	Young adults

Meningiomas
  Metastatic tumours
  Abscesses and haematoma
	Less common in the posterior fossa

Vascular lesions	Aneurysms of the superior cerebellar, posterior inferior cerebellar, and vertebral arteries
Developmental lesions	Arnold–Chiari malformation

Awake craniotomy

Procedure	Epilepsy surgery, excision of tumours in eloquent cortical areas
Time	1.5–4hr
Pain	+/+++
Position	See below
Blood loss	100–2000ml, G&S
Practical techniques	LMA, art line, consider monitoring for venous air embolism

Awake craniotomy allows intra-operative assessment of the patient's neurological status. It is mainly used to allow accurate mapping of the resection margins in epilepsy surgery, accurate location of electrodes in surgery for movement disorders, and excision of tumours from eloquent areas of the cortex (sensory, motor, speech areas). In tumour surgery the aim is to achieve maximal tumour resection with minimal neurological deficit. It is used most effectively in combination with modern imaging techniques such as 3D navigation systems. Awake craniotomy may be performed more frequently in the future since it is associated with a lower requirement for high-dependency care, shorter length of stay, and reduced costs. In the past a combination of local anaesthesia and sedation was used but the use of an asleep–awake–asleep technique with a laryngeal mask airway (LMA) is gaining popularity since it is associated with a lower incidence of complications such as over-sedation, airway obstruction, hypoventilation, and an uncooperative patient.

Preoperative
- As for craniotomy (p390).
- Both the neurosurgeon and neuro-anaesthetist must be experienced in awake craniotomy. Appropriate patient selection is essential. The patient must be well informed, motivated, and able to tolerate lying still for the duration of surgery. Confusion, anxiety, or difficulty in communication are contraindications. Obesity, oesophageal reflux, and highly vascular tumours may also cause problems.
- The patient should be given a full explanation of the procedures involved and what to expect.
- Premedication is generally avoided, but routine medication should be continued and administered on the day of surgery. Anticonvulsant prophylaxis should be prescribed routinely for all patients and dexamethasone for those undergoing tumour surgery.

Perioperative
- Aims are to ensure adequate sedation, analgesia, and cardio-respiratory stability as well as an awake and co-operative patient when required for intra-operative testing. Routine monitoring as for craniotomy should be used, including urinary catheterisation if the procedure is expected to be prolonged.

- IV anti-emetic prophylaxis is administered routinely (ondansetron 4mg IV). Anaesthesia is induced and maintained with a target controlled infusion of propofol and a remifentanil infusion (0.05–1µg/kg/min). The propofol dose is titrated against the patient's responses, haemodynamics, and possibly bispectral index monitoring. The patient's lungs are ventilated using an LMA, allowing monitoring and control of ventilation/$PaCO_2$. This minimises the risks of hypoventilation and airway obstruction, providing good operative conditions. Adequate local anaesthetic infiltration of the Mayfield fixator pin sites and the operative field must be ensured.
- When the tumour is exposed the remifentanil is reduced to 0.005–0.01µg/kg/min to allow return of spontaneous ventilation. When this occurs the LMA is removed and the propofol stopped. Once the resection is complete the patient is re-anaesthetised and the LMA reinserted until the end of the procedure.

Postoperative
- Morphine should be administered at the end of the procedure.
- Other aspects of postoperative care are as for craniotomy (p390).

Special considerations
- Ensure that a calm and quiet atmosphere is maintained in theatre. The patient should be draped in a fashion that allows constant access to the patient's airway and minimises the feeling of claustrophobia.
- Bispectral index monitoring may be useful in guiding the target controlled infusion.

Vascular lesions

Vascular lesions presenting for surgical management are usually either intracranial aneurysms or arteriovenous malformations.

Intracranial aneurysms

- Berry aneurysms occur at vessel junctions, cerebral arteries having a weaker, less elastic muscle layer than systemic vessels. They may occur in association with atherosclerosis, polycystic kidneys, hereditary haemorrhagic telangiectasia, coarctation of the aorta, Marfan's, Ehlers–Danlos, and Klinefelter's syndromes. Mycotic aneurysms may occur in rheumatic fever.
- The most common sites are the internal carotid system (41%), the anterior cerebral artery (34%), and the middle cerebral artery (20%).
- They are more common in females, 40–60yr olds and in 25% of cases they are multiple. In the UK, the incidence is 10–28:100 000 per year. The prevalence of aneurysm is 6% of the population in prospective angiographic studies.
- Aneurysms do not usually rupture until they are >5mm in diameter. They then present as a subarachnoid or intracerebral haemorrhage. Classic symptoms include sudden onset of severe headache with loss of consciousness that may be transient in mild cases. Occasionally a patient presents with a focal neurological deficit due to the pressure of an enlarging aneurysm on surrounding structures.
- Grading of subarachnoid haemorrhage (World Federation of Neurosurgeons): grade of SAH influences morbidity and mortality. It is also of value in deciding whether to operate or coil early (grades 1–3) or to wait (grades 4–5).

Grade	GCS (see p825)	Motor deficit
1	15	–
2	13–14	–
3	13–14	+
4	7–12	±
5	3–6	±

Arteriovenous malformations

- These are dilated arteries and veins with no intervening capillaries.
- They may present clinically with subarachnoid haemorrhage or seizures.
- High blood flow through such lesions may 'steal' blood from surrounding tissue leading to ischaemia.

Complications of aneurysmal subarachnoid haemorrhage (SAH)

Neurological complications

Re-bleeding

- The initial bleed and subsequent bleeds are the main cause of mortality. The highest risk period is in the first 24hr, during which there is a 4% risk of re-bleeding, followed by a further risk of 1.5% per day for the next 4wk.
- There is a 60% risk of death with each episode of re-bleeding. The main aim of management is to prevent re-bleeding by securing the aneurysm surgically by clipping it, or angiographically by obliterating it endoluminally.
- Surgery was previously delayed for up to 10d as early surgery is more difficult, and to wait for the peak of vasospasm to pass.
- The introduction of nimodipine has resulted in earlier surgery, ideally within 72hr. Grade 1–2 patients may be operated upon immediately.

Delayed neurological deficit (DND)

- DND may present as focal or diffuse deficits and is a major cause of morbidity. It is the second main cause of mortality.
- It is associated with vasospasm caused by substances released as the subarachnoid blood undergoes haemolysis. The most likely spasmogenic agent is oxyhaemoglobin.
- Although angiographic vasospasm occurs in up to 75% of studied patients, only half of these patients develop DND. Up to 20% of symptomatic patients will develop a stroke or die of vasospasm despite optimal management.
- DND peaks 3–14d after the initial bleed. With increasingly early surgery for aneurysms, it is now commonly seen postoperatively.

Treatment

- Calcium channel blockers: nimodipine is a relatively selective calcium channel antagonist with effective penetration of the blood–brain barrier. It is started at the time of diagnosis and continued for 3wk (60mg NG/PO 4-hourly). Alternatively it can be administered IV (1mg/hr increasing to 2mg/hr) either centrally or peripherally with a fast flowing IVI. Nimodipine may cause systemic hypotension, which should be managed aggressively with fluids and, if necessary, catecholamines.
- Hypertensive, hypervolaemic therapy with or without haemodilution ('*Triple H*' therapy): based on the theory that vasospasm can be prevented or reversed by optimising cerebral blood flow. Goals are to increase cardiac output and blood pressure using volume expansion and then vasoactive drugs. The resulting haemodilution may improve cerebral blood flow by reducing viscosity. Disagreement exists as to the fluids/drugs that should be used and which haemodynamic goals to aim for. Suggested values are normal MAP + 15%, CVP >12mmHg, Hct 30–35%. Some centres advocate the use of PA catheters to monitor therapy. Noradrenaline (0.025–$0.3\mu g/kg/min$) or dobutamine (2–$15\mu g/kg/min$) are used to increase MAP.
- In some centres balloon angioplasty or intra-arterial papaverine are also used.

Hydrocephalus
Blood in the subarachnoid space may obstruct drainage of CSF and result in hydrocephalus and raised ICP. Sudden reduction in pressure with the insertion of a ventricular drain may increase the risk of re-bleeding by reducing the transmural pressure across the aneurysm. Hydrocephalus must be ruled out by CT scan before attributing neurological deterioration to DND/vasospasm.

Other neurological complications
These include seizures and cerebral oedema.

Medical complications

Life-threatening associated medical problems occur in nearly 40% of patients and account for about 23% of deaths. Many of the cardiorespiratory complications following SAH are related to the massive sympathetic surge and catecholamine release that follow SAH.

- Severe LV dysfunction/cardiogenic shock: nearly 45% of patients have an ejection fraction <50% or regional wall motion abnormalities. Treat with dobutamine.
- ECG abnormalities: up to 27% of patients will have ECG changes— T wave inversion, ST segment abnormalities, and Q waves. Strongly associated with a poor neurological grade but not predictive of all cause mortality.
- Neurogenic pulmonary oedema: initially a hydrostatic pulmonary oedema resulting from an increase in pulmonary artery pressure, followed by damage to the pulmonary microvasculature and an increase in pulmonary capillary permeability.
- Hyponatraemia: many patients are hypovolaemic and hyponatraemic as a result of excessive atrial natriuretic peptide release. Fluid restriction is inappropriate and it should be managed with sodium repletion.
- Other complications include deep vein thrombosis, pneumonia, and hepatic, renal and GI dysfunction.

Outcome following subarachnoid haemorrhage

Approximately 20% of patients will die from SAH at the time of the initial bleed. Of those who survive to reach hospital a further 15% will die within 24hr, and 40% will make a good recovery.

Anaesthesia for vascular lesions

Procedure	Clipping of intracranial aneurysm, endovascular coiling of aneurysm
Time	3–6hr
Pain	++/+++
Position	Supine, head-up, lateral, or prone
Blood loss	200–2000ml; X-match 2U
Practical techniques	ETT, IPPV, art line, CVP

Clipping an aneurysm involves the use of microsurgery to apply a spring clip across the neck of the aneurysm. Aneurysms arising from branches of the vertebral or basilar arteries require a posterior fossa craniotomy, whereas others may be reached from a frontal or fronto-parietal approach. There is often a need to control the aneurysm prior to clipping by applying a temporary clip to a proximal vessel.

Preoperative

- Assess the effects of the haemorrhage and any pre-existing arterial disease on the brain and other organs. See p408.
- Ensure adequate fluid intake, and that fluid is not being unnecessarily restricted.
- Nimodipine treatment should be instituted.
- Ensure graduated compression stockings are fitted.
- Phenytoin (15mg/kg followed by a single daily dose of 3–4mg/kg) should be prescribed prophylactically for the majority of patients.
- Discuss the anticipated difficulty of the surgical approach with the surgeon as it influences the decision to use induced hypothermia, barbiturates, and other forms of cerebral protection.

Perioperative

As for craniotomy (p370) but note the following:
- Standard monitoring including invasive blood pressure monitoring should be instituted prior to induction. A CVP line can be inserted after induction. It will be useful not only intra-operatively but also in the postoperative period to help guide 'Triple H' therapy (p408).
- Ensure adequate venous access with a large bore cannula.
- Aim to avoid increases in arterial pressure that may result in aneurysm rupture, but maintain adequate cerebral perfusion pressure. Aim for the pre-induction BP ± 10%.
- Hypocapnia can result in cerebral ischaemia after SAH and must be avoided. Ventilate to a normal $PaCO_2$.
- Maintain core temperature at 36–37°C for all grade I–III patients.

- Modern neurosurgical practice is to use temporary spring clips rather than induced hypotension. The latter may still be required in difficult cases or if rupture occurs. In this situation aim for a systolic BP of 60–80mmHg. Moderate hypotension may be achieved using isoflurane (up to 1.5 MAC). Further hypotension is achieved using labetalol (5–10mg increments). Sodium nitroprusside is rarely used. Hypotension must not be induced in the presence of vasospasm.
- If rupture occurs:
  - Call for help.
  - Increase IV infusions and start blood transfusion.
  - Inducing hypotension helps to reduce bleeding.
  - Ipsilateral carotid compression.
- Other cerebral protection measures should be considered electively if temporary clipping of a major cerebral vessel is planned or in case of aneurysm rupture. This includes inducing the administration of thiopental (3–5mg/kg bolus followed by 3–5mg/kg/hr), in which case EEG monitoring should ideally be used to allow titration of the dose to burst suppression. It may be necessary to use a vasopressor to support MAP when infusing thiopental. Inducing hypothermia to a temperature of 32°C is reserved for complex surgical vascular procedures. The patient is cooled using surface devices and rewarmed once the cerebral circulation is restored.

Postoperative

- ICU/HDU care is required postoperatively for patients with a poor grade preoperatively, those who had a stormy perioperative course, and those requiring treatment for vasospasm.
- Codeine phosphate and regular paracetamol may be prescribed for analgesia.
- A decrease in the GCS may indicate vasospasm, intracranial haematoma, or hydrocephalus—perform a CT scan.

Special considerations

It is becoming increasingly common to control intracranial aneurysms by the insertion of platinum Guglielmi detachable coils (GDCs) via catheters inserted in the femoral artery. This approach is associated with a better 1yr outcome in many aneurysms than craniotomy.

- The procedure is undertaken in the angiography suite by neuroradiologists. Ensure skilled anaesthetic assistance and the same anaesthetic and monitoring facilities that would be available in theatre for a clipping procedure.
- Patients require general anaesthesia using techniques similar to that described for clipping aneurysms except that a CVP line is not commonly used.
- It is important to maintain MAP and a normal $PaCO_2$.
- Aneurysm rupture during the procedure occurs in ~1:300 cases and is almost invariably fatal.
- The overall mortality of the procedure is 8.1% at 1yr. Many are due to re-bleeding.

Arteriovenous malformations (AVMs)

- Surgery is not urgent unless the AVM or a resulting haematoma is causing pressure effects.
- The procedure may be associated with significant blood loss—crossmatched blood and adequate IV access are essential.
- Blood may be shunted through the AVM, resulting in relative ischaemia to the surrounding tissue. When the lesion is excised, a relative hyperperfusion of surrounding tissue may occur, resulting in cerebral oedema and increased ICP.
- There is no risk of vasospasm and when indicated hypotension may be induced with relative safety. This is achieved using isoflurane ± labetalol as outlined for SAH (p408).
- In children AVMs can cause high output failure due to intracerebral shunt. CCF may be precipitated by excision of the lesion.

Venous air embolism (VAE)

- VAE can occur whenever the operative site is higher than the right atrium. Its incidence is particularly high during craniotomy in the sitting position, and when the surgeon is dissecting tissues that do not allow veins to collapse despite a negative pressure within them (e.g. the emissary veins in the posterior fossa).
- VAE causes pulmonary microvascular occlusion, resulting in increased physiological dead space. Bronchoconstriction may also develop. A large volume of air causes frothing within the right atrium, leading to obstruction of the right ventricular outflow tract and a reduction in cardiac output.
- Signs of VAE include hypotension, arrhythmias, increased PA pressure, decreased $ETCO_2$, and hypoxia.
- N_2O does not increase the risk of VAE but may worsen its outcome.

Detection of VAE

- End-tidal CO_2 is generally the most useful monitor as it is widely available and sensitive. Air embolism results in a *sudden* reduction in $ETCO_2$. Hyperventilation, low cardiac output, and other types of embolism will also result in reduction in $ETCO_2$.
- Doppler ultrasound is the most sensitive non-invasive monitor. It uses ultrahigh-frequency sound waves to detect changes in blood flow velocity and density. Unfortunately, it is not quantitative and does not differentiate between a massive or physiologically insignificant air embolism. Positioning the probe and diathermy interference can prove problematic.
- Trans-oesophageal echo allows determination of the amount of air aspirated but is more invasive, difficult to place, and needs expertise to interpret.
- Pulmonary artery catheters are invasive but sensitive monitors for VAE. However, an increase in PA pressure is not specific for air.
- The least sensitive monitor is a precordial or oesophageal stethoscope to detect a 'millwheel' murmur. This is apparent only after massive VAE, which is usually clinically obvious.

Prevention

- Avoid the sitting position unless essential.
- Elevate the head only as much as necessary.
- Ensure adequate blood volume to maintain a positive CVP.
- Small amounts of PEEP (5–10cmH$_2$O) may reduce the risk of air entrainment.
- A 'G-suit' or medical anti-shock trousers may be used to increase venous pressure and reduce hypotensive episodes in patients in the sitting position.

Treatment

- Treatment is supportive.
- Inform the surgeon, who should flood the operative field with fluid. This stops further entrainment of air and allows the identification of open veins that can be cauterised or waxed if within bone.
- Stop N_2O if in use and increase the FiO_2 to 1.0.
- If possible position the operative site below the level of the heart to increase venous pressure.
- Aspirate air from CVP line. The tip should be placed close to the junction of the SVC and the right atrium.
- Support the blood pressure with fluid and vasopressors.
- If a large volume of air has been entrained and surgical conditions permit, turn the patient into the left lateral position to attempt to keep the air in the right atrium.
- Commence CPR if necessary.

Paradoxical air embolism

- Air emboli may enter the systemic circulation through the Thebesian veins in the heart, the bronchial vessels, or a patent foramen ovale. Such defects may be small and not picked up preoperatively.
- Small volumes of air in the systemic circulation can have disastrous consequences.
- Intra-cardiac septal defects are an absolute contraindication to surgery in the sitting position.

Brainstem death

The most common causes of brainstem death are head injury, cerebrovascular accidents (including SAH), cerebral tumours, and hypoxic brain injury. To diagnose brainstem death the patient needs to fulfil certain preconditions and have absent brainstem reflexes.

Preconditions

- The patient is apnoeic and dependent on mechanical ventilation.
- The coma must be caused by a known and irreversible structural cause of brain injury (most commonly traumatic brain injury or intracranial haemorrhage).
- Reversible causes for brainstem depression have been excluded: sedatives, muscle relaxants, alcohol, hypothermia, and metabolic or endocrine disturbances.

Absence of brainstem responses

Tests of brainstem reflexes should be performed only when the preconditions are fulfilled.

- Pupils are fixed and there is no direct or consensual response to light. The pupils are usually dilated, but this is not essential for the diagnosis.
- Corneal reflex is absent.
- There is no motor response within the cranial nerve distribution to painful stimuli applied centrally or peripherally. Spinal reflexes may persist in brainstem-dead patients, and may even return after an initial absence.
- Oculo-vestibular reflex is absent. There is no eye movement in response to the injection of 50ml ice-cold water into the external auditory meatus—direct access to the tympanic membrane should be verified using an auroscope. The eyes should be observed for at least 1min after each injection.
- There is no gag or cough reflex in response to a suction catheter passed into the pharynx or down the endotracheal tube.
- Apnoea is present on disconnection from mechanical ventilation. This test is done last, to avoid unnecessary hypercarbia should any of the other reflexes be present. The patient should be preoxygenated by ventilating with 100% O_2 for 5min. The patient is then disconnected and observed for any respiratory movement for 10min. The $PaCO_2$ should be measured and should be high enough to ensure an adequate stimulus to ventilation (>6.7kPa (50mmHg) in a previously normal individual). Hypoxia is avoided during apnoea by passing a suction catheter down the endotracheal tube and supplying 5–10l/min of oxygen while monitoring the SaO_2.

Other considerations

- Diagnosis of brainstem death should be made by two medical practitioners trained and experienced in the field. One must be a consultant and the other could be a second consultant or a doctor who has been registered for a minimum of 5yr. Neither should be a member of the transplant team.

- The tests must be performed on two occasions separated by an adequate time interval to satisfy all concerned.
- The diagnosis should not normally be considered until at least 6hr after the onset of apnoeic coma or 24hr after the restoration of circulation if the cause was cardiac arrest.
- Death is certified after the second set of tests but the time of death is recorded as the completion of the first set of brainstem death criteria.
- No additional tests are required in the UK, but other countries may require EEG, carotid angiography, or brainstem evoked potentials.
- The coroner (Procurator Fiscal in Scotland) needs to be informed of most of these patients due to the underlying diagnosis, and if organ donation is contemplated.
- Care of the relatives is essential at this time irrespective of whether the patient is to be an organ donor or not.

Organ retrieval from a beating heart donor

Procedure	Procurement of donor organs via long midline incision and median sternotomy
Time	Up to 6hr depending on number of organs retrieved
Pain	n/a
Position	Supine
Blood loss	Large fluid losses likely, X-match 4U
Practical techniques	Usually from ICU IPPV, CVP, and art line

Demand for donor organs continues to exceed supply and the criteria for suitable organs are constantly changing. Currently the only absolute contra-indication to donation is the existence of a transmissible fatal disease. Donor organ management cannot begin before confirmation of brainstem death.

Pathophysiology of brainstem death

- Early, short-lived massive sympathetic outflow occurs during brainstem herniation, causing hypertension, tachycardia, myocardial dysfunction, impaired organ perfusion, and tissue ischaemia.
- Paralytic autonomic collapse follows with a fall in cardiac output, hypotension, and atropine-resistant bradycardia. Circulatory collapse will ensue within 24–72hr without intervention.
- Deterioration in lung function is common due to neurogenic pulmonary oedema, acute lung injury, or pre-existing disease.
- Reduced circulating T_3 and T_4 with increased peripheral conversion of T_4 to reverse T_3 causes depletion of myocardial energy stores, myocardial dysfunction, and a global shift to anaerobic metabolism.
- Hyperglycaemia due to reduced circulating insulin and insulin resistance.
- Reduced ADH output leads to neurogenic diabetes insipidus with hypovolaemia and electrolyte disorders (hypernatraemia, hypermagnesaemia, hypokalaemia, hypophosphataemia, hypocalcaemia).
- Systemic inflammatory response with increased serum and organ cytokines and upregulation of endothelial adhesion molecules.
- Release of tissue fibrinolytic agents and plasminogen activators from necrotic brain causes a coagulopathy.
- Temperature regulation is lost due to hypothalamic dysfunction resulting in poikilothermia.

Preoperative

- Confirm brainstem death certification and status as organ donor— check that consent has been obtained from the relatives and the deceased discussed with the coroner.

- Emphasis in management changes from cerebral resuscitation to optimal organ perfusion and oxygenation.
- Ensure intravascular volume resuscitation with blood and gelatin based colloids using continuous CVP monitoring. Avoid over-hydration (especially in potential lung donors) which may precipitate pulmonary oedema, increase A–a oxygen gradients, cause cardiac over-distension and liver congestion.
- If optimal adjustment of preload fails to achieve target values (see box) inotropes should be started (use dopamine up to 10µg/kg/min as first choice, then adrenaline 0.01–0.05µg/kg/min if necessary).
- PAFC and transoesophageal echocardiography should be considered for heart donors with high inotrope requirements. They allow assessment of cardiac structure and function, and prevent intravascular overload.
- Lung toilet should continue with regular chest physiotherapy and suctioning.
- If desmopressin (DDAVP) has been used to control diabetes insipidus it should be changed to vasopressin (ADH)—restores vascular tone and arterial pressure without a direct myocardial effect
- Although debate continues on the value of T_3 replacement, hormone resuscitation (see table) is often commenced empirically soon after diagnosis of brainstem death and continued throughout organ procurement to stabilise haemodynamics. Usually marked effect on donors with poor cardiac function.
- Correct hypernatraemia with 5% dextrose (Na^+ <155mmol/l). Dextrose 4%/saline 0.18% with potassium chloride should be used to replace normal urinary water and electrolyte losses. Clotting abnormalities should be corrected with clotting factors and platelets.
- Central venous access via the right internal jugular vein and left radial arterial access are preferred due to early ligation of the left innominate vein and right subclavian artery respectively.
- CXR, ECG, echocardiography, and 4-hourly ABGs for potential heart/lung donors.

Target parameters	
CVP	4–10mmHg
MAP	60–80mmHg
PCWP	10–15mmHg
CI	>2.1l/min/m^2
Hb	10g/dl (Hct 30%)
SaO_2	>95% (with lowest FiO_2 and PEEP)
Tidal volume	<10ml/kg
$PaCO_2$	4.5–5.5kPa
Urine output	1–3ml/kg/hr
Peak inspiratory pressure	<30cmH$_2$O

Hormone resuscitation

	Bolus	Infusion	Action
Liothyronine (tri-iodothyronine, T_3)	4µg	3µg/hr	Reverses myocardial dysfunction and reduces inotrope requirements
Vasopressin (ADH)	1U	0.5–2U/hr	Treats diabetes insipidus and restores vascular tone. Titrated to MAP >60mmHg or SVR 800–1200 dyn.s/cm⁵
Insulin		Sliding scale	To maintain blood sugar 4–6mmol/l
Methylprednisolone	15mg/kg		Improves oxygenation and increases donor lung procurement by reducing cytokine-mediated cellular injury

Perioperative

- Standard monitoring plus CVP, arterial line, core temperature, urine output. Maintain core temperature >35°C. Frequent analysis of ABGs, electrolytes, Hct, glucose, and clotting. Large bore IV access (right upper limb) is mandatory for replacement of fluid losses (up to 8 litres) with crystalloid, colloid, or blood (keep Hct >30%).
- Need for general anaesthesia is controversial. Many use up to 1 MAC isoflurane or fentanyl (5–7µg/kg) to control reflex pressor responses during surgery. Labetolol or GTN can also be used to control hypertensive episodes intra-operatively.
- Non-depolarising neuromuscular blocking agents are administered to obtund reflex muscular contractions due to the preserved spinal arc and improve surgical access. Pancuronium and vecuronium are cardiostable and preferred.
- Large and frequent haemodynamic fluctuations occur due to compression of the inferior vena cava, manipulation of the adrenals, and blood/fluid loss. Hypotension is treated with colloid titrated to CVP, vasopressin infusion, or metaraminol (0.5mg increments).
- Broad spectrum antibiotics are given as per local transplant protocol.
- Full heparinisation (300IU/kg) should be administered centrally prior to surgical cannulation of the major vessels.
- Prostacyclin (5–20ng/kg/min) may be needed for 10min via pulmonary artery if lungs are to be harvested.
- PAFC/CVC withdrawn before ligation of SVC.
- Note time of aortic cross-clamp as beginning of organ ischaemic time.
- At the end discontinue mechanical ventilation/monitoring and remove the ETT after lung inflation and trachea cross-clamp.
- The abdominal surgical team continues to operate in circulatory arrest.

Special considerations

- Emotive, challenging area of critical care. Empathy and sensitivity is paramount throughout the management of the organ donor.
- The quality of care afforded the multi-organ donor could impact more than six recipients.
- In event of cardiac arrest CPR should be commenced, procurement of liver and kidneys should proceed rapidly with cross-clamping of the aorta at the diaphragm and infusion of cold preservation solution into the distal aorta and portal vein.

Further reading

Cottrell JE (1996). Trends in neuroanaesthesia. *Canadian Journal of Anaesthesia*, **43**, R61–R74.

Guidelines for adult organ and tissue transplantation (2004). The Intensive Care Society's Working Group on Organ and Tissue Donation. http://www.ics.ac.uk

International Subarachnoid Aneurysm Trial (ISAT) Collaborative Group (2002). International Subarachnoid Aneurysm Trial (ISAT) of neurosurgical clipping versus endovascular coiling in 2143 patients with ruptured intracranial aneurysms: a randomised trial. *Lancet*, **360**, 1267–1274.

Joshi S, Dash HH, Ornstein E (1997). Anaesthetic considerations for posterior fossa surgery. *Current Opinions in Anaesthesiology*, **10**, 321–326.

Porter JM, Pidgeon C, Cuningham AJ (1999). The sitting position in neurosurgery: a critical appraisal. *British Journal of Anaesthesia*, **82**, 117–128.

Sneyd JR, Whaley A, Dimpel HL, Andrews CJH (1998). An open, randomized comparison of alfentanil, remifentanil and alfentanil followed by remifentanil in anaesthesia for craniotomy. *British Journal of Anaesthesia*, **81**, 361–364.

Todd MM, Hindman BJ, Clarke WR, Torner JC (2005). For the intra-operative hypothermia for aneurysm surgery trial (IHAST). Mild intraoperative hypothermia during surgery for intracranial aneurysm. *New England Journal of Medicine*, **352**, 135–145.

Young PJ, Matta BF (2000). Anaesthesia for organ donation in the brainstem dead—why bother? *Anaesthesia*, **55**, 105–106.

Vascular surgery

General principles

Most vascular surgery involves operating on arteries diseased or damaged by atherosclerosis, causing poor peripheral blood flow (ischaemia) or emboli. Mortality is high (elective AAA surgery = 7%,[1] emergency AAA >50%). This is markedly increased in the presence of uncontrolled cardiovascular disease. Operations may be long and involve blood transfusion, marked fluid shifts, and significant impairment of lung function.

- Vascular patients are usually elderly arteriopaths with significant associated disease. Hypertension (66%), ischaemic heart disease (angina, MI), heart failure, diabetes mellitus, and COPD (50% are current or ex-smokers) are common. Many patients are taking aspirin, β-blockers, diuretics, heart failure medications, and, perhaps, insulin or oral hypoglycaemics.
- Some patients are anticoagulated, others will receive anticoagulants perioperatively, so consider the pros and cons of regional techniques carefully (see p1058). However, regional techniques can reduce morbidity and mortality (see below).
- Vascular patients tend to have serial operations, so there may be several previous anaesthetic records to review. 30–40% of vascular operations occur out of hours.
- Measure NIBP in both arms—there may be differences due to arteriopathy (use the higher of the two values clinically).
- All patients receiving synthetic vascular grafts require prophylactic antibiotic cover.
- Develop a working relationship with your vascular surgeon—you will have a better chance of being warned of untoward events (e.g. aortic clamping/unclamping, sudden massive blood loss, etc.).

Preoperative assessment

- Quantify the extent of any cardiorespiratory disease, both in terms of the planned surgical procedure and the postoperative period. Carefully consider (and document) whether regional anaesthesia is appropriate.
- Include direct questions about exercise tolerance (distance on the flat, ability to climb stairs) and ability to lie supine. Look for signs of cardiac failure.
- Investigations: FBC, U&Es, ECG, CXR, coagulation, and LFTs.
- A dynamic assessment of cardiac function is required for elective aortic surgery and for patients with symptomatic/new cardiac disease. Echocardiography, which also gives the left ventricular ejection fraction (EF), is simple and non-invasive. Patients with new ECG abnormalities or symptomatic heart disease need exercise ECG, stress echocardiography, radionuclide thallium scan or multigated acquisition scan (MUGA) (see p42). Patients with critical ischaemic heart disease should be referred for cardiological opinion for angiography and possible coronary revascularisation before aortic surgery.[2] Emergent vascular patients may have to undergo surgery before such dynamic investigations can be performed.
- Lung function tests (including ABG analysis while breathing air) should be performed in patients with significant respiratory disease presenting for AAA repair.

Premedication

There is some evidence that β-blockers (atenolol, bisoprolol) given preoperatively may reduce cardiovascular mortality following major vascular surgery.[3] This may even be true for a single dose; however, this is still controversial and is not routinely done. Patients already taking β-blockers should continue throughout the perioperative period.

Regional anaesthesia and analgesia in vascular surgical patients

Regional anaesthesia may be used alone for distal vascular surgery and is increasingly used for carotid surgery. Epidural analgesia is commonly used to supplement general anaesthesia for AAA. The advantages of regional techniques include:

- Improved patient monitoring (carotid endarterectomy)
- Improved blood flow, reduced DVT, reduced re-operation (peripheral revascularisation)[4]
- Postoperative pain relief (AAA, distal revascularisation, amputation)
- Reduced pulmonary complications (AAA surgery)
- Pre-emptive analgesia for amputations—possible reduction in phantom limb pain
- Treatment of proximal hypertension during aortic cross-clamp

Epidural catheters and anticoagulation

See p1058.

1 Bayly PJ et al. (2001). In-hospital mortality from abdominal aortic surgery in Great Britain and Ireland. British Journal of Surgery, **88**, 687–692.
2 McFalls EO, Ward HB, Moritz TE (2004). Coronary artery revascularization before elective major vascular surgery. New England Journal of Medicine, **352**, 2795–2804.
3 Poldermans D et al. (1999). The effect of bisoprolol on perioperative mortality and myocardial infarction in high-risk patients undergoing vascular surgery. New England Journal of Medicine, **341**, 1789–1794.
4 Christopherson R et al. (1993). Perioperative morbidity in patients randomized to epidural or general anaesthesia for lower extremity vascular surgery. Perioperative Ischemia Randomized Anesthesia Trial Study Group. Anesthesiology, **79**, 422–434.

Aortic aneurysm repair

Procedure	Excision of aortic aneurysmal sac and replacement with synthetic graft (tube/trouser graft)
Time	2–4hr
Pain	++++
Position	Supine, arms out (crucifix)
Blood loss	500–2000+ml (X-match 6U). Suitable for auto-transfusion
Practical techniques	ETT + IPPV, art + CVP lines. Epidural if possible

Preoperative

- Elderly, often multiple coexisting diseases.
- Mortality for elective surgery is 5–10% (predominately MI and multiorgan failure).
- Careful preoperative assessment is essential. Scrutinise ECG for signs of ischaemia and check for any renal impairment. Patient needs dynamic cardiac assessment preoperatively (see p424). Check access sites for CVP and arterial line.
- HDU/ICU for postoperative care. Alert the patient to this plan especially if a period of postoperative IPPV is planned. Preoptimisation is performed in some units—patients are admitted to the HDU/ICU a few hours preoperatively to have lines etc. inserted and to have haemodynamic status 'optimised'. This is controversial.
- Continue the usual cardiac medications. Consider adding a β-blocker (e.g. atenolol 25mg) to the premedication.

Perioperative[1]

- Have available vasoconstrictors (ephedrine and metaraminol), vasodilators (GTN), and β-blockers (labetalol).
- Two 14G or greater IV access. A hot-air and IVI warmer are essential. Monitor intra-operative temperature.
- A Level-1® fluid warmer or equivalent is extremely useful. Cell savers are indicated in cases where blood loss is expected to be >1000ml.
- Arterial line and thoracic epidural (T6–T11) pre-induction. Take a baseline blood gas sometime before cross-clamping.
- Have at least two syringe drivers present—inotropes, vasodilators, and eventually the epidural will all need them.
- Use a five-lead ECG (leads II and V5)—this increases the sensitivity for detection of myocardial ischaemia.
- Triple lumen CVP after induction. Consider inserting a PA introducer in complex cases as this will allow rapid fluid administration and facilitates PA catheter insertion if necessary (use right internal jugular or left subclavian vein to facilitate easier insertion of PA catheter if required).
- Consider PA catheter if severe CVS/RS disease, e.g. ejection fraction <25%, FVC <2 litres. Continuous cardiac output monitoring is useful during the cross-clamp period.

- Consider isovolaemic haemodilution pre-induction (see p1009). AAA is ideal for this as you can return the patient's blood (with platelets and clotting factors) when the aortic cross-clamp comes off. As a rough guide: Hb 10–12g/dl take 1U, Hb 12–14g/dl take 2U, Hb 14–16g/dl take 3U.
- Careful induction with monitoring of invasive arterial blood pressure. Use moderate/high-dose opioid, e.g. remifentanil (0.1–0.2μg/kg/min) or high-dose fentanyl (5–10μg/kg). Treat hypotension with fluids at first and then cautious vasoconstriction (metaraminol 0.25–0.5mg).
- Hypothermia is likely unless energetic efforts are made to maintain temperature during induction, line insertion, and perioperatively. Warming blankets should not be placed on the lower limbs while the aortic cross-clamp is in place as this may worsen lower limb ischaemia.
- Insert a urinary catheter for hourly measurement of urine output.
- Heparin will need to be given just before cross-clamp—3000–5000U is usual. This may be reversed after unclamping with protamine 0.5–1mg per 100U heparin IV slowly—causes hypotension if given too quickly.
- Proximal hypertension may follow aortic cross-clamping and is due to a sudden increase in SVR, increased SVC flow, and sympatho-adrenal response. Treat by deepening anaesthesia and/or a bolus of β-blocker (labetalol 5–10mg), GTN infusion, or epidural LA.
- While the aorta is clamped, metabolic acidosis will develop due to ischaemic lower limbs. Maintaining minute ventilation will cause a respiratory alkalosis to develop which will minimise the effects of this metabolic acidosis when the aorta is unclamped. Check arterial blood gases to assess haematocrit, metabolic acidosis, respiratory compensation, and ionised calcium.
- Cross-clamp time is usually 30–60min. During this time, start giving fluid, aiming for a moderately increased CVP (5cmH$_2$O greater than baseline) by the time the unclamping occurs. This helps cardiovascular stability, reduces sudden hypotension, and may help preserve renal function. Release of the cross-clamp one limb at a time also helps haemodynamic stability.
- Hypotension following aortic unclamping is caused by a decreased SVR, relative hypovolaemia, and myocardial 'stunning' due to return of cold metabolic waste products from the legs. Treat with IV fluids and/or lighten anaesthetic depth and/or small doses of inotropes, e.g. adrenaline 10μg aliquots (1ml of 1:100 000) and/or a bolus of calcium gluconate (up to 10ml 10%). Inotropes may be needed postoperatively.
- For fluid replacement, give isotonic crystalloid or colloid to replace insensible, third space, and initial blood loss. Give blood products when a deficiency is identified, e.g. haematocrit <25%, platelets <100 × 10^9/l. Check the activated clotting time (normal <140s) if you suspect coagulopathy. Thromboelastography will give you the whole coagulation picture. Consider the use of aprotinin (see p346).

1 Shine TS, Murray MJ (2004). Intraoperative management of aortic aneurysm surgery. *Anesthesia Clinics of North America*, **22**, 289–305.

Postoperative

- ICU/HDU is essential postoperatively. HDU may be appropriate for otherwise fit patients who can be extubated at the end of the case. Extubate if warm, haemodynamically stable, and with a working epidural. Otherwise transfer to ICU intubated.
- Opioid infusion and/or PCA if no epidural. Routine observations including invasive arterial and central venous pressure monitoring and urine output should be continued postoperatively to assess haemodynamic stability. Potential for large fluid shifts which need replacement. Assess distal pulses.
- Hypothermia should be treated aggressively.

Special considerations

- Management of epidural: a bolus of epidural diamorphine 2–5mg at induction will last for 12–24hr. Use epidural LA sparingly until the aorta is closed. It is easier to treat the hypotension of aortic unclamping with a functioning sympathetic nervous system.
- Renal failure occurs in 1–2% and is multifactorial in origin—but is associated with a mortality of 50% following AAA repair. It is more likely if the cross-clamp is suprarenal. There is no evidence that dopamine prevents renal failure, merely acting as an inotrope. Mannitol is used routinely by some (0.5g/kg during cross-clamp) as a free-radical scavenger and osmotic diuretic. Avoid hypovolaemia and monitor urine output hourly.

Emergency repair of AAA

A true anaesthetic and surgical emergency. May be:
- Acute: presents with cardiovascular collapse. Death is likely unless rupture is contained in the retroperitoneal space.
- Dissecting: dissects along the arterial intima—presents with back/abdominal pain.

Prehospital mortality for ruptured AAA is 50% and half of those reaching hospital also do not survive. Management is as for elective AAA, with the following additional considerations:
- Where doubt exists (and haemodynamically stable), diagnosis is confirmed by ultrasound or CT scan.
- If hypovolaemic shock present, resuscitate to a systolic pressure of 90mmHg. Avoid hypertension, coughing, and straining as this may precipitate a further bleed. Titrate IV morphine against pain.
- Pre-induction insert two 14G peripheral cannulae and (ideally) an arterial line. Use of the brachial artery may be necessary and some-times an arterial 'cut down' is indicated. Central venous access can wait until after the cross-clamp is applied. If peripheral IV access is difficult insert a 'Swan' sheath into the right internal jugular vein.
- Epidural analgesia is usually inappropriate.
- A urinary catheter can be placed before or after induction.
- Induction must be in the operating theatre, with the surgeons scrubbed, surgical preparation completed, drapes on, and blood available in theatre and checked. Rapid sequence induction is appropriate. Suitable induction agents include midazolam/remifentanil, etomidate, or ketamine. As soon as endotracheal intubation is confirmed, the surgeons can begin. Treat hypotension with IV fluids and small doses of vasopressors/inotropic agents.
- Hot-air warming and at least one warmed IVI are essential (a Level-1® blood warmer is invaluable).
- Use colloid or crystalloid depending on preference. Use a balanced crystalloid such as Hartmann's rather than 0.9% saline (helps prevent metabolic acidosis).
- Have both IV lines running maximally at induction. One assistant should be dedicated to managing IV fluid and ensuring an uninterrupted supply. Once the cross-clamp is applied there may be some degree of haemodynamic stability.
- Hypothermia, renal impairment, blood loss, and coagulopathy are common perioperative problems. Hypothermia is a particular hazard, as the patient will continue to bleed postoperatively—platelet function is markedly reduced below 35°C. Whilst there is no place for routine administration of platelets and FFP, consider early use when needed.
- Do not attempt to extubate at the conclusion of surgery—a post-operative period of ventilation on the ICU is essential to allow correction of biochemical/haematological abnormalities.
- Near patient testing (Hb and thromboelastograph) should be used if available to guide blood product administration. If the patient is exsan-guinating and crossmatched blood is not available, use type-specific.

Endovascular stenting of elective AAA

Procedure	Placement and deployment of bifurcated stent by interventional radiologists into aortic aneurysmal sac via femoral arteries
Time	2–4hr
Pain	+
Position	Supine
Blood loss	0–2000+ ml (X-match 6U)
Practical technique	Epidural + sedation, art + CVP lines

This technique is associated with lower operative morbidity and mortality than standard open AAA repair,[1] but it is still unproven whether it lowers the risk of aneurysm rupture; thus, postoperatively, patients must be kept under surveillance for the rest of their lives. Significant complications such as migration of the stent and endoleak can develop as well as frank rupture.

- The procedure is performed in the radiology/angio suite. The surgeons gain access to the aorta via the femoral arteries and the stent is inserted by an interventional radiologist.
- If aneurysm rupture does occur (incidence is 2% or thereabouts), mortality rises to >50%.
- Pre-assessment, monitoring, crossmatching are all exactly as for open repair. However, since the patient will not undergo aortic cross-clamping, patients who have been refused open surgery because of significant left ventricular impairment may tolerate endovascular repair.
- General or regional anaesthesia is appropriate, depending on preference.[2] One regime is an epidural/sedation technique consisting of an epidural bolus of diamorphine 2–3mg, followed by a bupivacaine 0.25% infusion (4–8ml/hr) in conjunction with propofol TCI (0.5–1µg/kg/min).
- Postoperatively, the patient may go to the high-dependency unit for overnight monitoring.
- A few centres stent ruptured AAAs. There is little data as yet on the efficacy or mortality of this procedure.

1 Prinssen M et al. (2004). A randomized trial comparing conventional and endovascular repair of abdominal aortic aneurysms. *New England Journal of Medicine*, **351**, 1677–1679.
2 Lippmann M et al. (2003). Anesthesia for endovascular repair of abdominal and thoracic aortic aneurysms: a review article. *Journal of Cardiovascular Surgery (Torino)*, **44**, 443–451.

Thoraco-abdominal aortic aneurysm repair

Procedure	Excision of aortic aneurysmal sac extending above the origin of the renal arteries and replacement with a synthetic graft. May involve thoracotomy and the need for one lung ventilation
Time	3–6hr
Pain	++++
Position	Supine, arms out (crucifix), may be R lateral if thoracotomy
Blood loss	1000ml–+++ (X-match 8U, plus platelets and FFP)
Practical techniques	DLT + IPPV, art + CVP lines. Thoracic epidural

Thoracic aneurysms of the ascending aorta require median sternotomy and cardiopulmonary bypass. Transverse aortic arch repair often requires hypothermic circulatory arrest as well.

Special considerations

As for infrarenal aortic aneurysm repair, with the following considerations:

- The aneurysm may compress the trachea and distort the anatomy of the upper vasculature.
- Intensive care is essential for postoperative ventilation and stabilisation.
- The aortic cross-clamp will be much higher than for a simple AAA. This means that the kidneys, liver, and splanchnic circulation will be ischaemic for the duration of the cross-clamp.
- Access to the thoracic aorta may require one lung ventilation—thus a left-sided double lumen tube (DLT) may be required (see p356). A Univent® tube is a possible alternative (p359).
- Proximal hypertension following aortic cross-clamping is more pronounced. Use aggressive vasodilatation with GTN (infusion of 50mg/50ml run at 10ml/hr until it starts to work) or esmolol (2.5g/50ml at 3–15ml/hr).
- Hypotension following aortic unclamping is often severe, requiring inotropic support postoperatively—use adrenaline (5mg/50ml) starting at 5ml/hr.
- Acidosis is a particular problem due to the metabolic acidosis during cross-clamping and an additional respiratory acidosis due to prolonged one lung ventilation. Ventilate adequately, use balanced crystalloids, consider using bicarbonate and ventilate postoperatively until it is resolved.
- Renal failure occurs in up to 25% of cases—principally related to the duration of cross-clamp. Monitor urine output, give mannitol 25g before cross-clamping, and maintain the circulating volume.

- Spinal cord ischaemia leading to paralysis may develop. This is related to the duration of cross-clamping and occurs because a branch of the thoracic aorta (artery of Adamkiewicz) reinforces the blood supply of the cord. Techniques used for prevention (none are infallible) include CSF pressure measurement and drainage through a spinal drain, spinal cord cooling through an epidural catheter, intrathecal magnesium, distal perfusion techniques, cardiopulmonary bypass, and deep hypothermic circulatory arrest. Surgeons performing this surgery have their own preferred techniques.
- Fluid balance is as for infrarenal AAA, although blood loss will be more extreme, blood transfusion will almost certainly be required, and platelets and FFP are more commonly used.
- Patients require ventilation postoperatively until acidosis and hypothermia are corrected and the lungs fully re-expanded.

Carotid endarterectomy

Procedure	Removal of atheromatous plaque from the internal carotid artery (ICA). The ICA is clamped, opened, the plaque stripped off, and then the artery closed either directly or with a Gore-Tex® vein patch
Time	1–3hr
Pain	++
Position	Supine, head up. Contralateral arm board
Blood loss	Minimal (G&S)
Practical techniques	Cervical plexus block + sedation, arterial line. ETT + IPPV, arterial line

An operation to reduce the incidence of stroke in symptomatic (TIA or CVA) patients with a 70% or greater carotid stenosis. Unfortunately it has a combined mortality and major stroke incidence of 2–5%. Patients are usually elderly arteriopaths similar to those presenting for aortic surgery. Dynamic cardiac assessment is not usually required.

- Monitoring cerebral perfusion during carotid cross-clamping is an important, but controversial, area. Advocates of regional anaesthesia cite the advantages of having a conscious patient in whom neurological deficits are immediately detectable and treatable by the insertion of a carotid shunt or pharmacological augmentation of BP.
- Under GA, other techniques may be used for monitoring cerebral perfusion, including measurement of carotid artery stump pressure, electroencephalograph (EEG) processing, monitoring somatosensory evoked potentials, transcranial Doppler of the middle cerebral artery, and, more recently, near-infrared spectroscopy. Individual units will have their own protocols.

Preoperative

- Elderly patients, often with severe cardiovascular disease. Most are hypertensive. At least 50% of deaths following carotid endarterectomy (CEA) are cardiovascular in origin; thus hypertension must be controlled preoperatively. Aim for 160/90.
- Determine the normal range of BP from ward charts. Measure BP in both arms.
- Document pre-existing neurological deficits so that new deficits may be more easily assessed.
- Have available vasoconstrictors (ephedrine and metaraminol) and vasodilators (GTN, labetalol).
- Consider cerebral monitoring techniques—there will be protocols in your unit.
- Premedication: sedative/anxiolytic, particularly if using GA.

Perioperative

- 20G and 14G IV access plus an arterial line in the contralateral arm (out on an arm board).
- Monitoring: five-lead ECG, arterial line, NIBP, SpO_2, $ETCO_2$.
- Maintain BP within 20% of baseline. During cross-clamping, maintain BP at or above baseline. If necessary use vasoconstrictors, e.g. metaraminol (10mg diluted up to 20ml, give 0.5ml at a time).

General anaesthesia for CEA

- Careful IV induction. Blood pressure may be labile during induction and intubation. Give generous doses of short-acting opioids and consider spraying the cords with lidocaine.
- Most anaesthetists use an endotracheal tube—the LMA cuff has been shown to reduce carotid blood flow but this is of unknown significance. Secure the tube and check connections very carefully (the head is inaccessible during surgery).
- Remifentanil infusion combined with superficial cervical plexus block gives ideal conditions, with rapid awakening. Otherwise isoflurane/ opioid technique. Maintain normocarbia.
- Extubate before excessive coughing develops. Close neurological monitoring in recovery until fully awake.

The 'awake carotid'

- Cervical dermatomes C2–C4 may be blocked by deep and/or superficial cervical plexus block or cervical epidural (rarely used in the UK). See also p1073.
- Patient preparation and communication are vital. A thorough explanation of the awake technique is invaluable.
- The site for the injection is the cervical transverse processes, which may be palpated as a bony ridge under the posterior border of sternocleidomastoid. For the deep block use three 5ml injections of 0.5% bupivacaine at C2, 3, and 4 or a single injection of 10–15ml 0.5% bupivacaine at C3. Reinforce this with 10ml 0.5% bupivacaine injected along the posterior border of the sternocleidomastoid (superficial block). Avoid the deep block in patients with respiratory impairment as they may not tolerate unilateral diaphragmatic paralysis. Infiltration along the jawline helps to reduce pain from submandibular retractor.
- Ensure the patient's bladder is emptied preoperatively. Give IV fluids only to replace blood loss—a full bladder developing while the carotid is cross-clamped can be tricky to manage.
- Sedation (e.g. propofol TCI 0.5–1µg/ml, remifentanil 0.05–0.1µg/kg/min) may be carefully employed during block placement and dissection. Once dissection is complete, patient discomfort is much reduced. No sedation during carotid cross-clamping will allow continuous neurological assessment. Give oxygen throughout.
- An L-bar angled over the patient's neck allows good access for both surgeon and anaesthetist.
- Despite an apparently perfect regional block, ~50% of patients will require LA supplementation by the surgeon, particularly around the carotid sheath. This is reduced using remifentanil sedation.

- Monitor the patient's speech, contralateral motor power, and cerebration.
- Neurological deficit presents in three ways:
  - Profound unconsciousness on cross-clamping
  - Subtle but immediate deficit following cross-clamping, e.g. confusion, dysphasia, delay in answering questions.
  - Delayed deficit—usually related to relative hypotension.
- Attentive monitoring of the patient is vital, particularly during cross-clamping. If neurological deficit develops, a shunt should be inserted immediately. Recovery should be rapid once the shunt is in place—if it is not, convert to general anaesthesia. Pharmacological augmentation of blood pressure may improve cerebration by increasing the pressure gradient of collateral circulation across the circle of Willis. Approximately 2.5% of patients will require conversion to general anaesthesia (use of an LMA is probably easiest).
- For patients who do not tolerate regional anaesthesia, GA is the best option.

Postoperative

- Careful observation in a well-staffed recovery room for 2–4hr is mandatory. HDU is optimal if available, particularly for those patients who develop a neurological deficit.
- Airway oedema is common in both GA and regional cases, presumably due to dissection around the airway. Cervical haematoma occurs in 5–10% of cases. Immediate re-exploration is required for developing airway obstruction (the regional block should still be working). Remove skin sutures in recovery as soon as the diagnosis is made to allow drainage of the haematoma.
- Haemodynamic instability is common postoperatively. Hyperperfusion syndrome, consisting of headaches and ultimately haemorrhagic CVA, is caused by areas of brain previously 'protected' by a tight carotid stenosis being suddenly exposed to hypertensive BP. Thus BP must be controlled. Careful written instructions should be given to staff about haemodynamic management.
  An example is
  - If systolic BP >160mmHg, give labetalol 5–10mg boluses IV or a hydralazine infusion.
  - If systolic BP <100mmHg, give colloid 250ml stat.
- New neurological symptoms and signs require immediate surgical consultation.
- Carotid stenting is a developing procedure for symptomatic carotid patients performed in the radiology suite in which a stent is placed under local anaesthetic into the stenotic carotid artery. Anaesthetic supervision may be required because of the complications, which include perioperative stroke and haemodynamic disturbances.

Peripheral revascularisation operations

Procedures	Bypass operations for patients with occlusive arterial disease of the legs. The long saphenous vein or a Gore-Tex® graft is used to bypass occluded arteries.
Time	1–6hr
Pain	+++
Position	Supine
Blood loss	Usually 500–1000ml (X-match 2U)
Practical techniques	Combined spinal/epidural with sedation, ?art line. ETT/IPPV, ?LMA

- Femoropopliteal bypass—femoral to above-knee popliteal artery
- Femorodistal bypass—femoral to anterior or posterior tibial artery
- Femorofemoral crossover graft—from one femoral artery to another

Preoperative

- Constitute a large proportion of elective vascular surgery. The duration of surgery is unpredictable—overruns are not uncommon.
- Assess cardiovascular system. Usually better tolerated than aortic surgery. A dynamic assessment of cardiac function is not usually necessary unless there have been new developments, e.g. unstable angina.
- The choice between general and regional anaesthesia is up to the individual. There is some evidence that regional anaesthesia is associated with lower re-operation rates.[1] Long operations (>3hr) may make pure regional techniques impractical, but they are still possible.

Perioperative

- IV access: ensure at least one large (14 or 16G) IV cannula.
- Insert arterial line for long cases (over 2hr), if haemodynamic instability is expected or in sicker patients. Otherwise standard monitoring with five-lead ECG. CVP monitoring is rarely necessary.
- GA techniques include ETT + IPPV or LMA + SV. The surgeon should be able to perform femoral nerve block perioperatively.
- Regional anaesthesia is an alternative offering good operating conditions and postoperative pain relief. Single-shot spinal may not allow enough time for some procedures. Combined spinal/epidural anaesthesia is better. Consider epidural diamorphine (2–3mg) and start an infusion of 0.25% bupivacaine at 5–10ml/hr. Always give supplemental oxygen. If the patient requests sedation propofol TCI is ideal.
- Heparin (3000–5000U) should be given before clamping—reverse with protamine 0.5–1mg/100U heparin slowly after unclamping.

Postoperative

Oxygen overnight.

1 Christopherson R *et al.* (1993). Perioperative morbidity in patients randomized to epidural or general anesthesia for lower extremity vascular surgery. Perioperative Ischemia Randomized Anesthesia Trial Study Group *Anesthesiology*, **79**, 422–434.

Axillobifemoral bypass

Procedure	Extraperitoneal bypass (trouser graft) from axillary artery to femoral arteries
Time	2–4hr
Pain	++++
Position	Supine
Blood loss	<1000ml
Practical techniques	GA—ETT, IPPV, art line, ?CVP

This is often a last-chance operation for patients with completely occluded aortic or iliac arteries. Some will already have had aortic surgery and have infected grafts. It is an extraperitoneal operation, so patients with severe cardiorespiratory disease who might be excluded from aortic surgery may tolerate it better. However, do not be misled—it is still a long operation which can involve significant blood loss, morbidity, and even mortality.

Preoperative

• Usual preoperative assessment of vascular patients (p424). Try to obtain recent information about cardiac function. An echocardiograph can easily be done at the bedside.
• Some of these patients will be very sick either from pre-existing cardiorespiratory disease or from infected aortic grafts. Surgery may be their only hope of life, although it can also be a rapid road to their demise. Provided the patient understands this, the operation may be appropriate despite high risk. These are not cases for inexperienced trainees to undertake alone.

Perioperative

• General anaesthesia with ETT and IPPV is appropriate. An arterial line and large-gauge cannula are mandatory, CVP monitoring is optional.
• Heparin/protamine will be required at clamping/unclamping.

Postoperative

• Extubation at the end of surgery is usually possible, but a period of time on the HDU is recommended if possible.
• PCA for postoperative analgesia.

Amputations

(below/through/above knee, Symes, digits, etc.)

Procedures	Removal of necrotic or infected tissue due to vascular ischaemia
Time	30–120min
Pain	++++
Position	Supine
Blood loss	Usually 200–500ml
Practical techniques	Spinal or epidural with sedation. Sciatic/femoral blocks ± GA

Preoperative

- Commonly sick, bed-bound diabetics with significant cardiovascular disease who have had repeated revascularisation attempts previously.
- Many will be in considerable discomfort preoperatively (less so the diabetics) and may be on large doses of enteral or parenteral opioids. Regional analgesia may give more predictable postoperative relief.

Perioperative

- Spinal anaesthesia ± sedation offers excellent anaesthesia, which can be directed unilaterally. The duration of block (and postoperative pain relief) can be extended with intrathecal diamorphine (0.25–0.5mg). Clonidine 15µg intrathecally has also been used.
- Epidural analgesia offers better postoperative analgesia and can be sited preoperatively if required (pre-emptive analgesia).
- General anaesthesia with LMA/SV or ETT/IPPV is an option, but additional regional blockade is advisable (combined sciatic/femoral blocks will ensure analgesia for up to 24hr). An epidural catheter can be placed alongside the sciatic nerve by the surgeon, for postoperative infusion of local anaesthetic, e.g. bupivacaine 0.25% 5ml/hr.
- Occasionally these patients are septic due to the necrotic tissue. The only way they will improve is to have the affected part amputated.

Postoperative

- Regional analgesia is the best option, otherwise PCA.
- Phantom limb pain is a problem for 60–70% amputees at some time. It must be distinguished from surgical pain and often requires chronic pain team input.
- Pre-emptive analgesia (preoperative siting of epidural) is believed by some to reduce the incidence and severity of chronic pain.[1]
- Combined sciatic/femoral nerve blocks are an alternative to epidural, particularly when the patient is receiving anticoagulation.
- Even with perfect regional analgesia you may need to continue enteral opioids postoperatively.

1 Bach S, Noreng MF, Tjellden NU (1988). Phantom limb pain in amputees during the first 12 months following limb amputation after preoperative lumbar epidural blockade. *Pain*, **33**, 297.

Thoracoscopic sympathectomy

Procedures	For patients with sweaty palms/axillae. The sympathetic trunk is divided via a thoracoscope inserted through a small axillary incision
Time	30–60min
Pain	++
Position	Supine, affected arm on arm board
Blood loss	Minimal
Practical techniques	IPPV via double lumen tube
	SV via LMA

- Patients are usually young and fit with hyperhidrosis (sweaty palms and axillae).
- Surgical technique involves cutting the thoracic sympathetic trunk at T2 or T3 thoracoscopically.
- Traditionally this is done using one lung anaesthesia (double lumen tube), with the patient in the reverse Trendelenburg position.
- A simpler technique involves the patient breathing spontaneously through an LMA. When the surgeon insufflates CO_2 into the pleural cavity, the lung is pushed away passively, allowing surgery to take place. The degree of shunt produced is less dramatic than with one lung ventilation. Assisted ventilation must be avoided, except to re-inflate the lung manually at the end. The CO_2 insufflator machine regulates intrapleural pressures.
- With either technique, at the conclusion of the procedure, the lung must be re-expanded (under the surgeon's direct vision) to prevent pneumothorax.
- Local anaesthetic can be deposited by the surgeon directly onto the sympathetic trunk and into the pleural cavity.
- A postoperative chest radiograph is required to confirm lung reinflation.
- Synchronous bilateral sympathectomy is a much more challenging operation. This can lead to profound hypoxia when the second lung is collapsed, due to persistent atelectasis in the first lung. It is certainly inappropriate for all but the very fittest patients. The mortality of this procedure has been recently highlighted.[1]

1 Collin J (2004). Uncovering occult operative morbidity and mortality. *British Journal of Surgery*, **91**, 262–263.

First rib resection

Procedures	Resection of the first/cervical rib in patients with thoracic outlet syndrome
Time	1–2hr
Pain	++
Position	Supine, affected arm on arm board
Blood loss	Minimal
Practical techniques	IPPV via COETT, avoid muscle relaxants

- Patients are usually young and fit.
- The position is similar to that for thoracoscopic sympathectomy.
- Muscle relaxants should be avoided, as the surgeon needs to be able to identify the brachial plexus perioperatively. Intubate under opioid/induction agent alone or use mivacurium/opioid and then hyperventilate with isoflurane/opioid or similar.
- At the conclusion of surgery, the wound is filled with saline and manual ventilation performed with sustained inflation pressures >40cmH$_2$O. This is to check for a lung leak and exclude pleural injury.
- A superficial cervical plexus block provides good postoperative analgesia. See p1073.
- A postoperative CXR is required in recovery.

Varicose vein surgery

Procedures	Removal of tortuous veins of the lower extremities:
	High tie and strip—long saphenous vein removal (sometimes bilateral)
	Short saphenous vein surgery—tied off in popliteal fossa
Time	30min to 3hr
Pain	++
Position	Supine or prone for short saphenous surgery
Blood loss	Up to 1000ml
Practical techniques	LMA/SV for most; ETT/IPPV for prone

- Patients are usually young and fit.
- The main operation is usually combined with multiple avulsions to remove varicosities. These are minute scars, which can, however, bleed profusely.
- Blood loss can be minimised by elevating the legs.
- Patients may need combined long and short saphenous surgery (i.e. two operative incisions on the same leg) and may require turning during the operation. In selected slim patients without aspiration risk, this can be done with the patient breathing spontaneously through an LMA.
- A combination of NSAIDs and local anaesthetic into the groin wound gives good postoperative analgesia. Caudal anaesthesia is possible for prolonged re-explorations.
- Bilateral surgery is common and takes 30–60min per incision.
- Redo surgery is also common and can be very prolonged.

Further reading

Caldicott L, Lumb A, McCoy D (2000). *Vascular Anaesthesia: A Practical Handbook*. Oxford: Butterworth Heinemann.

Mukherjee D, Eagle KA (2003). Perioperative cardiac assessment for noncardiac surgery: eight steps to the best possible outcome. *Circulation*, **107**, 2771–2774.

O'Connor CJ, Rothenburg DM (1995). Anesthetic considerations for descending thoracic aortic surgery: Parts 1 and 2. *Journal of Cardiothoracic and Vascular Anesthesia*, **9**, 581–588, 734–747.

Stoneham MD, Knighton JD (1999). Regional anaesthesia for carotid endarterectomy. *British Journal of Anaesthesia*, **82**, 910–919.

Chapter 18

Orthopaedic surgery

Ralph Worms and Richard Griffiths

General principles

Approximately 110 000 major joint replacements are performed annually in England and Wales.[1] Emphasis is now shifting to longer, more minimally invasive surgery permitting shorter hospital stays.[2] A diverse population of mostly elderly patients presents many challenges to the anaesthetist. Many operations are amenable to regional anaesthesia.

Frequent problems include arthritis, obesity, co-morbidity/polypharmacy, long procedures, major blood loss, and specific problems related to tourniquets, bone cement, and venous thromboembolism.

Preoperative

- Liaison with the surgeon is essential, particularly if undertaking regional techniques.
- Severe arthritis may make assessment of cardiorespiratory fitness difficult.
- Patients with rheumatoid disease are at risk of atlanto-axial instability.
- If planning a regional technique (particularly a central block), it is important to consider factors affecting clotting (timing of the last dose of anti-coagulant) and discuss specific risks and benefits with the patient (see p1058).
- A high risk of venous thromboembolism occurs with certain operations requiring antithromboembolism measures, e.g. LWMH, stockings, foot pumps (p10).

Perioperative

- Give IV antibiotic prophylaxis (p1163).
- Utmost care with positioning is essential to avoid soft tissue or nerve injuries. This is a shared responsibility between anaesthetist and surgeon.
- Blood loss may be significant (use a large-bore cannula with an extension) and may be increased by certain types of bone, e.g. Pagets.
- Monitor blood loss accurately. Consider cell salvage including drain salvage.
- Consider invasive monitoring for those patients with CVS disease.
- A urinary catheter should be inserted for long procedures, or when epidurals/spinal opioids are used.
- Maintenance of normothermia with blood warmers and warm-air blankets can reduce both morbidity and mortality.[3]

Postoperative

- Good analgesia will have a positive effect on recovery, mobility, and discharge.
- Liaise with the surgeon if prescribing NSAIDs—some surgeons may use indometacin to reduce new bone growth.

---

1 National Joint Registry; http://www.njrcentre.org.uk.
2 Connolly D (2003). Orthopaedic anaesthesia. *Anaesthesia*, **58**, 1189–1193.
3 Kirkbride DA (2003). Thermoregulation and nickel peri-operative hypothermia. *BJA CEPD Reviews*, **3**, 24–28.

Fat embolism syndrome (FES)[1]

FES is associated with trauma or surgery and has an extremely variable presentation—diagnosis is often made by exclusion. Although embolisation of fat occurs frequently, the syndrome is comparatively rare (1%). Early surgery and avoidance of intramedullary fixation have both reduced the incidence. Current treatment is supportive (early mortality 1–20%), but serious long-term complications are uncommon.

Classically seen in patients with long bone fractures who develop sudden tachypnoea and hypoxia. Although sometimes a petechial rash is seen (check conjunctiva), firm diagnosis is frequently difficult.

Features (as defined by Gurd[2])

Major

- Respiratory symptoms—tachypnoea, dyspnoea, bilateral crepitations, haemoptysis, diffuse shadowing on CXR
- Neurological signs—confusion, drowsiness
- Petechial rash.

Minor

- Tachycardia
- Retinal change—fat or petechiae
- Jaundice
- Renal—oliguria or anuria.

Laboratory

- Thrombocytopenia
- Sudden decrease in Hb by 20%
- Raised ESR
- Fat macroglobulaemia.

Treatment

- Early resuscitation and stabilisation are vital.
- Early O_2 therapy may prevent onset of syndrome.
- May require mechanical ventilation (10–40% of patients).
- Steroid use is controversial.[3]
- FES usually resolves within 7d.

1 Mellor A, Soni N (2001). Fat embolism. *Anaesthesia*, **56**, 145–154.
2 Gurd AR, Wilson RL (1974). The fat embolism syndrome. *J Bone Joint Surg Br*, **56**, 408–416.
3 National Joint Registry; http://www.njrcentre.org.uk.

Cement implantation syndrome

Methylmethacrylate bone cement is an acrylic polymer that has been used extensively in orthopaedic surgery for 30yr. Its use is associated with the potential for hypoxia, hypotension, and cardiovascular collapse. Fatal cardiac arrest is a reported complication. There are many suggested aetiologies of which fat embolisation appears to be the most likely. Air embolisation (Doppler evidence in 30% patients) or direct effects of the cement are also possible.

Severe embolic events (up to 85% of patients) and pulmonary dysfunction (mean reduction in SaO_2 7%) are most common with femoral cement insertion.[1] The ability of the patient to withstand these should be considered before use.[2]

Problems typically occur shortly after cement insertion. Hypotension is common (10–30%), independent of anaesthetic technique and worsened if there is any degree of hypovolaemia.

Prevention and treatment

- Suction applied to the bone cavity to evacuate air and fat during cement insertion dramatically reduces the incidence of complications.
- Measure blood pressure frequently during this time.
- Ensure adequate blood volume prior to cementing.
- Increase FiO_2 (hypoxia common).
- Stop N_2O.

It has been suggested that α-agonists might be superior to adrenaline when resuscitating these patients.[3]

1 Pitto RP, Koessler M, Kuehle JW (1999). Comparison of fixation of the femoral component without cement and fixation with use of a bone-vacuum cementing technique for the prevention of fat embolism during total hip arthroplasty. *Journal of Bone and Joint Surgery*, **81**, 831–843.

2 Parry G (2003). Sudden deaths during hip hemi-arthroplasty. *Anaesthesia*, **58**, 922–923.

3 McBrien ME, Breslin DS, Atkinson S, Johnston JR (2001). Use of methoxamine in the resuscitation of epinephrine-resistant electromechanical dissociation. *Anaesthesia*, **56**, 1085–1089.

Tourniquets[1]

Tourniquets are commonly used to produce a bloodless field.

- Only pneumatic tourniquets should be used as mechanical tourniquets can cause areas of unpredictably high pressure in the underlying tissues.
- Small tourniquets on fingers and toes are dangerous because they are easily forgotten. It is best to use a rubber strip with artery forceps.
- Expressive exsanguination using an Esmarch bandage is contraindicated in cases of tumour or severe infection because of the risks of dissemination. It is also contraindicated if DVT is suspected—fatal pulmonary embolism has been reported.[2] It also represents a potential risk of left ventricular failure from fluid overload if compression of both legs is carried out (adds 15% to the circulating volume); therefore limit to one leg only in patients at risk. Effective exsanguination can be achieved by arm or leg elevation for 5min at 90°, without mechanical compression.
- Peripheral arterial disease is a relative contraindication to use.
- Avoid in severe crush injuries.
- Sickle cell disease: use of tourniquets is controversial. Sickling of red blood cells under anoxic conditions causes thrombosis, but some surgeons use limb tourniquets after *full* exsanguination. If employed, use for as short a time as possible (see also p200).

Site of application

The upper arm and thigh have sufficient muscle bulk to distribute the cuff pressure evenly and are the recommended sites. For short operations (<1hr) in fit patients, a calf tourniquet is preferred by some surgeons.

Cuff width

The American Heart Association concluded that if a sphygmomanometer cuff has a width of 20% greater than the diameter of the upper arm or 40% of the circumference of the thigh (to a maximum of 20cm), then the pressure in the underlying central artery will be equal to that in the cuff. This avoids the need for excessively high cuff pressures. Modern silicone cuffs tend to be smaller than this, measuring 90mm width (bladder 70mm) for the arm and 105mm (bladder 75mm) for the leg. Cuff length should exceed the circumference of the extremity by 7–15cm. The cuff should be positioned at the point of maximum circumference of the limb. The tissues immediately underlying the cuff should be protected with cotton wool. This is not necessary with a correctly applied modern silicone cuff.

Pressure

- Based on the unsedated patient's blood pressure measured on the ward preoperatively.
- Upper limb: systolic BP + 50mmHg. Lower limb: twice systolic BP. This higher pressure is needed because there is often not enough room above the operating site for a full-sized cuff.
- The use of lower inflation pressures may minimise complications following the use of tourniquets and speed up postoperative recovery. In a normotensive patient a pressure of 200mmHg should be ideal for the upper limb and 250mmHg for the lower limb.

Tourniquet time

The minimum time possible should be the aim. Notify the surgeon at 1hr and remove as soon as possible after that. If the operation is difficult, time can be extended to 1.5hr. 2hr should be regarded as a maximum, but this will not be safe for all patients. Pulmonary emboli can occur following tourniquet release. When monitored using transoesophageal echocardiography the rate was increased with increased tourniquet time.[3]

Tourniquet pain

After 30–60min of cuff inflation a patient may develop an increase in heart rate and diastolic blood pressure. This response results from 'tourniquet pain'. This also occurs under anaesthesia, although the response is usually abolished by spinal or epidural techniques. In volunteers when a tourniquet is inflated, a dull pain, associated with an increase in blood pressure, occurs after 30min. Often the physiological changes are resistant to analgesic drugs and increased depth of anaesthesia. Small doses of ketamine given IV (0.25mg/kg) before tourniquet inflation can attenuate these blood pressure rises.[4]

1 Kam PC, Kavanaugh R, Yoong FF (2001). The arterial tourniquet: pathophysiological consequences and anaesthetic implications. *Anaesthesia*, **56**, 534–536.

2 Boogaerts JG (1999). Lower limb exsanguinations and embolism. *Acta Anaesthesiologica Belgica*, **50**, 95–98.

3 Hirota K, Hashimoto H, Kabara S, *et al.* (2001). The relationship time between pneumatic tourniquet time and the amount of pulmonary emboli in patients undergoing knee arthroscopic surgeries. *Anaesthesia and Analgesia*, **93**, 776–778.

4 Satsumae T, Yamaguchi H, Sakaguchi M, *et al.* (2001). Preoperative small dose ketamine prevented tourniquet induced arterial pressure increase in orthopaedic patients under general anesthesia. *Anesthesia and Analgesia*, **92**, 1286–1289.

Total hip replacement

Procedure	Prosthetic replacement of femoral head and acetabulum
Time	90–120min
Pain	+++
Position	Lateral or supine
Blood loss	300–500ml, G&S
Practical techniques	Spinal with sedation or GA/LMA ± nerve block

Total hip replacement is one of the most frequently performed orthopaedic operations. Regional anaesthesia offers several advantages and can be supplemented with sedation or general anaesthesia. Prevention of thromboembolic complications is of the utmost importance.[1]

Preoperative
- Careful preoperative evaluation of the patient is essential.
- It may be appropriate to avoid the use of cement in patients with severe cardiac disease, and this should be discussed with the surgeon beforehand.
- Antithrombotic measures should commence on admission to hospital.

Perioperative
- Place 16G or larger cannula in the upper arm (if a lateral position is anticipated).
- Ensure adequate hydration prior to performing a spinal and during cement insertion.
- For single-shot spinal ~3ml bupivacaine 0.5% depending on patient size. Diamorphine (0.25–0.5mg) may be added for more prolonged analgesia.
- When using spinal anaesthesia in the lateral position, intermittent doses of midazolam or TCI propofol are useful sedation techniques, with facemask supplemental oxygen. On occasions induction of general anaesthesia is required. For the supine position, consider an LMA with light general anaesthesia.
- For longer cases, a combined spinal/epidural technique can be used. Postoperative analgesic requirements rarely require this approach for an uncomplicated primary hip replacement.
- GA (rather than sedation) ± epidural or suitable block should be considered for any complex operation because of the prolonged surgical time.
- Using an epidural postoperatively will necessitate inserting a urinary catheter (which also helps monitor fluid balance) at some stage in the majority of patients. This is best performed at the time of surgery.

- If central neuraxial blockade is contraindicated, a psoas lumbar plexus block (or a femoral 3 in 1 block) provides comparable analgesia and can be used to supplement general anaesthesia.
- Aim to maintain BP at an adequate level based on preoperative readings; hypotension is not indicated.
- Intra-operative antibiotic prophylaxis will be required.
- Actively warming the patient reduces intra-operative blood loss significantly[2] and reduces morbidity and mortality.
- Blood recovery and autologous transfusion should be considered for complex surgery.

Postoperative

- Surgeons usually prefer the patient to be placed on their bed in the supine position with the legs abducted using a pillow to prevent dislocation of the prosthesis.
- Anti-thromboembolic prophylaxis is important—at least 1% of patients develop DVT even with measures in place.
- Oxygen therapy for up to 24hr is advisable in most patients.
- Haemoglobin should be checked 24hr postoperatively and treated either with transfusion or iron supplements as indicated.
- Patients are mobilised at 24–48hr and simple IM opioids with regular paracetamol or NSAIDs are usually sufficient for postoperative analgesia. If an epidural has been inserted, a postoperative infusion can be used but is rarely necessary and needs to cease prior to mobilisation.

Special considerations

- Blood loss varies significantly. It is also affected by anaesthetic technique. The average loss is 300–500ml (reduced by centroneuraxial techniques). A similar amount may be lost in the drain and tissues postoperatively.
- The decision to transfuse is multifactorial and includes general fitness, continuing surgical losses, and local practice.
- The benefits of epidural analgesia may be limited to the early postoperative period (up to 6hr).[3]
- Bone cementation is associated with a 3-fold higher risk for PE.[4]
- Unfractionated heparin is associated with a 6-fold higher risk for DVT compared with LMWH.[5]

1 Winkler M, Marker E, Hetz H (1998). The peri-operative management of major orthopedic procedures. *Anaesthesia*, **53**, S2, 37–41.

2 Winkler M, Akca O, Birkenberg B, Hetz H, *et al.* (2000). Aggressive warming reduces blood loss during hip arthroplasty. *Anesthesia and Analgesia*, **91**, 978–984.

3 Choi PT, Bhandari M, Scott J, Douketis J (2004). Epidural analgesia for pain relief following hip or knee replacement (Cochrane Review). In: The Cochrane Library, Issue 2, 2004. Chichester, UK: John Wiley & Sons, Ltd.

4 B Borghi, A Casati (2002). Thromboembolic complications after total hip replacement. *International Orthopedics*, **26**, 44–47.

5 Kirkbride DB (2003). *BJA CEPD Reviews*, **3**, 24–28.

Bilateral total hip replacement
- Preferred by some surgeons in younger, fit patients.
- This is major operation; careful patient selection is vital. Significant CVS disease increases mortality.
- GA with epidural is most practical.
- Consider invasive monitoring (arterial line ± CVP).

Regional anaesthesia
- Regional anaesthesia may be used for most joint replacements, (alone, with sedation, or as an adjuvant to GA). Central neuraxial blockade and major nerve blocks are commonly performed.
- In major orthopaedic surgery, blocks may provide postoperative pain relief and may reduce PONV.
- There is some evidence that regional anaesthesia, either alone or in combination with general anaesthesia, may reduce the incidence of thromboembolic complications, particularly in hip and knee surgery.[1]
- Good fixation of cement and joint prosthesis requires a dry, bloodless surgical field. Regional anaesthetic (particularly spinal/epidural) reduces bleeding at the surgical site without the need for other pharmacological hypotensive anaesthetic techniques.
- Surgeons often prefer the operating conditions produced by regional techniques.[2]

1 Rodgers A, Walker S, Schug S, *et al.* (2000). Reduction of postoperative mortality and morbidity with epidural or spinal anaesthesia: results from overview of randomized trials. *British Medical Journal,* **321**, 1493–1505.
2 Oldman M, McCartney CJL, Leung A, *et al.* (2004). A survey of orthopedic surgeons' attitudes and knowledge regarding regional anesthesia. *Anesthesia and Analgesia,* **98**, 1486–1490.

Revision of total hip replacement

Procedure	Revision of previous total hip replacement Revision may include one or both components
Time	2–6hr depending on complexity
Pain	++++
Position	Lateral or supine
Blood loss	1 litre, occasionally considerably more, X-match 2U
Practical techniques	GA ± epidural/nerve block

Essentially the same as primary hip replacement except for the length of surgery, blood loss, and postoperative pain. The complexity of surgery is very variable. These operations can be prolonged, with substantial blood loss, so discuss the anticipated operation with the surgeon beforehand.

Preoperative

General principles as for total hip replacement, except:
- Patients are more elderly and usually have more medical problems.
- The operation takes longer, at least 2–3hr, often more. This is too long for a single-shot spinal.
- Blood loss can be significant, with 1 litre or more commonly lost perioperatively.
- Postoperative pain can be a significant problem.

Perioperative

- Generally as for primary hip replacement, including a urinary catheter.
- If significant blood loss is anticipated, or the patient's CVS status indicates it, insert an arterial line and consider a CVP line.
- Technique should be planned on the length of surgery, the operative position, and patient factors.
  - For complex revisions anticipated to take >3hr, an IPPV technique with epidural supplementation may be most appropriate.
  - If central neuraxial block is contraindicated, consider supplementing GA with nerve blocks (femoral 3 in 1 or psoas compartment lumbar plexus).
- Blood recovery and autologous transfusion should be used wherever possible.
- Perioperative blood transfusion is frequently required and blood loss may be substantial. 2U of crossmatched blood should be available in theatre with the ability to obtain more within 30min.

Postoperative

- Mobilisation varies with the complexity of the revision and the strength of reconstruction.
- For pain relief, an epidural infusion is useful. PCA is a suitable alternative.
- Supplemental oxygen is required for 24hr or longer, particularly if significant blood loss or underlying cardiorespiratory disease.
- Prevention of thromboembolic complications is of the utmost importance.

Total knee replacement

Procedure	Prosthetic replacement of the knee joint
Time	1–2hr
Pain	++++/+++++
Position	Supine
Blood loss	Minimal with tourniquet, 250–500ml without. G&S
Practical techniques	Sciatic/femoral blocks ± spinal/LMA
	Spinal ± GA
	Epidural or combined spinal/epidural ± LMA

Similar patient population to hip surgery. Generally a shorter operation with less blood loss or cement hypotension. A tourniquet is commonly used. Postoperative pain can be extreme and must be anticipated; tourniquet pain often occurs despite nerve blocks.

Preoperative
As for hip surgery.

Perioperative
- The patient is always supine and therefore airway control under sedation can be a problem.
- Combination femoral and sciatic nerve blocks give good postoperative analgesia and mobilisation (see below). They are easiest to combine with a light GA. Epidural anaesthesia/analgesia may delay mobilisation. If nerve blocks are contraindicated postoperative PCA should be considered.
- A tourniquet is commonly used, therefore perioperative blood loss is not problematic, although expect to lose up to 500ml (and frequently more) from the drains in the first hour postoperatively. There is a trend to reduce use of the tourniquet.
- If a tourniquet is used one may see 'breakthrough' of tourniquet pain after about 1hr, causing CVS stimulation and hypertension. This is more common with leg blocks and is treated by deepening anaesthesia or adding IV opioid. Ketamine (0.25mg/kg) is effective at preventing the associated rise in blood pressure. Ensure the patient is well preloaded before the tourniquet is released. A short-lived reperfusion event is common (fall in BP and SaO_2, rise in $ETCO_2$) and is usually best prevented by fluid loading before and during tourniquet release.

Postoperative
- Postoperative pain is usually the most significant problem and this is the main determinant of the anaesthetic technique, as discussed below.
- When blood loss into the drains continues to be brisk after the first 500ml, the surgeon will often clamp the drains for a period of time.

Special considerations

- Femoral and sciatic nerve blocks have the following advantages:
  - Good postoperative pain relief in the first 12–24hr. Supplement with regular NSAID and oral analgesics plus parenteral opioid (PCA or IM).
  - Avoids the need for a urinary catheter.
  - Allows the patient more mobility in bed.
  - If possible, perform blocks 30min prior to surgery to allow onset time for surgical anaesthesia. This technique usually gives very good postoperative pain relief. Needs to be combined with spinal or GA as surgical anaesthesia is not produced.
- Spinal anaesthesia supplemented with diamorphine (0.25–0.5mg) followed by PCA is used by some.
- Patients undertake exercises in the operated leg at 24hr and are mobilised at 48hr. Nerve blocks fit well with this requirement, although some surgeons believe that an epidural gives better analgesic cover for the exercises. If used, it needs to be removed prior to mobilisation.

Bilateral total knee replacement

- Bilateral knee replacements should only be considered in young, fit, motivated patients.[2,3] Elderly patients and those with significant CVS disease are high risk.
- Advantage is that two admissions/operations are avoided.
- Disadvantage is that bilateral TKR is a major CVS stress and is associated with unpredictable blood loss and fluid requirements.
- GA + epidural is probably the most practical technique.
- Invasive monitoring should be considered (arterial line).

Revision of total knee replacement

Same as primary knee replacement except it takes longer, ≥2hr.

- The technique is as for primary knee replacement.
- If done without a tourniquet then 2U of blood should be crossmatched.

1 Satsumae T, Yamaguchi H, Sakaguchi M, *et al.* (2001). Preoperative small dose ketamine prevented tourniquet induced arterial pressure increase in orthopaedic patients under general anesthesia. *Anesthesia and Analgesia*, **92**, 1286–1289.
2 Ritter MA, Harty LD (2004). Debate: simultaneous bilateral knee replacements: the outcomes justify its use. *Clinical Orthopaedics & Related Research*, **428**, 84–86.
3 Oakes DA, Hanssen AD (2004). Bilateral total knee replacement using the same anesthetic is not justified by assessment of the risks. *Clinical Orthopaedics & Related Research*, **428**, 87–91.

Arthroscopic lower limb procedures

Arthroscopy with or without excision of cartilage	
Procedure	Arthroscopy, EUA, and washout ± excision of torn cartilage, removal of loose body
Time	10–60min
Pain	++
Position	Supine with leg over side of table
Blood loss	Nil
Practical techniques	GA/LMA or spinal

General principles
- The patient population is generally younger than those having joint replacements.
- Smaller procedures are done as day cases and therefore require a technique that allows early ambulation and discharge home. The main procedures undertaken are EUA, meniscal surgery/loose body removal, synovectomy, and ligament reconstruction.
- Virtually all are done on the knee, though arthroscopy is also performed on the ankle.
- Arthroscopy for knees with osteoarthritis is not supported by evidence of effectiveness.[1]

Technique
- Pre-med with paracetamol and NSAID.
- GA/LMA, a 'standard' day-case anaesthetic with IV opioids.
- A tourniquet is often used.
- Prescribe NSAIDs and strong oral analgesics to take home.
- Many surgeons instil 10–20ml of 0.5% bupivacaine ± morphine (10mg) into the joint cavity for postoperative pain relief.
- Ketamine in low dosage (IV) has been suggested to enhance analgesia (0.15mg/kg).[2]
- Ideally IV morphine should be avoided in day case arthroscopic procedures due to the high incidence of PONV.
- EUA ± washout can be performed under intra-articular and infiltration LA alone. Nerve blocks have been used but are limited by the long duration of action of anaesthesia and the failure to block the site of the arterial tourniquet.

1 http://www.jr2.ox.ac.uk/bandolier/band102/b102-3html.
2 Menigaux C, Guignard B, Fletcher D, et al. (2001). Intraoperative small-dose ketamine enhances analgesia after outpatient arthroscopy. *Anesthesia and Analgesia*, **93**, 606–612.

Cruciate ligament repair

Procedure	Arthroscopic reconstruction of anterior cruciate ligament using patellar tendon ± hamstrings
Time	1.5–2hr
Pain	+++/++++
Position	Supine
Blood loss	Nil
Practical techniques	Patellar tendon and hamstring repair: LMA + GA with combined femoral/sciatic blocks
	GA + PCA

Technique

- These operations are of two main types: using the patellar tendon only for the repair and using both the patellar tendon and hamstring ligaments.
- Usually 12hr of analgesia is required prior to mobilisation.
- If the patellar tendon only is used, postoperative pain is less of a problem and a femoral nerve block is very effective for 12–24hr.
- If the hamstrings are used, the operation takes longer and there is more postoperative pain. Consider GA with femoral and sciatic nerve blocks performed prior to induction.
- Use weaker concentrations of bupivacaine (0.125–0.25%) for nerve blocks, so that mobilisation/discharge is not delayed.
- Alternatively, combine LMA/femoral nerve block/PCA.

Ankle surgery

General principles

- Four main types of procedure: tendon transfers, open reduction and internal fixation (ORIF) of fractures, joint arthrodesis, and prosthetic joint replacement.
- Ankle arthrodesis takes 1–2hr. Tendon transfer is generally quicker than this and joint replacement may take longer.
- These operations are amenable to regional anaesthetic techniques, either alone or combined with GA.
- Tourniquets are often used and tourniquet pain has to be considered.
- Patients may be supine, prone, or, occasionally, on their side.
- In the case of ORIF following trauma, surgery may need to be undertaken urgently if distal circulation is compromised. Beware of the risk of aspiration from a full stomach and also take time to ensure that any other significant injury has been properly considered and dealt with.
- If regional block is considered for ORIF, check that there is no concern about the development of compartment syndrome postoperatively as the symptoms will be masked by the block (see p490).

Technique

- Local, regional, general, or a combination of techniques can be used for all procedures on the ankle.
- Nerve blocks are popular and for ankle surgery require sciatic and femoral nerve blockade—the saphenous nerve (terminal branch of the femoral nerve) supplies skin down to the medial malleolus of the ankle.
- Nerve blocks following a spinal anaesthetic improve analgesia well into the first postoperative day. General anaesthesia can also be combined with nerve blocks.
- Care must be taken in trauma cases with fractured ankles as nerve blocks may mask compartment syndrome. Always discuss your proposed technique with the surgeon. The general rule is that nerve blocks are best avoided in trauma cases. Local infiltration is useful.
- Tendon transfers last up to 1hr and are not particularly painful postoperatively.
- ORIF may be an emergency if the vascular supply is compromised, and a rapid sequence induction is the best anaesthetic option in this situation.
- A good alternative for ORIF is a spinal. The addition of intrathecal opioid (e.g. diamorphine 0.25–0.5mg) prolongs the period of analgesia.
- Ankle joint replacement is a procedure that is increasing in popularity. Usually the procedure is accomplished within 2hr.

Procedure	Time	Pain (+ to +++++)	Position	Blood loss	Practical technique
Tendon transfer/repair	~1hr	++	Supine (ruptured tendo-achilles—prone)	Nil with tourniquet	GA + LMA with infiltration of LA by surgeon. Spinal if supine. IPPV if prone
ORIF of ankle fracture	Variable 1.5–2hr	++/+++	Supine, occasionally on side or prone	Nil with tourniquet	GA (if in doubt RSI) or spinal. Generally avoid nerve blocks
Arthrodesis of ankle joint	1.5–2hr	+++	Supine	Nil with tourniquet	GA or spinal with nerve blocks PCA. Spinal + nerve blocks
Prosthetic replacement of ankle joint	2hr plus	++/+++	Supine	Nil with tourniquet	GA + nerve blocks. Spinal + nerve blocks

Foot surgery

General principles
- Most operations are on the forefoot and toes, e.g. first metatarsal osteotomy, Keller's, excision of ingrowing toenails, and terminalisation of toes. Other operations are in the midfoot, such as tendon transfers and some osteotomies.
- The patient population varies and many are elderly. Those for terminalisation of toes may well have concomitant problems such as diabetes and/or CVS disease.
- Osteotomies tend to be painful postoperatively.
- Surgical time is 30min to 1hr.
- Many are done as day cases and require early ambulation and discharge with adequate pain relief.
- Many operations are amenable to regional anaesthesia. Nerve blocks make a valuable contribution to postoperative analgesia, particularly in osteotomies or nail bed excision, and promote early ambulation. However, onset time is relatively long and they need to be performed a full 40min prior to surgery if planned without supplemental GA. With experience this can work well, but for the less experienced it is best to undertake them primarily for postoperative pain relief in combination with LMA and GA.
- Adrenaline must not be used for 'ring' or 'web-space' blocks and is best avoided in ankle blocks if peripheral circulation is poor.
- Breakthrough pain from the tourniquet can be a problem, especially if surgery is longer than 45min. Place the tourniquet as distally as possible to reduce this effect.

Technique
- Regional blocks useful for foot surgery include ring/web-space or ankle blocks for toe surgery, ankle block for forefoot surgery, and sciatic nerve block for operations on the midfoot. Most commonly these blocks are performed for postoperative pain relief and are combined with GA.
- An alternative in all cases is spinal anaesthesia.

Site	Procedure	Time (min)	Pain (+ to +++++)	Position	Blood loss/ X-match	Technique
Toes	Excision of nail bed, terminalisation	30	+++	Supine	Nil	Ring or toe web-block with sedation or GA/LMA + block
Forefoot	Tendon transfers	30–60	+/++	Supine	Nil	GA/LMA + local infiltration Ankle block with sedation or GA/LMA
Forefoot	First metatarsal osteotomy, Keller's	30–60	+++	Supine	Nil	GA/LMA with ankle block or infiltration
Midfoot	Tendon transfers	30–60	+/++	Supine	Nil	GA/LMA + local infiltration
Midfoot	Osteotomy	30–60	+++	Supine	Nil	GA/LMA ± sciatic nerve block at knee

Spinal surgery[1]

Definition

- Surgery on the spinal column between the atlanto-occipital junction and the coccyx.
- May be performed by orthopaedic or neurosurgeons depending on expertise.
- Can be loosely divided into four categories:
  - Decompression of the spinal cord and nerves
  - Stabilisation and correction of spinal deformity
  - Excision of spinal tumours
  - Trauma.

General principles

Children present for scoliosis surgery, young and middle-aged adults for decompressive surgery, and older patients for stabilisation.

- Most procedures are in the prone position, although anterior and lateral approaches are used. Some procedures will involve turning the patient during the operation.
- Airway access will be limited during surgery and so must be secure prior to starting.
- Prevent excessive abdominal or thoracic pressure due to incorrect patient positioning, which may compromise ventilation and circulation.
- Surgical blood loss can be considerable. Ensure good vascular access, accurate measurement of blood loss. Consider cell salvage.
- Long procedures necessitate active prevention of heat loss.
- Assessment of spinal function may be required during the procedure.

The prone position

A specially designed mattress allowing unhindered movement of the abdomen and chest (e.g. a Montreal mattress) should be used to minimise complications as outlined below.

- Turning the patient from prone to supine requires log rolling by a trained team to avoid applying twisting forces in the axial plane. This is especially important for the poorly supported cervical spine, which may be unstable due to fractures or degenerative disease. The surgeon should be present as part of the team for this manoeuvre. Specially designed mechanical hoists can be used to transfer patients from trolley to operating table.
- Pressure on the abdomen applies pressure to the diaphragm and increases intra-thoracic pressure, which in turn decreases thoracic compliance. This can lead to basal atelectasis and the need for higher lung inflation pressures, particularly in obese patients.
- Raised intra-abdominal pressure also compresses veins and decreases venous return, which may result in hypotension or increased venous bleeding from the surgical site.
- Accurate assessment of the circulation with invasive arterial monitoring and an indwelling urinary catheter is recommended for all major procedures. Central venous pressure may be difficult to interpret in the prone position and is rarely required.

- Peripheral pressure areas are at particular risk in the prone position. Pillows and silicone pads should be used judiciously to protect all areas. Ensure that the breasts and genitalia are not trapped. During long cases it may be necessary to move the patient's limbs and head every hour to avoid stagnation of peripheral blood and the development of pressure necrosis. Pay particular attention to the nose, eyes, chin, elbows, knees, and ankles.
- The arms are usually placed 'above the head' which puts the brachial plexus at risk of stretching or being pressed against the mattress. Ensure that the axillae are not under tension after positioning.

Anaesthesia

- Plans for the recovery period should be made in advance and will be dictated by local experience. Long cases, those involving excessive blood loss, and major paediatric cases will need postoperative care in the HDU. Few patients require postoperative ventilatory support.
- Secure venous access is vital. It may be difficult to access the cannula so an extension with a three-way tap is recommended.
- Choice of anaesthetic will be dictated by personal experience but most will choose an IV induction with muscle relaxation and opioid supplementation. Both low-flow volatile anaesthesia and TIVA are frequently used. Remifentanil is useful perioperatively.
- If spinal cord integrity is at risk during surgery, it may be necessary to use spinal cord monitoring. This is a specialist service provided by a neurophysiologist but will require that muscle relaxation is allowed to wear off. It may be necessary to deepen anaesthesia during this phase, but in reality this is rarely a problem. Somatosensory evoked potentials monitoring is the most commonly employed technique. Intra-operative monitoring has superseded the 'wake-up test' when patients were woken in the middle of surgery and asked to perform simple motor functions before being re-anaesthetised.
- In patients with paraplegia or other large areas of muscle denervation (2d–8 months), suxamethonium should be avoided (see p240).
- Airway access is likely to be limited once the procedure has started, so securing oral endotracheal intubation with a non-kinking tube is usual. Patients with unstable necks due to trauma or rheumatoid arthritis can be intubated using awake fibre-optic intubation or with manual in-line stabilisation depending on the degree of instability and the anticipated difficulty of intubation (p948). The tube should be moulded around the face with no bulky joints adjacent to the skin. A throat pack may be used to decrease the flow of secretions onto the pillow and the tube then secured with adhesive tape or film. Attention to detail and the use of padding is vital to protect pressure areas.

1 Raw DA, Beattie JK, Hunter JM (2003). Anaesthesia for spinal surgery in adults. *British Journal of Anaesthesia*, **91**, 886–904.

- Most patients will be paralysed and ventilated for these procedures with positional considerations noted above. Check that ventilation is adequate without excessive inflation pressures before surgery starts, as the only recourse may be to return the patient to the supine position if problems develop. Check the position of the endotracheal tube when the patient has been turned.
- Blood loss may be significant, with venous oozing proving hard to control. The use of cell salvage techniques (p1009) is advisable for long procedures involving instrumentation of multiple levels. All patients should have samples grouped and saved and more major procedures should have blood crossmatched even if cell salvage is employed (see below).
- Hypotensive anaesthesia may reduce blood loss during major spinal surgery. The mean arterial pressure should be maintained at a safe level—for normotensive patients >60mmHg. Direct arterial monitoring is mandatory when the blood pressure is being manipulated.
- The type of analgesia required will vary depending on the magnitude of surgery. Minor procedures (e.g. microdiscectomy) may manage with NSAIDs alone in association with infiltration of the operative site with local anaesthetic. Most procedures will necessitate opioids. PCA morphine is effective after adequate IV loading. The use of regional analgesia is encouraged where there is no need to assess neurological function, and the use of epidural and paravertebral analgesia is growing in popularity for major procedures such as correction of scoliosis. The catheter is usually placed by the surgeon at the end of the procedure and infusions of local anaesthetic or opioids continued for several days postoperatively.
- Effective analgesia is particularly important for surgery to the thoracic spine where postoperative respiratory function will be compromised if analgesia is inadequate. Consider using incentive spirometry and chest physiotherapy.

Summary of spinal surgery procedures

Operation	Description	Time (hr)	Position	Blood loss/ X-match	Pain (+ to +++++)	Notes
Discectomy or microdiscectomy	Excision of herniated inter-vertebral disc	1–2	Prone	Not significant	+/++	Microdiscectomy can be done as day case
Cervical discectomy	Excision of herniated cervical intervertebral disc	2	Prone/head on horseshoe or halo traction pins	Not significant	++/+++	May be an emergency with neurological deficit
Spinal fusion ± decompression	Correction of spondylolisthesis or spinal stenosis for pain or instability—often several levels	1–2 (then 1 per level)	Prone	500–2000ml, X-match 4U	+++/+++++	May take bone graft from pelvis. Metal instrumentation
Cervical fusion ± decompression	Fusion of unstable neck (e.g. arthritis, trauma)	2–3	Supine or prone. Cervical traction in place or applied at start	300–1000ml, G&S	++/+++	Neck can be very unstable and need fibre-optic intubation. Application of traction pins very stimulating

Table contd.

Operation	Description	Time (hr)	Position	Blood loss/ X-match	Pain (+ to +++++)	Notes
Excision of spinal tumour (e.g. vertebrectomy)	Tumours may be primary or secondary from any part of the spine	2–6+	Supine, prone, or lateral tilt	Potentially massive, X-match 6U + clotting factors available	+++/ ++++	Often difficult surgery with potential for excessive blood loss and neurological damage
Kyphoscoliosis surgery	Correction of major spinal deformities in patients who may have severe physical disability	3–6+	Supine and/or prone	Potentially massive, X-match 6U + clotting factors available	+++/ +++++	Often in children with severe restrictive respiratory disease and co-existing abnormalities. May involve surgery in abdominal and thoracic cavities. Spinal nerve monitoring used in some centres. May need postop ICU for IPPV
Repair of vertebral fracture	Repair for neurological deficit or instability	2–6	Supine and/or prone	500–2000ml, X-match 4U	++/ ++++	Often associated with other major injury (esp. rib fracture). May be in ICU/IPPV. Neurological deficit often not reversible. Note: suxamethonium may be contraindicated

Shoulder surgery

General considerations

Soft tissue operations around the shoulder are often extremely painful. This pain is not predictable and may last for several days, although it is certainly worst within the first 48hr.

Anaesthesia

- The patient is usually positioned with the head distal to the anaesthetist, requiring particular attention to the security of the airway. It is often easier to intubate the patient (south-facing RAE or armoured tube) except for shorter procedures, where an LMA may be suitable. Long ventilator and gas sampling tubes are required.
- Venous access should be placed in the opposite arm (with a long extension) or at the ankle/foot.
- The patient may be placed supine with head-up tilt, lateral, or in a deck-chair position. When using steep head-up tilt in patients with compromised cardiovascular function, change posture slowly and consider direct arterial pressure monitoring.
- Although blood loss is rarely significant, patients may be unable to take oral fluids for some hours postoperatively.
- Regional anaesthesia is a useful adjunct in shoulder anaesthesia and an interscalene block is the method of choice (p1077). Although procedures may be performed under regional anaesthesia alone, local anaesthetic is more commonly used to supplement general anaesthesia and to provide postoperative analgesia. When planning an interscalene block, inform the patient that their whole arm may go numb, and that they may sense that full inspiration is not possible when they wake up (phrenic nerve blockade). Interscalene block is contraindicated in patients with contralateral phrenic nerve/diaphragmatic palsy, or recurrent laryngeal nerve damage. Interscalene catheters can be used for prolonged postoperative analgesia.[1]
- When an interscalene block is impractical infiltration of local anaesthetics in reasonable quantities by the surgeon may also provide postoperative analgesia. A catheter can be placed in the subacromial space and used to instil further quantities of local anaesthetic in the postoperative period.[2] This is particularly effective in Bankart's and capsular shift operations.
- For rotator cuff repairs an epidural catheter placed during surgery over the repair can be used to supplement postoperative analgesia. Regular boluses (10ml 0.25% bupivacaine 2–4hourly) appear to work better than a continuous infusion.
- Potent analgesia is often required for 1–2d. The combination of PCA opioid/NSAIDs/paracetamol is usually effective. Good posture (sitting up with the elbow supported on a pillow) is also important.

1 Denny NM, Barber N, Sildown DJ (2003). Evaluation of an insulated Tuohy needle system for the placement of interscalene brachial plexus catheters. *Anaesthesia*, **58**, 554–557.
2 Axelsson K, Nordenson U, Johanzon E, *et al.* (2003). Patient-controlled regional analgesia (PCRA) with ropivacaine after arthroscopic subacromial decompression. *Acta Anaesthesiologica Scandinavica*, **47**, 993–1000.

Total shoulder replacement

Procedure	Prosthetic shoulder replacement
Time	2–3hr
Pain	+++/++++
Position	Supine, head up, or deck-chair
Blood loss	250–500ml
Practical techniques	ET + IPPV, interscalene block

Preoperative

- Many patients are elderly; severe rheumatoid disease is common.
- Ask about respiratory function/reserve if planning an interscalene block (some diaphragmatic function will be lost for several hours).
- Check the airway (particularly in rheumatoid arthritis) and range of neck movement. Some patients will need fibre-optic intubation.

Perioperative

- Consider performing an interscalene block before inducing anaesthesia (see p1077).
- Place IV infusion and blood pressure cuff on the opposite arm with a long extension.
- Intubate with a preformed 'south-facing' ETT.
- Hypotension is common when changing to head-up position.
- If interscalene block has been performed, anaesthesia is usually unremarkable. Sometimes breakthrough stimulation occurs during the glenoid phase (may receive fibres from T2 which are not always covered by the block).
- If no interscalene block, load the patient with morphine and ask the surgeon to infiltrate with local anaesthetic (20–30ml of 0.25% bupivacaine).
- Antibiotic prophylaxis.

Postoperative

- Pain is worst in the first 24hr postoperatively. PCA/intermittent morphine are usually satisfactory.
- NSAIDs are useful.

Special considerations

- Air/fat embolism is a rare event.
- In poor-risk patients direct arterial monitoring is advised.

Other shoulder operations

- Most shoulder surgery may be carried out using the anaesthetic guidelines above. Arthroscopic surgery is generally less painful and patients get effective postoperative analgesia if the surgeon injects 10–20ml bupivacaine 0.5% within the joint space at the end of surgery.
- Bankart's and capsular shift operations for recurrent dislocations are more painful for larger, muscular patients but not generally as painful as cuff repairs or open acromioplasties.
- Massive cuff repairs are often extremely painful and an interscalene block is useful. PCA should be considered and a loading dose of morphine should be administered during surgery. Consider interscalene catheter with infusion of LA.
- Pain following any operation around the shoulder is unpredictable and some patients who have had short procedures suffer severe pain for several days. A flexible approach is required for analgesia.
- Beware the pain-free patient following major shoulder surgery and connected to PCA morphine. When the regional block wears off, effective analgesia may take some time to establish.

Elbow replacement surgery[1]

Procedure	Prosthetic elbow replacement
Time	Variable
Pain	+/++
Position	Supine, arm out on table
Blood loss	Minimal
Practical techniques	GA, tourniquet

Total elbow arthroplasty is performed in patients with an ankylosed or a very stiff elbow (e.g. rheumatoid). The operation aims to provide an increase in the range of motion of the joint and pain relief. Complications, including reoperation, are frequent.

Technique

- Assess the patient for other manifestations of rheumatoid disease. (See p186.)
- LMA/GA and IV opioids.
- A tourniquet is often used.
- Careful poisoning to prevent tissue injury, and to reduce postoperative pain from other arthritic areas.
- Regional techniques—vertical infraclavicular block (VIB—see p1079) is probably block of choice.
- Postoperative ulnar nerve compression is common and may necessitate further surgery.

1 Mansat P, Morrey BF (2000). Semiconstrained total elbow arthroplasty for ankylosed and stiff elbows. *J Bone Joint Surg Am*, **82**, 1260–1268.

Anaesthesia for hand surgery

Procedure	Various
Time	Variable
Pain	+/+++
Position	Supine, arm out on table
Blood loss	Minimal
Practical techniques	Regional analgesia ± GA, tourniquet

The majority of hand surgery procedures are suitable for local or regional anaesthesia as a day case. This can be combined with general anaesthesia or additional sedation if required. Some procedures such as carpal tunnel release or trigger finger release can be done under local infiltration alone. Intravenous regional anaesthesia (IVRA) is suitable for procedures below the elbow of 30min or less.

An upper arm tourniquet is almost always used for any type of hand surgery. Positioning and duration of use will be an important determinant of whether the patient is able to tolerate regional or local anaesthesia alone. Patients with a good brachial plexus block will usually tolerate 60–90min of arm ischaemia.

An axillary brachial plexus block can provide excellent anaesthesia to the hand, arm, and forearm, although tourniquet pain may be a problem. Other approaches include infra- and supraclavicular approaches.

Preoperative

- Full assessment as for GA. The patient may request a GA and regional anaesthesia may fail.
- Check that patients can lie flat for the proposed duration of operation if planned to be awake.
- Assess movement of the operative arm. Can the patient achieve the necessary position for regional block or the surgery planned?

Perioperative

- Make sure the patient's bladder is empty.
- Use full monitoring whether or not GA/sedation is to be used.
- Perform local block with the patient awake or lightly sedated.
- Choose an appropriate and familiar block for the planned site of surgery ± tourniquet.
- Augment plexus anaesthesia with elbow or wrist blocks as necessary to improve success rates.
- Provide sedation or GA depending on safety and the patient's wishes. Have equipment and drugs ready to convert to sedation or GA if necessary during the operation.

Postoperative

- Surgery involving soft tissues and skin is generally less painful than surgery to the bones and joints.
- Simple analgesic combinations are usually adequate for the less painful procedures.
- Opioids or regional catheter techniques may be required for the more painful operations.
- Some patients dislike the postoperative 'dead arm' following brachial plexus block.

Special considerations

- Tourniquet pain can be reduced by blocking the intercostobrachial nerve subcutaneously on the medial aspect of the upper arm above the level of the tourniquet.
- Adrenaline-containing solutions should be avoided near digits.

Other hand surgical procedures

Operation	Description	Time (min)	Pain (+ to ++++)	Notes
Trigger finger release and carpal tunnel release	Tendon or nerve release	5–15	+	These procedures can usually be carried out under local infiltration anaesthesia
Dupuytren's contractures (simple)	Usually confined to ulnar and median distribution. Usually <30min tourniquet time	<60	+	GA with wrist block or infiltration. Brachial plexus block with upper arm tourniquet ± GA. Quick procedure: wrist block with wrist tourniquet
Dupuytren's contracture (complex)	Severe disease or redo procedure may need skin grafting	60–120	+	Prolonged tourniquet time means that a brachial plexus block or a GA with local block is often required
Swanson's joint replacement	MP joint replacement usually for rheumatoid	30 per joint	++/+++	Generally frailer patients with systemic disease
Tenolysis, capsulotomies, tendon grafts	These procedures may need patient participation to assess the adequacy of the procedure	15–60	+/++	If hand movement is required then any block must be distal. A wrist block with sedation is usually adequate
Digit re-implantation	Microvascular surgery	Hours	++	Regional anaesthesia for the sympathectomy is helpful. A GA is usually required because of the prolonged procedure
Ulnar head excision or trapeziectomy	Surgery for wrist pain in rheumatoid disease	30–60	++/+++	As pain is severe a single-shot brachial block or catheter technique is ideal with or without a GA

Anaesthesia for major trauma

Major trauma presents many challenges to the anaesthetist. Multiple injuries can cause significant physiological disturbance and may require urgent and/or prolonged surgery from different specialties. Significant injuries may be unrecognised, or not present until surgery. All patients should be resuscitated according to ATLS guidelines.

General considerations

- Major trauma cases often require a number of procedures. Life-saving surgery clearly takes priority, but it may be possible to perform several procedures at once.
- The patient should be personally fully reviewed preoperatively. Major injuries are easily missed in A&E. Check the CXR for missed pathology.
- Immediately prior to anaesthesia, every patient should have a minimum of an ATLS primary survey (airway, breathing, circulation, and disability).
- A high index of suspicion should exist for injuries that may not have been apparent at the initial assessment but may cause cardiorespiratory compromise—pneumothorax, spinal cord injury, cardiac tamponade, fat embolism, and occult haemorrhage.
- Hypothermia causes significant morbidity and should be rigorously avoided and treated.
- Life-saving surgery should not be delayed by unnecessary investigations.

Management of anaesthesia

Team work

It is important to use all members of the medical staff efficiently. Effective communication is an important determinant of outcome.

Airway

- Endotracheal intubation is usual.
- Intubation is more likely to be difficult; all the usual equipment should be available before starting induction of anaesthesia.
- Always assume a full stomach. Place a gastric tube during surgery to attempt gastric decompression. The tube should be placed orally if there are associated nasal/mid-face or base-of-skull fractures.

Ventilation

- Ventilator settings may have to be adjusted from 'normal' values to take into account problems that are particular to trauma patients.
- Patients with actual or potentially raised ICP should have their $PaCO_2$ kept at 4.5–5kPa (35–38mmHg) to maintain a stable ICP.
- Patients with chest trauma may require the use of special ventilator settings. It may be necessary to use an ICU ventilator.

Circulatory access

- Ensure adequate venous access—preferably two 14–16G cannulae. If venous access is difficult consider a cut-down/femoral line/external jugular line, or intraosseous access in children.

- Continue resuscitation during transfer to theatre, 'permissive hypovol-aemia' or 'hypotensive resuscitation' to a systolic BP of 80mmHg may be preferable for the trauma victim with ongoing uncontrolled haemorrhage.[1]
- Do not delay life-saving surgery with attempts to fully resuscitate hypovolaemia.
- Attach one IV line to a high-performance warming system, preferably with an automatic pressurisation system. This line should be dedicated to fluid resuscitation, unless haemorrhage is massive: this ensures adequate heating of all infused fluid. Ideally one person should be solely responsible for checking and dealing with all fluid on this line.
- An arterial line should be inserted when practical. They are not normally required immediately and should not delay surgery.
- Central venous access is not usually a priority and may be difficult due to injuries to the vasculature and hypovolaemia. It is best carried out after fluid resuscitation. A femoral line may be the most practical (and quickest) option if infusions of vasopressors/inotropes are required—however, avoid in abdominal trauma.

Temperature

Use a temperature probe and peripheral nerve stimulator. Try to maintain body temperature.

Regional anaesthesia

Regional anaesthesia may be considered as an adjunct, although preoperative urgency, haemodynamic instability, coagulopathy, and the possibility of compartment syndrome often make it impractical.

Problems

- Unexplained hypotension and tachycardia: consider hypovolaemia, pneumothorax, pericardial tamponade, fat/air embolism.
- Unexplained hypoxia is often associated with a rise in inflation pressure: consider tension pneumothorax and fat embolism.
- Unexplained hypertension: consider pain, raised ICP (search for associated neurological signs, obtain brain CT scan), or rarely traumatic disruption of thoracic aorta.

Changing anaesthetic teams

Major trauma cases often involve prolonged surgery by multiple teams; you may need to hand over the patient to different anaesthetist(s). This handover should be as detailed as possible. The anaesthetist should document the time and details of the handover on the anaesthetic record.

---

1 Stern SA (2001). Low-volume fluid resuscitation for presumed hemorrhagic shock: helpful or harmful? *Current Opinions in Critical Care*, **7**, 422–430.

Cervical spine fracture

Surgery for cervical spine fracture may comprise application of stabilising devices (halo traction, skull tongs, plaster jacket) or definitive fixation of the bony column (usually performed as a semi-elective procedure).

General considerations

- Patients have usually suffered major trauma, although fractures can occur following minor injury if pre-existing cervical spine disease.
- Controversy exists as to the best method of securing the airway. Awake intubation is considered safer in trained hands; however, it may result in coughing, and can be difficult and unpleasant for the patient. Direct laryngoscopy under general anaesthesia with manual in-line neck stabilisation (MILNS) may be associated with more neck movement.

Anaesthesia

- Patients for halo traction, skull tong application, or other stabilising procedures will usually be in full neck immobilisation. This is removed following application of the stabilising device—usually under local anaesthetic. Sedation may be required. General anaesthesia is occasionally required for more complex stabilisation or in confused/agitated patients. It should be performed as per anterior cervical stabilisation (p486).
- Patients for open cervical spine stabilisation require either an anterior or posterior approach and, in a few patients, both.
- Perform a full neurological examination before anaesthesia to assess the level and extent of any spinal cord injury. This is particularly important for patients who are to be turned prone.
- Anterior approaches are usually performed in the supine head-up position, through an oblique incision across the anterior aspect of the neck. The posterior approach is performed in the prone position, using a longitudinal incision. Occasionally, fractures to C1/C2 may require an approach through the mouth.
- Arterial and venous lines should be placed, and must be well secured to prevent kinking. A forced-air warming system should be used and urinary catheterisation is required. Nasogastric decompression is usual for prolonged surgery, or those with pre-existing spinal cord injury.
- For prone positioning, extreme care is needed during turning (involve the surgeon). The surgeon should control the head/neck, while at least three people perform the turn. The anaesthetist should hold the ET tube in situ and should be in charge of coordinating the turn. Some centres use awake intubation, followed by awake positioning prior to induction of anaesthesia.
- Blood loss is rarely significant for these procedures, and so deliberate arterial hypotension is not usually required.

Anaesthesia for repair of cervical spine fracture

Procedure	Anterior/posterior repair of cervical fracture
Time	2–6hr
Pain	++/+++
Position	Supine head up or prone for posterior approach
Blood loss	250–1 000ml, X-match 4U
Practical techniques	GA, art line, awake FOI

Preoperative

- Mostly trauma patients, often with other injuries. Sometimes older patients with fractures in a previously diseased cervical spine. Check for other manifestations of the underlying disease (e.g. rheumatoid).
- Check presence/degree of cervical spine injury, level of lesion, and likely approach.
- Check the need for postoperative ventilation and HDU care. Commoner with high lesions, which may need aggressive chest physiotherapy.
- Consider the technique of intubation. The patient may be in skull traction, which does not limit mouth opening but does limit neck movement. Full neck immobilisation (with a hard cervical collar and sandbags/tape) limits both neck movement and mouth opening.

Perioperative

- Insert arterial and venous lines, preferably in the same arm.
- Intubation: awake nasal intubation is commonest,[1] but a smaller tube size results. Awake oral intubation is harder to perform, but gives a larger tube size. If the surgeon is planning an intra-oral approach, check whether an oral or nasal ETT is preferred.
- Suxamethonium is contra-indicated in patients with spinal cord lesions that are >72hr old. In practice, it is rare to need suxamethonium.
- Positioning should be in combination with the surgeon. Some request check of residual neurological function following awake intubation and after turning prone.
- Check all pressure areas before draping. Procedures are prolonged.
- Bone graft may be required, and is usually taken from the iliac crest.

Postoperative

- PCA morphine is usually satisfactory.
- NSAIDs are useful.

Special considerations

- Patients with acute spinal cord lesions may demonstrate signs of neurogenic shock including bradycardia and hypotension (see p240). This is best treated with judicious use of fluids and pressor agents, guided by CVP monitoring. Cervical spine surgery is rarely performed in the first few hours after injury, which makes these problems uncommon. However, spinal hyper-reflexia may occur in patients with longer-standing lesions, and these should be treated symptomatically (p240).
- Tracheostomy is not advisable in patients scheduled for anterior fusion. Discuss with the surgeon if this is a likely option.

1 Sidhu VS, Whitehead EM, Ainsworth QP, Smith M, Calder I (1993). A technique of awake fibre-optic intubation. Experience in patients with cervical spine disease. *Anaesthesia*, **48**, 910–913.

Anaesthesia for limb fractures

Procedure	Closed or open reduction of limb fractures
Time	5min to many hours
Pain	Variable
Position	Usually supine
Blood loss	Minimal, but can be up to 2000ml for open procedures
Practical techniques	GA ± block, regional block alone

Discuss with the surgeon the nature and duration of the likely repair (MUA may become ORIF). If planning a regional block, you should also discuss the risk of compartment syndrome (p490).

Preoperative

- Check that no additional surgery is likely.
- Ensure the absence of other significant chest/abdominal/head injuries.
- Patients with recent (<24hr) moderate or severe head injury require very careful consideration before proceeding to non-life-saving surgery.
- Check the state of cervical spine clearance where relevant.
- Check the state of hydration of the patient and the time of the last food/drink in relation to the time of injury.
- In practice, the stomach may never empty in some patients, particularly children, and if in doubt consider the patient at risk of a full stomach.
- Check a chest radiograph for all major trauma patients.

Perioperative

- Ensure at least one large-gauge infusion/IVI warmer for all open reductions involving proximal limb fractures.
- Do not site IV on an injured limb.
- Blood loss is very variable. Proximal limb fractures (femur, humerus) and use of bone grafting cause considerable blood loss.
- The use of a tourniquet will reduce bleeding, but may be contraindicated because of the fracture type/site.
- Antibiotic prophylaxis prior to commencement of surgery/application of tourniquet.
- Patients are at risk of fat embolism (p447).
- Patients with pre-existing head injury may require ICP monitoring and postoperative ventilation. General anaesthesia can obscure the signs of deterioration in conscious level, and anaesthesia may also contribute to a rise in ICP.

Postoperative

- Postoperative analgesia requirements depend on the nature of the surgery.
- Closed reductions can often be managed with a combination of perioperative opioid together with NSAIDs/paracetamol/opioid orally.
- More complex repairs, including external fixation, may require the use of a PCA.

Special considerations

Regional anaesthesia can be a useful addition for the provision of analgesia, and may also be used as the sole anaesthetic for some fracture reductions. However, a local anaesthetic block may obscure neurological signs of a developing compartment syndrome. The best strategy is to discuss the problem with the surgeon beforehand.

In humeral fractures where surgical wire banding is planned, avoid regional blocks. The radial nerve is easily trapped during surgery and the diagnosis is delayed with a regional block.

Compartment syndrome[1]

Compartment syndrome arises when the circulation and tissues within a closed space are compromised by increased pressure. Ischaemia, necrosis, and loss of function result, further increasing compartmental pressure. Damage can become irreversible after only 4hr.

Compartment syndrome is thus a serious limb-threatening condition, which may also lead to systemic organ dysfunction if incorrectly managed. It should be anticipated in any significant limb injury, with or without fracture, especially in crush situations. It can also be caused by tourniquets, malpositioning in theatre, systemic hypotension, haemorrhage, oedema, and direct injection of drugs. In obtunded patients, where clinical signs may be masked, or in the presence of spinal cord injuries measurement of the compartmental pressure may be indicated. Early diagnosis and treatment are vital. Urgent fasciotomy may be required.

Signs and symptoms of compartment syndrome include:

- Pain mainly over the affected compartment, worsened by passive stretching of the muscles.
- Tense swelling over the compartment, with drum-tight fascia/skin.
- Paraesthesia in the distribution of nerves traversing the compartment.
- Weakness or paralysis of the limb is a late sign.
- Distal pulses are usually present.

Measuring compartment pressures

- This can be undertaken using a pressure transducer (as in an arterial line) attached to a needle placed into the suspect compartment.
- If the compartmental pressure is within 30mmHg of the diastolic pressure, diagnosis is confirmed.

Special considerations

- Compartment syndrome can occur with open fractures—some compartments may not be able to decompress through the open wound.
- Keep the limb at the level of the heart. Avoid elevation as this may decrease perfusion below critical levels.
- Release all constricting bandages, dressings, or casts encircling the limb. If this does not rapidly relieve symptoms, urgent surgical fasciotomy will be required to save the limb.
- After fasciotomy the limb should be splinted to prevent contractures and the fracture stabilised to prevent further bleeding.
- Ensure the patient is well hydrated and has a good urine output. Myoglobinuria is maximal after reperfusion.

Regional anaesthesia

Avoid local blocks or epidurals if the patient is at risk of developing compartment syndrome as the analgesia will mask early signs. The cardinal symptom is pain, and this occurs early in the syndrome. The risk is especially high in tibial and forearm fractures, so avoid blocks in these situations.

1 Martin JT (1992). Compartment syndromes: concepts and perspectives for the anaesthesiologist. *Anesthesia and Analgesia*, **75**, 275–283.

Anaesthesia for femoral neck fracture

Procedure	Cannulated screws, dynamic hip screw (DHS), cemented/uncemented hemi-arthroplasty
Time	10–120min
Pain	+/+++
Position	Supine (?on hip table), occasionally lateral
Blood loss	250–750ml
Practical techniques	SV LMA and regional block
	Spinal ± sedation
	ETT + IPPV

Hip fractures are common——~49 000 per annum in England (80% female). Average age is 80yr and 80% occur in those >75yr. In Western society the lifetime risk is 18% (women) and 6% (men).[1] 3-month mortality is ~12%, increasing to 21% at 1yr.[2]

Preoperative

- Physiological reserve is reduced and co-morbidity is common. Ideally resuscitation should start as soon as the patient is admitted to hospital. Thorough preoperative assessment must take place and surgery should be scheduled for the earliest possible daytime session.
- Surgical treatment can be either fracture fixation or femoral head replacement, depending on the nature of fracture, surgical preference, previous mobility, and life expectancy. Conservative (non-operative) management is always one option for the grossly unfit.
- Determine which procedure is to be performed. Cannulated hip screws are quick, largely non-invasive procedures with a small incision and little blood loss. Cemented/uncemented hemiarthroplasty is a longer procedure, similar to a primary hip replacement. Dynamic hip screw/Richard's screw and plate are intermediate procedures.
- A decision to delay surgery should be based on a realistic attempt to improve the patient's medical condition, rather than a fruitless pursuit of 'normal' values. A mild chest infection is unlikely to improve in a bed-bound elderly patient, whereas frank pneumonia with sepsis and dyspnoea may respond to rehydration, antibiotics, and chest physio-therapy. Good communication between surgeons and anaesthetists is important.
- An attempt should be made to control atrial fibrillation preoperatively to prevent severe perioperative hypotension.
- Dehydration is common as oral intake is often much reduced.

Perioperative

- For fracture fixation the patient is usually positioned supine on a 'hip table'. This involves placement of a groin prop, with the table supporting the upper body only. Feet are tied into shoe supports, and the table is then elevated to allow radiographic screening. The anaesthetist should be aware that the patient may slide off the lower end of the table. For hemi-arthroplasty the patient is lateral or supine on an ordinary operating table.
- Blood loss is variable. Much of the measured loss is old haematoma, but significant haemorrhage may occur and necessitate transfusion.
- Choice of anaesthetic technique: regional and general anaesthesia are both advocated, but there is little evidence to support one technique over another.[3] Options include:
  - Regional anaesthesia: epidural, spinal, psoas plexus (p1086), and 3 in 1 nerve block (p1088) have all been used for operative anaesthesia and postoperative analgesia. Sedation may be necessary.
  - Spinal anaesthesia may decrease the incidence of postoperative confusion and DVT, but can be associated with perioperative hypotension. A small dose of IV ketamine or alfentanil may be useful as analgesia when turning the patient before performing the block, but avoiding all sedatives is preferable.
  - General anaesthesia with opioid supplementation.
  - Regurgitation and aspiration occasionally occurs with LMAs in this group—if patient is at risk use endotracheal intubation.
- Check pressure points after placement on the 'hip table' as these patients are prone to pressure damage.
- Use some form of passive or active warming device to prevent hypo-thermia. Insulate the head and secure a warming blanket/polythene sheet around the chest and lower abdomen.
- Cemented hemiarthroplasty may be associated with a marked drop in arterial pressure, $ETCO_2$, and heart rate during cement insertion. Take the same precautions as with a total hip replacement (p448).

Postoperative

- Pain is often only due to the incision, which is small for cannulated screws and DHS, but larger for hemiarthroplasty. Fracture pain will be reduced, but is still present on rolling and turning in bed.
- Postoperative analgesia can be provided by regular IM or SC morphine. Most patients will require some postoperative analgesia, although some do not. Take care with NSAIDs because of the increased risk of gastrointestinal and renal complications.

Special considerations

- In poor-risk patients, procedures can be undertaken with local anaesthesia alone. Morbidity and mortality risks should be understood by the patient or relatives and in some patients, resuscitation status should be reviewed.

1 Gillespie W (2001). Hip Fracture. *British Medical Journal*, **322**, 968–975.
2 Parker MJ, Pryor GA, Myles J (2000). 11 year results in 2,846 patients of the Peterborough hip fracture project: reduced morbidity, mortality and hospital stay. *Acta Anaesth Scand*, **71**, 34–38.
3 Urwin SC, Parker MJ, Griffiths R (2000). General versus regional anaesthesia for hip fracture: a meta-analysis of randomized trials. *British Journal of Anaesthesia*, **84**, 450–455.

Procedures for fractured neck of femur

Operation	Description	Time (min)	Pain (+ to +++++)	Position	Blood loss/ X-match	Notes
Cannulated screws	Screws across femoral neck (previously 'Garden screws')	20	+	Supine, hip table	Nil	Minimally invasive, small thigh incision. Can be done with local/nerve block and sedation if necessary. X-ray guided
Richards screw and plate (RSP)	Plate along femur with compression screw into femoral head	30–45	++	Supine, hip table	<400ml	Somewhat larger thigh incision/blood loss. X-ray guided
Dynamic hip screw (DHS)	As RSP	30–45	++	Supine, hip table	<400ml	As RSP
Dynamic compression screw (DCS)	As RSP	30–45	++	Supine, hip table	<400ml	As RSP

Girdlestone osteotomy	Removal of femoral head. No prosthesis	30–45	++	Supine	<400ml	More extensive incision, but no prosthesis, hence quicker than below. Limited mobility afterwards
Austin Moore hemiarthroplasty	Replacement of femoral head. No cement	60–90	+++	Supine	400–600ml	Similar to total hip replacement, without acetabular component
Thompson's hemiarthroplasty	Replacement of femoral head. Cemented	60–90	+++	Supine	400–600ml	Similar to total hip replacement, without acetabular component
Exeter bipolar	Replacement of femoral head and acetabular component. Cemented	60–90	+++	Supine	400–800ml	Similar to total hip replacement, with acetabular component

Plastic surgery

Jon Warwick

General principles

Complexity of anaesthesia ranges from the routine to the challenging. Some extensive procedures (e.g. free flap repairs, craniofacial reconstruction) may involve invasive monitoring, extensive blood loss, and postoperative intensive care support.

Regional techniques

Minor body surface procedures may be performed under local anaesthetic infiltration alone. Upper or lower limb surgery is especially suitable for regional or peripheral nerve block. Sedation to supplement a regional technique may be required in anxious patients or for longer procedures. Propofol(0.5–1.0μg/ml TCI, or 10–15ml/hr of 1% solution) supplemented with a small dose of midazolam(1–2mg) is effective. Significant body surface procedures (e.g. excision and grafting of skin tumours) can be accomplished in those unfit for general anaesthesia using extensive infiltration of local anaesthesia and IV sedation. Incremental sedation with ketamine(10mg) and midazolam(1mg) is a safe and potent analgesic/ sedative combination in the elderly.

The difficult airway (see also p930)

Patients with head and neck pathology causing airway difficulty are often encountered. Airway difficulty may arise from anatomical deformity due to tumour, trauma, infection, previous operation, or scarring. Competence in difficult airway techniques (e.g. fibreoptic intubation) is required. The 'shared airway' is regularly a feature of head and neck surgery. Discuss with the surgeon which tube you propose to use, and by which route to achieve the best surgical access (oral, nasal, conversion to tracheostomy). How will the tube be secured (tied, taped, stitched)?

Poor access to patient

The operating site may be extensive (e.g. burns debridement) or multiple (e.g. free flap procedures). This may produce added difficulty with:
- Heat conservation. It may be difficult to achieve enough access to the patient's body surface area to maintain temperature. Heated under-blankets are useful.
- Monitoring. ECG leads, the pulse oximeter probe, and blood pressure cuff may all be difficult to position adequately.
- Vascular access. Position cannulae away from the operative field. Use femoral vessels or the foot if necessary. Long extension sets may be required.

Smooth emergence

Avoid the patient coughing and straining at the end of the procedure. This will put tension on delicate suture lines and increase bleeding and haematoma formation, especially for facial procedures. The combination of propofol maintenance and the laryngeal mask airway produces a particularly smooth emergence.

Attention to detail

Successful anaesthesia for plastic surgery requires thoroughness and careful attention to detail. Patients for aesthetic surgery will have high expectations and will be well informed.

Analgesia

Pain relief is always a challenge—in practice, effective pain control may be more readily achievable in patients recovering from plastic surgery for several reasons:

* Most procedures are performed on the body surface. These tend to be less painful than procedures involving the body cavities and are usually amenable to local anaesthetic infiltration. Continuous catheter techniques may be useful in limb procedures.
* Patients recovering from head and neck procedures are often surprisingly comfortable despite extensive surgery.
* Major body cavities and abdominal musculature are usually not involved. The pain experienced after abdominoplasty is significantly less than pain following laparotomy.
* Plastic surgery procedures seldom involve new fractures of long bones.
* The gastrointestinal tract is usually unaffected. The oral route for drugs is frequently available which may make dosing and administration of analgesics simpler.

Long operations

Patients undergoing complicated reconstructive procedures may be in theatre for many hours. Give careful consideration to:

* Vascular access. Check that line placement will not interfere with the site of surgery. Invasive arterial monitoring is desirable. A central venous line will assist with estimations of intravascular volume and provide dependable venous access in the postoperative period. Site at least one large-bore peripheral (14–16G) cannula for fluid administration and a small cannula (20–22G) for other infusions such as TCI or PCA.
* Blood loss. Ensure blood has been crossmatched. The initial dissection is usually the period of most blood loss and a moderate hypotensive technique may help to limit this. Thereafter losses may be insidious and ongoing. Aim to keep track by swab weighing, visual estimation, regular haemoglobin, or haematocrit estimations.
* Fluid balance. Urinary catheterisation is essential. Ensure careful monitoring of fluid balance, especially in children and patients with poor cardiorespiratory function.
* Body temperature. Monitor core temperature (e.g. rectal, nasopharyngeal, or oesophageal). Maintain temperature by using low fresh gas flows, a heat-moisture exchange (HME) filter, warmed IV fluids, a warm ambient theatre temperature (e.g. 24°C), a heated mattress, or external warming blankets (e.g. 'Bair Hugger®'). Take care not to overheat.
* Positioning. Ensure that structures such as the cervical spine or brachial plexus are not in positions of stress. Take care with pressure areas. Make liberal use of cotton wool padding ('Gamgee') over bony prominences. Raise the heels off the table using foam pads or boots.

- DVT prophylaxis. Venous thromboembolism is often initiated during surgery. All patients should receive daily low molecular weight heparin, thromboembolism ('TED') stockings, and intermittent calf compression whilst in theatre.
- Nasogastric tube. Consider emptying the stomach. Children are especially prone to gastric distension during prolonged procedures.
- Eye care. Lightly tape and pad the eyes for protection. Avoid excessive padding, since this may negate the natural protection afforded by the bony orbit. Prophylactic antibiotic ointment is unnecessary. Do not allow corneal abrasion to develop from surface drying.
- ET tube cuff pressure. Cuff pressure will gradually increase if N_2O is used. Where possible, recheck the cuff pressure at intervals during the case. Alternatively, fill the cuff with saline.
- Postoperative care. Discuss the preferred site of postoperative care with the nursing staff and surgical team. Surgeons often prefer patients to return to the plastic surgery ward where wound care and nursing observation may be more attuned to the specifics of the operation. Closer patient observation, invasive monitoring, and regular blood gas estimation may be more achievable in an intensive care/high-dependency unit. The site for immediate postoperative care is principally dictated by the general condition of the patient.

Breast reduction

Procedure	Reduction of breast size by glandular resection. Usually bilateral
Time	3hr
Pain	++
Position	Supine, 30° head up. Arms may be positioned on boards, or with elbows flexed and hands placed behind the upper part of the buttocks
Blood loss	500ml, G&S
Practical techniques	IPPV via ETT or LMA

Preoperative

- Bilateral breast reduction is not primarily an aesthetic procedure. These patients may suffer from severe neck and back pain. Participating in exercise and sport is not possible. There may be symptoms of emotional disturbance.
- Patients are usually fit—aged 20–40yr. Many surgeons exclude patients with a body mass index >30 due to a higher incidence of wound breakdown, infection, and haematoma formation.
- A mastopexy is a surgical procedure for correcting breast ptosis when breast volume is adequate. Anaesthetic implications are similar. Blood loss is less.
- FBC and group and save. Crossmatching is generally unnecessary except for larger reductions.
- Timing in relation to the menstrual cycle is unimportant.
- All patients should receive DVT prophylaxis (TED stockings, daily low molecular weight heparin).

Perioperative

- Balanced GA—IPPV may be preferable since the surgeon often puts pressure on the chest wall during surgery. IPPV will maintain satisfactory chest expansion with good aeration, control of $PaCO_2$ and help minimise blood loss. An LMA may be satisfactory for IPPV.
- Place ECG electrodes on the patient's back. Lie the patient on 'incontinence pads' to absorb blood loss.
- Take care to position the patient carefully on the operating table. The anaesthetic machine is usually at the head end. Ensure that the chest and arms are symmetrical. Confirm that cannulae are firmly positioned and their plastic caps covered with 'Gamgee' if the hands are to be positioned behind the buttocks. Local pressure damage to skin may otherwise ensue. Drip extension sets are needed and ensure that the drip runs freely.
- Blood loss depends on surgical technique. Use of cutting diathermy causes less bleeding than a scalpel. Infiltration with dilute adrenaline-containing LA helps reduce blood loss. All surgeons have their own recipe. Check the dosage being used, in practice this is seldom a concern (see liposuction p512).

- Fewer than 5% of patients require transfusion. Mild falls in haemoglobin are well tolerated in this young patient group.
- Moderate reductions may involve removal of 500g of tissue per breast.

Postoperative

- Bilateral breast reduction does not cause significant postoperative pain. Following a dose of morphine towards the end of surgery, regular simple analgesics and NSAIDs are adequate. IV PCA is generally unnecessary. An occasional dose of IM opioid may be required.
- Haematoma formation is an early complication. Occasionally nipple perfusion may be compromised and require decompression of the pedicle. Return to theatre may be indicated. Later complications include wound infection, dehiscence, and fat necrosis.

Special considerations

Occasionally patients for massive breast reduction are encountered (>1kg tissue removal per breast). 2 to 4U of blood should be cross-matched. The complication rate is higher. Older patients may have coexisting cardiopulmonary disease and require further investigation. Intubation and IPPV is the preferred technique.

Breast augmentation

Procedure	Bilateral or unilateral augmentation of breast size
Time	90min
Pain	++/+++
Position	Supine, 30° head up. Arms may be out on boards, or with elbows flexed and hands placed behind the upper part of the buttocks
Blood loss	Minimal
Practical techniques	Spontaneous ventilation or IPPV via LMA

Preoperative
- Breast augmentation may be performed for:
  - Reconstruction following mastectomy.
  - Correction of breast asymmetry.
  - Aesthetic bilateral augmentation.
- Patients are usually fit and well. Check FBC.

Perioperative
- Position on the operating table as for breast reduction.
- Conventional augmentation involves creation of a SC pocket for a silicone implant via an inframammary incision.
- Modern techniques involve pocket formation by the insertion of an inflatable capsule mounted on an introducer via a small incision in the anterior axillary line. This is then removed and the implant inserted.

Postoperative
- Postoperative discomfort may be related to the size of the implants. Large implants cause more tissue stretching and postoperative pain. In general, breast augmentation appears to cause more discomfort than breast reduction. Give regular NSAIDs and simple analgesics. Opioid analgesia may be needed but PCA techniques are seldom required.
- Haematoma formation may require early return to theatre. Later complications include infection, capsule formation, and rupture.

Special considerations
- An association between silicone breast implants and development of systemic symptoms of connective tissue diseases has been suggested. This association has not been proven following data from large studies.
- Soybean-oil-filled implants have been withdrawn from use in the United Kingdom. There are insufficient data concerning the long-term consequences of soybean oil breakdown. Saline implants are not perceived as sufficiently realistic and are unpopular with many women.
- Breast reconstruction following mastectomy is common. Options include insertion of a breast implant, reconstruction with a pedicled myocutaneous flap (e.g. latissimus dorsi or transverse rectus abdominis muscle 'TRAM'), or a free flap repair (usually TRAM).

Correction of prominent ears

Procedure	Surgical correction of prominent ears, usually caused by the absence of an antehelical fold.
	May be unilateral
Time	1hr
Pain	+
Position	Supine, 30° head up
Blood loss	Minimal
Practical techniques	Day case anaesthesia, flexible LMA and spontaneous ventilation

Preoperative
- Patients are usually children (4–10yr) and fit. May not present for surgery until teenage or early adulthood.
- Surgery is offered as child grows older and is aware of prominent ears. Often precipitated by teasing at school. Child may be self-conscious and anxious.
- Obtain consent for suppositories.

Perioperative
- Day case anaesthetic technique.
- Anaesthetic machine usually at the foot end.
- PONV is common. Propofol maintenance is well tolerated.
- Avoid morphine. Use shorter-acting opioids (fentanyl or alfentanil) and NSAIDs.
- The surgeons use extensive LA/adrenaline infiltration to aid surgery. This provides good analgesia.
- 20ml/kg crystalloid IV may improve the quality of early recovery.

Postoperative
- NSAIDs (e.g. ibuprofen syrup 20–30mg/kg/day) and paracetamol.
- Dressings should be firm without being excessively tight. Scalp discomfort and itching can be a source of discomfort.
- Excessive pain may be due to haematoma formation and requires a return to theatre for drainage.

Special considerations
Allow time for extensive bandaging at the end of the operation. If a COETT is used early reduction in anaesthetic depth will lead to coughing when the head is manipulated for bandage application. An LMA is ideal.

Facelift (rhytidectomy)

Procedure	Surgical reduction of facial folds and wrinkles to create a more youthful appearance
Time	3–4hr. More extensive procedures 6–8hr
Pain	+
Position	Supine, 30° head up
Blood loss	Minimal
Practical techniques	IPPV via LMA or ETT, hypotensive technique, facial nerve blocks

Preoperative
- Most patients are aged 45–65yr. Patients are usually fit and well. They may have high expectations of anaesthesia and surgery and may have undergone previous facelift procedures.
- NSAIDs should be discontinued for at least 2wk prior to surgery.

Perioperative
- Many surgeons in the United States perform routine facelift procedures under LA infiltration alone. Cost constraints in patients who are self-funding have contributed to this practice. Standard practice in the United Kingdom is for GA. Facelifts should always be regarded as major procedures.
- Incisions are placed in concealed areas (e.g. preauricular, extending up to the temporal region within the hair). The skin is mobilised by SC undermining and wrinkles/skin folds are improved by traction. Redundant skin is excised. Surgery is adapted to suit the needs of the patient and may include forehead lift, upper and lower blepharoplasty, and removal of sub-mental/submandibular fat. It is occasionally combined with septorhinoplasty.
- Discuss the choice of airway device with the surgeon (e.g. oral tube or nasal north-facing). Consider using a throat pack if there is nasal surgery.
- The anaesthetic machine is usually at the patient's foot end. Long breathing system tubing and drip extension sets are required.
- A moderate hypotensive technique (70–80 systolic) and 30° head up tilt will help minimise blood loss and improve surgical conditions. Remifentanil is ideal.
- Routine antiemetics.
- LA infiltration and specific nerve blocks provide good postoperative pain relief.
- Use a warming blanket.

Postoperative

- A smooth emergence is important to avoid bleeding beneath delicate suture lines. Propofol maintenance and flexible LMA are ideal. Avoid postoperative shivering (treat with pethidine 25mg IV). Bleeding and haematoma formation may require an early return to theatre.
- Pain is not a prominent feature. Discomfort is attributed to platysma tightening. Postoperative NSAIDs and simple analgesics are required. Marked pain should raise the suspicion of haematoma formation.

Special considerations

- The observed benefits from facelift procedures may only last 3–5yr. Repeat operations are common. Some patients may undergo several facelifts during their lifetime.
- Recent advances have involved more extensive procedures with deeper tissue undermining. These are all performed under GA. The composite facelift mobilises platysma, cheek fat, and orbicularis oculi muscle. This flap is then repositioned *en bloc* with the overlying skin. Complications are more frequent.

Free flap surgery

Procedure	The transfer of tissue from a donor site and microvascular anastomosis to a distant recipient site
Time	Variable depending on procedure. Minimum 4hr, often 6–8hr or longer
Pain	+++
Position	Variable. Usually supine. May require position change during surgery
Blood loss	Often 4–6U
Practical techniques	ETT + IPPV, arterial + CVP lines, urinary catheter, epidural catheter for lower limb flaps

Preoperative

- Free flaps are most commonly used to provide tissue cover following trauma or resection for malignancy. This is a widely used reconstructive technique. Understand what operation is proposed and what the aims of surgery are. Typical procedures are:
  - Free transverse rectus abdominis muscle (TRAM) myocutaneous flap to reconstruct a breast following mastectomy.
  - Free gracilis muscle flap to cover an area of lower limb trauma with tissue loss.
  - Free radial forearm fasciocutaneous flap to the oropharynx following tumour excision.
- The aim of anaesthesia is to produce a hyperdynamic circulation with high cardiac output, adequate vasodilation, and wide pulse pressure. Patients with lower limb trauma are often young and fit. Patients with head and neck cancer are often smokers with ischaemic heart disease. The elderly or patients with limited cardiorespiratory reserve may not be suitable for surgery.

Perioperative

- Be prepared for a long surgical procedure. All patients should receive a balanced GA. Regional anaesthesia alone is seldom appropriate for these long procedures.
- Isoflurane is the inhalational agent of choice due to its beneficial effects on systemic vascular resistance (SVR). Propofol maintenance is also ideal since it lowers SVR, is rapidly metabolised, anti-emetic, and may avoid postoperative shivering (there is also some *in vitro* evidence that propofol may be more favourable for microvascular flow by avoiding the effect of volatiles on red cell membrane stiffness). Remifentanil is used by many.
- A regional block is helpful to supplement anaesthesia. The sympathetic block and dense analgesia produce excellent conditions for graft survival. Lower limb flaps are especially suitable. Surgery on multiple sites may not all be covered by the block. Skin grafts are often taken from the leg to cover a muscle flap.

- Anaesthetic management requires a good practical knowledge of circulatory physiology. Blood flow through the microvasculature must be optimal to help ensure flap survival. Blood flow is primarily influenced by changes in perfusion pressure, calibre of vessel, and blood viscosity (Hagen–Poiseuille formula). We only have a superficial understanding of the physiology of the microcirculation. Much of our anaesthetic management is based on perceived wisdom, rather than on the results of randomised controlled trials.

- Monitor core (e.g. rectal, oesophageal) and peripheral temperature. Insulate the skin probe from any overlying warming blanket. Aim for a normal or even supranormal core temperature and a core-peripheral difference of <2°C. This must be achieved by the time that microvascular anastomosis is commenced. A widening of the core—peripheral temperature difference may herald vasoconstriction. Local vascular spasm may jeopardise the surgery.

- Correct any preoperative fluid deficit and commence volume loading. Continue maintenance crystalloid, and add 10ml/kg colloid bolus (e.g. Gelofusine or Hetastarch) as required to expand the intravascular volume. Aim for CVP 12mmHg (or 2–4mmHg above baseline), urine output 2ml/kg/hr, widened pulse pressure, and low SVR. Colloid will expand the intravascular volume more effectively than crystalloid. Transplanted tissue lacks intact lymphatics and excess crystalloid may contribute to flap oedema. Take care to avoid excessive volume loading in the elderly who are more prone to develop pulmonary oedema.

- Moderate hypotension and haemodilution during the early phase of dissection may help limit blood loss. Thereafter, maintain systolic arterial pressure (SAP) at >100mmHg or higher depending on preoperative blood pressure recordings.

- Viscosity is closely related to haematocrit (Hct). Viscosity rises dramatically when Hct >40%. Aim for 30%, which in theory gives the best balance between blood viscosity, arterial oxygen content, and tissue oxygen delivery.

- Dextran reduces platelet adhesiveness and factor VIII concentration. It may help maintain graft patency. Depending on surgical preference, give 500ml Dextran 40 during the procedure, and include 500ml in the daily IV fluid for 2–3d.

- Potent vasodilators (e.g. sodium nitroprusside, hydralazine, and phenoxybenzamine) are unnecessary. Sufficient vasodilation can be produced by the anaesthetic agent provided that the patient is warm, volume loaded, pain free, and normocarbic. Nifedipine 10mg given with the premed and continued three times a day for 5d in high-risk patients such as smokers, diabetics, and arteriopaths may improve flap survival. Chlorpromazine 1–2mg IV (dilute a 50mg ampoule to give a 1mg/ml solution for injection) is useful to narrow a widened core—peripheral temperature difference when all other factors have been corrected. The surgeon may use papaverine directly on the vessels to prevent local spasm.

- Prophylactic antibiotics are given at induction and may be repeated during the procedure.

Postoperative

- Aim for a smooth emergence.
- Continue meticulous care well into the postoperative period. Flap observation is a specialised nursing skill and care is often best provided on the plastic surgical ward. The need for HDU/ITU may be dictated by patient factors.
- Vasoconstriction from cold, pain, low circulating volume, hypotension, or hypocarbia will put the flap at risk and needs prompt correction.
- Treat shivering with pethidine 25mg IV. Continue with warming blanket in recovery.
- The health of the flap is monitored clinically. Hourly observations include a 'flap chart' where temperature, colour, and arterial pulses (using a Doppler probe if possible) are monitored. A pale, pulseless flap with sluggish capillary filling may indicate problems with the arterial supply. A swollen, dusky flap, which blanches easily with a brisk capillary return, indicates a venous outflow problem. An early surgical decision needs to be made concerning re-exploration.
- Analgesia by continuous epidural is ideal for lower limb flaps. An axillary brachial plexus catheter (e.g. continuous infusion of 0.25% bupivacaine 5ml/h for 2–3d) is useful for procedures on the forearm and hand.
- Careful consideration should be given as to whether more invasive analgesic techniques are justified for procedures on the upper torso (e.g. thoracic epidural or intrapleural analgesia). Potential risks may outweigh the benefits. These patients often do very well with IV patient controlled analgesia (PCA). For head and neck procedures IV PCA is best.
- Attitudes vary concerning perioperative NSAIDs. They are valuable analgesics and reduce platelet adhesiveness. They may produce increased oozing following lengthy and extensive surgery. Administration postoperatively when clot is more established may be preferable.

Special considerations

- The reimplantation of severed digits or limbs should be managed as for a free flap.
- A 'pedicle flap' is constructed when arteriovenous connections remain intact but the raised flap is rotated to fill a neighbouring defect. Examples include rotation of rectus abdominus muscle to fill a sternal wound, rotation of pectoral muscle to reconstruct a defect in the side of the neck following tumour excision, or pedicled latissimus dorsi breast reconstruction. Whilst the procedure may be technically more simple than free tissue transfer, anaesthesia requires similar attention to detail.
- Overall free flap survival is >95%. Flap failure will result in further reconstructive procedures. Patients in poor general condition with coexisting disease have the highest risk of flap failure.

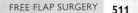

Liposuction

Procedure	Vacuum aspiration of SC fat via a small skin incision and a specialised blunt-ended cannula
Time	Variable 30–90min
Pain	+
Position	Variable, depending on site. Usually supine
Blood loss	1–40% of the volume of fat aspirated, depending on infiltration technique
Practical techniques	Local infiltration with IV sedation/LMA and spontaneous ventilation

Preoperative
- Procedure may be used for:
  - Lipoma removal.
  - Gynaecomastia.
  - Reducing the bulk of transplanted flaps to make them more closely contour the surrounding skin.
  - Cosmetic removal of SC fat ('liposculpture') in the abdominal wall, thighs, buttocks, and arms.
- Patients presenting for aesthetic surgery are often fit and well.

Perioperative
- The total amount of fat aspirated depends on patient requirement and surgical judgement.
- Fat is infiltrated with dilute local anaesthetic with adrenaline. Back and forth movement of the cannula disrupts fatty tissue which is then aspirated either by suction apparatus or syringe.
- Injection of fluid helps fat breakdown and aids aspiration. There are several recipes for SC infiltration solutions: 1000ml warmed Hartmann's containing 50ml 1% lidocaine and 1ml 1:1000 adrenaline is popular. 1ml infiltrate per 1ml aspirate is commonly used (superwet technique).
- The tumescent technique refers to a large volume of LA/adrenaline infiltrate to produce tissue turgor. Developed as an outpatient technique and performed without additional anaesthesia or sedation. 3ml infiltrate per 1ml aspirate are often used. There is little evidence that this technique is superior to the superwet technique, and may produce more complications. It may provide unsatisfactory anaesthesia when used alone. Additional sedation or general anaesthesia may be necessary.
- Blood loss depends on the volume of LA/adrenaline infiltrate used. Loss is approximately 1% of the volume of the aspirate for the tumescent technique. This may increase to 40% without SC infiltration.
- Extensive liposuction physiologically resembles a burn injury and large fluid shifts result. Commence IV infusion for aspirates >1500ml. Replace aspirate 1:1 with IV crystalloid.

Postoperative
- Pressure dressings are usually applied.
- Encourage oral fluids, monitor urine output.
- Check Hct following extensive liposuction (>2500ml aspirate).
- Bruising can be considerable.
- Use NSAIDs and simple analgesics for pain relief.

Special considerations
- Dose safety limits for large-volume LA infiltration are controversial. Doses significantly higher than the conventional lidocaine toxic dose (5mg/kg) are often used, e.g. 30–70mg/kg. This may be possible due to the adrenaline producing slower drug absorption, the poor vascularity of fat, and the aspiration of much of the infused solution before the drug has been absorbed.
- Complications are associated with excessive liposuction. In the United Kingdom aspiration is restricted to approximately 2 litres of fat. Considerably higher volume procedures have been reported especially in the United States (in excess of 10 litres). Deaths have occurred from pulmonary oedema and lidocaine toxicity. Morbidity is related to high aspiration volume and high lidocaine dosage.

Skin grafting

Procedure	Free skin grafts applied to surgically created raw surfaces following debridement, or to granulating wounds
Time	Variable 30min–2hr
Pain	++/+++ (especially the donor site)
Position	Variable. Depends on the area to be grafted. Usually supine
Blood loss	Nil for simple grafts. Extensive debridement and grafting of burns may require 6–8U
Practical techniques	GA/LMA spontaneous respiration (with lateral cutaneous nerve of thigh or femoral 3 in 1 block if thigh donor site). Spinal for lower limb surgery

Preoperative
- Patients for simple excision and grafting of isolated lesions may be otherwise well.
- Elderly patients for excision/grafting of skin lesions or pretibial lacerations may be in poor general health. A local or regional technique may be preferable to a GA.
- Patients with extensive burns for debridement and grafting require careful assessment—see below

Perioperative
- Full thickness skin graft (FTSG). Consists of epidermis and dermis. Used in small areas where the thickness, appearance, and texture of skin are important. Usually harvested with a scalpel. FTSG can be harvested using SC LA infiltration with a 27G needle. Addition of hyaluronidase aids spread (e.g. 1500IU to 100ml of LA solution). The donor site needs to be closed directly:
  - postauricular skin for grafts to the face
  - groin or antecubital fossa to the hand for management of flexion contractures.
- Split skin graft (SSG). Consists of epidermis and variable portion of dermis. Much wider usage than FTSG. Usually harvested with a skin graft knife or power-driven dermatome. Donor sites will heal spontaneously within 2wk. Donor sites are chosen according to the amount of skin required, colour and texture match, and local convenience. Meshing is used to expand the extent of the area that the graft is required to cover. Common donor sites are thigh, flexor aspect of forearm, upper arm, or abdomen. SSG can be harvested using LA cream. It should be applied at least 2hr in advance and covered with an occlusive dressing. Anaesthesia does not extend into the deeper dermis so the technique is unsuitable for FTSG. Lateral cutaneous nerve of thigh (LCNT) or femoral 3 in 1 block provides useful analgesia of a thigh donor site. Excess harvested skin can be stored at 4°C for 2–3wk.

Postoperative

- The SSG donor site is a potentially painful wound. Supplement with local anaesthesia (LCNT or femoral block) where possible. The type of dressing is important for donor site comfort. 'Kaltostat' alginate dressing impregnated with LA (e.g. 40ml 0.25% bupivacaine) is commonly used. Dressings are difficult to secure on the thigh and frequently slip when the patient mobilises. A thin adhesive fabric dressing (e.g. sterile 'Mefix') is used by some surgeons and may afford better protection and donor site comfort. The dressing is soaked off after 2wk. NSAIDs and simple analgesics are usually required for 3–4d. Itching follows when the acute pain settles and healing is under way.

Special considerations

Burns Patients (see also p838)

- Extensive debridement and grafting of burns is a major procedure. These patients should receive a balanced GA. Current management is to aim to debride burnt tissue and cover with SSG at the earliest opportunity (often within 48hr). This converts the burn to a healthy surgical wound. Potential sources of sepsis are eradicated, fluid shifts are less, and intensive care management tends to be more stable.
- Two anaesthetists may be required. Two surgical teams will considerably speed up the procedure and help minimise complications.
- Blood loss. Ensure 6–8U are crossmatched. Debrided tissue bleeds freely. Losses can be difficult to estimate, particularly in small children. Regularly check Hct and maintain at approximately 30%.
- Temperature control. A large exposed body surface area will lose heat rapidly by radiation and evaporation. Measure core temperature. Use all methods available for heat conservation. Little body surface area may be available for warming blankets. Maintain the operating theatre at 25°C.
- Monitoring. Placement of non-invasive monitoring devices may be difficult. An arterial line facilitates measurement of blood pressure and blood sampling. A central venous line is valuable to provide reliable venous access for this and future procedures, and help in the management of intravascular volume. Maintain strict asepsis during line insertion. Cannulae may need to be stitched. Try to place through intact skin. A urinary catheter is essential.
- Suxamethonium is contraindicated except in the first 24hr following burn. Massive K^+ release may cause cardiac arrest.
- Postoperative care. Return to the burns unit. Large body surface area burns (e.g. >40%) or those with additional injury (e.g. smoke inhalation) may need continued ventilation on ICU until warm and stable.
- Analgesia is best provided by IV opioids either as PCA or continuous infusion. Suggest early intervention of the acute pain team. Dressing changes may be helped by Entonox or ketamine/midazolam sedation.
- Antibiotics and early nutrition are important to increase survival.

Other plastic surgical procedures

Operation	Description	Time (min)	Pain (+ to +++++)	Position	Blood loss/ X-match	Notes
Abdominoplasty	Excision of redundant lower abdominal skin	120	++ to +++	Supine	G&S	LMA or ETT, IPPV
Carpal tunnel release	Release of flexor sheath at the wrist to relieve median nerve entrapment	30	+	Supine, arm board	Nil (tourniquet)	LA infiltration, or brachial plexus block, or day case GA
Dupuytren's contracture	Excision of contracted palmar fascia	60–90	+	Supine, arm board	Nil (tourniquet)	Brachial plexus block, or day case GA
External angular dermoid	Excision of congenital dermoid cyst usually from lateral supraorbital ridge	30	ns	Supine, head ring	Nil	LMA and spontaneous ventilation
Flexor/extensor tendon repair	Repair of hand tendons following trauma. Often multiple. May be extensive. May involve nerve/vessel repairs	30–120+	+ to ++	Supine, arm board	Nil (tourniquet)	Brachial plexus block ± GA, LMA and spontaneous ventilation, IPPV for extensive repairs
Gynaecomastia	Excision or liposuction of excess male breast tissue	45	+ to ++	Supine	Nil	LMA and spontaneous ventilation

Hypospadias repair	Correction of congenital abnormality of male urethra. Usually infant	90	++	Supine	Nil	LMA and spontaneous ventilation. Caudal or penile block
Insertion of tissue expander	SC insertion of saline-filled silastic bags, often scalp	45	+ to ++	Supine, head ring	Nil	LMA and spontaneous ventilation
Neck, axilla, or groin dissection	Block dissection of regional lymph nodes to excise secondary malignant disease	90–120	++	Supine, head ring	2U	LMA or ETT, IPPV
Preauricular sinus	Excision of congenital sinus tract, often bilateral	45	+	Supine, head ring	Nil	LMA and spontaneous ventilation
Pretibial laceration	Excision of pretibial wound and SSG	45	+ to ++	Supine	Nil	Spinal or GA
Syndactyly	Release of congenital fusion of two or more digits. May be bilateral. May require FTSG	60–180	++	Supine	Nil (tourniquet)	LMA and spontaneous ventilation. ETT + IPPV for extensive repairs

General surgery

Matt Rucklidge

Anaesthesia for elective laparotomy

General considerations
Anaesthesia for laparotomy is generally straightforward in a fit young adult, but is associated with significant morbidity/mortality in the elderly or compromised patient.

Major surgery generates a strong inflammatory response which leads to an increase in oxygen demand which in the healthy patient is met by increasing cardiac output; however patients who do not have the physiological reserve to compensate for this increase in stress are at high risk of complications after surgery.

Preoperative
- History, examination, ECG, FBC, U&Es, and coagulation screen.
- Antithrombotic measures (see p10).
- Optimise cardiac and respiratory function.
- Consider overnight IV fluid prior to surgery if inadequate fluid intake, impaired renal function or if there is evidence of jaundice or dehydration. Preoperative bowel preparation can result in significant dehydration.
- Discuss analgesia options. If neuraxial block is planned and the patient is receiving low molecular weight heparin ensure this is administered at least 12hr in advance of the scheduled time of surgery.
- Discuss invasive monitoring, including arterial and central venous pressure lines if appropriate.
- Discuss rapid sequence induction if indicated. Consider premedication with H_2 antagonist or proton pump inhibitor.
- Consider whether HDU/ICU care is indicated postoperatively and ensure bed is booked before surgery.

Perioperative
- Large bore IV access with long extension if access to arms likely to be restricted.
- Site epidural if consent obtained and administer test dose (see below).
- Rapid sequence induction if evidence of abdominal obstruction or risk of aspiration.
- Insert nasogastric tube if required by surgeons.
- Prophylactic antibiotics (see p1163).
- Avoid prolonged exposure during preparation for surgery and establish active patient warming (fluid warmer, hot air blanket, insulation) as soon as possible. Monitor central temperature with a rectal or naso-pharyngeal temperature probe.
- Urinary catheter.
- Postoperative nausea and vomiting are common after gastro-intestinal surgery. Administer an antiemetic in theatre and prescribe postoperatively.

- Procedures may be prolonged; pay special attention to pressure areas whilst positioning. Be prepared for lithotomy or Lloyd-Davies position with head down tilt. Prolonged surgery in this position may require higher FiO_2 and PEEP to maintain oxygenation.
- Pay close attention to fluid balance. Significant fluid losses take place from an open abdomen and during intra-peritoneal dissection.
- Provide muscle relaxation until the abdomen is closed.
- Aspirate the nasogastric tube prior to waking and extubation.

Postoperative

- Continue active patient warming in recovery.
- Prescribe supplemental oxygen for up to 72hr.
- Arrange a chest radiograph if CVP line sited.
- Continue close monitoring of fluid balance. Consider on-going losses from abdominal drains, ileostomy, NG aspirate, and blood. In high-risk patients and following major surgery measure urine output hourly for at least 48hr.
- Consider daily FBC/U&Es until return of normal bowel function.
- Close management of postoperative pain; effective analgesia may reduce respiratory complications.

Intra-operative invasive monitoring

- Balance the pre-existing health of the patient with the planned complexity and duration of the surgical procedure and consider the additional information invasive monitoring will provide against risks involved in its placement and interpretation.
- The oesophageal Doppler provides a minimally invasive means of real time continuous cardiac output monitoring as well indicating preload, afterload, and myocardial contractility. It is increasingly used to guide fluid titration during major bowel surgery. (See p984.)

Suggested indications for invasive monitoring

Central venous pressure	Large fluid shifts, major blood loss, CVS or renal compromise, prolonged surgery, vasopressors required.
Arterial line	CVS ± respiratory compromise, major blood loss, need for blood gas sampling.
Oesophageal Doppler	Major abdominal surgery with large fluid shifts, CVS compromise, patient likely to require perioperative inotropes.

Analgesia

Abdominal incisions are painful for several days and associated with reduced ability to cough and a reduction in FRC. There are three main approaches to analgesia:

- Simple IM/SC opioids for less invasive procedures, e.g. appendicectomy, reversal of colostomy.
- Opioids by continuous IV infusion or by PCA e.g. lower abdominal procedures, open cholecystectomy following failed laparoscopy or for any laparotomy when an epidural is contra-indicated or refused. Continuous infusion techniques may be preferable in the elderly population who may become confused postoperatively and unable to use a PCA effectively. Ensure additional oxygen therapy and hourly sedation/pain scoring.
- Epidural analgesia (see p1038): provides better analgesia especially for upper abdominal incisions, although there is a 10–30% failure rate over three days of infusions.

Regular paracetamol should be administered concurrently to reduce opioid or epidural requirements. Rectal administration if impaired bowel function prohibits oral administration. Prescribe NSAIDs with caution in the elderly population undergoing major surgery; this group may be very susceptible to the side effects of these drugs.

Epidural analgesia

This is commonly used for patients undergoing laparotomy.

Advantages include

- Improved pain relief. Thoracic epidurals provide superior analgesia to systemic opioids for laparotomy.
- Improved postoperative respiratory function resulting in reduced incidence of respiratory failure.
- Improved postoperative gastrointestinal motility.
- Improved myocardial function. By providing superior analgesia, stress induced increases in heart rate, coronary vasoconstriction, and myocardial workload are reduced.
- Potentially improved postoperative patient mobilisation.
- Reduction in thromboembolism.
- Reduced sedation and postoperative nausea and vomiting.

Disadvantages include

- Risks related to insertion including postdural puncture headache, epidural haematoma or abscess.
- Risk related to misplaced catheter e.g. intrathecal, intravascular.
- Perioperative hypotension.
- Epidural failure (can be as high as 30% for postoperative analgesia).
- Postoperative motor blockade impeding patient mobilisation.
- Itch associated with epidural opioids.
- Urinary retention.

Epidural analgesia and outcome after abdominal surgery

Whilst improved analgesia is well established, the influence of epidural analgesia on mortality/morbidity following major abdominal surgery is controversial. A meta-analysis of randomised controlled trials found neuraxial block was associated with significantly decreased perioperative morbidity and mortality;[1] however a large randomised controlled trial, the MASTER Anaesthesia Trial demonstrated no significant improvement in major morbidity or mortality between control or epidural groups in the trial[2] or in selected subgroups at increased risk of respiratory or cardiac complications.[3]

Practical considerations for epidural analgesia

- The catheter should be sited at an appropriate level. A useful guide is to place the catheter at a level corresponding to the dermatome innervating the middle of the planned abdominal incision. In general, site at T10–T11 for lower abdominal procedures and T8–T9 for upper abdominal procedures. Failure of analgesia is common if the catheter is placed too low.
- Placement whilst awake or anaesthetised is controversial. Inserting the epidural awake is probably safer in adults (especially if thoracic) since it enables patient feedback during insertion and test dosing.
- Intra-operatively epidural loading dose of 8–10ml of 0.25–0.5% bupivacaine with 50–100µg fentanyl (divide into 3–4ml boluses) and assess response.
- Bupivacaine takes 15–20min to achieve its maximum spread and top ups should be performed cautiously. An extensive sympathetic block may develop with relatively low volumes of local anaesthetic in thoracic epidurals.
- If extensive bleeding is expected, or in cardiovascularly unstable patients, it is often wise to avoid epidural local anaesthetic until bleeding is controlled and the patient has stabilised. Epidural opioids alone may be a safer option.
- Epidural block for AP resection (which requires analgesia and anaesthesia across thoracic, lumbar, and sacral dermatomes) can be difficult. Effectiveness of the epidural may be improved by the addition of epidural opioid and larger volumes of weak anaesthetic solution, e.g. 0.125% bupivacaine. Consider supplementing general anaesthesia with a short-acting opioid, e.g. remifentanil/alfentanil. The epidural is usually effective for postoperative (mainly incisional) pain.
- Treat hypotension with fluids and vasopressors to ensure end-organ perfusion.
- An appropriate regime for postoperative analgesia consists of a mix of LA and opioid, e.g. bupivacaine 0.167% + diamorphine 0.1mg/ml (2–8ml/hr), bupivacaine 0.125% + fentanyl 4µg/ml (2–8ml/hr).

1 Rodgers A et al. (2000). Reduction of post-operative mortality and morbidity with epidural or spinal anaesthesia: results of overview from randomized trials. British Medical Journal, 321, 1493–1497.
2 Rigg JRA et al. (2002). Epidural anesthesia and analgesia and outcome of major surgery: a randomized trial. Lancet, 359, 1276–1282.
3 Peyton P et al. (2003). Perioperative epidural analgesia and outcome after major abdominal surgery in high risk patients. Regional Anesthesia, 96, 548–554.

Temperature control

Patients undergoing general anaesthesia become hypothermic due to impairment of thermoregulatory control and surgical heat loss.[1] Patients undergoing laparotomy are at high risk due to prolonged procedures, an open abdomen, and limited access for external body warming. Even mild hypothermia is associated with a number of adverse outcomes:
- Myocardial ischaemia or arrhythmias.
- Increased intra-operative blood loss and requirement for transfusion.
- Increased surgical wound infection.
- Prolonged duration of action of neuromuscular antagonists.
- Increased duration of recovery and possible increased hospital stay.

Hypothermia develops in a characteristic three-phase pattern.
- Phase 1: rapid reduction in core temperature of 1–1.5°C within first 30–45min as the tonic vasoconstriction that normally maintains core to periphery temperature gradient is inhibited.
- Phase 2: more gradual reduction in core temperature of a further 1°C over the next 2–3hr due to heat loss by radiation, convection, and evaporation exceeding heat gain determined by metabolic rate. Evaporative heat loss is exacerbated during major abdominal surgery.
- Phase 3: a plateau phase where heat loss is matched by metabolic heat production. Occurs when anaesthetised patients become sufficiently hypothermic that vasoconstriction is triggered. If a thoracic epidural is used, compensatory vasoconstriction is lost.

Cutaneous warming
- Passive insulation. A single layer of insulation (e.g. space blanket) traps a layer of air and may reduce cutaneous heat loss by 30%. Insulation to exposed areas, e.g. wrapping the head, may further reduce heat loss.
- Active warming. Forced air warming devices are more effective than passive insulation. They reduce heat loss through radiation and may increase heat gain if forced air is warmer than the skin. Active warming by a circulating water mattress is less efficient.

Internal warming
- Airway humidification. A heat and moisture exchange filter (HME) humidifies and warms inhaled gases; however <10% of heat loss occurs via the respiratory tract.
- Fluid warming. Prevents conductive heat loss associated with the administration of cold fluids. Use fluid warming devices when large amounts of fluid or blood are anticipated.
- Invasive internal warming techniques. Cardiopulmonary bypass and peritoneal dialysis are very effective at transferring significant heat but are not relevant for management of mild perioperative hypothermia. The use of irrigation fluids in the bladder or abdomen which have not been warmed to body temperature may induce significant heat loss.

1 Sessler DI (2000). Perioperative heat balance. *Anesthesiology*, **92**, 578–596.

Fluid management

Patients undergoing laparotomy are at risk of significant fluid loss. Appropriate fluid administration maintains cardiac output and oxygen delivery permitting development of an appropriate stress response preserving end organ function. There is some evidence that outcome following major surgery can be improved by effective IV fluid therapy optimising cardiovascular filling. Inotropes or vasopressors will also be needed in some patients.

Causes of fluid loss include

- Preoperative: reduced fluid intake secondary to underlying disease process and preoperative fasting. Increased fluid losses due to vomiting, bowel preparation, and sequestration into an obstructed bowel.
- Intra-operative: large evaporative losses from the peritoneal cavity through the abdominal incision, sequestration of fluid into the omentum and bowel lumen (third space loss), blood loss, nasogastric loss, evaporative loss from the respiratory tract, urine production.
- Postoperative: ongoing sequestration of fluid into the omentum and bowel (paralytic ileus), ongoing nasogastric loss, urine production, ongoing blood loss.

Losses must be replaced with an individualised fluid regime. Those with large preoperative fluid deficits should have IV fluids instigated well before surgery and CVP monitoring considered. During surgery with an open abdomen, crystalloid maintenance rates are between 10 and 30ml/kg/hr. Significant fluid shifts may affect serum electrolyte concentrations and these should be monitored throughout the perioperative period.

Postoperative paralytic ileus

- Bowel function begins to return 24–36hr postoperatively, but may not return to normal until 72hr or longer. Prolonged ileus leads to collection of fluid and gas in the bowel resulting in distension, pain, nausea, vomiting, and delayed mobilisation/discharge. The aetiology of ileus is multifactorial and includes manipulation of the bowel at surgery, hormonal stress response, increased sympathetic activity, postoperative pain, immobility, opioids, hypokalaemia, and other electrolyte imbalances.

Operation	Description	Time (hr)	Pain (+ to +++++)	Position	Blood loss (l)	Notes
Hemicolectomy	Resection of right or left hemicolon	1–3	++++	Supine	0.5	Low thoracic epidural or opioid infusion/PCA
Sigmoid colectomy	Resection of sigmoid colon with bowel anastomosis	1–3	++++	Supine. Head down. May need Lloyd-Davies	0.5–1.0	Low thoracic epidural or opioid infusion/PCA
Hartmann's procedure	Resection of sigmoid colon with colostomy	1–3	++++	Supine. Head down. May need Lloyd-Davies	0.5–1.0	Low thoracic epidural or opioid infusion/PCA
Anterior resection	Resection of rectum	2–3	++++	Head down. Lloyd-Davies	0.5–1.5	Low thoracic epidural
AP resection	Resection of rectum and anus	2–4	+++++	Head down. Lloyd-Davies	0.5–2.0	Low thoracic epidural. Can be difficult to block sacral nerve roots. CVP line
Gastrectomy	Resection of stomach	2–3	+++++	Supine	0.5–1.0	Thoracic epidural, consider CVP/art line
Cholecystectomy (open)	Resection of gall bladder	1	+++/++++	Supine	0.5	Right upper quadrant incision. PCA
Closure of loop colostomy or loop ileostomy	Local closure of colostomy or loop ileostomy	0.5–1	++	Supine	Nil	Still requires muscle relaxation. May need PCA
Reversal of Hartmann's	Laparotomy. Bowel ends re-anastomosed	1–2	++++	Supine. Head down. May need Lloyd-Davies	0.5–1.5	Low thoracic epidural

The sick laparotomy

(See also 'Septic shock' p848–851)

Patients for emergency abdominal surgery are at greater risk of perioperative complications than those presenting electively. Poor outcome is associated with inability to mount a physiological response to the systemic inflammatory response, poor cardiac function, and reduced DO_2. The time available for preparation is often limited and it is important to balance the benefits of preoperative resuscitation with those of timely surgery. Whatever the underlying pathology, disordered cellular metabolism results in generalised organ system dysfunction including:

- Cardiovascular—widespread vasodilatation, loss of reactivity to catecholamines, depressed myocardial function, arrhythmias.
- Pulmonary—acute lung injury or ARDS, fluid extravasation into pulmonary interstitium, alveolar collapse, hypoxaemia, shunting, reduced compliance and FRC, and increased work of breathing.
- Haematological—DIC with low platelets, hypofibrinogenaemia, prolonged clotting times.
- Renal—hypoperfusion due to relative hypovolaemia and systemic vasodilatation may result in renal failure and altered drug clearance.
- Metabolic—impaired glucose tolerance, altered drug metabolism.
- Hepatic—impaired hepatic oxygen delivery at a time of increased hepatic oxygen consumption resulting in liver dysfunction.

Preoperative assessment

- Discuss the probable diagnosis with the surgical team. Different abdominal problems have different implications for anaesthetic management:

Surgical problem	Anaesthetic implications and management
Upper intestinal perforation	Often haemodynamically stable. Early surgery improves outcome.
Lower intestinal perforation	With heavy faecal soiling mortality is high. Postoperative ICU/HDU should be routine as deterioration is common.
Bowel obstruction	May be hypovolaemic due to third space losses. Usually time for preoperative resuscitation. Beware risk of perforation.
Ischaemic bowel	May be painless and sometimes difficult to diagnose. Frequently acidotic and warrants urgent laparotomy. Consider postoperative ICU/HDU.
Haematemesis/malaena	Often difficult to assess blood loss. Hypovolaemic shock common. Consider immediate transfer to theatre for laparotomy or endoscopy to locate bleeding point.

- Investigations: FBC, electrolytes (include magnesium if possible), LFTs, amylase, clotting, ECG, chest radiograph, and crossmatch.
- ABGs and lactate are useful to assess the degree of metabolic derangement and may indicate severity of illness, impact of resuscitation, and the appropriate environment for perioperative care.
  An unresponsive metabolic acidosis is a poor predictor of outcome.

Perioperative haemodynamic optimisation

Pre-optimisation has been shown to improve survival in high risk elective surgery and the same principles apply to the compromised emergency patient. The ultimate goals are to restore effective tissue perfusion and oxygen delivery. In addition, there is increasing evidence that early attempts to restore tissue perfusion and oxygen delivery may reduce mortality in patients with sepsis and septic shock.[1]

Haemodynamic support[2]

- Fluid infusion should be the initial step. Crystalloids or colloids are equally effective.
- Haemoglobin concentrations should be maintained above 8g/dl.
- Once adequate fluid resuscitation use vasopressors to achieve adequate tissue perfusion. Noradrenaline and dopamine are both effective. Dopamine use may be limited by tachycardia.
- Administration of low dose dopamine to maintain renal perfusion is not recommended.
- Dobutamine is the first choice inotrope in patients with low cardiac index despite fluid resuscitation ± vasopressor.
- Patients with hypotension refractory to vasopressors may benefit from addition of replacement dose of steroids, e.g. hydrocortisone 200–300mg/d for 7d.

Monitoring

- Invasive arterial and CVP monitoring are advisable and should be established preoperatively.
- The oesophageal Doppler allows real time estimation of stroke volume and cardiac output and may be a useful monitor to guide fluid therapy, vasopressor, and inotrope use in the sick laparotomy patient.
- Central venous oxygen saturation ($ScvO_2$) may be a useful marker of cardiac performance and its measurement may help guide haemodynamic therapy. Aim for $ScvO_2 \geq 70\%$.[3]

Preoperative preparation

- Finding the correct balance between preoperative resuscitation and surgical urgency is critical, though often difficult. Preoperative admission to ICU/HDU, invasive CVP and arterial pressure, aggressive rehydration, and occasionally inotropic support may be appropriate.

1 Rivers E et al. (2001). Early goal-directed therapy in the treatment of severe sepsis and septic shock. N Engl J Med, **345**, 1368–1377.
2 Hollenberg S et al. (2004). Practice parameters for haemodynamic support of sepsis in adult patients: 2004 update. Crit Care Med, **32**, 1928–1944.
3 Sessler DI (2000). Perioperative heat balance. Anesthesiology, **92**, 578–596.

- Oxygen should be administered preoperatively to all sick patients.
- Initial resuscitation should aim to restore intravascular volume and perfusion with colloid or blood depending on haematocrit. Once an adequate circulating volume is achieved, prescribe crystalloid and/or colloid to maintain hydration and perfusion.
- Fluid resuscitation should be guided by the response to fluid challenges of heart rate, blood pressure, urine output, CVP, peripheral perfusion, and in some cases oesophageal Doppler indices and $ScvO_2$.
- A nasogastric tube should be inserted in patients presenting with intestinal obstruction.
- Electrolytes will often be deranged and should be corrected as far as possible prior to surgery.
- Monitor blood sugar closely. Known diabetics are likely to demonstrate poorer blood sugar control and non-diabetics may develop impaired glucose tolerance due to the septic process. Tight control of blood sugar using intensive insulin therapy may reduce morbidity and mortality among critically ill patients.[1]
- Metabolic acidosis should improve with aggressive fluid and cardiovascular manipulation. If the pH does not respond and remains low (<7.2) the patient is at high risk. Tissue hypoxia is the likely cause of acidosis if blood lactate is high. If acidotic with normal lactate, exclude renal failure and underlying metabolic disorders e.g. diabetic ketoacidosis. If surgery is indicated and the pH unresponsive, 1mmol/kg(1ml/kg) of 8.4% sodium bicarbonate IV should be considered.
- Thrombocytopenia and coagulopathies should be anticipated and treated appropriately, especially in the septic patient and following transfusion of large volumes of stored blood. Liaise with the haematologists for transfusion of blood products. Increased INR indicates septic coagulopathy (unless on warfarin) and may require administration of vitamin K (5–10mg slow IV).
- Use IV morphine for pain control prior to surgery and avoid NSAIDs in the critically ill due to risk of renal damage, decreased platelet function, and gastroduodenal ulceration in an already stressed patient.
- Check that appropriate antibiotics have been given if indicated.

Perioperative care

- Consider anaesthetising all sick patients on the operating table in theatre, and in some cases insist the theatre team are scrubbed and prepared for surgery.
- Aspirate nasogastric tube prior to induction.
- Have a large-bore IV infusion running connected to pressurised fluids.
- Anticipate hypotension following induction. Have vasopressors (ephedrine and metaraminol) and vagolytics (atropine, glycopyrronium) drawn up and to hand.
- Preoxygenate and perform rapid sequence induction.
- Choice of induction agent and dose depends on cardiovascular stability. Thiopental is commonly used for rapid sequence induction; propofol is probably best avoided in the hypotensive patient. Etomidate causes less hypotension on induction however may temporarily interfere with steroid synthesis so its use in critically ill patients (already at

risk of adrenocortical insufficiency) is controversial.[2] If etomidate is used, administer steroid cover with 50–100mg hydrocortisone. Ketamine (1–2mg/kg IV) may be useful in the severely compromised patient, but avoid in those with pre-existing cardiovascular disease.

- Relaxants. Suxamethonium for rapid sequence then use drugs metabolised independently of liver and renal function, e.g. atracurium.
- Analgesia. Centroneuraxial blockade should be used cautiously in this group of compromised patients. Disadvantages include the risk of infective complications, excessive hypotension, and potential complications due to coagulopathy. If an epidural is used, local anaesthetic agents should be restricted until cardiovascular stability is achieved. In some patients this may be postoperatively on the ICU.
- Fentanyl/morphine for intra-operative analgesia. Give with induction and supplement as needed. Caution with remifentanil; may cause significant hypotension if hypovolaemic.
- Patients who require repeated doses of vasopressors (ephedrine or metaraminol) despite an adequately restored circulating volume, should be commenced on an infusion of vasopressor/inotrope early. The choice of agent may be difficult. Noradrenaline is the first choice for the vasodilated septic patient. Dopamine may be useful in patients with compromised systolic function but causes more tachycardia and may be more arrhythmogenic. Dobutamine may be useful in patients with measured or suspected low cardiac output in the presence of adequate fluid resuscitation but may worsen hypotension if fluid resuscitation is inadequate. In the emergency situation an infusion of adrenaline (make up 1:10 000 and start at 5ml/hr) can be commenced and continued until the most appropriate agent is determined.
- Active warming should be strenuously undertaken with the aim of maintaining normothermia (see p524).

Postoperative

- Wherever possible, compromised patients who have undergone major surgery should be nursed in HDU/ICU for a period of stabilisation. Patients who are cold, cardiovascularly unstable, acidotic, or hypoxic should be kept intubated and ventilated until stable. If inotropes/vasopressors have been needed in theatre they should be continued postoperatively. If an ICU/HDU bed is unavailable, patients should be kept in recovery for ongoing observation and support.
- Frequent review of postoperative fluid balance guided by vital signs ± CVP measurement.
- Urine output should be measured hourly throughout the perioperative period maintaining an output >0.5ml/kg/hr.
- Postoperative CXR to check CVP line position.
- Administer oxygen for a minimum of 72hr postoperatively.
- Regular chest physiotherapy.

1 Van den Berghe G et al. (2001). Intensive insulin therapy in critically ill patients. N Engl J Med, **345**, 1359–1367.
2 Morris C, McAllister C (2005). Etomidate for emergency anaesthesia; mad, bad and dangerous to know? Anaesthesia, **60**, 737–740.

Anaesthesia for laparoscopic surgery

Laparoscopic surgery is widely established for a range of increasingly complex procedures including cholecystectomy, fundoplication, hernia repair, appendicectomy, and nephrectomy. There is also an increase in the number of emergency operations performed laparoscopically. Benefits of laparoscopy over laparotomy include:

- Reduced tissue trauma, wound size, and postoperative pain.
- Improved postoperative respiratory function, reduced postoperative ileus.
- Earlier mobilisation, shorter hospital stays.
- Improved cosmetic results.

Surgical requirements

- Insufflation of gas (usually carbon dioxide) into the peritoneal cavity creates a pneumoperitoneum and separates the abdominal wall from the viscera.
- Carbon dioxide, being non-combustible, allows the use of diathermy or laser.
- Carbon dioxide is insufflated at a rate of 4–6l/min to a pressure of 10–20mmHg.
- The pneumoperitoneum is maintained by a constant gas flow of 200–400ml/min.

Physiological effects of pneumoperitoneum

Respiratory
Airway pressure	↑
FRC	↓
Pulmonary compliance	↓
V/Q mismatch	↑

Cardiovascular
Venous return	↓
Systemic vascular resistance	↑
Cardiac output	↔↓
Risk of arrhythmias	↑

Gastrointestinal
Risk of regurgitation	↑

Neurological
ICP	↔↑
CPP	↔↓

Patient Positioning

- Upper abdominal procedures, place head up (reverse Trendelenburg). Lower abdominal procedures, place head down (Trendelenburg). Some left tilt is usual with cholecystectomy.
- Patients placed head down are at greater risk of reduction in FRC, V/Q mismatch and atelectasis. Cephalad movement of the lungs and carina in relation to a fixed endotracheal tube increases the risk of endobronchial intubation.
- Patients placed head up are at increased risk of reduced blood pressure and cardiac output due to decreased venous return. Those most at risk include the hypovolaemic patient, the elderly, and patients with pre-existing cardiovascular disease.

Effects of gas insufflation

- Carbon dioxide is the most frequently used gas—being colourless, non-flammable, non-toxic and highly soluble.
- Stretching of peritoneum may cause vagal stimulation resulting in sinus bradycardia, nodal rhythm, and occasional asystole. Anticipate and treat with vagolytics.
- CO_2 is readily absorbed from the peritoneum and may cause hypercarbia and acidosis.
- Extra-peritoneal gas insufflation may occur through a misplaced trocar or insufflation needle, via an anatomical defect (e.g. between pleura and peritoneum), or when gas under pressure within the abdomen dissects through tissue planes. This may result in subcutaneous emphysema, pneumomediastinum, pneumopericardium, or pneumothorax.
- Venous gas embolism may rarely occur when gas is inadvertently insufflated directly into a blood vessel. Physiological effects are less with CO_2 than air due to its greater plasma solubility; however a significant embolism may be fatal. Signs of venous gas embolism include reduced $ETCO_2$, desaturation, arrhythmias, myocardial ischaemia, hypotension, and elevated CVP (see p415).
- Sympathetic response. Hypertension and tachycardia are often observed.
- CVS depression with a fall in cardiac output. Treat with fluids, vasodilators, inotropes.

Trauma

- Introduction of trocars may cause damage to organs (e.g. spleen, bladder, liver, bowel, stomach). Organ damage may not always be apparent at the time of injury.
- Damage to blood vessels may result in massive haemorrhage necessitating rapid conversion to an open procedure.

Preoperative

- Contraindications to laparoscopic surgery are relative; risks are increased with ischaemic heart disease, valvular heart disease, increased intracranial pressure, and hypovolaemia.
- NCEPOD 1996/1997 recommended caution in patients who were ASA >3, age >69yr, those with a history of cardiac failure, and widespread ischaemic heart disease. Minimally invasive surgery may not be minimally stressful to the patient.
- All patients scheduled must be considered at risk of conversion to an open procedure.
- Laparoscopic procedures are increasingly performed in obese patients due to improved postoperative recovery when compared to an open procedure.
- Premedication with H_2-antagonists or proton pump inhibitors if at risk of aspiration (e.g. obesity, hiatus hernia). Simple analgesics (paracetamol, NSAIDs) may be beneficial.

Perioperative

- General anaesthesia with endotracheal intubation, muscle relaxation, and controlled ventilation is considered the safest technique as it protects against pulmonary aspiration, enables control of $PaCO_2$, and aids surgical exposure.
- Avoid gastric distension during bag-mask ventilation. A gastric tube may be required to deflate the stomach to reduce risk of gastric injury during trocar insertion and to improve surgical view.
- For lower abdominal procedures a urinary catheter may be required to decompress the bladder and reduce risk of injury.
- Systemic absorption of CO_2 and raised intra-abdominal pressure will require increased minute volume and result in higher intrathoracic pressure.
- Aim for normocarbia but beware of adverse affects of high intrathoracic pressure. Controlling $ETCO_2$ during prolonged procedures, especially in the obese and head down position can be difficult and may occasionally necessitate intermittent release of intraperitoneal gas or tolerance of a degree of hypercarbia.
- Nitrous oxide is controversial due to possible associations with bowel distension and increased postoperative nausea and vomiting.
- Analgesia: dictated by the procedure. Pain may be intense but short-lived and short acting opioids, e.g. fentanyl, alfentanil may be effective for short procedures. Remifentanil infusion can be useful for longer procedures. Longer acting opioids may be required for extensive laparoscopic operations.
- Fluids: avoid hypovolaemia as this exaggerates the deleterious CVS effects of laparoscopy.

- Anti-emetics: high incidence of nausea and vomiting following laparo-scopic surgery. Give prophylactic antiemetic and prescribe postoperatively.
- Monitoring: Pay close attention to $ETCO_2$ and airway pressure. In addition to standard monitoring with neuromuscular monitoring, invasive arterial blood pressure and CVP monitoring may be required for extensive procedures, or for patients with CVS or respiratory compromise.

If hypoxia occurs consider:
- Hypoventilation—inadequate ventilation due to pneumoperitoneum, head down position etc.
- Reduced cardiac output—IVC compression, arrhythmias, haemorrhage, myocardial depression, venous gas embolism, extra-peritoneal gas.
- V/Q mismatch—reduced FRC, atelectasis, endobronchial intubation, venous gas embolism, pulmonary aspiration, and rarely pneumothorax.
- Subcutaneous emphysema during the procedure should arouse suspicion—stop gas insufflation immediately and check for the source of the problem.

Postoperative
- At the end of the operation encourage the surgeon to expel as much intra-peritoneal gas as possible to reduce postoperative pain.
- Intra-peritoneal local anaesthetic ± infiltration of port sites may reduce postoperative analgesia requirements. 20–30ml of 0.25% bupivacaine on the gallbladder bed may reduce postoperative analgesic requirements for laparoscopic cholecystectomy.
- Pain varies and is often worst in the first few hours. Shoulder tip pain due to diaphragmatic irritation may be troublesome but is usually short-lived. Significant pain extending beyond the first day raises the possibility of intra-abdominal complications.
- Prescribe regular paracetamol and NSAIDs with opioid PRN for more extensive procedures. Postoperative antiemetic.

Special considerations
- LMA: some anaesthetists use an LMA for laparoscopic procedures. This is an individual choice but should be avoided with a history of reflux or obesity, an anticipated difficult or prolonged procedure or an inexperienced surgeon. An LMA may be useful for short procedures (e.g. laparoscopic sterilisation) provided that the anaesthetist is experienced and patient selection appropriate. The proseal LMA has a drainage tube to permit drainage of gastric secretions, provides a higher seal pressure than the standard LMA and may offer theoretical advantages.
- Regional anaesthesia is not generally used as the sole anaesthetic technique because of the high level of block required to cover the pneumoperitoneum.
- Laparoscopic appendicectomy: may aid diagnosis of patients with right lower quadrant pain and prevent unnecessary laparotomy. Less useful if perforated appendix is suspected.

Anaesthesia for breast surgery

See also Breast reduction (p496) and Breast augmentation (p498).

General considerations

Breast cancer accounts for 30% of all new cancer cases in women in the UK. Mortality from breast cancer has fallen steadily since 1990, probably because of earlier detection and improved treatment. However it accounts for 15% of all female cancer deaths. The last decade has seen the development of more extensive combined procedures of breast resection and reconstruction. Patients are often anxious and management of postoperative pain and nausea/vomiting may be difficult.

Preoperative

- Anxiety often high. Important to gain patient's confidence at the preoperative visit, discuss analgesia, and prescribe anxiolysis (e.g. temazepam 10–20mg) if necessary.
- Patients who have recently undergone chemotherapy may be immuno-compromised. Check FBC for evidence of bone marrow suppression and anticipate potentially difficult venous access.
- Reconstructive procedures, mastectomy following radiotherapy, mastectomy where breasts are large, and breast reduction surgery increase the risk of blood loss. Check Hb and ensure blood is grouped and saved.

Perioperative

- Standard monitoring is appropriate for most procedures. Longer procedures will require active warming and temperature measurement.
- Avoid venous access on the side of surgery.
- Additional invasive monitoring may be required for prolonged reconstructive procedures including free flap surgery (see p508).
- LMA and spontaneous ventilation is often appropriate for short to medium length procedures. Intubation and mechanical ventilation for prolonged procedures, the obese and patients at risk of aspiration.
- Balanced analgesia including NSAID if tolerated, systemic opioid or regional techniques if necessary (see below).
- Breast surgery patients are at high risk of PONV. Avoid causative agents and administer prophylactic anti-emetic.

Regional analgesia

- Regional techniques may offer advantages in some cases; however the risks in healthy women undergoing minor procedures often outweigh the benefits.
- Consider for more radical procedures, e.g. radical mastectomy/axillary clearance or breast reconstruction.
- Four types of regional analgesia can be used: paravertebral block, thoracic epidural, intercostal blocks, and intrapleural block. Beware of complications of each technique.

Postoperative
- HDU may be required after extensive procedures.
- If paravertebral catheter or thoracic epidural sited continue infusion postoperatively.

Special considerations
- Patients may present with previous breast surgery and axillary clearance. Cannulation should be avoided in the arm on the affected side due to the risk of infection and potential development of lymphoedema.
- Chronic pain typically presenting in the affected anterior chest wall, ipsilateral axilla or upper arm may occur following breast surgery. Intensity of pain following extensive surgery, postoperative radiotherapy, and chemotherapy are risk factors.

Laparoscopic cholecystectomy

Procedure	Laparoscopic removal of gall bladder
Time	40–80min
Pain	+++/++++
Position	Supine, 15–20 degree head up, table tilted towards surgeon
Blood loss	Not significant
Practical techniques	GA, ETT, IPPV

Preoperative
- Patients classically 'female, forty, fair, fat, and fertile'.
- The procedure is potentially painful.
- Consider NSAID and paracetamol premedication.

Perioperative
- The stomach may need deflating; insert a large bore naso/oro-gastric tube following intubation and remove at the end of surgery.
- 16G IV access—haemodynamic changes may be profound and potential for sudden blood loss.
- Combination of pneumoperitoneum and obesity may make ventilation difficult.
- Surgical time is variable and operator dependent.
- Ask the surgeon to infiltrate port sites with local anaesthetic at the end.
- Conversion to open procedure typically about 5%. This is usually due to difficulty identifying the cystic duct, suspected common bile duct injury, uncontrolled bleeding from the cystic artery, stones present in the common bile duct or acute inflammatory changes. see p527.

Postoperative
- High incidence of PONV.
- Pain can be severe and often requires opioids.

Special considerations
- This can be a very stimulating procedure, particularly during diathermy around the liver.
- Local anaesthetic applied to the gall bladder bed may reduce postoperative analgesic requirements (20ml 0.25% bupivacaine).
- Laparoscopic cholecystectomy, on appropriately selected patients, is now being performed on a day surgical basis in some centres.

Appendicectomy

Procedure	Resection of appendix
Time	20–40min
Pain	++/+++
Position	Supine
Blood loss	Not significant
Practical techniques	Rapid sequence induction, ETT, IPPV, ±ilioinguinal block

Preoperative
- Patients are usually aged 5–20yr and are often fit unless appendix ruptured.
- Occasionally present in the elderly. May be the presenting condition of caecal adenocarcinoma requiring right hemicolectomy.
- Check fluid status and replace deficit prior to surgery if possible.
- Consent for suppositories.
- If considering ilioinguinal block, warn of possible associated femoral nerve blockade.

Perioperative
- Rapid sequence induction.
- Muscle relaxation required for surgery.
- Consider rectal NSAID and paracetamol.
- Ask the surgeon to infiltrate locally or perform right ilio-inguinal nerve block.
- Extubate awake on left side.

Postoperative
- Prescribe regular simple analgesics, PRN opioid, antiemetic, and IV fluids until tolerating oral fluids.

Inguinal hernia repair

Procedure	Repair of inguinal muscular canal defect through which bowel protrudes
Time	30–60min
Pain	++/+++
Position	Supine
Blood loss	Not significant
Practical techniques	GA, SV, LMA, inguinal field block
	Spinal
	Local infiltration and/or sedation

Preoperative
Patients are usually adult males or young children.

Perioperative
- Likely to need opioid if not using a local technique.
- Inguinal hernia field block may be used as sole technique for surgery or to complement general anaesthesia (see p1096).
- Iliohypogastric and ilioinguinal nerves are easily blocked 2cm caudal and medial to the anterior superior iliac spine (see p1096). Genitofemoral nerve is located 1–2cm above the midpoint of the inguinal ligament, deep to the aponeurosis of external oblique. This may be left to the surgeon to block, reducing the risk of vascular or peritoneal puncture.

Special considerations
- Often performed as a day case procedure.
- If day case, prescribe adequate analgesia to take home, e.g. NSAID, paracetamol ± tramadol 50–100mg qds.
- Repair using inguinal hernia field block is probably the technique of choice in the high-risk patient if operator is experienced in local anaesthetic techniques.
- Mesh insertion usually requires administration of prophylactic antibiotics.

Haemorrhoidectomy

Procedure	Excision of haemorrhoids
Time	20min
Pain	++/+++
Position	Supine, lithotomy, head down
Blood loss	Not significant
Practical techniques	GA, SV LMA ± caudal Spinal ('saddle block')

Preoperative
Assess suitability for LMA/lithotomy/head down position. Consider ETT if the patient is obese or history of reflux.

Perioperative
- Opioid analgesia (fentanyl or alfentanil)—short but intensely painful stimulus.
- Caudal anaesthesia is useful for postoperative analgesia (bupivacaine 0.25% 20ml), but beware risk of urinary retention. Infiltration by the surgeon during the procedure is usually as effective.
- Potential for bradycardia/asystole as surgery starts. Anticipate and have vagolytics to hand.

Postoperative
Avoid PR route of drug administration.

Special considerations
- Avoid spinal followed by head down tilt.
- Anal stretch is an intense stimulus. There is a risk of laryngospasm and coughing if anaesthesia too light. Anticipate and deepen the anaesthetic, e.g. increase volatile and give a bolus of short acting opioid e.g. alfentanil (500µg). The anal stretch can also produce an increase in vagal tone.
- A sacral only spinal block ('saddle block') using heavy bupivacaine is a useful alternative with little effect on cardiovascular dynamics.
- Antibiotic prophylaxis for patients at risk of endocarditis.

Testicular surgery

Procedure	Removal/biopsy of testis, marsupialisation of hydrocele, vasectomy, testicular torsion
Time	30min–1hr
Pain	++/+++
Position	Supine
Blood loss	Not significant
Practical techniques	GA, LMA ± spermatic cord block
	RSI/ETT if emergency (e.g. torsion)
	Spinal
	LA infiltration

Preoperative
- May be suitable for day surgery.

Perioperative
- Beware vagal responses—have atropine ready.

Special considerations
- Innervation of testes and scrotum: somatic innervation is via ilioinguinal, genitofemoral, pudendal, and posterior scrotal nerves (branches of posterior cutaneous nerve of the thigh) with nerve root contributions from L1–S3. Autonomic innervation is from the sympathetic chain T10–L4 and the parasympathetic plexus S1–S3. Local techniques therefore need to cover T10–S3.
- A spermatic cord block can be used as an adjunct to GA or as part of a local technique for scrotal surgery. The block covers all nerves except the pudendal and posterior scrotal branches. If used as part of a local anaesthetic technique supplemental infiltration of the scrotal skin is also required.
- Spermatic cord is best blocked under direct vision by the surgeon. However, if a local technique is planned, feel for the spermatic cord as it enters the top of the scrotum and infiltrate 5–10ml local anaesthetic around it.

Chapter 21

Liver transplantation and resection

Mark Bellamy

General principles

Patients presenting for liver transplantation have either acute hepatic failure or end-stage liver disease. The majority of transplants are performed semi-electively in those with end-stage disease. Wordwide, the commonest indication for hepatic transplantation is post-hepatitis C cirrhosis. This is likely to change in the future as more effective anti-viral therapies become available.

Preoperative assessment includes investigation/treatment of:
- Jaundice, hyponatraemia, ascites, pleural effusions, diabetes
- Renal failure
- Systemic vasodilatation with hypotension, cardiac failure
- Poor nutritional state and decreased muscle mass
- Portopulmonary syndromes (associated severe portal and pulmonary hypertension leading to right ventricular failure and potential cardiac arrest intra-operatively)
- Hepatopulmonary syndromes (hypoxia and intrapulmonary shunting occurs in 0.5–4% of patients with cirrhotic liver disease)
- Varices (oesophageal, gastric, rectal, abdominal wall)
- Coagulopathy (prolonged prothrombin time, low platelet count, fibrinolysis)

Haemodynamic instability can result from cardiac involvement in the underlying process (e.g. alcoholic cardiomyopathy), from pericardial effusions, or from circulatory failure due to dilatation and low SVR. Anaemia resulting in a low plasma viscosity further reduces SVR.

Surgical techniques vary, but there are a number of common features:
- Stage 1 of the operation is dissection (which involves laparotomy) and haemostasis (including ligation of varices). The liver is exposed, its anatomy defined, and slings placed around the major vessels.
- Stage 2 of the operation is the anhepatic phase during which the hepatic artery, portal vein, hepatic veins, and bile duct are divided. The liver, together with its included portion of vena cava, is then removed and the donor liver implanted. Anastomoses are made between donor and recipient vena cava, and recipient and donor portal vein. Venous return during this phase is severely compromised leading to haemodynamic instability. Venovenous bypass is employed in some centres to facilitate venous return from the lower part of the body (femoral vein to right internal jugular or brachiocephalic vein). During this stage, patients with acute liver failure may become profoundly hypoglycaemic, although this is less common in patients being transplanted for chronic liver disease.
- Stage 3 of the procedure is the post-reperfusion phase, beginning with the re-establishment of blood flow through the liver (portal vein to vena cava). This may be accompanied by a massive reperfusion syndrome, comprising release of cytokines, complement activation, transient reduction in core temperature, arrhythmias, and hypotension. Immediately after reperfusion, there is a rapid elevation in plasma K^+ as it is washed out of the liver graft (up to 8–9mmol/l). Preservation solution constituents, including adenosine, may also have a clinically important effect (bradycardia, hypotension).

As the cell membranes of the graft begin to function normally, electrolyte gradients are restored and a fall in plasma K^+ ensues (sometimes producing ventricular ectopic beats). Hypotension at this stage results from myocardial depression and subsequently from vasodilatation. Myocardial depression usually resolves within 2 or 3min, but the vasodilatation may persist for several hours. Following reperfusion, the hepatic artery is re-anastomosed and finally the bile duct reconstructed, either by direct duct-to-duct anastomosis, or by construction of a Roux loop.

Liver transplantation

Procedure	Transplantation of entire liver
Time	4–10h
Pain	Variable, but less than other comparable procedures (e.g. gastrectomy, thoracotomy). Back pain/shoulder pain may be a feature. PCA (occasionally epidural) effective
Position	Supine, arms out
Blood loss	0–4000ml, X-match 10U (initially, then use uncrossmatched if necessary) and FFP 12U. Cell saver mandatory (typically reinfuse 2000ml)
Practical techniques	ET, IPPV—details below

Preoperative

- Includes investigation and correction of the factors mentioned above.
- Usual tests include: FBC, U&Es, clotting, ECG, echocardiogram, stress ECG/dobutamine stress echo, chest radiograph, liver/chest CT, spirometry, immunology, virology, and hepatic angiographic MRI scan.
- Preoperative fluids are not routinely administered except in patients with renal impairment or hyperacute liver failure (dextrose-based solutions).

Perioperative

- Establish peripheral venous and arterial access before induction.
- Induce anaesthesia (propofol, thiopental, or etomidate) and relaxant (atracurium, vecuronium). Vasopressors may be required.
- Ventilate to normocarbia using oxygen-enriched air and volatile agent (isoflurane or sevoflurane). Establish infusion of an opioid agent (alfentanil, remifentanil, or fentanyl). Patients undergoing transplantation for fulminant liver failure are at risk of raised intracranial pressure. In this patient group volatile agents must be avoided and TCI propofol used. ICP monitoring may be used depending upon the jaundice–encephalopathy interval (0–7d always—raised ICP in 70% of cases, 7–28d occasionally—raised ICP in 20%, 28–90d seldom—raised ICP in 4%).
- Establish central venous monitoring. Transoesophageal echocardiography (TOE) may be used in some centres. Insert a large-bore nasogastric tube. In patients with suspected pulmonary hypertension there may be a role for pulmonary artery catheterisation.
- Lines for venovenous bypass can either be placed by the surgical team using femoral cut downs, or inserted percutaneously, using extra corporeal membrane oxygenation lines (21Fr in the right internal jugular and right femoral veins). These are used both for venovenous bypass and large vascular access. Venovenous bypass uses heparin–Carmeda bonded circuitry, so systemic anticoagulation is unnecessary.

- The patient's temperature must be rigorously maintained as hypothermia quickly develops especially during the anhepatic phase, or with massive transfusion. A forced warm air blanket should be placed over the patient's head, upper chest and arms, and another over the legs.
- Fluids are administered by a rapid infusion system and are warmed through a counter-current heating mechanism (e.g. Level-1® system with high-flow disposables and high-flow taps, allowing transfusion of 600ml/min at body temperature). Perioperatively and postoperatively, the Hct is maintained between 0.26 and 0.32 by infusion of blood, and the right ventricular end-diastolic volume index maintained at 140ml/m^2 by infusion of other colloidal fluids as appropriate.
- FFP is transfused approximately 2U per unit of blood transfused. Clotting is monitored and fine-tuned by thromboelastography.
- Antifibrinolytic agents are commonly administered—tranexamic acid (15mg/kg bolus then 5mg/kg/h by infusion) is given during the anhepatic phase.
- A dextrose-containing solution is infused continuously to maintain blood sugar.
- K^+ and Ca^{2+} should be monitored regularly during surgery and supplemented when required to maintain normal values. Hypocalcaemia is common during the anhepatic phase as a result of chelation with un-metabolised citrate. This can lead to cardiac depression and poor clotting. Recheck electrolytes immediately prior to graft reperfusion.
- Severe metabolic acidosis is common but rarely needs correction. At the start of reperfusion, a bolus dose of 10mmol of calcium is administered to protect the patient against the cardiac effects of potassium released from the liver graft. Progressive hypotension follows reperfusion. This may be severe and require small incremental IV doses of adrenaline (50μg) to maintain mean arterial pressure at a clinically acceptable value (above 70mmHg). In severely ill patients, an infusion of noradrenaline may subsequently be required.
- Coagulopathy with defibrination and thrombocytopenia may also occur at graft reperfusion. Treatment includes bolus doses of antifibrinolytic drugs and platelets, as guided by the thromboelastograph. The haemodynamic and biochemical mayhem of graft reperfusion should resolve rapidly in the event of a functioning liver graft. Persisting acidosis or hypocalcaemia are suggestive of graft primary non-function, which represents a transplantation emergency. This may necessitate urgent retransplantation.
- There is no proven strategy for avoiding renal failure, other than optimising fluid balance and avoiding any nephrotoxins.

Postoperative

- Patients should be managed on the ICU. Early extubation is often feasible. As a result of improved techniques, the mean intensive care stay post-transplant can be reduced to 6hr.
- Analgesia: PCA/epidural/paravertebral blocks have all been used to good effect. Epidural analgesia is possible in only a minority of cases because of coagulopathy. Avoid NSAIDs (interaction with calcineurin inhibitors to induce renal failure).

- Postoperative fluids: maintenance fluid/nasogastric feed at 1.5ml/kg/h. Give blood/HAS/FFP to maintain CVP at 10–12mmHg, Hct at 0.26–0.32, and PT <23s.
- Bleeding postoperatively is relatively uncommon (5–10%).
- Graft primary non-function occurs in up to 5% of cases, requiring retransplantation.
- Hepatic artery thrombosis occurs in 0.5–5% of cases. Thrombectomy may be attempted, but super-urgent re-transplantation may be necessary.
- Other postoperative problems include sepsis (10–20%) and acute rejection (up to 40%). These are managed medically with good results.
- Immunosuppression is usually started with standard triple therapy (steroid/azathioprine/tacrolimus) and then tailored to the individual. Other drugs in current use include ciclosporin, mycophenolate mofetil, sirolimus and basiliximab.
- Long-term results of liver transplantation are encouraging. One-year survival figures in major centres now run between 85–95%, with a good long-term quality of life.

Hepatic resection

Procedure	Resection of liver tissue
Time	3–12hr
Pain	As for transplantation
Position	Supine, arms out
Blood loss	1000ml, X-match 10U
Practical techniques	ET, IPPV. Details below and p546

The major indication for hepatic resection is metastatic colorectal ade-nocarcinoma. Most patients presenting for hepatic resection are other-wise relatively fit. Stigmata of liver disease and significant jaundice are unusual except in those presenting for radical hepatic resection for cholangiocarcinoma, where some patients require biliary stenting or drainage preoperatively to reduce jaundice prior to major surgery. The principles underlying anaesthesia for this group of patients are similar to those for any patient undergoing a major laparotomy.

Major liver resection usually results in 75% of the functional hepatic tissue being removed. As the remaining hepatocytes function poorly for some days following surgery, short-acting drugs should be used. Drugs which might compound postoperative hepatic encephalopathy, or which rely on hepatic metabolism, should be avoided (e.g. benzodiazepines). Most resections are accomplished with minimal blood loss but unex-pected catastrophic haemorrhage may occur.

Liver resection operations commence with perihepatic dissection and identification of the vascular anatomy. Once this has been defined (in particular the relationship of lesions to the hepatic veins), resection of the liver can take place. Intra-operative diagnostic ultrasound is often used to pinpoint lesions requiring resection. Bleeding occurs either from vascular inflow to the liver (portal vein, hepatic artery), or by venous back bleeding from the hepatic venous system. Usually, branches of the hepatic artery and portal vein to the segment of liver to be resected have been ligated, so inflow bleeding should not be a major problem. In practice, the line of resection often passes through a watershed area, between vital and devitalised tissue, and remaining inflow bleeding may require additional control by intermittent cross-clamping of vascular inflow to the rest of the liver (the so-called Pringle manoeuvre). This results in a degree of ischaemia-reperfusion injury to the remaining liver tissue, and potentially poor postoperative liver function. This can be minimised by ischaemic preconditioning and the use of intermittent rather than continuous clamping.

Very radical liver resections are now possible where the liver is totally excised, along with its included portion of vena cava, and dissected *ex vivo* on the bench following perfusion with ice-cold preservation solu-tion. Healthy parts of the liver are then attached to a Gore-Tex® vena cava graft and reimplanted. The anaesthetic technique for this prolonged and difficult procedure is very similar to that for liver transplantation.

Preoperative

As for any major abdominal surgery, but including screening of liver function and coagulation.

Perioperative

- All patients undergoing major liver resection should be invasively monitored and have large venous access. Either a 12Fr high-flow central line or a pair of 7.5Fr Swan–Ganz introducer catheters may be substituted.
- Thoracic epidural analgesia is utilised to good effect postoperatively.
- The anaesthetic technique employed should be aimed at preserving hepatic blood flow and minimising liver injury. Artificial ventilation of the lungs with oxygen-enriched air and a volatile agent is the best way of achieving this. Isoflurane and desflurane are associated with the best preservation of hepatic blood flow.

Fluid management

- Maintenance of a high central venous pressure used to be common to reduce the risk of air embolism but it is associated with an increased risk of venous back bleeding.
- A reduced central venous pressure substantially reduces bleeding. This approach has dramatically reduced transfusion requirements, with no reported adverse consequences, despite the theoretically increased risk of air embolus. Techniques for reducing the central venous pressure include epidural boluses and head up (reverse Trendelenburg) tilt. Aim for CVP of 0–2mmHg and systolic BP of 70–80mmHg.
- Intra-operative blood sampling allows accurate transfusion replacement. Fresh frozen plasma is occasionally also required in cases of massive haemorrhage, in cases where there is a prolonged hepatic inflow cross-clamp time, or where very little hepatic tissue remains. However, intra-operative coagulopathy is relatively uncommon. Peak disturbances in clotting are seen on postoperative days 2–3. As with patients undergoing liver transplantation, active warming measures should be taken to maintain the patient's temperature and minimise any coagulopathy.

Postoperative

- Patients should initially be managed in a HDU.
  Coagulopathy and encephalopathy may develop postoperatively in those who have undergone very major resections. This has practical implications for the timing of removal of epidural catheters etc.—which may require FFP cover.
- The overall results of radical hepatic resection are very encouraging with many cases treated that were previously considered inoperable. Many remain disease free 5yr following resection. In those cases where recurrences arise, further hepatic resection is often possible.

Further reading

Anesthesia and Intensive Care for Patients with Liver Disease (1995). Park GR and Kang Y (Eds). London, Butterworth Heinemann.

Chapter 22

Endocrine surgery

Anna Batchelor

Thyroidectomy

Procedure	Removal of all or part of the thyroid gland
Time	1–2hr depending on complexity
Pain	+/++
Position	Bolster between shoulders with head ring. Head-up tilt
Blood loss	Usually minimal. Potentially major if retrosternal extension
Practical techniques	IPPV + reinforced ETT

General considerations (see also p158)
- Complexity can vary from removal of a thyroid nodule to removal of long-standing retrosternal goitre to relieve tracheal compression.
- Retrosternal goitre is usually excised through a standard incision, but occasionally a sternal split is required.
- Recurrent laryngeal nerves and parathyroid glands may be damaged or removed.
- Straightforward unilateral surgery can be performed under superficial and deep cervical plexus block but general anaesthesia is usual (see p1073).

Preoperative
- Ensure that the patient is as near euthyroid as possible—see p158.
- Check for complications associated with hyperthyroidism: AF, tachycardia, proptosis.
- Some preoperative regimes for thyrotoxicosis involving iodine preparations have a narrow window for surgery, discuss with surgeon and endocrinologist.
- Check biopsy histology for malignancy.
- Ask about duration of goitre. Longstanding compression of the trachea may be associated with tracheomalacia.
- Ask about positional breathlessness. Make a routine assessment of the airway.
- Examine the neck. How big is the goitre? Can you feel below the gland (retrosternal spread)? Is there evidence of tracheal deviation (check radiograph)?
- Look for signs of SVC obstruction.
- Listen for stridor.
- Check the range of neck movements preoperatively and do not extend them outside of their normal range during surgery.
- Preoperative paracetamol/NSAIDs (oral or rectal) helps postoperative pain control.

Investigations
- FBC, U&Es, Ca^{2+}, and thyroid function tests are routine.
- Chest radiograph. Check for tracheal deviation and narrowing. Thoracic inlet views may be necessary if retrosternal extension is suspected, and to detect tracheal compression in the anterior-posterior plane (retrosternal enlargement may be asymptomatic).

- CT scan accurately delineates the site and degree of airway encroachment or intraluminal spread. Advisable if there are symptoms of narrowing (e.g. stridor, positional breathlessness), or more than 50% narrowing on the radiograph. Plain radiographs overestimate diameters due to magnification effects and cannot be relied on when predicting endotracheal tube diameter and length.
- ENT consultation to document cord function for medicolegal purposes is not routine in all units unless abnormality is likely e.g. previous surgery and malignancy. Pre-existing cord dysfunction may be asymptomatic. Fibre-optic examination also defines any possible laryngeal displacement (useful in airway planning).

Airway planning

- The majority of cases are straightforward even when there is some tracheal deviation or compression. A reinforced ETT will negotiate most distorted tracheas and permit optimal head positioning. Preoxygenation should be followed by IV induction and a neuromuscular blocking drug (after checking that the lungs can be inflated manually).
- The following features should lead to a more considered approach and may require discussion with the surgeon and radiologist:
  - Malignancy. Cord palsies are likely. Distortion and rigidity of surrounding structures. Possibility of intraluminal spread. Larynx may be displaced. Tumour can produce obstruction anywhere from glottis to carina.
  - Significant respiratory symptoms or >50% narrowing on chest radiograph or lateral thoracic inlet view.
  - Coexisting predictors of difficult intubation.

Options to secure the airway for complicated thyroid surgery

- Teamwork between anaesthetist and surgeon is the key to successful and safe airway management.
- Inhalational induction with sevoflurane or halothane in patients with stridor and suspected difficult upper airway. Stridor and decreased minute ventilation delay the onset of sufficiently deep anaesthesia for intubation. Topical local anaesthetic may be useful. Be prepared for rapid lightening of consciousness whilst attempting intubation.
- Fibre-optic intubation (p948). Attempts to pass a fibre-optic bronchoscope in an awake patient with stridor are difficult as the narrowed airway may become obstructed by the instrument. May be useful where there is marked displacement of the larynx or coexisting difficulties with intubation, e.g. ankylosing spondylitis.
- Tracheostomy under local anaesthetic. This will only be possible if the tracheostomy can be easily performed below the level of obstruction.
- Ventilation through a rigid bronchoscope is a backup option when attempts to pass an ETT fail. The surgeon and necessary equipment should be immediately available for complex cases, particularly involving significant mid to lower tracheal narrowing.

Perioperative

- Eye padding and tape are important, especially if exophthalmos.
- Full relaxation is required to accommodate tube movements. Local anaesthetic spray on the ETT reduces the stimulation produced by tracheal manipulation during surgery.
- Securely fix the ETT with tape, avoiding ties around the neck. Access to check tube is difficult during procedure.
- Head and neck extension with slight head-up tilt.
- Consider a superficial cervical plexus block for postoperative analgesia. Some surgeons infiltrate subcutaneously with local anaesthetic and adrenaline before starting. Local anaesthesia at the end can produce spurious nerve palsies (see p1073).
- Arms to sides, IV extension.
- Communicate with the surgeon if there are excessive airway pressures during manipulation of the trachea. Obstruction may be due to airway manipulation distal to the tube or the bevel of the tube abutting on the trachea.
- Monitor muscle relaxation on the leg.
- In cases of longstanding goitre some surgeons like to feel the trachea before closing to assess tracheomalacia. They may ask for partial withdrawal of the endotracheal tube so that the tip is just proximal to the operative site.
- At end of surgery reverse muscle relaxant and extubate. Any respiratory difficulty should lead to immediate reintubation. The traditional practice of inspecting the cords immediately following extubation is difficult and unreliable. Possible cord dysfunction and postoperative tracheomalacia is better assessed with the patient awake and sitting up in the recovery room.

Postoperative

- Intermittent opioids with oral/rectal paracetamol and NSAIDs.
- The opioid requirement is reduced with SC infiltration or superficial cervical plexus blocks.
- Use fibre-optic nasendoscopy if there is doubt about recurrent laryngeal nerve injury.

Postoperative stridor

- Haemorrhage with tense swelling of the neck. Remove clips from skin, and sutures from platysma/strap muscles to remove the clot. In extremis this should be done at the bedside. Otherwise return to theatre without delay.
- Tracheomalacia. Longstanding goitre may cause tracheal collapse. Immediate reintubation followed by tracheostomy may be necessary.
- Bilateral recurrent laryngeal nerve palsies. This may present with respiratory difficulty immediately postoperatively or after a variable period. Stridor may only be obvious when the patient becomes agitated. Assess by fibre-optic nasendoscopy. May require tracheostomy.

Other postoperative complications

Hypocalcaemia

- Hypocalcaemia from parathyroid removal is rare. Serum calcium should be checked at 24hr and again daily if low.
- Presentation—may present with signs of neuromuscular excitability, tingling around the mouth, or tetany. May progress to fits or ventricular arrhythmias.
- Diagnosis—carpopedal spasm (flexed wrists, fingers drawn together) may be precipitated by cuff inflation (Trousseau's sign). Tapping over the facial nerve at the parotid may cause facial twitching (Chvostek's sign). Prolonged QT interval on ECG.
- Treatment: serum calcium below 2mmol/l should be treated urgently with 10ml 10% calcium gluconate over 3min plus oral alfacalcidol or dihydroxycholecalciferol 1–5g orally. Check level after 4hr and consider calcium infusion if still low. If hypocalcaemic but level above 2mmol/l treat with oral calcium supplements (see also p163).

Thyroid crisis

- This is rare as hyperthyroidism is usually controlled beforehand with antithyroid drugs and β-blockers. May be triggered in uncontrolled or undiagnosed cases by surgery or infection.
- Diagnosis: tachycardia and rising temperature. May be difficult to distinguish from MH. Higher mixed venous $PvCO_2$ and higher CPK in MH.
- Treatment: see p159.

Pneumothorax

Pneumothorax is possible if there has been dissection behind the sternum.

Further reading

Farling PA (2000). Thyroid disease. *British Journal of Anaesthesia*, **85**, 15–28.

Parathyroidectomy

Procedure	Removal of solitary adenoma or four glands for hyperplasia
Time	1–3hr
Pain	+/++
Position	Bolster between shoulders with head ring. Head-up tilt
Blood Loss	Usually minimal
Practical techniques	IPPV + ETT

General considerations (see also p162)

- Usual indication for operation is primary hyperparathyroidism from parathyroid adenoma.
- With preoperative localization, removal of simple adenoma has been described using sedation and local anaesthesia. General anaesthesia is more usual.
- Carcinoma may require *en bloc* dissection.
- Total parathyroidectomy may also be performed in secondary hyperparathyroidism associated with chronic renal failure.
- Hypercalcaemia may produce significant debility, particularly in the elderly.

Preoperative

Hypercalcaemia is usual. With moderate elevation ensure adequate hydration with 0.9% saline. Levels over 3mmol/l should be corrected before surgery as follows:

- Urinary catheter.
- 0.9% saline 1 litre in first hour then 4–6 litres over 24hr.
- Pamidronate 60mg in 500ml saline over 4hr.
- Watch for fluid overload. CVP measurement may be necessary in some patients. Monitor electrolytes including magnesium, phosphate, and potassium.
- Severe hypercalcaemia may occasionally necessitate emergency surgery. Benefits usually outweigh risks as long as managed as above.
- Preoperative imaging using ultrasound and unilateral exploration may be performed for adenoma.
- Secondary hyperparathyroidism occurs secondary to low serum calcium in chronic renal failure. In this situation:
  - Total parathyroidectomy may be required. Control afterwards is easier if no functioning parathyroid tissue is left.
  - Dialysis will be required preoperatively.
  - The risk of bleeding is increased.
  - Alfacalcidol is usually started preoperatively.
- Primary hyperparathyroidism has been associated with increased risk of death from cardiovascular disease, hypertension, left ventricular hypertrophy (LVH), valvular and myocardial calcifications, impaired vascular reactivity, alterations in cardiac conduction, impaired glucose metabolism and dyslipidaemia. Parathyroid hormone has serious consequences on cardiac function in renal failure.

- Methylene blue may be used to highlight parathyroid glands. Most useful in four gland hyperplasia, parathyroids are highly vascular and take up the dye faster than surrounding tissues. If given too far in advance the effect is lost as surrounding tissue colours. The usual dose is 5mg/kg diluted into 500ml given over 1hr prior to surgery. Complications of methylene blue use include restlessness, paraesthesia, burning sensation, chest pain, dizziness, headache, and mental confusion. Pulse oximetry will not be accurate if infusion is too fast.

Perioperative
- Similar anaesthetic considerations as for thyroid surgery.
- Airway encroachment is not usually a problem.
- Operation times may be unpredictable, especially if frozen section or parathyroid assays are performed.
- Consider active heat conservation.

Postoperative
- Serum calcium checked at 6 and 24hr. Hypocalcaemia may occur (for diagnosis and treatment see p557, 'Thyroidectomy' and also p163). Continuation of alfacalcidol in secondary hyperparathyroidism lessens the chance of hypocalcaemia postoperatively.
- Perform fibre-optic nasendoscopy if recurrent laryngeal nerve damage is suspected.
- Pain not usually severe, especially with local anaesthetic infiltration or superficial cervical plexus blocks. Rectal paracetamol is useful. Avoid NSAIDs in patients with poor renal function.

Further reading
Mihai R, Farndon JR (2000). Parathyroid disease and calcium metabolism. *British Journal of Anaesthesia*, **85**, 29–43.

Phaeochromocytoma

Procedure	Removal of 1 or 2 adrenals or extra-adrenal tumour
Time	1–2hr open, possibly longer if laparoscopic
Pain	+/++ (depending if open or laparoscopic)
Position	Lateral or supine for open, lateral for laparoscopic
Blood loss	Variable
Practical techniques	IPPV + ETT, art & CVP lines, ± cardiac output monitor

- Tumours of chromaffin cells secreting noradrenaline (commonest), adrenaline, or dopamine (least common). May secrete more than one amine.
- May secrete other substances e.g. VIP, ACTH.
- 90% occur in adrenals, 10% bilateral, may be anywhere along the sympathetic chain from base of the skull to pelvis.
- Most are benign, a few are malignant.
- Occur in all age groups, less commonly in children.
- Can occur in association with **m**ultiple **e**ndocrine **n**eoplasia 2A (MEN2A—medullary thyroid carcinoma, parathyroid adenomas), or MEN2B (medullary thyroid carcinoma and Marfanoid features). Both have abnormalities of the RET oncogene on chromosome 10 (see p314).
- Also found in patients with neurofibromatosis and Von Hippel–Lindau syndrome (see p308).

Presentation

- Hypertension can be constant, intermittent, or insignificant.
- Association of palpitations, sweating, and headache with hypertension has a high predictive value.
- Anxiety, nausea and vomiting, weakness and lethargy also common features.
- Acute presentations include pulmonary oedema, myocardial infarction, and cerebrovascular episodes.
- Can present perioperatively. Unless the diagnosis is considered and appropriate treatment instituted the mortality is high—up to 50%.

Diagnosis

- Clinical suspicion.
- With increased genetic testing of families more patients are being diagnosed before they become symptomatic.
- Urinary catecholamines or their metabolites (metadrenaline and nor-metadrenaline) measured either over 24hr or more conveniently overnight.
- CT radiocontrast may provoke phaeo crises and its use must be avoided in unblocked patients. Modern contrast agents may be used.
- MIBG (meta-iodobenzylguanidine) scan—a radio-labelled isotope of iodine taken up by chromaffin tissue.
- MRI.
- Search in the abdomen first and widen the search if tumour not located. MIBG is particularly helpful in revealing unusual sites.

Investigations relevant to anaesthesia

- CVS including cardiac echo (patients with persistent hypertension, those with any history of ischaemia or evidence of heart failure). Patients can present with a catecholamine cardiomyopathy.
- Blood glucose—excess catecholamines result in glycogenolysis and insulin resistance—some patients become frankly diabetic.

Preoperative

- Refer the patient to an experienced team. It is not acceptable to manage on an occasional basis.
- Usual management is sympathetic blockade with first α and then β-blocker if required for tachycardia (phenoxybenzamine and then atenolol).
- Preoperative blockade allows:
  - Safe anaesthesia for the removal of the tumour,
  - Prevents hypertensive response to induction of anaesthesia,
  - Limits the surges in BP seen during tumour handling.
- Avoid unopposed β-blockade—theoretical risk of increasing vasoconstriction and precipitating crisis. Although this has been reported, many patients will already have received β-blockers for hypertension before presentation without adverse effects.
- Prazosin and doxazosin have been used. These are competitive selective α_1 blockers. They do not inhibit presynaptic NA re-uptake and thus avoid the tachycardia seen with non-selective α-blockade. The literature contains reports both in favour and against the use of selective blockade.
- Calcium channel blockers (particularly nicardipine) have been used. This inhibits noradrenaline mediated calcium influx into smooth muscle, but does not affect catecholamine secretion by the tumour.
- Metyrosine is an inhibitor of catecholamine synthesis. It is toxic and not widely used.
- It has been suggested that modern cardiovascular drugs, along with invasive monitoring and better understanding of the physiology, should allow safe removal of the tumours without preoperative preparation. Patients with phaeochromocytoma are very varied, as are their tumours; some patients may have a smooth intra-operative course whilst others may develop acute pulmonary oedema, heart failure and die. Any study inevitably has small numbers of patients. Caution should be exercised in discarding a safe, tried, and tested regime of α- ± β-blockade.

Assessment of sympathetic blockade

- 24hr ambulatory BP monitoring. Aim for BP <140/90 throughout the 24hr period, with heart rate <100bpm.
- Erect and supine BP and heart rate. Should exhibit a marked postural drop with compensatory tachycardia.
- The duration of blockade is determined by the practicalities of tumour localization and scheduling of surgery.
- Blockade is started to treat symptoms as well as to prepare for surgery.

Perioperative

- Laparoscopic or open adrenalectomy through a midline, transverse, or flank incision (introduction of gas for laparoscopic resection can result in hypertension in normal subjects and this may be exaggerated in patients with phaeochromocytomas).
- Premedication as required (e.g. temazepam 20–30mg).
- Monitoring to include direct BP and CVP (triple lumen to allow drug infusions). Consider cardiac output monitoring in patients with CVS disease or catecholamine cardiomyopathy.
- Large-bore IV access.
- Monitor and maintain temperature, particularly during laparoscopic resection which can be prolonged.
- Induction: avoid agents which release histamine and thus catecholamines (use etomidate or propofol, alfentanil or remifentanil, and vecuronium).
- Hypotension is unlikely, but may be treated with adrenaline infusion.
- Maintenance: isoflurane.
- Epidural with opioid and local anaesthetic if appropriate to surgical approach (sympathetic blockade will not prevent catecholamine-induced vasoconstriction), otherwise fentanyl/alfentanil/remifentanil until tumour removal, when morphine can be substituted for postoperative analgesia.
- Fluctuations in BP tend to be transient and medication needs to respond in a similar fashion. SNP is effective and is preferred to phentolamine, because it provides rapid control with no prolonged effects. The doses required are unlikely to lead to toxicity.
- Nicardipine, or magnesium also useful (blocks catecholamine release, blocks receptors, direct vasodilator and possibly myocardial protective).
- Control heart rate at <100bpm with metoprolol or esmolol.
- Once the tumour is resected BP takes several minutes to decline. Prevent hypotension by ensuring an adequate preload. Maintain a high CVP of 10–15mmHg. Several litres of crystalloid may be needed.
- Hypotension following resection can be due to low cardiac output or a low SVR. Treat the first with adrenaline and the latter with noradrenaline. Vasopressin has been used in resistant hypotension. Terlipressin 1mg bolus, followed if required by vasopressin starting at 0.04U per minute then titrated to effect.
- It is unusual to require inotropic support by the time the patient is ready to leave theatre unless there are coexisting medical problems.

Postoperative

- Patient should be nursed in an HDU or ICU for 12hr.
- Monitor blood glucose. Catecholamines cause an increase in glucose levels: in their acute absence blood glucose may drop. Residual β-blockade may limit response to this.
- If both adrenals are resected the patient will require steroid support immediately. Hydrocortisone 100mg bolus in theatre decreasing to maintenance dose after surgical stress. Fludrocortisone 0.1mg daily may be commenced with oral intake.

- Even when only one adrenal is removed patients may occasionally be relatively hypoadrenal and require support. If this is suspected (e.g. unexpectedly low BP) a small dose of hydrocortisone (50mg) will do no harm whilst the result of cortisol estimation is awaited.

Special considerations

Pregnancy

- There are many reports of the combination of a newly diagnosed phaeochromocytoma and pregnancy. Overall mortality is up to 17%.
- Phenoxybenzamine and metoprolol are safe.
- If phaeochromocytoma is diagnosed before midtrimester it should be resected at this stage.
- There is a high mortality associated with normal delivery; consider LSCS with or without resection of the phaeochromocytoma at the same procedure.

Management of an unexpected phaeochromocytoma

- Any patient who has unexplained pulmonary oedema, hypertension, or severe unexpected hypotension should prompt consideration of the diagnosis; however, it can be very difficult. There is no quick available test to support the diagnosis in the acute situation.
- Once the diagnosis has been considered, if possible, surgery should be discontinued to allow acute treatment, investigation, and blockade prior to definitive surgery. Attempts to remove the tumour during a crisis may result in significant morbidity or even mortality.
- Treatment acutely should consist of vasodilators and IV fluid; this may be counterintuitive in a patient with severe pulmonary oedema. The circulating volume in patients with phaeochromocytoma may be markedly reduced and vasodilatation will result in a profound drop in BP. Glyceryl trinitrate can usually be successfully titrated in this situation.
- Patients who present with hypotension have an acutely failing heart due to profound vasoconstriction. These are the most difficult ones in whom to make the diagnosis and to treat. Additional catecholamines in this situation merely fuel the fire but are difficult to resist. The mortality rate is very high.

Further reading

Hull CJ (1986). Phaeochromocytoma—diagnosis, preoperative preparation and anaesthetic management. *British Journal of Anaesthesia*, **58**, 1453–1468.

O'Riordan JA (1997). Pheochromocytomas and anesthesia. *International Anesthesiology Clinics*, **35**, 99–127.

Prys-Roberts C (2000). Phaeochromocytoma—recent progress in its management. *British Journal of Anaesthesia*, **85**, 44–57.

Chapter 23

Urological surgery

Julia Munn

Cystoscopic procedures

- Includes cystoscopy, transurethral resection of the prostate (TURP), bladder neck incision, transurethral resection of bladder tumour, ureteroscopy, and/or stone removal or stent insertion.
- The majority of patients are undergoing procedures for benign prostatic hypertrophy or carcinoma of the bladder. The incidence of both these conditions increases markedly over 60yr and bladder cancer is smoking-related, so patients frequently have coronary artery disease and chronic obstructive airways disease.
- FBC, creatinine, and electrolytes should be checked preoperatively because bladder cancers can bleed insidiously. Both bladder cancer and benign prostatic hypertrophy can cause an obstructive uropathy/renal impairment and drugs and technique should be chosen accordingly.
- Flexible cystoscopy is largely used for diagnostic purposes, does not require full bladder distension, and can normally be performed under local anaesthetic. Biopsies can be taken this way with only a small amount of discomfort and skilled surgeons can perform retrograde ureteric catheterisations. Occasional patients insist on sedation/GA for flexible cystoscopy. Midazolam or propofol is ideal.
- Rigid cystoscopy requires general anaesthesia, due to scope diameter and the use of irrigating solution to distend the bladder and allow visualisation of the surgical field. If large volumes of irrigant are absorbed systemic complications due to fluid overload can result (see TURP syndrome p570).
- Spinal anaesthesia works well for rigid cystoscopic procedures, and is commonly used for TURP. Sensory supply to the urethra, prostate, and bladder neck is from S2–S4. Sensory supply to the bladder however, is from T10–T12 so a higher block is required. Many patients will request sedation. In the elderly population 1–2mg midazolam (± fentanyl 50µg) is usually adequate. Higher doses may result in loss of airway control, confusion, and restlessness. A low-dose propofol infusion is an alternative. Spinal anaesthesia is advantageous for severe COAD, as long as the patient can lie flat without coughing.
- Hyperbaric bupivacaine usually produces a higher block than the isobaric solution, especially when the injection is performed with the patient in the lateral position and then turned supine. 2.5–3ml 'heavy bupivacaine' 0.5% usually gives a block to T10. Do not tilt the patient head down unless the block is not sufficiently high. Alternatively 2.5–3ml plain bupivacaine will give an adequate block for TURP, with less hypotension, but may not be adequate for transurethral bladder surgery.
- Patients with chronic chest disease tend to cough on lying flat. During surgery under regional block coughing can seriously impair surgical access. Sedation can help to reduce the cough impulse.
- Patients with spinal cord injuries (see p240) often require repeated urological procedures. Bladder distension during cystoscopy is very stimulating and prone to cause autonomic hyperreflexia so a GA or spinal is advisable-check previous anaesthetic charts.

- Take particular care positioning elderly patients in lithotomy, especially those with joint replacements.
- Penile erection can make cystoscopy difficult and surgery hazardous. It usually occurs due to surgical stimulation when the depth of anaesthesia is inadequate and can usually be managed by deepening anaesthesia. If the erection still persists small doses of ketamine can be useful.
- Routine antibiotic prophylaxis (single dose of an agent with Gram-negative cover) at induction of anaesthesia has been shown to significantly reduce bacteraemia after TURP, even when preoperative urine is sterile. Patients at risk of acquiring deep-seated infection, i.e. those with abnormal or prosthetic heart valves, prosthetic joints, or aortic grafts will need prophylaxis routinely, with the addition of Gram-positive cover (see p1163).
- DVT prophylaxis: graduated compression stockings are generally considered adequate in low-risk patients undergoing cystoscopic procedures, as most will mobilise rapidly following surgery. However, low-dose heparin should also be used in patients with additional risk factors or those who have recently undergone other surgery and a period of immobility.

Postoperative complications of rigid cystoscopic procedures

- Perforation of the bladder can occur and can be difficult to recognise, especially in the presence of a spinal block, which may mask abdominal pain. Perforations are classified as extraperitoneal, when pain is said to be maximal in the suprapubic region, and intraperitoneal when there is generalised abdominal pain, shoulder tip pain due to fluid tracking up to the diaphragm, and signs of peritonism. Intraperitoneal perforations need fluid resuscitation and urgent surgery to prevent progressive shock.
- Bacteraemia can have a very dramatic onset with signs of profound septic shock. If the diagnosis is made quickly, there is usually a rapid response to IV fluids and appropriate antibiotics (gentamicin-single dose 3–5mg/kg followed by cefuroxime 750–1500mg usually suitable—modify according to sensitivities on preoperative MSU). Always suspect this diagnosis with unexplained hypotension after a seemingly straightforward urinary tract instrumentation.
- Bladder spasm is a painful involuntary contraction of the bladder occurring after any cystoscopic technique, most commonly in patients who did not have an indwelling catheter preoperatively. Diagnosis is supported by the failure of irrigation fluid to flow freely in and out of the bladder. It responds poorly to conventional analgesics but is often eased by small doses of IV benzodiazepine, e.g. diazepam 2.5–5mg or Buscopan (hyoscine butylbromide) 20mg IV or IM.
- Bleeding and fluid overload are dealt with under anaesthesia for TURP (p568).

Transurethral resection of prostate (TURP)

Procedure	Cystoscopic resection of the prostate using diathermy wire
Time	30–90min, depending on the size of the prostate
Pain	+
Position	Lithotomy ± head down
Blood loss	Very variable (200–2000ml), can be profuse and continue postop. G&S
Practical techniques	Spinal ± sedation GA, LMA, and SV GA, ETT, and IPPV

Preoperative

- Patients are frequently elderly with coexistent disease.
- Check for renal impairment.
- Uncontrolled heart failure presents a particularly high risk due to fluid absorption.
- Assess mental state and communication—spinal anaesthesia is difficult if the patient is confused or deaf.

Perioperative

- Insert a large cannula (16G) and use warmed IV fluids as rapid transfusion is occasionally necessary.
- Spinal anaesthesia: in theory easier to detect signs of fluid overload (see below); shown in some, but not all, studies to reduce blood loss; 2.5–3ml bupivacaine (plain or hyperbaric) is usually adequate; frequent BP check—hypotension unusual with the above doses but can occur suddenly; check BP at end when the legs are down (unmasks hypotension).
- GA: consider intubation if the patient is very obese or has a history of reflux; intra-operative fentanyl or morphine plus diclofenac 100mg PR provides adequate analgesia; unusual to need opioids postoperatively.
- Blood loss can be difficult to assess. In theory can be calculated from measuring Hb of discarded irrigation fluid. In practice it is commoner to visually assess the volume and colour, but this can be misleading. Checking the patient's Hb with a bedside device (e.g. HemoCue®) is useful. Blood loss is generally related to the size and weight of prostatic tissue excised (normally 15–60g), the duration of resection, and the expertise of the operator.
- Antibiotic prophylaxis (see p567).
- Obturator spasm (see p572).
- Fluid therapy: crystalloid can be used initially. Bear in mind that a significant volume of hypotonic irrigating fluid may be absorbed so do not give excessive volumes and never use dextrose. Consider switching to a colloid if hypotension results from the spinal. Replace blood loss with colloid and be ready to transfuse if the Hb falls below target.

Postoperative

- There is generally little pain, but discomfort from the catheter or bladder spasm may be a problem (see p567).
- Bladder irrigation with saline via a three-way catheter continues for approximately 24hr, until bleeding is reduced. Clot retention can give a very distended painful bladder and require washout, sometimes under anaesthetic.
- Bleeding can continue and require further surgery—resuscitation may be necessary preoperatively.
- Measure FBC, creatinine, and electrolytes the following day.

Special considerations

- Hypothermia may result when large volumes of irrigation fluid are used (the fluid should be warmed to 37° C)
- If the prostate is very large (>100g), a retropubic prostatectomy may carry fewer complications.
- The risk of complications increases with resection times of >1hr. If a resection is likely to take longer than an hour consider limiting the resection to one lobe only, leaving the other to be done at a later date.
- Laser prostatectomy and transurethral vaporisation of the prostate (TUVP)
    - Several 'minimally invasive' techniques using lasers and other forms of heat have been developed which reduce prostate size. These generally cause less bleeding and absorption of fluid so are sometimes chosen for patients perceived to be at higher risk from conventional TURP.
    - The few randomised controlled trials show a reduction in the need for transfusion, reduced need for bladder irrigation and reduced length of stay in hospital. However, no clear difference in complication rate or long-term urological outcome has yet been demonstrated.
    - Anaesthetic requirements and duration of surgery are similar to TURP.

TURP syndrome

- A combination of fluid overload and hyponatraemia,[1,2] which occurs when large volumes of irrigation fluid are absorbed via open venous sinuses. Irrigation fluid must be non-conductive (so that the diathermy current is concentrated at the cutting point), non-haemolytic (so that haemolysis does not occur if it enters the circulation), and must have neutral visual density, so that the surgeon's view is not distorted. For these reasons it cannot contain electrolytes but cannot be pure water. The most commonly used irrigant is glycine 1.5% in water, which is hypotonic (osmolality 220mmol/l).
- Some irrigation fluid is normally absorbed, at about 20ml/min, and on average patients absorb a total of 1–1.5 litres, but absorption of up to 4–5 litres has been recorded. In clinical practice it is almost impossible to accurately assess the volume absorbed.
- The amount of absorption depends upon the following factors:
  - Pressure of infusion—the bag must be kept as low as possible to achieve adequate flow of irrigant at minimum pressure, usually 60–70cm, never more than 100cm. Higher pressures increase absorption.
  - Venous pressure—more fluid is absorbed if the patient is hypovolaemic or hypotensive.
- Long duration of surgery and large prostate-problems are more common with surgery lasting more than an hour, or with a prostate weighing more than 50g.
- Blood loss—large blood loss implies a large number of open veins.
- TURP syndrome is more likely to occur in patients with poorly controlled heart failure. Do not increase the risks of fluid overload by giving an unnecessarily large volume of IV fluid.
- Glycine is a non-essential amino acid which functions as an inhibitory neurotransmitter and it is unclear whether glycine toxicity plays a part in the syndrome. Ammonia is a metabolite of glycine and may also contribute to CNS disturbance.
- Pulmonary oedema, cerebral oedema, and hyponatraemia are the usual presenting features. Signs will be detected earlier in the awake patient. Mortality is high unless recognised and treated promptly.
- Early symptoms include restlessness, headache, tachypnoea, and these may progress to respiratory distress, hypoxia, frank pulmonary oedema, nausea, vomiting, visual disturbances, confusion, convulsions, and coma. In the anaesthetised patient the only evidence may be tachycardia and hypertension. Rapid absorption of a large volume can lead to reflex bradycardia. Hypotension can also occur. The diagnosis can be confirmed by low serum sodium. An acute fall to <120mmol/l is always symptomatic. A quick check of Na^+ is often possible by checking an ABG (use venous blood unless concerned about acid/base balance).

- If detected intra-operatively bleeding points should be coagulated, surgery terminated as soon as possible, and IV fluids stopped. Give furosemide 40mg and check serum Na^+ and Hb. Support respiration with oxygen or intubation and ventilation if required. Administer IV anticonvulsants if fitting.
- Both severe acute hyponatraemia and over-rapid correction of chronic hyponatraemia can result in permanent neurological damage (most commonly central pontine myelinolysis).
- If the serum sodium has fallen acutely <120mmol/l, and is associated with neurological signs, consider giving hypertonic saline ($NaCl$ 1.8–3%) to restore Na^+ to around 125mmol/l. See p180.
- The volume of 3% saline (in ml) which will raise the serum Na^+ by 1mmol/l is twice the total body water (TBW) in litres. TBW in men is about 60% of body weight, i.e. for a 70kg man
  - Calculate TBW = 70 × 0.6 = 42 litre
  - Therefore 84ml 3% saline will raise serum Na^+ by 1mmol/l
  - 1008ml 3% saline over 24hr will raise serum Na^+ by 12mmol/l.
- In practice give 1.2–2.4ml/kg/hr of 3% saline until symptomatic improvement. This should produce a rise in serum Na^+ of 1–2 mmol/l/hr.
- Correction should ideally not be faster than 1.5–2mmol/l/hr for 3–4hr then 1mmol/l/hr until symptomatic improvement or Na^+ >125mmol/l. Maximum rise should not exceed 12mmol/l in 24hr.
- Beware of compounding effects on Na^+ by other simultaneous treatments (diuretics, colloids etc.).
- Admit to ICU/HDU for management including regular measurements of Na^+.

1 Adrogué HJ, Madias NE (2000). Hyponatremia *N Engl J Med*, **342**, 1581–1589.
2 Kumar S, Berl T (1998). Sodium. *Lancet*, **352**, 220–228.

Transurethral resection of bladder tumour

Procedure	Cystoscopic diathermy resection of bladder tumour
Time	10–40min
Pain	+/++ and bladder spasm
Position	Lithotomy
Blood loss	0–>500ml
Practical techniques	GA with LMA
	Spinal ± sedation

Preoperative
- Most common in smokers—check for IHD, COAD.
- Check Hb, chronic blood loss is common.
- Check renal function.
- Refer to previous anaesthetic charts, as many patients have repeated surgery.

Perioperative
- Obturator spasm occurs when the obturator nerve, which runs adjacent to the lateral walls of the bladder, is directly stimulated by the diathermy current. It causes adduction of the leg and can seriously impair surgical access and increase the risk of bladder perforation. It can usually be controlled by reducing the diathermy current.
- Antibiotic prophylaxis (see p561).
- If resection is limited and postoperative irrigation is not planned the surgeon may request a diuretic to 'flush' the bladder—check that the patient is not hypovolaemic.

Postoperative
- Pain can be a problem with extensive resections—NSAIDs are useful (check renal function).
- Bladder spasm is common (see p567).

Special considerations
- If using a spinal anaesthetic, ensure block to above T_{10} (see p566).

Open (retropubic) prostatectomy

Procedure	Open excision of grossly hypertrophied prostate
Time	60–120min
Pain	+++
Position	Supine
Blood loss	500–2000ml, X-match 4U
Practical techniques	ETT, IPPV, ± epidural

Preoperative
- Elderly men, as for TURP.
- Check renal function.

Perioperative
- Prepare for major blood loss with a large IV cannula, a blood warmer, heated blankets, etc.
- A Pfannenstiel type incision is used.
- Epidural should be used cautiously intra-operatively to avoid exacerbating hypotension due to blood loss.
- Cell salvage techniques can be useful where blood loss is expected to be substantial.

Postoperative
- An epidural is useful.
- Ensure adequate chest physiotherapy.

Radical prostatectomy

Procedure	Open complete excision of malignant prostate
Time	120–180min
Pain	++++
Position	Supine
Blood loss	1000–>3000ml, X-match 4U
Practical techniques	ETT, IPPV, ± epidural

Preoperative
- Patients are selected according to age and fitness.
- Consider booking an HDU bed depending on local practice.

Perioperative
- Prepare for the possibility of very large blood loss with a large IV cannula, blood warmer, etc.
- Consider using arterial and CVP lines, particularly in patients with cardiovascular disease.
- Epidural should be used cautiously intra-operatively to avoid exacerbating hypotension due to blood loss.
- Ensure blood is available and reorder intra-operatively as necessary.
- Take measures to prevent heat loss, e.g. warm air blanket.
- Air embolism is a possible complication.

Postoperative
Urine output is difficult to measure due to irrigation.

Nephrectomy

Procedure	Excision of kidney for tumour, other pathologies, or live donor
Time	1–2.5hr
Pain	+++/++++
Position	Supine or lateral (kidney position)
Blood loss	Depends on pathology, 300–>3000ml. G&S/X-match as required
Practical techniques	ETT + IPPV ± thoracic epidural

Preoperative

- Ascertain the pathology before deciding on the technique and monitoring.
- Check Hb—renal tumours can cause anaemia without blood loss.
- Check BP and renal function—'non-functioning' kidney or renovascular disease is associated with renal impairment and hypertension.
- Consider autotransfusion intra-operatively.
- Check serum electrolytes—renal tumour can cause inappropriate ADH secretion.
- Check the chest radiograph if there is a tumour—there may be metastases, pleural effusions, etc.
- Radiofrequency ablation is being developed for some tumours, and avoids the need for open surgery. Laparoscopic nephrectomy is also becoming more common.

Perioperative

- Common surgical practice in the United Kingdom is for laparotomy via a paramedian or transverse incision for a tumour and a loin incision with retroperitoneal approach for other pathologies or donor nephrectomy.
- Loin incision requires the 'kidney position', i.e. lateral with patient extended over a break in the table—a marked fall in BP is common on assuming this position due to reduced venous return from the legs and possible IVC compression. Further compression during surgery may result in a severe reduction in venous return and cardiac output.
- Ask the surgeon about the predicted extent of surgery—a large tumour may necessitate extensive dissection, possibly via a thoracotomy, or opening of the IVC to resect tumour margins, in which case sudden, torrential blood loss is possible. Occasionally the IVC is temporarily clamped to allow dissection and to control haemorrhage; this gives a sudden fall in cardiac output. Inform the surgeon if BP falls suddenly, have colloid and blood checked and available to infuse immediately under pressure, and have a vasoconstrictor or inotrope such as ephedrine prepared.

- Large IV cannulae, blood warmer, CVP and arterial line if the procedure is anything other than an uncomplicated, non-malignant nephrectomy.
- Heminephrectomy is occasionally performed for a well-localised tumour or in a patient with only one kidney (beware precarious renal function). Blood loss can be large, as vessels are more difficult to control.
- If an epidural is used a high block will be required postoperatively but use it cautiously intra-operatively until bleeding is under control.

Postoperative

- All approaches are painful—epidurals are useful but need to cover up to T7/8 for a loin incision. PCA or opioid infusion is an alternative.
- Intercostal blocks will give analgesia for several hours.
- NSAIDs are useful if renal function is good postoperatively and the patient is not hypovolaemic.
- Monitor hourly urine output.

Cystectomy

Procedure	Excision of bladder plus urinary diversion procedure (e.g. ileal conduit) or bladder reconstruction (orthotopic bladder formation)
Time	2–3hr (longer with bladder reconstruction)
Pain	++++
Position	Lithotomy + head-down
Blood loss	700–>3000ml, X-match 4U
Practical techniques	ETT, IPPV, arterial line + CVP ± epidural

Preoperative

- Check for IHD, COPD, renal function, and FBC.
- Book HDU bed depending on local practice/coexisting problems.
- Consider autotransfusion intra-operatively.
- Ensure thromboprophylaxis is prescribed.
- Consider preoperative IV hydration to compensate for hypovolaemia due to 'bowel prep'.

Perioperative

- Prepare for major blood loss: large IV cannulae, blood warmer, CVP, and direct arterial monitoring are routine.
- Ensure blood is available and reorder intra-operatively as necessary.
- A nasogastric tube is necessary for prolonged postoperative ileus.
- May need aggressive fluid replacement (guided by CVP) from the start to compensate for bowel prep and action of the epidural if used.
- Use epidural cautiously intra-operatively: there will be plenty of time after the main blood-losing episode to establish an adequate block.
- Take measures to prevent heat loss, e.g. warm air blanket.
- Antibiotic prophylaxis as for bowel resection.
- Blood loss can be insidious from pelvic venous plexuses: weigh swabs.
- If blood salvage is used discontinue it when the bowel is opened.
- Air embolism is a possible complication, as in any major pelvic surgery.

Postoperative

- Epidural or PCA is advisable for at least 2d.
- NSAIDs are useful, but ensure good renal function before prescribing.
- Use CVP to guide fluid replacement—requirements are usually very large due to intraperitoneal loss and ileus.
- Urine output via a new ileal conduit is difficult to monitor as drainage tends to be positional.
- Leakage from a ureteric anastomosis may present as urine in the abdominal drain—confirm by comparing biochemistry of the drainage fluid and urine from the conduit.
- HDU or ICU are ideal for the immediate postoperative period.

Laparoscopic urological surgery

- Increasingly common technique for many abdominal, retro-peritoneal and pelvic procedures in urology—including nephrectomy, live donor nephrectomy, pyeloplasty, prostatectomy, and cystectomy.
- Only a few controlled trials of adequate size comparing surgical outcomes from open and laparoscopic procedure. Tendency to show reduced pain/length of stay and faster return to oral diet after laparoscopic nephrectomy, compared to open operation.
- Preoperative investigation and preparation as for equivalent open procedure.
- Time taken will depend on procedure but may take considerably longer than open operation when surgeon is new to technique, so prepare for prolonged procedure with heat conservation etc.
- Positioning will depend on procedure—retro-peritoneal approach to kidney will be in lateral position. Cystectomy and prostatectomy will require head-down position, possibly for many hours.
- Prolonged increase in intra-abdominal pressure can reduce renal function with theoretical risk of postoperative renal dysfunction, or of poor transplant kidney function in the case of donor nephrectomy. Possibly helped by perioperative fluid loading to maintain a diuresis and by limiting insufflation pressures.
- Significant CO_2 absorption can occur so end tidal CO_2 must be monitored, and ventilation may need to be adjusted accordingly throughout case.
- It is possible that prolonged steep head-down position may increase intra-cranial pressure, which could be exacerbated by hypercarbia.
- Rates of surgical complications are reported as low, and are of the same nature as for the equivalent open operation, plus a small but significant risk of diaphragmatic tear during retroperitoneal nephrectomy.
- Postoperative pain is considerably less than for open procedures but can still be severe enough to require opioid analgesia in addition to simple analgesics.

Percutaneous stone removal

Procedure	Endoscopic excision of renal stone via nephrostomy
Time	60–90min
Pain	++/+++
Position	Prone oblique
Blood loss	Variable, 0–1000ml
Practical techniques	ETT and IPPV

Preoperative
- Usually healthy young and middle-aged adults, but stones may be due to underlying metabolic problem or due to bladder dysfunction from neurological disability.
- Check renal function.

Perioperative
- Patient initially in the lithotomy position to insert ureteric stents, then turned semiprone to place nephrostomy posterolaterally below the twelfth rib, under radiographic control—potential to dislodge lines and for pressure area damage.
- Consider an armoured ETT to prevent kinking, and secure well.
- Tape and pad the eyes.
- Support the chest and pelvis to allow abdominal excursion with ventilation.
- Support and pad the head, arms, and lower legs.
- Check ventilation during and after position changes.
- May need to temporarily interrupt ventilation for radiographs.
- Antibiotic prophylaxis required.

Postoperative
- Pain from nephrostomy is variable.
- NSAIDs (check renal function), IM morphine, or oral codeine/paracetamol.

Special considerations
- Hypothermia can occur if large volumes of irrigation fluid are used.
- Insertion of nephrostomy is often close to the diaphragm with possibility of breaching the pleura, causing pneumothorax or hydrothorax—if in doubt perform a CXR postoperatively.
- Rupture of the renal pelvis is a recognised complication when large volumes of irrigant may enter the retroperitoneal space.
- Postoperative Gram-negative septicaemia is a significant risk, after any urinary tract surgery for stones.

Extracorporeal shock wave lithotripsy

Procedure	Non-invasive fragmentation of renal stones using pulsed ultrasound
Time	20–40min
Pain	+/++
Blood loss	Nil
Practical techniques	Sedation for adults GA, LMA for children

In the early days of extracorporeal shock wave lithotripsy patients were suspended in a water bath in a semi-sitting position, which produced a number of problems for the anaesthetist. Developments in the 1980s meant that a water bath was no longer required and more recent refinements of the ultrasound beam have made it less uncomfortable so that with most current lithotriptors only a few patients need anaesthesia or sedation.

Preoperative
- Patients often undergo repeated lithotripsy, so refer to previous treatment records where possible.
- Premedication with oral diclofenac + IM pethidine is usually effective for treatment.

Perioperative
- Lateral position with arms above the head.
- Renal stones are located using ultrasound or an image intensifier and the shock wave focused on the stones.
- Antibiotic prophylaxis required due to significant risk of postoperative bacteraemia.

Postoperative
Mild discomfort only, oral analgesics or NSAIDs (beware renal function) are adequate.

Special considerations
- Shock wave can cause occasional dysrhythmias, which are usually self-limiting. If persistent the shock waves can be delivered in time with the ECG (refractory period). Judicious use of anticholinergics (glycopyrronium 200µg) will increase the heart rate and increase the frequency of delivered shock.
- Pacemakers can be deprogrammed by the shock wave—seek advice from a pacemaker technician.
- Energy from shock waves is released when they meet an air/water inter-face, it is advised to use saline, rather than air, for 'loss of resistance' if siting an epidural.

Renal transplant

Procedure	Transplantation of cadaveric or live donor organ
Time	90–180min
Pain	++/+++
Position	Supine
Blood loss	Not significant—500ml
Practical techniques	ETT and IPPV, CVP

Preoperative

- Usual problems related to chronic renal failure and uraemia (see p123).
- Chronic anaemia is common (Hb usually around 8g/dl).
- There has usually been recent haemodialysis, therefore some degree of hypovolaemia and possibly residual anticoagulation.
- Check postdialysis potassium.
- Note sites of any A-V fistulae and avoid potential sites when placing the IV cannula.

Perioperative

- Fluid load prior to induction—wide swings in arterial pressure are common.
- Commonly used agents include isoflurane, atracurium, fentanyl (or morphine) due to renal disease.
- Insert a triple lumen central line with strict aseptic technique and monitor central venous pressure.
- Prior to graft insertion, gradually increase CVP to 10–12mmHg (using colloids or crystalloids) to maintain optimal graft perfusion and promote urine production.
- Maintain normothermia.
- Most centres use a cocktail of drugs once the graft is perfused to enhance survival (e.g. hydrocortisone 100mg, mannitol 20% 60ml, furosemide 80mg or more). Have these prepared.

Postoperative

- PCA morphine is a suitable analgesic. Epidural is also possible, but there is a danger of bleeding on insertion (residual anticoagulation from haemodialysis, poor platelet function, etc.) and problems with fluid loading and maintaining blood pressure postoperatively.
- Avoid NSAIDs.
- Monitor CVP and urine output hourly. Maintain mild hypervolaemia to promote diuresis.

Other urological procedures

Other urological procedures

Operation	Description	Time (min)	Pain (+ to +++++)	Position	Blood loss/ X-match	Notes
Ureteroscopy	Investigate obstruction, remove stones	20–60	+	Lithotomy	Nil	LMA + SV. Check renal function. Antibiotic prophylaxis
Insert ureteric stent	To relieve ureteric obstruction, using image intensifier	20	+	Lithotomy	Nil	LMA + SV. Antibiotic prophylaxis
Remove ureteric stent	Cystoscopy to retrieve stent	10–20	+	Lithotomy	Nil	Awake or LMA + SV. Usually possible with flexi scope and LA
Insert suprapubic catheter	Transcutaneous insertion of catheter into full bladder	15	+	Lithotomy or supine	Nil	Sedation + LA or LMA + SV. Often patients with neurological disease
Bladder neck incision	Transurethral diathermy incision of prostate at narrowed bladder neck	15	++	Lithotomy	Nil	LMA + SV. Younger patients than TURP
Urethroplasty	Reconstruction of urethra narrowed by trauma or infection-very variable procedure	90–240	++++	Lithotomy	300–2000ml	ETT + IPPV ± epidural. Beware prolonged lithotomy. Consider epidural for postoperative pain
Nesbitt's procedure	Straightening of penile deformation from Peyronie's disease	60–120	+++	Supine	Nil	LMA + SV. Consider caudal or penile block

Circumcision	Excision of foreskin	20	++	Supine	Nil	LMA + SV + LA. Penile block or caudal useful. Topical lidocaine gel to take home. LA alone possible in frail elderly
Urethral dilatation	Stretching of narrowed urethra with serial dilators	10	+	Lithotomy or supine	Nil	LMA or spinal
Urethral meatotomy	Incision to widen urethral meatus	10	+	Supine	Nil	LMA + SV
Orchidectomy	Remove testis/es—through groin or scrotum depending on pathology	20–45	++	Supine	Nil	LMA + SV + ilioinguinal block. Need to block to T9/10 if using regional technique due to embryological origins
Vasectomy	Division of vas deferens via scrotal incision	20–40	++	Supine	Nil	LMA + SV. Often under LA
Pyeloplasty	Refashioning of obstructed renal pelvis via loin incision. Children and young adults	90–120	++++	Lateral 'kidney position'	300–500ml	ETT + IPPV + epidural/PCA. Similar considerations as nephrectomy. May be significant blood loss in children

Further reading

Conacher ID, Soomro NA, Rix D (2004). Anaesthesia for laparoscopic urological surgery. *British Journal of Anaesthesia*, **93**, 859–864.

Gravenstein D (1997). Transurethral resection of the prostate syndrome: A review of the pathophysiology and management. *Anesthesiology and Analgesia*, **84**, 438–446.

Hoffman RM, MacDonald R, Wilt TJ. (2004) *Cochrane Database Systemic Review* (1) CDOO1987. Laser Prostatectomy for Benign Prostatic Hypertrophy.

Peterson GN, Kreiger JN, Glauber DT (1985). Anaesthetic experience with percutaneous lithotripsy. *Anaesthesia*, **40**, 460–464.

Rabey PG (2001). Anaesthesia for renal transplantation. *British Journal of Anaesthesia CEPD Reviews*, **1**, 24–27.

Roberts FL, Brown EC, Davis R, Cousins MJ (1989). Comparison of hyperbaric and plain bupivacaine with hyperbaric cinchocaine as spinal anaesthetic agents. *Anaesthesia*, **44**, 471–474.

Anon (2004) Antibiotic prophylaxis in surgery: 2 – Urogenital, obstetric and gynaecological surgery. *Drugs and therapeutics Bulletin*. **42**, 9–11.

Gynaecological surgery

John Saddler

General principles

Many gynaecological patients are fit and undergo relatively minor procedures as day cases. Others are inpatients undergoing more major surgery. Elderly patients often require operations to relieve pelvic floor prolapse.

- Many patients are apprehensive, even for relatively minor surgery.
- Postoperative nausea and vomiting (PONV) is a particular problem. With high-risk patients use appropriate techniques and give prophylactic anti-emetics.
- Pelvic surgery is associated with deep vein thrombosis (DVT)—ensure that adequate prophylactic measures have been taken.
- Prophylactic antibiotics reduce postoperative wound infection rates for certain operations—check your hospital protocol.
- Patients on the OCP should be managed according to local protocol; guidelines are suggested on p10.
- Vagal stimulation may occur during cervical dilatation, traction on the pelvic organs or the mesentery, or during laparoscopic procedures.
- Take care during patient positioning. Patients are often moved up or down the table, when airway devices can be dislodged and disconnections can occur. Pre-existing back or joint pain may be worsened in the lithotomy position, and if the legs are supported in stirrups there is a potential for common peroneal nerve injury.
- During laparotomies ensure that patients are kept warm.
- During major gynaecological surgery considerable blood loss may occur, and surgery may be prolonged.

Minor gynaecological procedures

Procedure	D&C, hysteroscopy, oocyte retrieval
Time	20–30min
Pain	+
Position	Supine, lithotomy
Blood loss	Nil
Practical techniques	LMA, SV, day case

Minor operations that enable access to the endometrial cavity through the cervix include:
- D&C (dilatation and curettage). Largely superseded now by hysteroscopic examination.
- Hysteroscopy: the surgeon is able to visualise the endometrial cavity using a rigid scope. The hysteroscope is flushed with crystalloid to enable better visualisation. Fluid volume is measured to ensure there is no uterine perforation (suspect if volume recovered less than the volume infused).
- A brief general anaesthetic may be requested for an oocyte retrieval procedure. Patients will have received prior hormonal stimulation to induce the production of oocytes in the ovaries. These are removed with the aid of ultrasound through a transvaginal approach. This may also be performed with sedation.

Preoperative
- Many patients will be treated as day cases.
- Consider prescribing diclofenac and ranitidine, or obtain permission for rectal administration perioperatively.

Perioperative
Spontaneous ventilation using a facemask or LMA, propofol (infusion or intermittent bolus) or volatile.

Postoperative
Simple oral analgesics, plus anti-emetic of choice.

Special considerations
- Vagal stimulation may occur with cervical dilatation, anticholinergic drugs should be immediately available.
- Stimulation may also induce laryngospasm—ensure adequate depth of anaesthesia.
- There is a risk of uterine perforation through the fundus whenever surgical instruments are introduced through the cervix and into the endometrial cavity. Antibiotics are usually prescribed if this is thought to have occurred. A small perforation can be treated expectantly; larger perforations may require a laparoscopy to evaluate the extent of the perforation.

ERPC, STOP (VTOP)

Procedure	ERPC (evacuation of retained products of conception). STOP/VTOP (suction or vaginal termination of pregnancy)
Time	10–20min
Pain	+
Position	Supine, lithotomy
Blood loss	Usually minimal
Practical techniques	LMA, SV, day case

Preoperative

- ERPC: remaining products of conception may have to be surgically removed after an incomplete miscarriage. This usually occurs between 6–12wk gestation. Substantial blood loss may have occurred preoperatively, and may continue perioperatively. IV access and crystalloid/colloid infusion are required if haemorrhage appears anything more than trivial.
- STOP/VTOP is a procedure undertaken up to 12wk gestation.

Perioperative

- LMA or FM. Intubate unfasted emergency patients.
- Avoid high concentrations of volatile agents due to the relaxant effect on the uterus. Propofol induction followed by intermittent boluses or TIVA and an opioid (fentanyl), is appropriate.
- A drug to help contract the uterus and reduce bleeding is usually requested. Oxytocin (Syntocinon) 5U is usually given. This may cause an increase in heart rate. The use of ergometrine, a vasoconstrictor, is declining because it raises arterial pressure.

Postoperative

Oral analgesics and anti-emetic.

Special considerations

- Pregnancies beyond 12 weeks can be terminated surgically by dilatation and evacuation (D + E). The procedure is similar to a STOP/VTOP, but there is greater potential for blood loss. Larger doses of oxytocin may be required.
- If there are symptoms of reflux oesophagitis, ranitidine premedication and intubation are indicated.
- If a pregnancy has gone beyond 16wk, it may be terminated medically with prostaglandin. These patients may still require an ERPC, and should be managed similarly to a retained placenta (see p726).

Laparoscopy/laparoscopic sterilisation

Procedure	Intra-abdominal examination of gynaecological organs through a rigid scope ± clips to Fallopian tubes
Time	15–30min
Pain	+/++
Position	Supine, lithotomy, head down tilt
Blood loss	Nil
Practical techniques	ETT, IPPV
	LMA, SV, day case

Preoperative
- Usually fit young adults.
- Obtain consent for suppositories.

Perioperative
- Use a short-acting non-depolarising muscle relaxant. 'Top-ups' may be required. Monitor with a nerve stimulator and use reversal agents if necessary at the end.
- Endotracheal intubation.
- Give a short-acting opioid (e.g. fentanyl) and PR NSAID (e.g. diclofenac 100mg).
- Encourage the surgeon to infiltrate the skin incisions with local analgesia.
- An alternative technique for uncomplicated short procedures is to use spontaneous ventilation and an LMA. This is only suitable for non-obese patients and the potential for gastric regurgitation and aspiration must be assessed carefully. If gas insufflation is hampered by abdominal muscle tone, deepen anaesthesia or use a small dose of mivacurium, and assist ventilation until the return of SV.

Postoperative
Opioids (morphine) may be required.

Special considerations
- As many of these procedures are short and may only take 10–15min, mivacurium is a logical muscle relaxant to use. Intermittent use of suxamethonium has unwanted side-effects.
- Bradycardias are common, due to vagal stimulation. Atropine should be readily available. Many anaesthetists administer glycopyrronium prophylactically at induction.
- Shoulder pain is common postoperatively due to diaphragmatic irritation. Although self-limiting, it can be difficult to treat, and is reduced by expelling as much carbon dioxide from the abdomen as possible at the end of the procedure.

- Occasionally, surgical instruments damage abdominal contents, and a laparotomy is required. This may result in severe blood loss.
- Very rarely carbon dioxide gas may be inadvertently injected intra-vascularly, resulting in gas embolus. This results in ventilation/perfusion mismatch, with a fall in $ETCO_2$, impaired cardiac output, hypotension, arrhythmias, and tachycardia. If this is thought to have occurred, the surgeon should be alerted, nitrous oxide should be discontinued, and the patient should be resuscitated (p415).
- If an LMA is used, consider premedication with oral ranitidine (150–300mg).

Tension-free vaginal tape (TVT)

Procedure	Tape insertion for stress incontinence
Time	20min
Pain	+
Position	Lithotomy
Blood loss	Minimal
Practical techniques	Various (see below)

Preoperative
- Consent for suppositories.

Perioperative
- Several anaesthetic techniques are currently employed.
- Some surgeons are happy with a spontaneous breathing technique with LMA.
- Many require the patient to cough, so that the tension in the tapes can be adjusted. Here, a spinal or local anaesthetic technique can be employed, usually with sedation.
- PR NSAID (e.g. diclofenac) is advisable
- Take care with positioning (lithotomy position).

Postoperative
- Patients may be day cases, but some stay overnight.
- Opioids (e.g. morphine) are only rarely required.

Special considerations
- Anaesthetic technique is largely determined by the surgical approach. Liaise carefully with the surgeon before induction of anaesthesia .

Abdominal hysterectomy

Procedure	Removal of uterus through abdominal incision (may also include ovaries as bilateral salpingo-oophorectomy)
Time	1hr, often longer
Pain	+++
Position	Supine, head down
Blood loss	250–500ml, G&S
Practical techniques	ETT, IPPV, PCA

Preoperative
- Patients may be anaemic if they have had menorrhagia or postmenopausal bleeding.
- Renal function may be abnormal if an abdominal mass has been compressing the ureters.
- Many patients are anxious and require premedication.
- Postoperative nausea and vomiting (PONV) is common.
- Ensure prophylaxis for deep vein thrombosis (DVT) has been initiated.

Perioperative
- Oral intubation and ventilation.
- If a Pfannenstiel ('bikini line') incision is anticipated, consider bilateral ilioinguinal blocks with bupivacaine. The patient should be warned about the possibility of femoral nerve involvement.
- Deep muscle relaxation is required to enable the surgeon to gain optimal access.
- Antibiotic prophylaxis is usually required.
- Head down positioning is often requested which may cause ventilation pressures to rise with diaphragmatic compression. Central venous pressure will increase and gastric regurgitation is also more likely.
- Blood loss is variable; some hysterectomies bleed more than expected. Crossmatch blood early if bleeding appears to be a problem.
- Heat loss through the abdominal incision can be significant. Use a warm air blanket over the upper body during the operation.

Postoperative
- Pain is usually reasonably well controlled with a PCA. This can be supplemented with local anaesthetic blocks or wound infiltration, regular paracetamol and NSAIDs. Regular administration of anti-emetics may be required. They can also be added to the opioid mix e.g. cyclizine (up to150mg) can be added to a 50ml syringe with 50mg morphine.
- Oxygen therapy is indicated for 24hr postoperatively or longer. Patients usually tolerate nasal cannulae better than face masks.

Special considerations

- Epidural analgesia is effective for post-hysterectomy pain, particularly in patients who have had midline ('up and down') incisions, and may also reduce the incidence of PONV. However, because of the potential for morbidity, many anaesthetists avoid using them for routine hysterectomies.
- Wertheim's hysterectomy is undertaken in patients who have cervical and uterine malignancies. The uterus, Fallopian tubes, and often the ovaries are removed but, in addition, the pelvic lymph nodes are dissected out. These operations take much longer and there is a potential for substantial blood loss. Invasive monitoring, in the form of central venous access and direct arterial pressure monitoring, should be considered particularly for compromised patients. Epidural analgesia is useful for postoperative pain.

Vaginal hysterectomy

Procedure	Removal of the uterus through the vagina
Time	50min
Pain	+/++
Position	Lithotomy
Blood loss	Variable, usually less than 500ml
Practical techniques	LMA, SV, caudal
	Spinal

Preoperative
A degree of uterine prolapse enables the operation to be performed more easily. Patients are therefore usually older and may be frail with underlying cardiac or respiratory problems.

Perioperative
- A spontaneous breathing technique with LMA is usual. Give a longer-acting IV opioid (e.g. morphine 5–10mg or pethidine 50–100mg) and supplement with NSAIDs.
- A caudal with 20ml bupivacaine 0.25% improves postoperative analgesia, but beware toxic levels (see below).
- Spinal anaesthesia (3ml bupivacaine 0.5%) with or without supplemental sedation is a satisfactory alternative.
- The surgeon usually infiltrates the operative field with a vasoconstrictor to reduce bleeding. Local analgesia infiltration at the same time will aid postoperative analgesia. Monitor the cardiovascular system carefully during this period, and ensure that safe doses of these drugs are not exceeded.
- Take care with positioning. Many patients will have hip and/or knee arthritis, and may have had surgery to these joints. Lloyd-Davies leg slings may be preferable to leg stirrups if leg joints articulate poorly. The common peroneal nerve may be compressed in leg stirrups.
- Keep the patient warm, preferably with a warmed air blanket.

Postoperative
- This operation is less painful than an abdominal hysterectomy. If opioids, NSAIDs and local analgesia infiltration/caudal have been given intra-operatively, further analgesia needs are often very modest (IM opioids).
- Elderly patients will require supplemental oxygen for at least 24hr postoperatively.

Special considerations

- The procedure is often supplemented by either an anterior or posterior repair which reduces bladder or bowel prolapse through the vagina.
- It is usually not possible to remove the fallopian tubes and ovaries during a vaginal hysterectomy because of the restricted surgical field.
- Laparoscopically-assisted vaginal hysterectomy (LAVH) is designed to enable the uterus, Fallopian tubes, and ovaries to be removed through the vagina. The operation begins with a laparoscopy, at which the broad ligament is identified and detached. There is a risk of haemorrhage and ureteric damage at this stage. The anaesthetic principles for laparoscopy apply except that a longer-acting muscle relaxant and an endotracheal tube should be used. Once satisfactory mobility of the gynaecological organs has been achieved at laparoscopy, they are then removed through a vaginal incision. PCA analgesia should be considered postoperatively.

Ectopic pregnancy

Procedure	Laparotomy to stop bleeding from ruptured tubal pregnancy
Time	40min
Pain	++/+++
Position	Supine
Blood loss	Can be massive, X-match 2U
Practical techniques	ETT, IPPV, PCA

Preoperative
- The presentation is variable. A stable patient may have ill-defined abdominal pain and amenorrhoea, others may present with life-threatening abdominal haemorrhage. At least one large-bore IV cannula should be inserted prior to theatre, and crystalloids, colloids, or blood products infused according to the clinical picture.
- FBC, crossmatch, and possibly a clotting screen should be requested on admission.
- Seek help from a second anaesthetist if the patient is unstable.

Perioperative
- Rapid sequence induction.
- Careful IV induction if blood loss is suspected. Use etomidate or ketamine if shocked.
- Continue IV fluid resuscitation.

Postoperative
- Clotting abnormalities are not uncommon if large volumes of blood have been lost. Send a clotting screen for analysis if necessary, and organise fresh frozen plasma and platelet infusions if indicated.
- Actively warm the patient in the recovery room with heated blankets if possible.
- PCA for postoperative analgesia.

Special considerations
- Stable patients may undergo a diagnostic laparoscopy. Be aware that the pneumoperitoneum may impede venous return resulting in hypotension.
- Many centres now perform the whole operation through the laparoscope as a routine, and only convert to a laparotomy if there are any complications.

Other gynaecological procedures

Operation	Description	Time (min)	Pain (+ to +++++)	Position	Blood loss/ X-match	Notes
Colposuspension	Abdominal procedure for stress incontinence	40	+++	Supine	G&S	ETT, IPPV
Cone biopsy	Removal of the terminal part of the cervix through the vagina	30	++	Supine	G&S	May bleed postoperatively. LMA, SV
Laparotomy, investigative	Abdominal assessment of pelvic mass	150	++++	Supine	2U	Ovarian tumours may be adherent to adjacent structures. Potentially large blood loss
Myomectomy	Abdominal excision of fibroids from uterus	60	+++	Supine	G&S	Blood loss may be greater than expected. ETT, IPPV
Oophorectomy	Removal of ovaries	40	+++	Supine	G&S	ETT, IPPV
Repair, anterior	Repair of anterior vaginal wall	20	++	Lithotomy	Nil	Often combined with vaginal hysterectomy. LMA ± caudal

Table contd.

Operation	Description	Time (min)	Pain (+ to +++++)	Position	Blood loss/ X-match	Notes
Repair, posterior	Repair of posterior vaginal wall	20	++	Lithotomy	Nil	Often combined with vaginal hysterectomy. LMA ± caudal
Sacrocolpopexy	Abdominal repair of vault prolapse	60	+++	Supine	G&S	ETT, IPPV
Sacrospinous fixation	Vaginal operation for vault prolapse	40	++	Lithotomy	Nil	
Shirodkar suture	Insertion of suture around cervix to prevent recurrent miscarriage	20	++	Lithotomy	Nil	May need antacid prophylaxis (see p752)
Thermoablation	Thermal obliteration of endometrium	20	++	Lithotomy	Nil	May require opioids
TCRE	Endoscopic resection of endometrium	30	+	Lithotomy	Nil	Systemic absorption of water may occur from the glycine solution Treat as for TURP syndrome
Vulvectomy, simple	Excision of vulva	90	+++	Lithotomy	G&S	
Vulvectomy, radical	Excision of vulva and lymph nodes	150	++++	Lithotomy	2U	Epidural analgesia recommended

Ear, nose, and throat surgery

Fred Roberts

General principles

Airway problems are the major concern in ear, nose, and throat (ENT) surgery, related both to the underlying clinical problem and the shared airway.

Presenting pathology may:
- Produce airway obstruction
- Make access difficult or impossible.

Surgeons working in or close to the airway can:
- Displace or obstruct airway equipment
- Obscure anaesthetist's view of patient
- Limit access for anaesthetist during operation
- Produce bleeding into the airway (intra- and postop).

The surgeon and anaesthetist should plan together to use techniques/equipment that provide good conditions for surgery whilst maintaining a safe, secure airway. Whenever an airway problem is suspected intra-operatively, correcting it is the first priority, stopping surgery if necessary. Other structures around the head are inaccessible during surgery and need protection—especially the eyes. Ensure they are kept closed with appropriate tape, padded as necessary, and that pressure from equipment is prevented, especially for long cases.

Airway/ventilation management

ETT or LMA

- Traditionally an endotracheal tube (ETT) has been used for airway protection for the majority of ENT work.
- Preformed RAE (Ring, Adair, Elwyn) tubes provide excellent protection with minimal intrusion into surgical field.
- An oral (south-facing) RAE tube is used for nasal and much oral surgery, although a nasal tube (north-facing) allows better surgical access to the oral cavity.
- The laryngeal mask airway (LMA) is increasingly being used, usually of the reinforced flexible type. It offers adequate protection against aspiration of blood or surgical debris and reduces complications of tracheal intubation/extubation. It restricts surgical access to a greater degree, however, and is more prone to displacement during surgery (with potentially catastrophic results).

SV or IPPV

- Neuromuscular blockade (NMB) is not required for most ENT surgery.
- Many ENT anaesthetists still favour spontaneous ventilation (SV), regarding movement of the reservoir bag as a valuable sign of airway integrity.
- If SV is used via an ETT, suxamethonium produces the best conditions for intubation, but side-effects can be troublesome, particularly myalgia in a population where early ambulation is likely. Alternatives include mivacurium, combinations of high-dose propofol and alfentanil/remifentanil or deep inhalational anaesthesia.
- IPPV enables faster recovery and return of airway reflexes.

Deep or light extubation

- Many ENT procedures create bleeding into the airway. Suction (and pack removal) under direct vision before extubation is essential in such cases, taking care not to traumatise any surgical sites.
- One particular danger site for blood accumulation is the nasopharynx behind the soft palate, an area not readily visible. Blood pooling here can be aspirated following extubation, with fatal results ('Coroner's clot'). It is best cleared using either a nasal suction catheter or a Yankauer sucker rotated so its angled tip is placed behind the uvula.
- Laryngospasm can follow extubation, particularly in children, from recent instrumentation of the larynx or irritation by blood. The risk is minimised by extubating either deep or light (not in-between).
- Deep extubation is best suited to SV. At the end of surgery, increase the volatile agent concentration, but discontinue nitrous oxide (to increase the FRC oxygen store). After careful suction, insert a Guedel airway, turn patient left lateral/head down (tonsil position), check respiration is regular (turning can produce transient coughing/breath holding) then extubate.
- Check airway/respiration are fine, and keep patient in this position until airway reflexes return.
- Because of the risk of airway complications, high quality recovery care is essential for all ENT work, but particularly so if deep extubation used.
- In the early recovery period, continuous low suction can be done via a catheter just protruding from the Guedel airway.
- Light extubation is best suited to IPPV. After careful suctioning, any residual NMB is reversed, inhalational agents discontinued and the trachea extubated after laryngeal reflexes have returned.
- Light extubation often produces a brief period of coughing/restlessness initially.
- Light extubation is recommended in all patients with a difficult airway.

Throat packs

- A throat pack (wet gauze or tampons) is often used around the ETT/LMA to absorb blood that might otherwise pool in the upper airway.
- A throat pack is particularly useful during nasal operations where bleeding can be substantial and is not cleared during surgery.
- The pack must be removed before extubation, as it can lead to catastrophic airway obstruction if left. Systems to ensure removal include:
  - Tie or tape the pack to the ETT.
  - Place an identification sticker on the ETT or patient's forehead.
  - Include the pack in the scrub nurse's count.
  - Always perform laryngoscopy prior to extubation.

Nasal vasoconstrictors
- Vasoconstriction is used to reduce bleeding in most nasal surgery. Cocaine (4–10%) and adrenaline (1:100 000–1:200 000) are the most commonly used agents, administered by:
  - Spray
  - Paste/gel
  - Soaked swabs
  - Infiltration (not cocaine).
- The recommended maximum dose of cocaine is 1.5mg/kg, though absorption from topical application is only partial. Sympathomimetic activity can result transiently after cocaine absorption.
- Moffett (1947) described a mixture for topical nasal vasoconstriction, consisting of:
  - 2ml cocaine 8%
  - 1ml adrenaline 1:1000
  - 2ml sodium bicarbonate 1%.
- Moffett's solution is still used with assorted modifications, e.g. cocaine 10%, bicarbonate 8.4% or mixed in aqueous gel.

Remifentanil
- The intense opioid action of remifentanil, combined with its rapid recovery profile, has led to its growing popularity amongst ENT anaesthetists.
- Normally given by infusion, clinical applications include:
  - Middle ear surgery/major head and neck resections (controlled arterial hypotension reduces bleeding)
  - Parotidectomy (facilitates IPPV without relaxant)
  - Laryngoscopy/pharyngoscopy (attenuates hypertensive response).
- Beware of bradycardia/hypotension on induction, particularly in the elderly: give a 5–10ml/kg IV preload and glycopyrronium if heart rate drifts down.
- Inter-patient variability greatly limits the value of predetermined infusion schemes.
- For major surgery, to prevent postoperative rebound hypertension/ agitation in recovery, give morphine 15–20min before the end of surgery: clonidine up to 150µg IV is also useful.

Preoperative airway obstruction

(see also p938)

Assessment

- Patients with preoperative airway obstruction usually present for surgery either to establish the diagnosis or to relieve the obstruction.
- The most common level for obstruction is the larynx, producing stridor (high-pitched, inspiratory) and markedly reduced exercise tolerance. Classified as supraglottic, glottic, or subglottic.
- In adults, tumours are the commonest cause of upper airway obstruction, though haematoma or infection (including epiglottitis) is also possible. In children, infection (croup/epiglottitis) or foreign body is more likely, though in the UK Hib vaccination has made epiglottitis in children very rare.
- Extreme airway obstruction will cause obvious signs of respiratory distress at rest. Exhaustion or an obtunded conscious level indicate the need for immediate intervention.
- If obstruction has a gradual onset, patients can compensate very effectively and moderately severe obstruction can develop without gross physical signs. Features to help recognise a substantial degree of upper airway obstruction include:
  - Long, slow inspirations, with pauses during speech.
  - Worsening stridor during sleep (history from spouse/night nursing staff) or exercise.
- Oropharyngeal lesions rarely present with airway obstruction and assessment is normally straightforward on preoperative examination. Important features are limitation of mouth opening and tongue protrusion, and identification of any masses compromising the airway.
- Useful information may come from radiographs (plain films, CT/MRI) or ENT clinic flexible or indirect laryngoscopy.

Management

- For life-threatening airway obstruction emergency intervention may be needed, but usually surgery will be a planned procedure.
- For emergencies, avoid undue delays. Whilst preparing theatre, helium by facemask (FM) can improve flow past the obstruction (low density favourable for turbulent flow), though must not delay definitive management. Medical helium comes premixed (79%) with oxygen (21%): additional oxygen should be added via a Y connector.
- The main problems in securing airway access are:
  - Airway obstruction likely to be worsened by lying the patient flat, instrumenting the larynx, or general anaesthesia (all techniques).
  - Identifying the laryngeal inlet may be difficult because of anatomical distortion (especially supraglottic lesions).
  - Severe stenosis may make passage of tube difficult (particularly glottic or subglottic tumours).

- There is little evidence to support any one particular anaesthetic technique. However, the use of IV induction agents or NMB carries the catastrophic risk of 'can't intubate/can't ventilate' in a patient unable to breathe spontaneously.
- The three main options for establishing secure airway access are:
  - Direct laryngoscopy/tracheal intubation under deep inhalational anaesthesia using sevoflurane or halothane.
  - Tracheal intubation under local anaesthesia (LA) using fibreoptic laryngoscopy.
  - Tracheostomy under LA (or deep inhalational general anaesthesia with FM or LMA in less severe cases).
- Fibreoptic intubation under LA may be difficult with stenotic lesions as the airway may be completely blocked by the scope during the procedure.
- Mason and Fielder[1] reviewed the merits of each technique for airway obstruction at different levels, but concluded none is universally certain, safe, and easy and the final decision in each case will be strongly influenced by the particular skills and experience of the anaesthetist and surgeon concerned.
- Whichever technique is used, a full range of equipment should be prepared, including different laryngoscopes, cricothyroidotomy kit, and tubes in various sizes. An ETT kept on ice will be stiffer and may be useful to get past an obstructing lesion.
- In children, deep inhalational anaesthesia is the only realistic option. Delays in getting to theatre must be avoided because of rapid and unpredictable decline in condition. To minimise upset in a small child, it may well be best to delay IV cannulation until after induction—usually best undertaken with the child sitting, being comforted by a parent. A moderate degree of CPAP is very effective at keeping the airway patent as anaesthesia deepens. Once deep, and if stable, LA spray to the larynx can be helpful in extending the available time for laryngoscopy before airway reflexes return. In epiglottitis, distortion of the epiglottis can make recognition of the glottis very difficult; a useful aid is to press on the child's chest and watch for a bubble of gas emerging from the larynx.
- If complete airway obstruction occurs and all conventional attempts to secure the airway fail, emergency surgical access to the airway is the only option. Cricothyroidotomy is preferable to tracheostomy for emergency airway access, as it is quicker to perform, more superficial, and less likely to bleed (above the thyroid gland). (See p890.)

1 Mason RA, Fielder CP (1999). The obstructed airway in head and neck surgery. *Anaesthesia*, **54**, 625–628.

Obstructive sleep apnoea (see p118)

- Obstructive sleep apnoea (OSA)[1] is the most common form of sleep apnoea syndrome. The airway obstructs intermittently because of inadequate muscle tone/coordination in the pharynx. The problem usually occurs in association with other factors such as obesity.
- In adults surgery for OSA may include nasal operations or uvulopalatopharyngoplasty (UPPP), although the role of UPPP in OSA is controversial as it may render nasal CPAP less effective in the long term.
- In children OSA usually results from extreme adenotonsillar hypertrophy, and adenotonsillectomy is performed to relieve this.[2]
- OSA produces total obstruction with repeated episodes of hypoxia leading to arousal (though not awakening). Multiple episodes can occur each night, with oxygen saturation falling repeatedly to below 50%.
- Repeated interruptions to sleep produce daytime lethargy and somnolence whilst extensive nocturnal hypoxia can lead to pulmonary or systemic hypertension with ventricular hypertrophy and cardiac failure.
- A careful history (from the partner or parent) is the most valuable information initially. In OSA snoring is interrupted by periods of silent apnoea broken by a 'heroic' deep breath.
- Sleep studies reveal the extent of disease. If a history unexpectedly gives a clear picture of OSA the patient should be referred preop.
- In children with suspected OSA, features of chronic hypoxaemia should be sought. These include polycythaemia and right ventricular strain (large P wave in leads II and V1, large R wave in V1, deep S wave in V6). If features exist, echocardiography and referral for sleep studies should be considered. In severe cases, corrective otolaryngological surgery should be undertaken before unrelated elective surgery.
- Perioperatively the biggest danger is impairment of respiratory drive and hypoxic arousal mechanisms by the sedative action of drugs.
- Anaesthetic management is aimed at minimising periods of sedation and ensuring that ventilation and oxygenation are maintained until the patient is adequately recovered. Specific points include:
  - Avoidance of preoperative sedative drugs.
  - Intubation is usually not a problem unless other factors are present.
  - Long-acting opioids should be avoided if possible. Use NSAIDs, paracetamol, tramadol or local infiltration where feasible.
  - When needed, long-acting opioids should be given IV and titrated carefully against response.
  - Close overnight monitoring (including pulse oximetry). Admission to HDU or even ITU may be necessary.
  - For nasal surgery a nasopharyngeal airway can be incorporated into the nasal pack and left in place overnight.

---

1 Loadsman JA, Hillman DR (2001). Anaesthesia and sleep apnoea. *British Journal of Anaesthesia*, **86**, 254–266.
2 Warwick JP, Mason DG (1998). Obstructive sleep apnoea syndrome in children. *Anaesthesia*, **53**, 571–579.

Grommet insertion

Procedure	Myringotomy and grommet insertion, usually bilateral
Time	5–15min
Pain	+
Position	Supine, head tilted to side, head ring
Blood loss	Nil
Practical techniques	FM or LMA SV using T-piece

Preoperative
- Usually children (1–8yr), day case if sole procedure.
- Repeated ear infections, check for recent URTI.

Perioperative
- FM suitable if surgeon happy to work round it, but assistant needed to adjust vaporiser, etc. Insert Guedel airway before draping and ensure reservoir bag visible throughout (T-piece ideal if face mask used).
- LMA popular.

Postoperative
PRN paracetamol or diclofenac oral/PR—many need no analgesia.

Special considerations
- If FM airway difficult, change early to LMA.
- Reflex bradycardia occasionally seen related to partial vagal innervation of tympanic membrane.

Tonsillectomy/adenoidectomy: child

Procedure	Excision of lymphoid tissue from oropharynx (tonsils) or nasopharynx (adenoids)
Time	20–30min
Pain	+++
Position	Supine, pad under shoulders
Blood loss	Usually small, can bleed post-op
Practical techniques	South-facing uncuffed RAE tube or reinforced LMA, placed in groove of split blade of Boyle–Davis gag SV or IPPV

Preoperative
- Careful history to exclude OSA (see p610) or active infection.
- Topical local anaesthesia on hands (mark sites of veins).
- Consent for PR analgesia.

Perioperative
- IV or inhalational induction (sevoflurane)—Guedel airway useful if nasopharynx blocked by large adenoids.
- Intubate (uncuffed RAE) using relaxant or deep inhalational anaesthesia or insert LMA using propofol/opioid or deep inhalational anaesthesia.
- Secure in midline, no pack (obscures surgical field).
- Beware surgeon displacing/obstructing tube intra-op, particularly after insertion or opening of Boyle-Davis gag.
- T-piece ideal for SV, but ensure reservoir bag always visible.
- Reliable IV access essential, though IV fluids not routine.
- Analgesia with diclofenac/paracetamol PR, morphine or pethidine IV/IM.
- Careful suction of oropharynx and nasopharynx at end under direct vision (surgeon may do).
- Extubate left lateral/head down (tonsil position), with Guedel airway.

Postoperative
- Keep patient in tonsil position until airway reflexes return.
- High-quality recovery care essential.
- Analgesia with PRN paracetamol or diclofenac oral/PR, morphine or pethidine IV/IM.
- Leave IV cannula (flushed) in place in case of bleeding.

Special considerations
- In small children, a pillow under the chest can be used to provide necessary tilt.
- Avoid blind pharyngeal suction with rigid sucker as may start bleeding from tonsil bed.
- NSAIDs increase bleeding slightly (especially if given preop)—this needs to be balanced against benefits.

- LA infiltration of tonsil bed has been used, but is not routine.
- Beware continual swallowing in recovery, a sign of bleeding from tonsil/adenoid bed.
- Adenoidectomy increasingly done as day case, with extended stay and education of parents to recognise signs of bleeding. Tonsillectomy also being done as day case, but risks/problems greater.

Variant Creutzfeldt–Jakob disease (see p291)

- Prions, which accumulate in lymphoid tissue such as the tonsils and adenoids, are not reliably destroyed during standard methods of surgical sterilisation. Inter-patient transmission of prion-borne conditions, such as variant Creutzfeldt-Jakob disease, via theatre equipment contaminated during tonsillectomy/adenoidectomy is therefore a possible risk, although generally considered minimal.
- In January 2001 the UK Department of Health issued guidelines that all relevant surgical and anaesthetic equipment used for tonsillectomy/adenoidectomy should be single-use.
- An increased risk of haemorrhage associated with disposable instruments led to the removal of this guideline for surgical equipment.
- The single-use guideline remains in place, however, for all anaesthetic equipment that is placed in the mouth, such as ETTs and LMAs. The guideline also recommends sheathed or single-use laryngoscope blades, though it is difficult to see how a laryngoscope used solely at the start of a case represents a greater contamination risk in this context than for any other operation.

Bleeding after adenotonsillectomy

- May be detected in recovery or many hours later.
- Loss may be much greater than readily apparent (swallowed blood).
- Senior anaesthetist must be involved.
- Problems include:
  - Hypovolaemia
  - Risk of aspiration (fresh bleeding and blood in stomach)
  - Difficult laryngoscopy because of airway oedema and blood
  - Residual anaesthetic effect.
- Resuscitate preop, check Hb (HemoCue® ideal), crossmatch, and give blood as needed. Note: Hb will fall as IV fluids administered (dilution).
- Options:
  - Rapid sequence induction: enables rapid airway protection, but laryngoscopy may be difficult (blood, swelling)—generally preferred.
  - Inhalational induction left lateral/head down: allows time for laryngoscopy, but takes longer and unfamiliar technique to many.
- Use wide-bore gastric tube to empty stomach after bleeding stopped.
- Extubate fully awake.
- Extended stay in recovery for close monitoring.
- Nasopharyngeal pack occasionally needed (secured via tapes through nose) if bleeding from adenoids cannot be controlled. Usually very uncomfortable—patient may need midazolam/morphine to tolerate.
- Check postoperative Hb.

Tonsillectomy in adults

As for child, except:
- Nasal tube preferred by some surgeons.
- Usually more painful postop in adult—give morphine in theatre.
- IPPV-relaxant technique used more commonly. Mivacurium useful with quick surgeon.
- Preoperative oral NSAID avoids suppository use, though may increase bleeding risk.
- Occasionally patients present with peritonsillar abscess (quinsy). Now normally treated with antibiotics and tonsillectomy performed later. If drainage essential because of airway swelling, pus usually aspirated with syringe and large needle under LA infiltration.

Myringoplasty

Procedure	Reconstruction of perforated tympanic membrane with autograft (usually temporalis fascia)
Time	60–90min
Pain	++
Position	Supine, head tilted to side, head ring, head-up tilt
Blood loss	Minimal
Practical techniques	South-facing RAE tube or LMA (usually reinforced) SV or IPPV

Preoperative

Usually young, fit patients.

Perioperative

- Ensure coughing avoided during surgery: LA spray to larynx, monitor neuromuscular block if IPPV-relaxant technique used.
- Dry field improves the surgical view, though not as important as for stapedectomy—head-up tilt and avoiding hypertension/tachycardia normally sufficient.
- Remifentanil infusion suitable.
- Routine anti-emetic useful.

Postoperative

- PRN paracetamol or diclofenac oral/PR; may need morphine.
- PRN anti-emetic.

Special considerations

Using N_2O may produce diffusion into middle ear and risk graft lifting off: less important with advances in surgical technique—discuss with surgeon.

Stapedectomy/tympanoplasty

Procedure	Excision/reconstruction of damaged middle ear structures
Time	2–4hr
Pain	++/+++
Position	Supine, head tilted to side, head ring, head-up tilt
Blood loss	Minimal
Practical techniques	South-facing RAE tube or LMA (usually reinforced) IPPV normally Arterial line often used

Preoperative
- Check for cardiovascular disease, as will limit degree of hypotension possible.
- Oral premedication options include benzodiazepines, β-blockers and clonidine.

Perioperative
- Monitor to ensure adequate neuromuscular block.
- Bloodless field enables greater surgery accuracy—simple measures include: potent opioid pre-induction, ensure coughing avoided at intubation (LA spray to larynx helpful), head-up tilt to reduce venous pressure.
- Further benefit achieved by lowering arterial BP (mean of 50–60mmHg in healthy patients) and HR (<60bpm)
- Remifentanil infusion ideal to achieve this. Alternatively, use IV β-blocker (metoprolol 1mg increments, esmolol infusion) plus vasodilator (isoflurane, hydralazine, phentolamine): IV labetalol (combined α/β-blocker, 5mg increments) also used, though less individual control of HR and BP.
- Arterial line strongly advised with cardiovascular disease or if potent vasodilators used: head-up tilt further reduces perfusion pressure to brain.
- Give anti-emetic routinely.

Postoperative
- Regular anti-emetic for 24–48hr.
- PRN paracetamol or diclofenac oral/PR; may need morphine.

Special considerations
- N_2O diffusion into middle ear may disrupt surgery, though less important than in myringoplasty. If avoidance requested, can still be used until 20min before end of case, then discontinued.

Nasal cavity surgery

Procedure	Submucous resection (SMR) of septum, septo-plasty, turbinectomy, polypectomy, antral washout
Time	20–40min
Pain	++
Position	Supine, head ring, head-up tilt
Blood loss	Usually minor
Practical techniques	South-facing RAE tube or LMA (usually reinforced) SV or IPPV Throat pack

Preoperative
- Obstructive airways disease often associated with nasal polyps.
- Combination of above procedures frequently performed.

Perioperative
- Face mask ventilation often needs Guedel airway due to blocked nose.
- Nasal vasoconstrictor usually applied (LA/adrenaline infiltration, cocaine spray/paste, Moffett's solution).
- Leave eyes untaped for polypectomy (optic nerve can be close and surgeon needs to check for eye movement).
- Suck out pharynx (particularly behind soft palate—'Coroner's clot') before extubation: less easy with LMA.

Postoperative
- Left lateral/head down with Guedel airway in place until airway reflexes return.
- Analgesia with PRN paracetamol or diclofenac oral/PR.
- Nose usually packed producing obstruction of nasal airway—if disturbing to patient, or in cases of OSA, nasopharyngeal airway(s) can be incorporated into the pack.
- Sit up as soon as awake to reduce bleeding.

Special considerations
- Leave IV cannula in overnight, as can bleed postoperatively.

Microlaryngoscopy

Procedure	Examination of larynx using operating microscope (+ excision/biopsy)
Time	10–30min
Pain	+/++
Position	Supine, pad under shoulders, head extended
Blood loss	Nil
Practical techniques	Microlaryngeal tube and conventional IPPV
	TIVA and jet ventilation using Sanders injector (O_2 + entrained air) via:
	• injector needle on the operating laryngoscope
	• semi-rigid tracheal catheter
	• cricothyroidotomy needle/cannula

Ventilation during microlaryngoscopy

Microlaryngeal tube and conventional IPPV
- Microlaryngeal tube is a long 5.0mm ETT with a high-volume/low-pressure cuff.
- Enables maintenance of anaesthesia with inhalational agents.
- Protects against aspiration of blood/surgical debris but restricts surgeon's view.
- Use long, slow inspiration for IPPV because of the high resistance of tube. Measured inflation pressure will be high, but patient's airway pressures distal to tube will be lower.

Jet ventilation
- Ventilation achieved using a Sanders injector (O_2 + entrained air) via:
  - Injector needle attached to proximal end of operating laryngoscope and ventilation started when correctly aligned with larynx. Various needle sizes available with different flow rates. Technique not suitable if good view of larynx is unobtainable and has disadvantage of blowing debris/smoke into trachea with ventilation.
  - Semi-rigid tracheal catheter (ordinary suction catheter not suitable) with tip placed mid-way down the trachea. Special catheters available with gas sampling port or made from laser-proof material.
  - Cricothyroidotomy needle/cannula placed through cricothyroid membrane under LA before induction and aimed towards carina. Commercial versions available or Tuohy needle can be used: beware gas injected into tissues if needle misplaced/displaced.
- Induce in theatre or use microlaryngeal tube initially then remove and change to jet ventilation when all ready in theatre (not with cricothyroidotomy needle).
- Ensure anaesthetic machine in theatre situated close to enable easy FM ventilation at induction/recovery.
- TIVA needed for maintenance (propofol/remifentanil infusion).

- Ventilate using normal respiratory rate and adjust inspiratory flow (alter injector settings or change needle size) to produce appropriate degree of chest expansion.
- Accurate flow/pressure measurement not easy: barotrauma a potential risk.
- Stop ventilation intermittently during surgical work (clear communication essential).
- Provides minimal obstruction to surgical view.
- At end of case, either continue jet ventilation until SV re-established or discontinue and ventilate by FM until SV recommences.

Preoperative

- Patients often elderly, usually smokers; CVS/RS problems common.
- Carefully assess airway for evidence of obstruction. History, examination, ENT clinic assessment, plain films, and CT scan may all help, but if any degree of stridor present obstruction must be substantial (see p608).
- Ensure all equipment ready before induction, including cricothyroidotomy kit, and that surgeon is available for emergency tracheostomy if required.

Perioperative

- If airway obstruction suspected, secure airway initially using principles p608. Inserting a cricothyroid cannula under LA pre-induction provides a route for ventilation in event of total obstruction.
- Give short-acting opioid (alfentanil, remifentanil) to attenuate hypertensive response.
- Muscle relaxation usually essential: mivacurium or intermittent suxamethonium (+ glycopyrronium/atropine to prevent bradycardia).
- LA spray to larynx reduces risk of laryngospasm, though impairs airway protection, so recover left lateral, head down.

Postoperative

- Analgesia with PRN paracetamol or diclofenac oral/PR.
- May develop stridor postoperatively from oedema of an already-compromised airway—dexamethasone 8–12mg IV sometimes used to prevent.

Special considerations

- Jet ventilation preferable if laser work planned.
- Microlaryngoscopy can be used to inject inert material (Teflon) into paralysed vocal cords to improve phonation, though can lead to airway obstruction if overdone.
- High-frequency jet ventilation has been used, though complex, and assessment of ventilation difficult.

Tracheostomy

Procedure	Insertion of a tracheal tube via neck incision
Time	30min
Pain	++
Position	Supine, pad under shoulders, head ring, head-up tilt
Blood loss	Normally small, though can bleed from thyroid vessels
Practical techniques	IPPV, ETT with tubing going 'north', changed to tracheostomy tube during case LMA if airway not a problem, IPPV or SV Can be done under LA

Preoperative
- Normally done for long-term ICU ventilation or airway obstruction.
- ICU patients almost certainly already intubated. If ventilation difficult and oxygenation critical, set up ICU ventilator in theatre, using TIVA rather than inhalational agents.
- Stop NG feeds if applicable.
- If tracheostomy is for airway obstruction, secure airway initially using principles p608.
- Before induction ensure all equipment prepared (including cricothyroidotomy kit) and surgeon ready for emergency tracheostomy if required.

Perioperative
- Secure ETT with tape to allow easy removal during case, with pilot cuff readily accessible.
- Aspirate NG tube (if present) and clear oropharynx of secretions before draping.
- Drape patient to allow anaesthetist access to ETT for tube change.
- Long tubing needed for breathing circuit and gas sampling.
- Before changing to tracheostomy tube, preoxygenate for 3–4min (increasing volatile agent as necessary) and check neuromuscular blockade adequate.
- Ensure scrub nurse has correct tracheostomy tube and sterile catheter mount.
- Deflate ETT cuff before surgeons incise trachea, so it can be reinflated and ventilation continued if problems occur.
- Withdraw ETT slowly into upper trachea (do not remove from trachea until tracheostomy secure and certain) and connect breathing circuit and capnograph to new tracheostomy tube via sterile catheter mount.
- Beware false passage created during tracheostomy tube insertion, especially in the obese: check position with fibreoptic endoscopy if any doubt.
- If problems occur, remove tracheostomy tube and advance ETT back down trachea.

Postoperative
- Regular suction to new tracheostomy (blood, secretions).
- Humidify inspired gases.
- Analgesia in recovery with diclofenac PR or morphine IV. Usually little analgesia required thereafter.
- A new tracheostomy often produces protracted coughing—morphine, benzodiazepines, or low-dose propofol useful for control.
- Anti-emetic as required.
- If tube comes out, reinsertion can very difficult in first few days—orotracheal intubation often more practical. Two retraction sutures left in tracheal incision are useful for identifying and opening the stoma.

Special considerations
- Can be done under LA, though difficult in a dyspnoeic, struggling patient.
- In ICU tracheostomy now commonly done percutaneously using dilatational technique: theatre cases likely to be the difficult ones.
- Tracheostomy not the ideal route of approach for emergency airway access: cricothyroidotomy more accessible and less likely to bleed.
- LMA can be used if tracheostomy done at start of larger procedure and upper airway normal.

Tracheostomy tubes
- Specific features available include:
  - Fenestration: allows speech by occluding lumen with finger and exhaling through hole in back wall of tube.
  - Inner tube (eg. Shiley®): permits removal for cleaning.
  - Adjustable flange: length can be modified for short trachea or deep stoma.
  - Channel in obturator for guide-wire.
- Tube change:
  - New tube must be inserted with obturator in place to prevent stomal damage.
  - May be difficult to find trachea in new tracheostomy: guide-wire very useful.
  - Prepare for oro-tracheal intubation in case of problems.
  - Cannot be left in place longer than 28d (classified as an implant thereafter).

Laryngectomy

Procedure	Excision of larynx (epiglottis and glottis) with creation of and end-stomal tracheostomy
Time	3–4hr
Pain	+++
Position	Supine, pad under shoulders, head ring, head-up tilt
Blood loss	Moderate to substantial; X-match 2–4U
Practical techniques	IPPV, ETT with tubing going 'north', changed to tracheostomy during case Arterial line, urinary catheter, CVP line if surgery likely to be long/complicated or if indicated by cardiac disease

Preoperative
- Some degree of airway obstruction likely. Patient likely to have had recent GA (for diagnosis) to guide airway management: beware if some time has elapsed.
- If no recent GA, assess the airway as for microlaryngoscopy (p618)
- Usually smokers: CVS/respiratory system problems and malnutrition common.
- Discuss implications of tracheostomy preoperatively (communication, secretions, coughing produced by tube). Speech therapist will do much of this.

Perioperative
- Insert fine-bore NG feeding tube at induction and fix securely (can be sutured to nasal septum).
- Warming blanket and fluid warmer.
- Long tubing needed for breathing circuit and gas sampling tube.
- Remifentanil infusion ideal.
- Substantial blood loss can accumulate under drapes at back of neck and may not be apparent until end of case.
- For CVP access, all neck lines hinder surgery: femoral best, though antecubital fossa (ACF) or subclavian can be used.
- Antibiotic prophylaxis for at least 24hr.
- When changing to tracheostomy tube, see precautions for tracheostomy (p620), though end-stoma makes tracheal access safer and easier.
- During surgery, long tube (armoured or special preformed) via tracheostomy useful to enable surgical access round stoma—beware endobronchial intubation.

Postoperative
- HDU ideal.
- Humidification and regular suction essential (blood, secretions).
- New tracheostomy produces protracted coughing—morphine, benzodiazepines, or low-dose propofol useful for control.

- Analgesia with PRN diclofenac PR, morphine IV/IM. Suitable for PCA, although analgesic requirements surprisingly low. Paracetamol suspension (via NG tube) useful after initial postoperative period.
- Anti-emetic as required.

Special considerations

- Beware of air emboli during dissection—early detection by sudden fall in $ETCO_2$.
- For previous laryngectomy patients presenting for surgery, to ventilate via stoma use paediatric facemask turned through $180°$, LMA applied to neck, or intubate awake after LA spray to stoma. Tracheostomy tube insertion usually easy, though check stoma for stenosis or tumour recurrence and always preoxygenate.
- Partial laryngectomy, with laryngeal reconstruction and temporary tracheostomy, favoured by some as alternative to radiotherapy in early laryngeal tumours.

Pharyngectomy

Procedure	Excision of pharynx (includes glossectomy and radical tonsillectomy): may involve mandibular split for access and tissue transfer
Time	6–8hr
Pain	++++
Position	Supine, pad under shoulders, head ring, head-up tilt
Blood loss	Major; X-match 4U initially
Practical techniques	IPPV, ETT (nasal may be best) with tubing going 'north' initially, changed to tracheostomy during case
	Arterial line, CVP line, urinary catheter

Preoperative
- Discuss plans with surgeons to ensure what needs to be left untouched, e.g. forearm flap.
- Assess airway carefully: patient likely to have had recent GA (for diagnosis) to guide airway management.
- CVS/respiratory system problems and malnutrition common.
- Inform patient about lines, tracheostomy etc.
- Ensure ITU bed available.

Perioperative
- Insert fine-bore NG feeding tube at induction and fix securely (can be sutured to nasal septum).
- Femoral route best for CVP access.
- Long tubing needed for breathing circuit and gas sampling tube.
- Warming blanket and fluid warmer.
- Access to patient severely restricted: ensure all lines/tubes secure at start.
- Remifentanil infusion ideal.
- Substantial blood loss may be hidden under drapes: check regular HemoCue®.
- Ensure patient is well-filled, especially if free-flap used (aim for Hb of ~10g/dl)—see p508.
- Antibiotic prophylaxis for at least 24hr.

Postoperative
- ICU essential.
- Keep sedated and ventilated until stable and warm.
- Regular flap observations.
- Avoid tracheostomy ties round neck (may compromise flap blood supply).
- Humidification and regular suction (blood, secretions) to tracheostomy.
- Analgesia with PCA morphine once awake and PRN diclofenac/ paracetamol NG/PR.
- Anti-emetic as required.

Radical neck dissection

Procedure	Excision of sternomastoid, internal and external jugular veins and associated lymph nodes
Time	2–4hr
Pain	+++
Position	Supine, pad under shoulders, head on ring tilted to side, head-up tilt
Blood loss	Moderate to substantial, X-match 2–4U
Practical techniques	IPPV, ETT with tubing going 'north'
	Arterial line, urinary catheter, CVP line if surgery likely to be long/complicated or with cardiac disease

Preoperative
- Assess airway carefully, as may be an associated head and neck tumour or previous major surgery.
- May be performed with another procedure, e.g. laryngectomy.

Perioperative
- Warming blanket and fluid warmer.
- Long tubing is needed for the breathing circuit and gas sampling.
- Remifentanil infusion ideal.
- Can bleed briskly from large neck vessels, with substantial accumulation of blood under drapes (that may not be apparent until end of case).
- For CVP access femoral is best, though subclavian or antecubital fossa on opposite side from surgery can be used (if on same side can enter neck vein and become transfixed by surgeon). Must avoid remaining jugulars, as head and neck venous drainage dependent on them.

Postoperative
- Head and neck oedema likely for several days (impaired venous drainage). Keep head up as much as possible and avoid excessive IV fluids.
- To reduce chance of agitation/rebound hypertension and wound haematoma in recovery, give morphine 15–20min before end of surgery: clonidine up to 150µg IV also very useful. Treat any hypertension early.
- Analgesia with PRN paracetamol or diclofenac oral/PR, morphine IV/IM. Surprisingly low analgesic requirements normally.
- Anti-emetic as required.

Special considerations
- Beware of air emboli during dissection—early detection by sudden fall in $ETCO_2$.
- Surgical manipulation of carotid sinus can produce marked bradycardia.
- If neck dissection previously done on other side, oedema usually worse and can raise ICP. Dexamethasone 8–12mg IV preoperatively (then 4mg IV 6-hourly) used by many to reduce this.

Parotidectomy

Procedure	Excision of parotid gland, usually preserving facial nerve
Time	2–5hr
Pain	++/+++
Position	Supine, head ring, head tilted to side and moderately extended, head up tilt
Blood loss	Usually small/moderate, G&S. Greater for malignancy
Practical techniques	South-facing RAE tube and IPPV normally used, though SV possible for suitable patients Reinforced LMA and IPPV or SV also possible No NMB during dissection

Preoperative
- Check if suitable for SV—not if elderly, obese, or respiratory disease.
- Check mouth opening, especially if malignant.

Perioperative
- Warming blanket and fluid warmer, plus urinary catheter if prolonged.
- Avoid neuromuscular blockade (NMB) after initial dose (check recovery with PNS).
- Remifentanil infusion ideal to allow IPPV without NMB and also reduce blood loss.
- Alternatively suppress respiratory drive with other opioid, volatile agent, or propofol infusion combined with moderate hyperventilation.
- LA spray to larynx useful to prevent coughing.
- If SV used, ensure patient settled initially using high level of volatile agent.

Postoperative
- To reduce chance of agitation/rebound hypertension and wound haematoma in recovery, give morphine 15–20min before end of surgery, keep head up and treat hypertension early: clonidine up to 150µg IV very useful.
- Anti-emetic as required.
- Analgesia with PRN morphine IV/IM, paracetamol or diclofenac oral/PR.

Special considerations
- Surgeon normally uses nerve stimulator to identify facial nerve during dissection and may wish to leave ipsilateral eye exposed to monitor response. Avoid prolonged NMB—initial dose has usually worn off in time for surgical dissection.
- Large-bore IV access at start, as can bleed substantially (especially malignant tumours).

Other ENT procedures

Operation	Description	Time (min)	Pain	Position	Blood loss	Notes
Mastoidectomy	Clearance of cholesteatoma from mastoid cavity	90–120	++	Head-up tilt, head tilted to side on ring	Minimal	RAE tube or LMA, SV or IPPV. Bloodless field needed (see stapedectomy). If disease close to facial nerve, surgeon may request no relaxant used (see parotidectomy)
Drilling of ear exostoses	Excision of external auditory ('swimmers') exostoses	60–90	++	Head-up tilt, head tilted to side on ring	Minimal	RAE tube or LMA, SV or IPPV
BAHA	Application of bone-anchored hearing aid	90–120	++	Head-up tilt, head tilted to side on ring	Minimal	LA + sedation or GA with RAE tube or LMA, SV or IPPV
FESS	Functional endoscopic sinus surgery	45–60	++	Head-up tilt, head-ring	Small	RAE tube or reinforced LMA, SV or IPPV, throat pack. Moffett's normally used. Moderate hypotension useful to decrease bleeding
MUA # nose	Correction of nasal fracture	1–15	+	Supine	Small	If quick, preoxygenate + propofol only. If longer, RAE tube or reinforced LMA + throat pack. Occasionally bleeds dramatically
Removal of foreign body from nose	Removal of foreign body from nose, usually in child	5–10	Nil	Supine, head-ring		Gas induction, RAE tube or LMA, throat pack, SV. Avoid FM ventilation if possible (risk of pushing FB down into lower airway)

Rhinoplasty	Cosmetic alteration or reconstruction of nose using bone/cartilage graft	60–90	++	Head-up tilt, head-ring	Small	RAE tube or reinforced LMA, SV or IPPV, throat pack. Moderate hypotension useful to decrease bleeding
Lateral rhinotomy	Resection of nasal tumour via lateral rhinotomy	90	++	Head-up tilt, head-ring	Moderate	RAE tube or reinforced LMA, SV or IPPV, throat pack. Moderate hypotension useful to decrease bleeding
Uvulo-palato-pharyngoplasty (UPPP)	Excision of uvula and lax tissue from soft palate, sometimes using laser	20–30	+++	Supine, pad under shoulders	Small	RAE tube or reinforced LMA, SV or IPPV. Laser-proof tube if needed. Regular postop diclofenac + paracetamol. OSA precautions if indicated
Submandibular gland excision	Excision of blocked/diseased sub-mandibular gland	45–60	++	Supine, pad under shoulders, head-ring	Small	RAE tube or reinforced LMA on opposite side, SV or IPPV
Tracheo-bronchial foreign body removal	Removal of inhaled foreign body using rigid bronchoscope, usually in child (see also p810)	20–30	Ns	Supine, pad under shoulders	Nil	Deep inhalational anaesthesia using oxygen and halothane, allowing surgeon intermittent access. LA spray. Atropine useful to prevent bradycardia

Table contd.

Operation	Description	Time (min)	Pain	Position	Blood loss	Notes
Laryngoscopy in child	Examination of larynx in child, usually for recurrent stridor or aspiration	15–20	ns	Supine, pad under shoulders	Nil	Inhalational induction, LA spray to larynx. Either SV via rigid surgical laryngoscope (circuit connected to scope) or LMA with bars removed and fibreoptic laryngoscopy through it (ideal for small child and enables larynx to be viewed during emergence)
Direct pharyngoscopy	Examination of pharynx using rigid pharyngoscope	10–15	+	Supine, pad under shoulders	Nil	Check for reflux. Small (6.5–7) oral RAE tube secured on left, IPPV, mivacurium or intermittent suxamethonium. Risk of bleeding if biopsies done
Endoscopic stapling of pharyngeal pouch	Division of opening to pharyngeal pouch using staple gun endoscopically	15–20	+	Supine, pad under shoulders	Nil	Preoxygenate, avoid FM ventilation, small (6.5–7) oral RAE tube secured on opposite side, IPPV. NG tube at end and IV fluids as nil by mouth postop
Excision of pharyngeal pouch	Excision of pharyngeal pouch via external approach	45–60	++	Supine, pad under shoulders, head-ring	Nil	Preoxygenate, avoid FM ventilation, small (6.5–7) oral RAE tube secured on opposite side, IPPV. Surgeon may want oesophageal bougie inserted to help recognise anatomy. Antibiotic cover, NG tube at end and IV fluids as nil by mouth postop

Procedure	Description	Time	Pain	Position	Blood loss	Notes
Insertion of speaking valve (eg Provox®)	Insertion of speaking valve via tracheo-oesophageal puncture, following laryngectomy	15	+	Supine, pad under shoulders, head-ring	Nil	Microlaryngoscopy tube inserted via tracheostomy, IPPV, mivacurium or intermittent suxamethonium, remifentanil or alfentanil to reduce CVS response
Pharyngo-laryngo-oesophagectomy	Resection of larynx, pharynx and oesophagus for tumour of hypopharynx, usually with stomach pull-up. Involves laparotomy ± thoracotomy	6–8hr	++++	Supine, pad under shoulders, head-ring	Major, X-match 4–6U	No access to patient whatsoever! Prepare as for laryngectomy with all lines, plus double-lumen tube if doing thoracotomy. Consider epidural analgesia for laparotomy/thoracotomy (using plain LA) with PCA morphine to cover remaining surgical sites. ICU mandatory postop see also p378

Maxillofacial and dental surgery

Richard Telford

Babinder Sandhar

Oral/maxillofacial surgery

General principles

Anaesthesia for intraoral/maxillofacial procedures requires management of a shared airway and potentially difficult intubation. Nasal intubation is frequently used to improve access to the mouth. At the preoperative visit check nostril patency and ask about epistaxis and the use of anticoagulants. Discuss choice of airway with surgeon.

- Simple intraoral procedures are often possible using a reinforced laryngeal mask airway. However, access to the mouth is inevitably compromised. The LMA may be dislodged and vigilance is required. Similarly, for unilateral intraoral procedures an oral ETT placed on the opposite side of the mouth may be acceptable.
- If the nasal route is chosen for intubation, use a local anaesthetic and/or vasoconstrictor mixture (cocaine 5–10%, lidocaine 5%/ phenylephrine 0.5%—Co-phenylcaine®), or xylometazoline (Otrivine®). There are many varieties of nasal tube—the 'Polar Preformed North Nasal' from Portex® is ideal. These 'north-facing' tubes are made of soft material and cause little nasal trauma. Sizes of 6.0, 6.5, and 7.0mm should be available. Place in warm water before use to soften the material even further.
- Protect the eyes with tape and eye pads.
- Position the patient with the head at the opposite end to the anaesthetic machine—a long breathing circuit is normally required.
- Stabilise the head with a horseshoe or head ring. For operations on the roof of the mouth use a bolster under the shoulders to extend the neck further.
- Throat packs are used to minimise contamination of the airway with blood and debris. Ribbon gauze or tampons may be used. A robust system should be in place to ensure that throat packs are not inadvertently left in situ. They should preferably be included in the swab count (see p605).
- Careful laryngoscopy should always be performed at the end of the procedure.

Extubation

- There is a risk of aspiration of blood, pus, and debris. Patients are therefore best extubated in the left lateral position with head down tilt.
- Some anaesthetists extubate the patient 'deep,' having used a spontaneous breathing technique, whereas others use opioid/relaxant and prefer to extubate awake. The use of a nasotracheal tube, which does not stimulate the gag reflex as much as an oral tube, facilitates the latter approach.
- If a nasal tube has been used it is possible to convert it into a nasopharyngeal airway by withdrawing it until the tip lies in the oropharynx, cutting at the 15cm mark and inserting a safety pin at the proximal end (to prevent tube being lost into the nostril).

Cardiac arrhythmias

Cardiac arrhythmias are common during dental extraction if a spontaneously breathing technique is chosen. These are particularly common with halothane due to sensitisation of the myocardium to catecholamines. Contributory factors include hypercarbia, hypoxia, light anaesthesia, and injected sympathomimetic agents. Correction of the underlying problem is usually effective. Infiltration of local anaesthetic by the surgeon virtually abolishes them. Arrhythmias are less common with enflurane, isoflurane, desflurane, and sevoflurane.

Free-flap surgery

- Many major maxillofacial reconstructions are performed using tissue/bone free flaps (particularly from the radial forearm).
- These operations are lengthy, 6–18hr.
- The same principles apply as for plastic surgery free flaps (p508) with the added complication of a potentially difficult airway, both pre- and post surgery.
- Surgical tracheostomy may be indicated because of the potential for postoperative airway compromise.
- HDU or ICU care is usually indicated postoperatively.

Surgical extraction of impacted/buried teeth

Procedure	Removal of teeth
Time	3–45min
Pain	+
Position	Supine, head ring, bolster under shoulders if teeth to be extracted in the roof of mouth
Blood loss	Minimal
Practical techniques	Nasal tube and IPPV—extubate awake Nasal tube and SV—extubate deep LMA and SV

Preoperative
- Careful assessment of the airway. Check nostrils for patency.
- If the patient has a dental abscess there may be marked swelling of the face and severe trismus. Awake fibre-optic intubation may be necessary (see p948).
- Obtain consent for an NSAID suppository if planned.

Perioperative
- Consider LMA/oral tube for simple/unilateral extractions.
- Intubate with a warmed, preformed nasal tube after applying vaso-constrictor to the nasal mucosa (see p634).
- Protect the eyes with tape and pads.
- The surgeon should anaesthetise the appropriate terminal branches of the maxillary division (infraorbital, greater palatine, nasopalatine) and mandibular division (inferior alveolar, lingual, buccal, mental) of the trigeminal nerve with a long-acting local anaesthetic (bupivacaine 0.5% with adrenaline 1:200 000).
- Give an intra-operative opioid and NSAID.
- IV antibiotics are administered to minimise the risk of infection (benzylpenicillin 600mg).
- Steroids (e.g. dexamethasone 8mg IV) are given to minimise swelling.
- Extubate in the left lateral position with head down tilt.

Postoperative
- Balanced analgesia with regular paracetamol and NSAIDs. Prescribe rescue analgesia with PRN codeine phosphate/tramadol.

Special considerations
- Talk to the surgeon to ascertain the likely length of surgery. Remember that some patients require general anaesthesia only because they are 'dental phobic.' The surgical extractions may be simple and operative time consequently very short. A short-acting muscle relaxant may be required.

Maxillary/mandibular osteotomy

Procedure	Surgical realignment of the facial skeleton
Time	Lengthy, 4–6hr
Pain	++
Position	Supine, with head up tilt, head ring
Blood loss	Variable. Occasionally can be severe. X-match 2U
Practical techniques	Nasal tube and IPPV—extubate awake. Art line

Patients presenting for orthognathic surgery may have malformations isolated to one jaw or have multiple craniofacial deformities as part of a syndrome. They have often had prior dental extractions and preoperative orthodontic work. There are many surgical procedures performed to correct facial deformities. Patients are usually in their late teens or early twenties and are generally fit and healthy. When a mandibular osteotomy is performed, the bone is plated and often stabilised by wiring the maxilla and mandible together. If vomiting occurs postoperatively, or intraoral bleeding occurs, fatal airway obstruction may occur unless the fixation can be instantly removed. This requires expert trained staff and adequate facilities postoperatively.

Preoperative
- Assess the airway carefully. Check the nostrils for patency.
- Check Hb and crossmatch blood as per surgical blood ordering schedule (2U).
- Thromboembolic prophylaxis (TEDS, unfractionated or low-molecular-weight heparin). Consider the use of intermittent pneumatic compression boots in theatre.

Perioperative
- Intubate nasally using a preformed nasal tube (see p634).
- Good venous access. Consider invasive pressure monitoring due to length of surgery.
- Put Lacrilube® into the eyes and protect them with pads and tape.
- Position the patient carefully on the operating table. Place the head on a ring and tilt the table head up.
- Use a balanced anaesthetic technique and aim for an awake, co-operative patient who can maintain their airway at completion of surgery. Induced hypotension is useful to help minimise blood loss. Remifentanil infusion (0.04–0.25µg/kg/min) as part of a balanced anaesthetic may help control blood pressure.
- Give IV antibiotics and steroids (e.g. dexamethasone 8mg IV) to minimise swelling.
- Keep the patient warm. Measure core temperature, warm IV fluids, and use a heating mattress and/or hot air blower.

- Monitor blood loss carefully. The HemoCue® is an accurate way of tracking haemoglobin concentration in theatre.
- The patient's jaws will frequently be wired together on completion of surgery. Ensure that throat packs are removed and that the oro-pharynx is cleared of blood and debris before this is done.
- Administer prophylactic anti-emetics (granisetron + cyclizine ± haloperidol) to minimise the risk of nausea and vomiting. Dexamethasone is also effective.
- Extubate the patient once fully awake. Withdraw the nasal tube and cut (15cm mark at the nostril) to leave as a nasopharyngeal airway.
- Prescribe small doses of IV opioid to be administered in recovery.
- Ensure that you and the nursing staff are familiar with the position of the wires that hold the jaws together. Make sure wire cutters are with the patient at all times.

Postoperative

- Some units send these patients to HDU. Others send them to the ward after a lengthy period in recovery.
- Administer humidified oxygen.
- Ensure all oral analgesics are prescribed in a soluble form. PRN IM opioids should also be prescribed.
- Continue prophylactic antibiotics and steroids postoperatively as per your unit's protocol.
- Prescribe IV fluids. Encourage the patient to take fluid by the oral route as soon as possible.

Fractures of the zygomatic complex

Procedure	Elevation of fractured zygomatic complex ± fixation
Time	10–180min
Pain	+/++
Position	Supine
Blood loss	Minor (significant with internal fixation)
Practical techniques	Oral RAE tube and IPPV LMA/SV for simple elevation

These fractures may occur in isolation or may be associated with damage to other parts of the facial skeleton. There may be limitation of mouth opening due to interference with movement of the coronoid process of the mandible by the depressed zygomatic complex. Following elevation, the fracture may be stable or unstable and require internal fixation. Most surgery is carried out via a temporal approach or a percutaneous route through the cheek. Intraoral and transantral routes have also been described but are rarely used. Unstable fractures require plating or wiring via skin or intraoral incisions.

Preoperative

- Assess the patient carefully for associated injuries. Treatment of these fractures does not have high clinical priority. The operation is often easier if a period of time elapses (5–7d) to allow the associated facial swelling to disperse.
- Make a careful airway assessment.
- Obtain consent for an NSAID suppository if planned.

Perioperative

- Intubate the patient with an oral RAE tube. For simple fracture elevations a flexible LMA may be used, but discuss with surgeon whether open fixation of the fracture is planned.
- Lubricate and protect the eyes.
- Give antibiotics and steroids as requested.
- Extubate in the lateral position with the fractured side uppermost.

Postoperative

- IV opioids may be required in recovery.
- Balanced oral analgesia for the ward.

Mandibular fractures

Procedure	Reduction and fixation of a fractured mandible
Time	2–3hr
Pain	+
Position	Supine, with head up tilt, head ring
Blood loss	Variable. Consider G&S
Practical techniques	Nasal tube and IPPV
	Fibre-optic intubation may be required

Mandibular fractures can be treated by either closed reduction and indirect skeletal fixation (using interdental wires, arch bars, or splints) or by open reduction and direct skeletal fixation using bone plates. When indirect skeletal fixation is used the patient's jaws are wired together at the completion of surgery. When direct skeletal fixation is used this is not usually the case.

Preoperative
- Careful assessment for associated injuries.
- Make a meticulous assessment of the airway. There may be severe trismus and marked soft tissue swelling.
- Assess nostril patency. Check for evidence of basal skull fracture and CSF leak as these contraindicate nasal intubation.

Perioperative
- Trismus makes intubation look potentially difficult preoperatively as mouth opening may be markedly limited, but this tends to relax following induction.
- Bilateral mandibular fractures also allow increased anterior jaw displacement after induction, but airway maintenance by facemask may not always be easy due to increased jaw movement/swelling. A rapid sequence induction with suxamethonium is usually appropriate.
- Marked swelling may make intubation more difficult and an awake fibre-optic intubation may occasionally be required.
- Gas induction is often difficult due to pain when applying the facemask.

Postoperative
As for patients having maxillary/mandibular osteotomies.

Anaesthesia for dentistry

General considerations

- General anaesthesia for dental procedures should be reserved for patients unable to tolerate local anaesthesia (i.e. young children or adults with mental disability) and undertaken in a hospital setting by anaesthetists with appropriate postgraduate training.
- **Facilities** should be the same as for any other day surgery procedure.
- **Selection criteria.** Patients with significant intercurrent disease should be referred for in-patient treatment, as for any other day case procedure. Mentally disabled patients may have difficulty understanding the procedure and are often anxious. A short-acting anxiolytic agent, such as oral midazolam, and topical anaesthetic cream may be helpful. Mental disability may be part of a more complex medical disorder, such as Down's syndrome or other congenital abnormality. It is important to exclude any significant cardiac pathology and to give endocarditis prophylaxis when appropriate. Patients requiring extensive extractions or restoration work can be admitted to a day case unit for treatment, but may require overnight stay if medically compromised.
- **Positioning.** There is no longer a place for 'chair dental anaesthesia.' Postural hypotension can be easily overlooked and it is now standard practice to keep patients supine.
- **Arrhythmias.** Dental anaesthesia is associated with a high incidence of arrhythmias, usually related to hypoxia, hypercarbia, inadequate anaesthesia, and volatile anaesthetic agents. Arrhythmias are mainly ventricular and may progress (rarely) to ventricular fibrillation. Halothane is associated with an arrhythmia frequency of up to 75% in dental anaesthesia and should be avoided. The incidence of hypoxia can be reduced by using 100% oxygen for maintenance. End-tidal CO_2 is difficult to measure when using a nasal mask but can be monitored properly when using an LMA.
- **Local anaesthetic infiltration** should be used whenever possible— caution in very young children where it may lead to accidental biting/laceration.
- **Dental labelling.** Deciduous teeth are assigned letters A–E in each quadrant and adult teeth are numbered 1–8.
- **Simple extractions** are very quick procedures lasting only a few minutes. A nasal mask is commonly used, but laryngeal mask airways (plain or flexible) are preferable for multiple extractions. A prop/gag and a mouth pack are inserted by the dentist to prevent soiling of the lower airway—ensure that it does not obstruct the airway. When extractions are complete, a pack is positioned over the dental sockets to absorb any oozing blood. During extractions, patency of the airway must be maintained and may require support of the jaw.
- **Restoration work** can take over an hour and often requires intubation and ventilation.

Simple dental extractions

Procedure	Dental extractions
Time	2–10min
Pain	+/++
Position	Supine
Blood loss	Nil
Practical techniques	Nasal mask/LMA

Preoperative

- Usually children 3–12yr.
- Beware of undiagnosed pathology e.g. heart murmurs which may need prophylactic antibiotic therapy (see p1163).
- Obtain consent for analgesic suppositories.

Perioperative

- Give pre-emptive oral analgesia if possible e.g. paracetamol (20mg/kg), diclofenac (1mg/kg).
- Apply topical anaesthetic for cannulation if IV induction planned.
- Propofol for induction, sevoflurane for gas induction.
- Tape the eyes.
- Maintenance with volatile agent or IV agent.
- Use local anaesthetic infiltration (by dentist), avoid opioids except in longer cases or in-patients.
- Stabilise the head and neck manually during the procedure.
- Place in lateral position, slightly head down at the end.

Postoperative

- Regular paracetamol (15mg/kg) for 12–48hr.
- Diclofenac (1mg/kg) or ibuprofen (5–10mg/kg) as indicated.

Special considerations

- The dentist may apply considerable pressure during extraction and the anaesthetist should apply counter-pressure to support and stabilise the head and jaw.
- Beware of potential hypoxia. Give 100% oxygen for maintenance if necessary.
- When using a nasal mask, mouth breathing can occur around the dental pack resulting in decreased uptake of the anaesthetic agent and the patient becoming light. This can be a problem when using short-acting agents such as sevoflurane—use isoflurane for maintenance or give increments of propofol.
- Children with blocked noses can be safely anaesthetised using an LMA (provided there is no upper respiratory tract infection).

Sedation for dentistry

Patients who are unable to tolerate dental treatment under LA can often be managed by a combination technique using sedation. These procedures are usually performed by the dentist in the dental clinic. Oral or IV sedation can be provided by short-acting benzodiazepines such as midazolam, but the effects can be unpredictable, especially in children. Inhalational sedation can be provided by sub-anaesthetic concentrations of nitrous oxide (up to 50%) in oxygen using a nasal mask—termed 'relative analgesia.' Whichever route of administration is used, it is important to ensure that the patient *remains conscious throughout*.

General considerations
- Ideally patients should be ASA1 or 2.
- Patients will require an escort for the procedure and to care for them afterwards.
- Written instructions should be provided regarding limitations on driving (as for GA) and operating machinery postoperatively. The patients should also be told to avoid a heavy meal/alcohol prior to treatment.
- Inhalational sedation cannot be used in patients with nasal obstruction or those unable to co-operate with breathing through a nasal mask.
- LA is used in all patients after sedation has been established.
- The patient should be able to communicate throughout the procedure.

Suitable regimes include:
- For adults, midazolam 2mg IV, wait 90s, then give 1mg every 30s until sedated.
- Low dose propofol infusion (only with suitable training).
- 100% oxygen via nasal mask, add 10% nitrous oxide for 1min, then 20% for 1min. Continue increments of 5% until sedated (up to 50%).

Special considerations
- Do not use mouth props as the ability to keep the mouth open is an important indicator of consciousness.
- Have flumazenil available.
- Allow at least 1hr for recovery following IV sedation.
- Following nitrous oxide sedation, 100% oxygen must be administered to prevent diffusion hypoxia.
- The patient can be discharged once they are able to stand and walk unaided.

Further reading
Blayney MR, Malins AF, Cooper GM (1999). Cardiac arrhythmias in children during outpatient general anaesthesia for dentistry. *Lancet*, **354**,1864–66.
Holroyd I, Roberts GJ (2000). Inhalation sedation with nitrous oxide: A review. *Dent Update*, **27**,141–6.
Royal College of Anaesthetists (1999). Standards and guidelines for general anaesthesia for dentistry.
Standing Dental Advisory Committee (1990). Report of an expert Working Party (Chairman: Professor D Poswillo). General Anaesthesia, Sedation and Resuscitation in Dentistry.

Chapter 27

Ophthalmic surgery

Andrew Farmery

General principles

Intraocular pressure (IOP)

IOP normally ranges between 10–20mmHg, but transient changes occur with posture, coughing, vomiting or Valsalva manoeuvres. Such changes are normal and have no bearing on the intact eye. However, when the globe is open during surgery, such pressure changes may cause vitreous extrusion, haemorrhage or lens prolapse.

Factors affecting IOP (analogous to factors affecting ICP):

- Aqueous humour volume (determined by balance of production and drainage).
- Choroidal blood volume (determined by the balance of arterial flow and venous drainage).
- Head-up position (via its affect on the above).
- Tone in extraocular muscles.
- Mannitol and acetazolamide: Mannitol (0.5g/kg IV) reduces IOP by withdrawing fluid from the vitreous. Acetazolamide (500mg IV) reduces IOP by reducing aqueous production by the ciliary body. Both can be used in the medical management of glaucoma, but the anaesthetist may be required to give them intra-operatively to reduce IOP acutely. Both are mild diuretics, urinary catheterisation may be indicated.
- Anaesthetic factors:

Anaesthetic factors increasing IOP	Anaesthetic factors decreasing IOP
External compression of the globe by tightly applied face mask	Induction agents principally by reduction in arterial and venous pressure
Laryngoscopy—either pressor response, or straining in an inadequately relaxed patient	Non-depolarising muscle relaxants by reduction in tone of extraocular muscles
Suxamethonium increases IOP transiently by contracting extraocular muscles	Head-up tilt at 15°, assists venous drainage
Large volumes of local anaesthetic solution placed in the orbit. This effect is transient (2–3min)	Moderate hypocapnia: 3.5–4.0kPa (26–30mmHg) reduces choroidal blood volume by vasoconstriction of choroidal vessels

Oculomedullary reflexes

Oculocardiac, oculorespiratory and oculoemetic reflexes.

- Incidence: 50–80%. Commonly seen in paediatric squint surgery.
- Triggers: Traction on extraocular muscles, pressure on globe.
- Afferent arc: Fibres running with long and short ciliary nerves, via ciliary ganglion to trigeminal ganglion near floor of 4th ventricle.
- Efferent arc: Vagus, fibres to respiratory and vomiting centre.
- Effects: Bradycardia, sinus arrest, respiratory arrest, nausea.
- Prevention: All of these (bradycardia, respiratory arrest, nausea) can be moderated to some extent by use of local anaesthesia (to abolish the

afferent arc), avoiding hypercapnia (which appears to sensitise the reflex) and prophylactic glycopyrronium (200–400µg) or atropine (300µg).

Preoperative assessment

Many patients presenting for eye surgery are at the extremes of age. The majority of ophthalmic operations (predominantly cataract surgery) are performed as day cases under local anaesthesia (LA). Most patients are elderly and may have one or more serious systemic diseases. Patients scheduled for general anaesthesia should have routine investigations performed (see p4). Patients having cataract extraction under LA, however, do not warrant routine investigation. Many centres do not routinely fast such patients and a light meal, two to three hours preoperatively, may be less disruptive for this elderly population and facilitate better diabetic control. Light sedation is routinely used in these unfasted patients without harm.

Preoperative assessment for local anaesthetic cataract surgery should include:
- Axial length.
- INR/APPT if on warfarin or heparin.
- Blood glucose if diabetic.
- Ability to lie flat for 1hr (heart failure, arthritis etc).
- Hearing/comprehension—will they be able to hear and understand instructions?
- Anxiety level—will sedation be required?
- Ability to tolerate supplemental oxygen—is there a risk of CO_2 retention, requiring delivery of a precise concentration of oxygen?

General anaesthesia versus local anaesthesia

There are a number of advantages to avoiding general anaesthesia in this population. These include:
- Minimisation of physiological disturbance (including postoperative sleep disturbance).
- Reduced morbidity and mortality.
- Economic factors—increased patient throughput (ward admissions and theatre throughput), less demanding on nursing resources, portering etc.

There are situations when general anaesthesia is preferable:
- Patients who refuse the operation under LA. Unless there are overwhelming risks, such patients should be offered general anaesthesia providing they are fully informed about the risks and accept them.
- Children or patients with learning disabilities/movement disorders.
- Major and lengthy operations (oculoplastics and vitreoretinal) are commonly performed under GA since it may be unrealistic to expect patients to tolerate them otherwise.
- Patients unable to lie flat and remain motionless for up to 1hr (although some surgeons can operate in a 'deck chair' position rather than true supine for LA).

Local anaesthesia for intraocular surgery

Basic anatomy

The orbit is 40–50mm deep and pyramidal in shape with its base at the orbital opening and its apex pointing to the optic foramen. Its volume is approximately 30ml, 7ml of which is occupied by the globe and its muscle cone, and the remainder loose connective tissue through which local anaesthetic solutions can spread. The lateral walls of both orbits form an angle of 90° to each other and the angle between the medial and lateral wall of each orbit is 45°. The medial wall is parallel to the sagittal plane.

The globe lies in the anterior part of the orbit and sits high and lateral (i.e. nearer the roof than the floor and nearer the lateral than the medial wall). This relationship is important when considering needle access, which is usually achieved either medially or inferolaterally where the gap between globe and orbital wall is greatest. The sclera forms the fibrous bulk of the globe. It is 1mm thick and although tough, is easily penetrated by a sharp needle. Deep to the sclera is the uveal tract which comprises the ciliary body, iris and choroid layer. Superficial to, and enclosing the sclera is the membranous Tenon's capsule, lying directly underneath the conjunctiva. It is easily recognised, as it is white and avascular, unlike the vascular sclera below. The four recti and two oblique muscles control eye movement and influence IOP. The lateral rectus is innervated by the abducent nerve (VIth), the superior oblique by the trochlear nerve (IVth) and the rest by the occulomotor nerve (IIIrd) [$(LR_6SO_4)_3$]. The recti form the muscle 'cone' which encloses the sensory nerves, ciliary ganglion, optic nerve, retinal artery and vein. It is through this cone that peribulbar local anaesthetic drugs must flow or diffuse to effect their action.

The cranial nerves enter the cone and pierce the muscles on their intraconal surface. These are motor only. The sensory supply is via branches of the trigeminal (Vth) cranial nerve. The 1st division of the trigeminal (ophthalmic nerve, V_1) enters the orbit via the superior orbital fissure and supplies branches intraconally to the sclera/cornea, and extraconally to the upper lid and conjunctiva after leaving the orbit via the superior orbital notch. The 2nd division (maxillary nerve, V_2) enters the orbit via the inferior orbital fissure. Branches of this nerve are entirely extraconal and supply the lower lid and inferior conjunctiva after leaving the orbit via the inferior orbital foramen.

The ciliary ganglion, lying within the cone, relays sensory fibres from the globe to V_1, receives a parasympathetic branch from the (motor) IIIrd cranial nerve and sympathetic fibres from the carotid plexus.

Ocular block techniques

Retrobulbar block

Local anaesthetic is deposited **within** the muscle cone (retrobulbar intraconal), blocking the ciliary ganglion, sensory nerves to the sclera/cornea, and motor nerves to the extraocular muscles. This provides anaesthesia and akinesia with a rapid, predictable onset, using a small volume of solution. It is not now recommended because of the following potential complications:

- Globe perforation (0.1–0.7%)
- Intravascular injection
- Haemorrhage (1%)
- Penetration and injection of the optic nerve sheath (0.27%) with resultant optic nerve damage, subarachnoid spread, brainstem paresis, and cardiopulmonary arrest.

Retrobulbar anaesthesia is not further considered.

Peribulbar block

First described in 1986. Local anaesthetic solution is deposited within the orbit but outside the muscle cone (peribulbar periconal). The complication rate is therefore reduced.

Single injection techniques provide adequate anaesthesia although akinesia is not guaranteed. They are now preferred to two-site injections because the risks of complications are theoretically halved. In modern ophthalmic practice, a completely akinetic eye is seldom required. Discuss this requirement with the surgeon. The most commonly used single injection technique is an inferolateral injection.

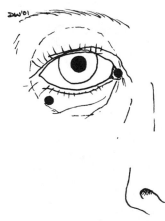

Peribulbar block I: inferolateral and medical canthus injection sites

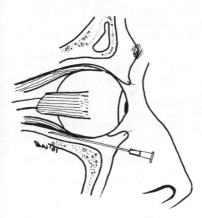

Peribulbar block II: inferolateral injection (side view)

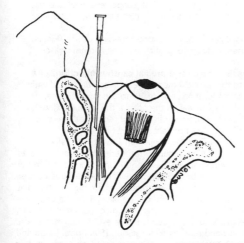

Peribulbar block III: medial canthus injection (top view)

Inferolateral injection
- Establish IV access and monitoring.
- When indicated use minimal sedation e.g. midazolam 0.5–1.5mg or propofol 20mg ± alfentanil 250μg or fentanyl 50μg.
- Instil topical local anaesthetic drops to anaesthetise the conjunctiva— proxymetacaine (0.5%).
- Patient lies supine and is asked to look straight ahead (primary gaze).
- Palpate junction of the medial 2/3 and lateral 1/3 of the inferior orbital rim with the non-dominant hand where a groove is felt at the junction of the maxilla and zygoma.
- Just lateral to this point, and 1mm above the rim, insert a 25G 25mm standard hypodermic needle ('long orange') mounted on a 10ml syringe, and pass slowly backwards perpendicular to all planes. Needle entry can be either transcutaneous, or, by retraction of the lower lid, transconjunctival.
- If the needle tip contacts the bone, it is redirected slightly superomedially, to follow the orbit floor once more.
- Advance the needle until its tip is about level with the posterior pole of the globe (i.e. until the hub reaches the plane of the iris). The globe should be observed carefully for any sign of rotation during insertion, indicating scleral contact. Avoid any temptation to 'wiggle' the needle to confirm that the sclera is unengaged. This is likely to increase the risk of haemorrhage.
- After aspiration, slowly inject 6–8ml of local anaesthetic. The globe can be palpated with the other hand to assess tension. Stop injecting if globe becomes tense/proptosed, or if the upper eyelid falls, as this is likely to indicate retrobulbar injection, requiring a smaller volume of agent.
- Following injection, digital massage or a compression device (Honan balloon) can be used to dissipate local anaesthetic and normalise intraocular pressure.
- If a further 'top-up' is needed use a **medial canthus injection.** At a point just medial to the caruncle the needle is passed backward with the bevel facing the globe, at an angle of 10° to the sagittal plane, directed towards the medial wall of the orbit. If the medial wall is contacted, the needle is withdrawn slightly and redirected laterally.
- If both medial and lateral injections are planned (Two Injection Technique), use 6ml for inferolateral injection and 4ml medially.

The larger volumes of solution required for peribulbar block tend to cause proptosis and a temporary increase in IOP. In the intact globe this has no consequence, but will be problematic when the globe is opened for surgery. The raised IOP usually disappears when the solution has dissipated, alternatively a Honan balloon can be used. This is a compression device applied to the eye at a set pressure (25mmHg), which reduces the volume of blood and aqueous in the eye. Upon release the eye becomes hypotonic and remains so for about 15min until blood and aqueous volumes are re-established.

Contraindications to peribulbar block

- INR >2.0. Whenever possible warfarin therapy should be adjusted to reduce the INR to < 2.0. If this is considered inappropriate then a sub-Tenon approach, topical anaesthesia or GA should be considered.
- Axial length >26mm. In severely myopic patients the globe often has a long antero-posterior diameter ('sausage shaped'). This increases the likelihood of globe perforation due to increased globe length, thinner sclera and increased likelihood of staphyloma (hernial outpouchings of the sclera). Where axial length is greater than 26mm, consider a sub-Tenon approach, topical anaesthesia or general anaesthesia.
- Perforated or infected eye.
- Inability to lie flat and still.

Complications

The risk of complications from peribulbar anaesthesia, although out-weighed by the benefits, are still appreciable—1:750 and 1:360 LA anaes-thetics have 'life-threatening' and 'serious' complications respectively.

- Globe perforation: <0.1%. Globe perforation is diagnosed by sudden pain on injection, loss of vision, poor red reflex or vitreous haemor-rhage. Globe perforation is not always obvious. It may be noted at the time of surgery if the eye becomes hypotonic in which case there is a serious risk of retinal haemorrhage and detachment which may require laser retinopexy or vitrectomy.
- Retrobulbar haemorrhage: incidence 0.07%. Recognised by rapid orbital swelling and proptosis. The surgeon should be informed immediately and the pulsation of the central retinal artery assessed. If this is com-promised, a lateral canthotomy may be required to relieve IOP.
- 'Systemic complications' (faints/bradycardia/epileptic seizure) occur with an incidence of 0.9%, although most of these are self-limiting.

Sub-Tenon block

Originally described in 1884 by Turnbull and in 1992 by Stevens, this technique is gaining popularity as a safe and effective alternative to retro and peribulbar anaesthesia. It avoids 'blind needling' to the orbit, and so has no appreciable risk of sharp needle complications. It effectively blocks the ciliary ganglion, long and short ciliary nerves. Larger volumes depos-ited more posteriorly are required to block the motor nerves and extra-conal branches of the ophthalmic and maxillary nerves.

- Apply topical proxymetacaine 0.5% to the conjunctiva and retract the lower lid using either an assistant or a lid speculum.
- In the inferonasal quadrant, the conjunctiva is lifted with Moorfield's forceps at a point 5–7mm from the limbus (awake patients are asked to look up and out).
- A small incision is made in the conjunctiva with (blunt ended) Westcott's spring scissors which are then used to blunt dissect inferonasally in a plane between the sclera and Tenon's capsule (Tenon's capsule is white and avascular which distinguishes it from the vascular sclera).

- Once in this plane, a blunt curved cannula (Southampton cannula or similar) is passed backwards beyond the equator and 3–5ml of local anaesthetic is deposited. Care must be taken to dissect in the correct plane. If the cannula is placed subconjunctivally most of the LA solution will escape or cause considerable chemosis.
- Sub-Tenon block can be used safely in patients with axial lengths >26mm. It is the block of choice in anticoagulated patients, since any bleeding point can be cauterised directly. It may be most easily performed by the surgeon, although it is increasingly being performed by anaesthetists.

Complications
- Conjunctival haematoma. Occurs rarely (less than 0.5%) and is usually easily treated by cautery.
- Mild chemosis and superficial haemorrhage, making for a less cosmetically appealing eye in the short term. This resolves completely in days.
- Isolated case reports of more serious complications have been reported (such as globe perforation and central retinal artery occlusion), but are less than a handful in number, and of uncertain causation. No large series exist.

Topical/infiltration anaesthesia

Anterior segment (principally cataract) surgery can be carried out under:
- Subconjunctival injection: A small volume of LA is injected near the superior limbus by the surgeon.
- Topical corneoconjunctival anaesthesia: Topical agents can be used to provide up to 15min of anaesthesia. Bupivacaine 0.75% is effective but can sting initially and cloud the cornea. Proxymetacaine 0.5% is superior.

For both these techniques, anaesthesia is not as complete as with formal ocular blocks. The iris and ciliary body retain their sensitivity and akinesia is not a feature. The surgeon and staff need to ensure that good communication is maintained with the patient at all times. A mild anxiolytic premedication may be useful.

- Intracameral anaesthesia is often used to supplement a topical 'block'. Here the surgeon injects a small quantity (~0.1ml) of isotonic, preservative-free lidocaine into the anterior chamber using the microscope at the start of surgery. This provides anaesthesia to the iris and ciliary body.

No local anaesthetic agent is ideal for topical anaesthesia. All are mildly toxic to corneal epithelium and cause slight temporary swelling and clouding, but satisfactory results can be achieved with an initial drop of proxymetacaine 0.5%, (causes less stinging than bupivacaine, and less clouding than amethocaine) followed by bupivacaine 0.5% to provide greater anaesthetic duration than proxymetacaine alone.

Local anaesthetic solutions

- The commonest solution is a 1:1 mixture of lidocaine 2% and bupivacaine 0.5% (or levobupivacaine 0.75%). Adrenaline adds little to block quality and is best avoided. For routine cataract extraction lidocaine 2% alone gives sufficient duration, but for vitreoretinal surgery levobupivacaine 0.75% is more suitable.
- Hyaluronidase can be added to promote spread and reduce IOP. Concentrations between 10–30U/ml are used. The drug data sheet suggests 15U/ml.
- Alkalinisation and warming of the LA (to 37°C) may reduce latency and decrease pain on injection.

Joint working party on anaesthesia in ophthalmic surgery

The Joint Report of the Royal Colleges of Anaesthetists and Ophthalmologists (2001) suggested that local anaesthesia should be administered by an 'appropriately trained' anaesthetist, ophthalmologist or nurse. The latter may give topical or sub-conjunctival (and occasionally sub-Tenon's) anaesthesia, but they are not recommended to undertake peri/retro-bulbar blocks. An anaesthetist is not required to be present for surgery proceeding under topical, subconjunctival or sub-Tenon's block without sedation. An anaesthetist must be 'available' when surgery is proceeding under retro- or peribulbar block without sedation, but must have 'sole responsibility' for a list in which sedation is used. Monitoring of patients having surgery under LA should include clinical observation of ventilation, and monitoring of the circulation with pulse oximetry by a suitable trained person. One person in the theatre team should have had training in advanced life support.

General anaesthetic technique

The aim is to minimise increases in IOP whilst maintaining cardiovascular stability and avoiding overly deep anaesthesia in a population which is likely to be elderly and have several co-morbidities.

Indications

- Patient preference
- Other patient factors (e.g movement disorders, dementia, claustrophobia)
- Long operations (e.g vitreoretinal)
- Multiple operation sites (e.g. oculoplastics with distant graft donor site).

Preoperative

In addition to routine consultation and investigations (see p4), the preoperative visit should identify patients with co-morbidities such as diabetes and cardiovascular disease. Insulin dependent diabetics will often have reduced their morning dose of insulin and will be fasted. Such patients will require close monitoring of blood glucose, and the institution of a euglycaemic control regimen.

ETT or LMA?

Unless contraindicated, the LMA is ideal. It obviates laryngoscopy and the possible adverse effects on IOP. It produces minimal stimulation once in place and permits lighter anaesthesia. The quality of emergence is also superior (see below).

IPPV or SV?

For extraocular and minor surgery (including cataract extraction) spontaneous ventilation is acceptable. Controlled ventilation has a number of advantages in intraocular and more major surgery. It allows control of CO_2 (reducing IOP and desensitising the oculomedullary reflex) and permits the other benefits of a balanced technique.

- Ventilating via an LMA is usually uneventful. Avoid high airway pressures (>15cmH$_2$O, with the risk of gastric insufflation) by adjusting the tidal volume and using a more symmetrical I:E ratio (1:1.5).
- Always monitor CO_2 waveform. Any change usually heralds a change in ventilation before it is clinically apparent (malpositioned LMA, inadequate muscle relaxation).
- Use a nerve stimulator routinely. Coughing and gagging are less well tolerated by ophthalmic surgeons than by their orthopaedic colleagues.

Nitrous oxide?

Nitrous oxide should be avoided in vitreoretinal surgery if intraocular gas bubbles of sulphur hexafluoride (SF_6) or similar are planned. Discuss this with the surgeon in advance.

Supplementary local block?

Probably the only indication for local block in addition to GA is for vitreoretinal surgery, in which case a sub-Tenon's block (with negligible risk) is the preferred technique—can be administered following induction.

Emergence without coughing

With an LMA, emergence and LMA removal are usually smooth. If a tracheal tube is used, spray the cords with lidocaine at intubation. Unfortunately the effect is short lived and may no longer be effective at extubation. Other techniques are to extubate in a deep plane or administer a bolus of IV lidocaine (1mg/kg) or propofol (30–40mg) 1min prior to extubation.

It is best not to lighten anaesthesia until the surgery is complete and the 'sticky-drapes' removed (if a block has been used, drape removal may well be the most stimulating part of the operation). Emergence hypertension (and the concomitant raised IOP), if it occurs, can be moderated by the use of IV lidocaine (up to 1mg/kg) 2min before emergence.

A standard technique: summary

- IV induction; propofol bolus or TCI.
- Airway: Reinforced LMA if appropriate.
- IPPV.
- Maintenance: Propofol infusion (~5mg/kg/hr or 2.5µg/ml if TCI) or volatile agent.
- Ventilate with oxygen/air.
- Analgesia provided ideally with a local anaesthetic block if indicated, or with either alfentanil or remifentanil for stimulating procedures.

General points

- Tape the non-operative eye.
- Access to the airway may be limited—have a low threshold for moving everyone out of the way to inspect the airway if you suspect difficulties.
- The use of glycopyrronium will reduce the volume of saliva pooling behind an LMA (which can otherwise spill from the corner of the mouth and soak through the surgical drapes). It may also reduce the incidence and severity of 'oculocardic' bradycardias.

Postoperative

Analgesia requirements are usually modest, especially if supplemental local anaesthesia is used. Nausea and vomiting is common in squint surgery, but less so in the majority of other cases. It is reasonable to use ondansetron (100µg/kg) for prophylaxis in squint surgery although it is only modestly effective.

Cataract extraction and IOL

Procedure	Phacoemulsification of opacified lens, removal and replacement with artificial intraocular implant
Time	20–40min
Pain	—
Position	Supine
Blood loss	Nil
Practical techniques	Local technique
	LMA (armoured), SV/IPPV
	ETT (RAE, armoured), IPPV

Preoperative

- Check axial length (less than 26mm for peribulbar block) and INR if necessary. For operations under LA, patient must be able to lie flat and still.
- Often 'Day-case'.

Perioperative

- Use supplemental oxygen (via nasal cannulae).
- Monitor BP, SpO_2 and nasal expired CO_2 if possible. The latter serves as an apnoea indicator and is useful if sedation is used. Be aware that the use of sedation may serve to disinhibit rather than sedate some patients.
- If sedation required use midazolam (0.25–1mg) with fentanyl (25–50µg), or propofol (20mg). This is best employed during block insertion. The patient should then be allowed to awaken when in theatre to gain cooperation and avoid sleeping, snoring and airway problems.

Postoperative

Simple oral analgesics only required.

Strabismus surgery

Procedures	Extraocular surgery for correction of squint—may be unilateral or bilateral
Time	60–90min
Pain	+
Position	Supine
Blood loss	Nil
Practical techniques	LMA (armoured), IPPV/SV ETT (RAE, armoured), IPPV

Preoperative
- Patient population mainly children (commonest ophthalmic operation in children).
- May be 'Day-case'.
- Preoperative analgesia (20mg/kg soluble paracetamol).

Perioperative
- Higher incidence of oculocardiac reflex; have atropine prepared. Prophylaxis with glycopyrronium has no proven benefit.
- Suxamethonium should be avoided because tone in the ocular muscles remains abnormal for up to 20min, making surgical assessment and correction difficult.
- Controlled ventilation, via LMA or tracheal tube is used (although not invariably). This allows control of CO_2 which reduces the incidence and severity of the oculocardic reflex.
- All anaesthetics affect eye movement and the position of neutral gaze (Guedel's signs). Propofol may affect this the least, and the rapid recovery it affords allows early assessment of the correction in recovery. Anaesthesia with volatile agents should be of sufficient depth to ensure neutral gaze.
- Rectal diclofenac (1mg/kg).
- Opioids may be avoided, thereby reducing incidence of PONV.

Postoperative
- Postoperative pain is mild and can be treated with oral analgesics and topical proxymetacaine eye drops.
- High incidence of PONV. It is reasonable to use ondansetron (100µg/kg) for prophylaxis in squint surgery although it is only modestly effective.

Vitreo-retinal surgery

Procedures	Intraocular surgery. Vitrectomy, cryotherapy, laser, plombage, insertion of oil and/or gas, scleral banding ('explant')
Time	90–180min
Pain	++/+++
Position	Supine
Blood loss	Nil
Practical techniques	LMA (armoured), IPPV
	ETT (RAE, armoured), IPPV
	Sub-Tenon's block ± GA

Preoperative
- Patient population generally aged 60–70yr. May have coexisting morbidities e.g. hypertension, ischaemic heart disease and diabetes.
- May be retinal detachments and therefore semi-urgent.

Perioperative
- Surgery is characterised by alternating periods of intense and minimal stimulation. Achieving a depth of anaesthesia and analgesia to accommodate these extremes is not easy without concurrent local block.
- Often prolonged operations, performed largely in the dark.
- Axial length is usually high (profound myopia causes retinal detachment) so retro/peribulbar blocks are relatively contraindicated. Sub-Tenon's block in addition to GA is ideal.
- If necessary, can be performed under block only, but duration of surgery makes this difficult in the majority of patients.
- Controlled ventilation is usual. LMA/propofol/remifentanil is ideal.
- A supplementary sub-Tenon's block improves intra-operative stability, obviates the need for opiates and reduces postoperative pain and nausea. Place after induction or ask the surgeon to perform periop.
- Avoid N_2O. Intraocular tamponade with gas (SF_6 or C_3F_8) may be used, usually towards the end of the case. It is recommended that nitrous oxide be discontinued 20min beforehand. It is probably better to omit altogether because surgeons seldom give notice and it is probably not wise to interfere with the equilibrium of the anaesthetic at a time when muscle relaxation is wearing off. If a supplementary block is not used, remifentanil should be used instead of nitrous oxide since cryotherapy and scleral indentation are very stimulating.
- Beware 'lightening' the patient too soon at the end of surgery. The other eye is often examined, and possibly cryo-cauterised.

Postoperative
- With block, postoperative analgesic requirement is minimal and PONV is rare.
- Otherwise, simple oral analgesics.

Dacrocystorhinostomy (DCR)

Procedures	Probing of tear duct, insertion of drainage tube, formation of stoma between tear duct and nasopharynx
Time	30–45min
Pain	+
Position	Supine, slight head-up
Blood loss	Can be relatively bloody, with soiling of nasopharynx
Practical techniques	ETT (RAE, armoured), IPPV LMA (armoured), IPPV

Perioperative
- Lacrimal surgery can range from simple probing of the tear ducts, to insertion of tubes or formal DCR. The latter is usually done under GA.
- DCR may be bloody. Blood will pass into the nasopharynx/oropharynx. Topical vasoconstrictor solutions (cocaine/Moffett's soaked pledgets) placed intranasally after induction may reduce this. Infiltrate the surgical field with LA containing vasoconstrictor to further reduce bleeding.
- Slight head-up tilt and deliberate moderate hypotension (or avoidance of hypertension) further improves the operative field.
- Intubation (oral RAE or reinforced) protects the lower airway definitively, but a reinforced LMA may be used where topical vasoconstriction, moderate hypotension and surgical co-operation are available. A throat pack should be used in either case.
- Controlled ventilation, by facilitating moderate hypocapnia, may also contribute to mucosal vasoconstriction and improved operative field. If using an LMA, positive pressure ventilation may reduce the likelihood of blood soiling the lower airway.

Postoperative
- Postoperative analgesia provided by oral NSAIDs and paracetamol/codeine.
- Ask the surgeon to irrigate the ducts with topical local anaesthetic.

Penetrating eye injury

Procedures	EUA, debridement, closure of punctum
Time	30–45min
Pain	+/+++
Position	Supine
Blood loss	—
Practical techniques	ETT (RAE, armoured), IPPV
	LMA (armoured), IPPV

Preoperative

- Although relatively straightforward in adults, this can be difficult to manage in children (in whom it is a common injury, representing more than a third of paediatric trauma cases). The essential danger is that elevation of IOP either pre- or perioperatively, risks extrusion of the vitreous, haemorrhage and lens prolapse.
- Pain, eye rubbing, crying, breath holding and screaming will elevate IOP. IV sedation may be required to control such a child.
- Give analgesia (oral/rectal paracetamol/NSAIDs). Opioids should be avoided if possible (or at least used cautiously and with an antiemetic) since vomiting will also affect IOP adversely.
- Patients may have a full stomach. Traumatised children may still have a full stomach several hours post injury.

Perioperative

- Suxamethonium causes a transient increase in IOP and there is good reason to avoid its use when the eye is open. However, induction agents *reduce* IOP and so moderate its effects. The risks imposed by suxamethonium should be balanced against the risks (specific to each case) imposed by a full stomach. If in doubt, use suxamethonium following a large dose of induction agent. There are, however, two practical alternatives to suxamethonium:
  - Wait. If immediate operative repair is not imperative (and it seldom is) the case can be deferred until the stomach is considered safe. Prokinetic agents may be of use.
  - If no airway problems are anticipated, use a rapid sequence technique with rocuronium (1mg/kg), or 'high' dose vecuronium (0.15mg/kg).
- The pressor response to intubation can be moderated by IV lidocaine (1mg/kg), IV esmolol or pre-priming with induction agent immediately prior to intubation.
- Opioids may be used as part of a balanced technique.

Postoperative

Analgesia provided by paracetamol/codeine preparations and oral/rectal diclofenac.

Further reading

Farmery AD, Shlugman D, Rahman R, Rosen P (2003). Sub-Tenon's block reduces both intraoperative and postoperative analgesia requirement in vitreo-retinal surgery under general anaesthesia. *European Journal of Anaesthesia*, **20**, 973–978.

Hamilton RC (1995). Techniques of orbital regional anaesthesia. *British Journal of Anaesthesia*, **75**, 88–92.

Local Anaesthesia for Intraocular Surgery. The Royal College of Anaesthetists and The Royal College of Ophthalmologists (2001). http://www.rcoa.ac.uk/docs/rcarcoguidelines.pdf.

Ripart J *et al.* (1996). Medial canthus (caruncle) single injection periocular anesthesia. *Regional Anesthesia and Pain Management*, **83**, 1234–1238.

Wong, DHW (1993). Regional Anaesthesia for intraocular Surgery. *Canadian Journal of Anaesthisia*, **40**, 635–657.

Other ophthalmic procedures

Operation	Description	Pain (+ to +++++)	Time (min)	Position	Blood loss	Notes
Trabeculectomy	Surgical correction of glaucoma	+	50–80	supine	Nil	Usually performed under LA block—peribulbar often preferred to sub-Tenon's. Axial length may not have been checked
Moh's reconstruction	Plastics procedure on eyelids after excision of BCC	+	45–60	supine	Nil	May be under local, but may require use of fat or fascia taken from the thigh so GA may be preferred
Enucleation	Removal of globe for tumour or chronic infection	++	60–90	supine	0–200ml	Anaesthetic technique as for vitreoretinal surgery. Local techniques not appropriate
Evisceration	Removal of globe contents for later replacement with prosthesis	+	60–90	supine	Nil	Anaesthetic technique as for vitreoretinal surgery. Local techniques not appropriate
Syringing of tear ducts in babies		+	30	supine		Straightforward technique. SV via LMA. Throat pack to absorb any 'wash'
EUA of eyes in babies		+	10–20	supine		Beware oculocardiac reflex. Have atropine 10µg/kg prepared

Day surgery

Peter Davies

Day surgery

A surgical day case is a patient who is admitted for investigation or operation on a planned non-resident basis.

- Organisation is the key to efficient good-quality day surgery and requires close cooperation between all agencies involved, including surgeons, anaesthetists, day case unit staff, general practitioners, and patients themselves.
- Facilities: an efficient organisation requires 'ring fenced' theatres and ward space. Day cases on inpatient wards or theatres will suffer cancellation when there are bed shortages and emergency operations. Self-contained units with their own facilities, within an acute hospital, probably offer the best option.
- Staff: senior staff should perform day case anaesthesia and surgery. Much of the surgery and anaesthesia may be viewed as routine or simple, but it must be performed to a high standard for day units to operate efficiently.

Patient selection

In theory all patients should follow a sequential pathway and should be pre-assessed by specially trained nurses, according to set day case criteria. However, pre-assessment should be approached flexibly as different methods work for different patient groups.

- With short waiting times, patients can be reviewed at the hospital on the day of their surgical outpatient appointment.
- Some patient groups can be telephone assessed; in particular those who have direct access surgery (not seeing a surgeon until the day of surgery).
- Older patients need earlier pre-assessment at the hospital so that tests can be performed and the results reviewed prior to surgery.
- In some hospitals surgeons book day cases after reviewing them and instructions are sent out by clerical staff. This can work well as long as the surgeon is senior and is fully conversant with the requirements of day surgery.
- Patients must agree/understand that they should not drive, cycle, operate machinery, or take alcohol for a minimum of 24hr after their anaesthetic.
- Some patients who fall outside the guidelines need to be discussed on an individual basis and may include ASA 3 patients who would do better in a day case environment rather than as an inpatient, e.g. chemotherapy patients, stable diabetics.
- Many paediatric anaesthetists will anaesthetise babies as young as 6wk on a day case basis (provided the infant was not premature).
- Moderate obesity in itself does not preclude day stay surgery, but does cause unpredictable problems in terms of length of surgery and anaesthesia. BMI is not the ideal tool for assessing fitness for day surgery, but provides pre-assessment nurses with guidance. Obese patients should be scheduled mid morning to allow preoperative antacid therapy time to work and still allow time for recovery. Remember that obesity may cause as many problems to the surgeon as to the anaesthetist. In general a BMI >35kg/m^2 is not suitable (BMI = weight (kg)/height^2 (m)).

Day case selection criteria

Health status: generally fit and healthy (ASA 1 and 2). Patients with significant cardiovascular or respiratory disease, insulin-dependent diabetics, or those with gross obesity are not suitable.

Age: patients should be older than 6 months. There is no upper age limit; physiological fitness should be considered rather than chronological age.

Complexity of surgery: operations lasting more than 60min and those associated with a risk of significant postoperative pain, haemorrhage, or prolonged immobility should not be performed.

Transport: all patients must be escorted home by a responsible, informed adult and be adequately supervised during their recovery at home for a minimum of 24hr.

Social support: patients must have suitable home conditions with adequate toilet facilities and a telephone should be readily available for advice in an emergency.

Geography: the patient should live within 1hr travelling distance from the hospital.

Common co-existing diseases

- Stable asthmatics are suitable for day surgery. Regular hospitalisation, oral steroid therapy, and poor control of symptoms would suggest unsuitability.
- Stable epileptics on medication are suitable for day surgery. Avoid propofol if they have a driving licence (see p230).
- Well-motivated, well-controlled diabetics having operations with a low incidence of postoperative nausea can be managed as day cases, with either general or local anaesthesia.

Cancellations and DNAs (did not attend)

Most cancellations on the day of surgery can be avoided by careful patient selection by experienced staff. It is often unavoidable to cancel patients who have an acute illness, e.g. a heavy cold, or an exacerbation of previously well controlled asthma. However, diseases such as undiagnosed hypertensive disease or uncontrolled atrial fibrillation should be discovered by pre-assessment at the day surgery unit.

Fassting instructions

- Morning lists: no solid food after midnight and free clear fluids up to 06.30hr.
- Afternoon lists: no solid food after 06.30hr and free clear fluids up to 11.30hr.
- Preoperative verbal and written instructions are important so that milky drinks are avoided. In practice, accept drinks with 1 to 2 teaspoons of milk but treat any more as solid food and require a 6hr fast.

Driving

Patients should not drive for at least 24hr postoperatively because of residual effects of the anaesthetic. Remember that some operations themselves will preclude driving for longer because of pain and limited movement, e.g. arthroscopy and inguinal hernia repair. This advice must be contained in the preoperative verbal and written instructions given to the patient.

Conduct of anaesthesia

Use local anaesthetic, or short-acting general anaesthetic drugs which have few residual psychomotor effects and a low incidence of postoperative nausea or vomiting (PONV).

Preoperative

- Nurses, surgeon, and anaesthetist will need to undertake an adequate history and examination as a full medical clerking is not usually performed by junior medical staff. This should include blood pressure measurement and cardiorespiratory examination.
- Avoid premedication if at all possible. If necessary use oral midazolam (up to 0.5mg/kg) in a little undiluted sweet fruit cordial (as it tastes awful) for children, or temazepam (10–20mg) in adults.
- There is no evidence for any increase in regurgitation/aspiration in day case patients so the routine use of antacid drugs is probably unnecessary. However, in those with a history of regurgitation, ranitidine (300mg PO) or omeprazole (40mg PO) is appropriate.
- NSAIDs, e.g. diclofenac 50–100mg, given orally or rectally, reach peak effect after 1–2hr and are a useful adjunct to anaesthesia, with very few side effects. Remember that slow release oral preparations do not reach steady state concentrations until after several doses, and are thus not useful for early analgesia.

Perioperative

- Total IV anaesthesia with propofol (without nitrous oxide) is widely used. Propofol induction with isoflurane/sevoflurane maintenance is an alternative.
- Incremental fentanyl, often 2–4µg/kg in divided doses.
- Diclofenac (PO/PR) and local anaesthetic for every suitable patient/operation.
- Whenever possible use a laryngeal mask airway, avoiding intubation, muscle relaxants and reversal agents. Laryngeal masks for gynaecological laparoscopy and armoured laryngeal masks for wisdom tooth extraction can be used safely in most circumstances.
- Antiemetics are not indicated routinely but should be reserved for treatment of any PONV or prophylaxis in those with a history of PONV.

Postoperative

- The inclusion of opioids, NSAIDs, and local anaesthetics should provide adequate analgesia. If more analgesia is needed it is imperative to treat it early (fentanyl 50–75µg).
- Give morphine if stronger analgesia is required. Remember that pain worsens nausea.
- Simple oral analgesics may be of help, as may physical therapies such as hot water bottles, particularly for the cramping lower abdominal pain following gynaecological surgery.

Postoperative nausea and vomiting (see also p1049)

- A multifactorial approach to the prevention of PONV should be used. Early ambulation is a risk factor so all day case patients should be treated as high risk. PONV must be fully controlled before discharge home.
- For high risk patients TIVA propofol, omitting nitrous oxide, multi-modal analgesic therapy, good hydration (IV fluids), and minimal (2hr) fluid fast are appropriate. Dexamethasone 8mg is an effective and cheap prophylactic agent. This is a recipe approach which works well and leaves a small number of patients requiring treatment, for which a 5-HT$_3$ antagonist such as granisetron would be suitable.

Regional anaesthesia

Regional anaesthesia is widely used in Europe and North America for day case anaesthesia. PONV is reduced. Timing and planning are important as blocks take longer to set up or wear off compared with general anaesthesia. Perform spinals early on the list to allow timely recovery. Spinals must have worn off completely before discharge to allow safe ambulation. However, it is reasonable to discharge patients with working plexus blocks thus allowing the benefit of prolonged postoperative analgesia. Remember that patients need special instructions on care of the anaesthetised part so as to avoid inadvertent damage. This would include a sling for patients with brachial plexus blocks.

Local anaesthesia and sedation

With increased use of local anaesthetics, short-acting sedative drugs will inevitably be used to increase tolerability. It must be noted that sedation is a poor adjunct to an imperfect local anaesthetic block. However, judicious use of intermittent midazolam or propofol infusions (TCI 1–1.5µg/ml) can provide good amnesia with few postoperative effects. If sedation is to be used it must be provided and monitored by someone other than the operating surgeon.

Specific blocks

- Field block: excellent for LA hernia repair as provides postoperative analgesia and obviates the need for general anaesthesia.
- Spinals: use 25/26G pencil point needles and 0.25% heavy bupivacaine (1:1 diluted 0.5% heavy bupivacaine and sterile saline). This gives a similar onset of anaesthesia with a shorter discharge time (4 versus 6hr). The addition of 10–25µg of fentanyl improves block quality whilst allowing local anaesthetic reduction.
- Epidurals are less suitable due to the time factor in achieving block.
- Caudals: use dilute solutions (0.125% bupivacaine) add preservative free ketamine 0.5mg/kg or clonidine 1µg/kg to prolong the block for up to 24hr. Warn patients about ambulation difficulties.
- Brachial plexus blocks: use axillary approach (low incidence of pneumothorax). If used with GA use dilute local anaesthetic (0.25% bupivacaine) to minimise motor block. If without GA, take onset time into account when planning the list.
- Femoral nerve block in adults is controversial as mobilisation is difficult.

Specific discharge criteria for regional techniques

Spinals
- Full recovery of motor power and proprioception.
- Passed urine.

Brachial plexus blocks
- Some regression of motor block.
- Understanding of protection of partially blocked limb.

Lower limb blocks
- Some regression of motor block.
- Adequate mobility demonstrated on crutches.
- Understanding of protection of partially blocked limb.

Discharge drugs

All patients should have a supply of suitable oral postoperative analgesics at home or be given them on discharge. Inguinal hernia repair, laparoscopic surgery, wisdom tooth extraction, etc. should be given at least 2 days supply of analgesics (diclofenac 50mg tds, co-codamol 30/500 2 tablets qds).

Discharge criteria

- Stable vital signs.
- Fully awake and orientated.
- Able to eat and drink.
- Passed urine (urological surgery) and after spinal/caudal.
- Ambulant.
- Pain and nausea well controlled.
- At least a 1hr wait postoperatively is a sensible condition of discharge.

Discharge organisation

- IV cannula removed and wound checked.
- Written and verbal discharge information.
- Discharge drugs.
- Suture removal organised if required.
- GP letter.
- Contact telephone number.
- Collected by responsible adult.

Postoperative admission

Reasons for overnight admission:
- Do not fulfil discharge criteria before unit closes.
- Observation after surgical or anaesthetic complications.
- Unexpectedly more extensive surgery.
- Inadequate social circumstances.
- Uncontrolled pain or PONV.

Overall, unanticipated admission occurs in 0.5–2.0% cases, depending on the mix of surgery. Gynaecology and urology have the highest admission rates. Surgical causes of hospital admission are three to five times greater than anaesthetic causes. Common anaesthetic reasons for hospital admission are inadequate recovery, nausea/vomiting and pain. Anaesthesia-related complications are more frequent with general anaesthesia than with local anaesthesia or regional anaesthesia. Surgical reasons include bleeding, extensive surgery, perforated viscus, and further treatment.

Further reading

Chung F, Mezei G (1999). Adverse outcomes in ambulatory anesthesia. *Canadian Journal of Anaesthesia*, **46**, RI8–R26.

Liu SS (1997). Optimizing spinal anesthesia for ambulatory surgery. *Regional Anesthesia*, **22**, 500–510.

Peng PWH, Chan VWS, Chung FFT (1997). Regional anaesthesia in ambulatory surgery. *Ambulatory Surgery*, **5**, 133–143.

Rowe WL (1998). Economics and anaesthesia. *Anaesthesia*, **53**, 782–788.

Ansell GL, Montgomery JE (2004). Outcome of ASA III patients undergoing day case surgery. *British Journal of Anaesthesia*, **92**, 71–74.

Watson BV, Allen J, Smith I. Spinal anaesthesia: a practical guide 2004: www.bads.co.uk

Website of the British Association of Day Surgery: www.bads.co.uk (for updates and new day surgery links).

Website of the US Society of Ambulatory Anesthesia: www.sambahq.org

Chapter 29

Laser surgery

John Saddler

General principles

- Laser is an acronym for Light Amplification by Stimulated Emission of Radiation. Laser light is an intense beam of energy capable of vaporising tissues. Lasers have numerous medical and surgical applications, but also create unique hazards to patients and staff.
- Light is a form of radiant energy that spans the mid-range of the electromagnetic spectrum. It is released as photons and travels as a wave.
- In a laser tube, the application of an energy source on a lasing medium creates stimulated emissions of photons. These bounce back and forth between carefully aligned mirrors, and are focused into a high-intensity beam. The light produced is monochromatic (all the same wavelength) and coherent (all the wave peaks moving synchronously at the same amplitude).
- Lasers are defined by their wavelengths, which also determines their colour. Some lasers are outside the visible spectrum and require a light guide to direct the laser beam to the surgical site.
- Fibre-optic bundles can be used to transmit visible and near-infrared wavelength lasers. Wavelengths out of this range usually require an articulated arm.

Laser wavelength and colour

Laser type	Wavelength (nm)	Colour
Dye laser	360–670	Blue to red
Argon	488–515	Blue/green
Helium–neon	633	Red
Ruby	694	Red
Nd–YAG	1064	Near-infrared
Carbon dioxide	10 600	Far-infrared

Laser light striking a tissue surface may be:
- Reflected. Reflection off shiny surfaces may damage the eyes of staff in the vicinity.
- Transmitted to deeper layers. Lasers pass through tissues to a variable depth, which is partially determined by the wavelength.
- Scattered. Shorter wavelengths induce greater scattering.
- Absorbed. This produces the clinical effect, when the absorbed light is converted to heat. Organic tissue contains various substances capable of absorbing light. These are termed chromophores, and include haemoglobin, collagen, and melanin. Each substance has a particular absorption spectrum, which is determined by its chemical structure. For example, oxyhaemoglobin, which is targeted in vascular lesions, has absorption peaks at 418nm, 542nm, and 577nm. Laser light at or close to these frequencies will be the most effective.

Safety aspects

- A designated laser safety officer should be present at all times when a laser machine is in use. An illuminated light should display outside the theatre when the laser is in operation.

- Laser light can be reflected off mirror-like surfaces. Medical instruments used with lasers should have matt, rather than shiny surfaces.

- The eye is the most susceptible tissue to injury. Retinal and corneal damage can occur, depending on the frequency of the beam. All operating room personnel must wear safety glasses appropriate for the laser in use. These should have side shields to protect the lateral aspect of the eye. If an anaesthetised patient is receiving laser radiation near the eyes, protective matt metallic eye covers can be applied.

- Damage to skin can occur, depending on the type of laser in use. Anaesthetised patients must have all exposed skin covered with drapes. These should be made of absorbable material and not plastic, which is potentially combustible. Tissue adjacent to the lesion can be protected with moistened pads or swabs. In all cases, the eyes should be taped closed and covered with moist swabs. Plastic tape is combustible and should be avoided.

- Some skin preparation fluids are flammable, and should not be used during laser surgery.

- Laser light can ignite plastic and rubber materials. Carefully consider the optimum method of airway maintenance if lasers are employed within the airway. The simplest approach is to use a Venturi system (Sanders injector). This uses a high-pressure oxygen source and entrainment of atmospheric air. The injector is placed in the lumen of a rigid laryngoscope or bronchoscope which is open at both ends, and permits entrainment of oxygen-enriched air during inspiration and escape of carbon dioxide and exhaust gases during expiration. This system of a 'tube within a tube' is safe, and reduces the chances of barotrauma-induced pneumothorax or pneumomediastinum. IV anaesthesia is usually employed to ensure an adequate depth of anaesthesia. It is also important to prevent the patient from moving or coughing, so a suitable muscle relaxant should be administered and neuromuscular transmission monitored with a nerve stimulator.

- If the use of an endotracheal tube is required, unmodified conventional tubes cannot be used because they support combustion and can potentially cause airway fires. Specifically-prepared non-flammable laser tubes are available, e.g Laser-Trach™ (Sheridan) or Laser-Shield™ (Medtronic Xomed). The cuffs of these tubes are vulnerable, and should be protected by damp pledgets. The cuff should be filled with saline, which can be mixed with methylene blue so that cuff puncture is obvious.

- If laser surgery is needed to the oropharynx a standard nasal ETT can be employed, but must be protected with saline-soaked gauze packing.

- Both nitrous oxide and oxygen support combustion. If using a circuit rather than an oxygen injector, 30% oxygen and air is a sensible choice. If air is not available, oxygen and nitrous oxide can be used, but take special care to protect the tube cuff.

- A laser plume, composed of smoke and gas, accompanies the use of medical lasers. Efficient smoke evacuation must be maintained close to the operative site.
- If a fire occurs in an airway during laser surgery, the flow of anaesthetic gases (including oxygen) should be stopped, and the tube removed. The area should be flooded with saline, followed by ventilation with 100% oxygen. Spontaneous breathing in a sitting position should be aimed for in recovery, but reintubation may be necessary if airway oedema is severe. A tracheostomy may also be necessary.

Examples of medical lasers

Pulsed dye laser

This uses light at a wavelength that targets red blood cells within blood vessels. The energy is dissipated within the dermis, and causes only minimal epidermal scarring. This is used mainly for treating port wine skin lesions. Children requiring laser therapy to these lesions will often be subjected to multiple treatments, usually under general anaesthesia. Postoperative pain may be a problem, particularly if large areas are treated. Combinations of paracetamol and NSAIDs may be effective, but occasionally opioid analgesics are required.

Carbon dioxide laser

These lasers have a long wavelength (10 600nm, outside the visible spectrum), and are preferentially absorbed by water. Target cells are heated to the point of vaporisation by the beam. They penetrate to only a very shallow depth, so tissue damage can be directly observed. They are used in aesthetic facial surgery, to reduce the wrinkling associated with ageing, and in ENT practice to vaporise vocal cord and airway lesions. Care must be taken to avoid eye and airway injury (see above).

Nd–YAG laser

This laser is also outside the visible range, and, unlike the CO_2 laser, is transmitted through clear fluids and absorbed by dark matter. It can penetrate to a depth of 1cm. It has multiple applications, including airway neoplasms, vascular malformations, and ophthalmic surgery.

Chapter 30

CT and MRI imaging

David Sanders

Anaesthesia for CT and MRI scanning

The anaesthetist working in the medical imaging department may be expected to use unfamiliar equipment in a potentially hazardous environment. Ensure that trained assistance, monitoring etc are available and familiarise yourself with the surroundings. Locate the nearest resuscitation facilities (self-inflating bag/mask, portable oxygen, 'crash' trolley and defibrillator)—confirm that your assistant and the radiographers also know where these are!

Indications for anaesthesia

- Infants or uncooperative children. Small babies (under 2 months) will often sleep through a scan if given a feed and wrapped up well.
- Older children or adults with psychological, behavioural, or movement disorders.
- Intubated patients such as acute trauma victims and patients receiving intensive care.
- Analgesia, sedation, or anaesthesia may also be required for interventional procedures performed under CT or possibly MRI guidance.
- Patients for elective scans commonly have a range of problems. Check the indications for scan and nature of the underlying pathology—developmental delay, epilepsy, malignancy, psychiatric, and movement disorders. Significant cardiovascular and respiratory problems are uncommon but beware of 'syndromes' with CVS manifestations.

Anaesthesia—general points

- Choice of sedation or GA and type of GA depends upon the needs of patient, the nature of the investigation, and the skills and experience of the anaesthetist (see later).
- Check whether the anaesthetic machines are using piped gases or cylinders. If using cylinders confirm that a full spare oxygen cylinder is immediately available.
- Plan the location of the anaesthetic machine, suction and monitoring, and the configuration and routing of the breathing system in advance.
- Decide where to induce the patient—a dedicated induction area may not be available or may be very small. It is usual to induce on a tilting trolley, then transfer to the scanner when anaesthetised.
- Certain equipment configurations (e.g. anaesthetic machine in scan room and monitors in control room) may require two anaesthetists to manage the patient safely.
- Ensure satisfactory recovery facilities are available—i.e. appropriately equipped recovery bay and an experienced recovery nurse near the scanner, or arrangements for safe transfer of the patient to an operating department recovery room.

Anaesthesia for computerised tomography (CT)

- The CT scanning environment does not restrict the type of equipment used but space is often limited so compact anaesthetic machines and monitors are more practical.
- Patient, anaesthetic machine, and monitors must all be visible from the control room.
- The patient's head is usually accessible during CT scanning so an LMA may be used if the patient does not require IPPV or airway protection.
- A variety of anaesthetic (and sedation) techniques can be used. The final choice should be determined by the equipment available and the patient's needs.
- Only 'light' anaesthesia to produce immobility and lack of awareness is required.

Hazards

- CT scanning generates potentially harmful ionising radiation so it is preferable for the anaesthetist to monitor the patient from outside the scan room. If it is necessary to remain near the patient wear appropriate radiation protection.
- Cannulae, catheters, drains, and endotracheal tubes can be pulled out during transfers and by movement of the patient through the scanner— ask the radiographer how far the table will move and check that lines and breathing system do not snag other equipment.

Contrast media

- Modern intravascular contrast media for X-ray imaging utilise highly iodinated, non-ionic, water soluble compounds.
- Common agents are iohexol (Omnipaque™) and iopamidol (Niopam™) which are monomeric, and the dimeric compound iodixanol (Visipaque™). Concentrations equivalent to 300–320mg of iodine per ml are typically used.
- You may be asked to administer IV contrast to anaesthetised patients. The volume required varies with the preparation, investigation, age, and body weight but may be up to 150ml (see table).

Investigation	Adult Volume (ml)	Child Volume (ml)
CT head	50–100	10 + 2ml/kg
CT body	100–150	(up to adult dose)
Aortography	100	–
Urography	2–3ml/kg	2–3ml/kg

- Check the timing of injection with the radiographer because some 'dynamic' investigations (e.g. aortography) require contrast to be administered as the scan is occurring.
- Contrast is viscous and can be difficult to inject through small cannulae or injection ports (take the bung off and inject via the hub of the cannula).
- Automated contrast injectors should not be connected to central venous lines. The high pressure developed by the rapid injection of viscous medium down a long narrow lumen can burst the line.
- IV iodine-containing contrast media occasionally trigger allergic reactions (ask about iodine sensitivity).
- These agents may cause renal failure in patients who are dehydrated or have impaired renal function so ensure adequate hydration in patients who have been starved for GA. Lactic acidosis can be precipitated in patients taking biguanides (metformin) and these should ideally be avoided for 48hr before and after the scan.

Practical considerations

- Metal containing objects (such as ECG leads, pressure transducer cables, or clips) lying in the X-ray beam can cause artefacts so route them away from the area to be scanned.
- Thoracic or abdominal scans may require 'breath-holds' to reduce respiratory movement artefacts. Both paralysed and spontaneously breathing patients can be ventilated manually and their lungs held in inspiration for the few seconds needed to perform each individual scan.
- The patient's arms usually need to be positioned above the head during thoracic or abdominal scans. Wide adhesive tape is useful for securing the limbs (keep a roll on the anaesthetic machine).
- Intensive care patients requiring CT scans should be managed like any inter-ICU transfer with full transport monitoring and ventilatory support. Ideally the ICU resident or consultant should supervise the patient and review the scan with the reporting radiologist. Getting such patients into and out of the scanner can be a slow process.

Anaesthesia for magnetic resonance imaging (MRI)

MRI is a versatile imaging tool free from the dangers of ionising radiation. A computer creates cross-sectional or three-dimensional images from minute radio-frequency signals generated as hydrogen nuclei are flipped in and out of alignment with a powerful magnetic field by high frequency magnetic pulses.

- Non-invasive but has unpleasant aspects—subject has to lie motionless in a long narrow noisy tunnel with the part of body to be imaged closely surrounded by an 'aerial coil'—creating a very claustrophobic environment.
- Typical sequence of scans lasts 15–25 minutes but complex scans may take much longer.
- Up to 3% of adults cannot tolerate scanning without sedation or anaesthesia.
- Provision of safe anaesthesia for MRI requires specialised equipment and careful organisation—unlike CT you cannot simply take a standard machine and monitor to the MRI scanner.

Hazards

- Most scanners use a super-conducting magnet to generate a high-density static magnetic field, which is always present. Field strength is measured in Tesla (T)—most scanners use 0.5–1.5T magnets (about 10 000 times the Earth's magnetic field).
- Near the scanner (> 5mT) the static field exerts a powerful attraction on ferromagnetic materials (e.g. scissors, gas cylinders, laryngoscopes) which can become projectiles. Electric motors (e.g. in syringe drivers) may run erratically and any information stored on magnetic media (credit cards, cassette tapes or floppy disks) will be erased. The magnetic field decreases as distance from the scanner increases— beyond the 0.5mT boundary or outside the scan room can be considered safe.
- Devices (e.g. hypodermic needles) made from non-ferromagnetic stainless steel can be taken into the scan room. If you are unsure about an object don't risk it!
- Oscillating magnetic fields induce eddy currents in electrical conductors (e.g. ECG leads, metallic implants). These currents may disrupt or damage electronic equipment (including pacemakers) and cause heating effects that can result in burns.
- Large masses of metal (e.g. anaesthetic machines, gas cylinders) near the scanner or small amounts of non-ferrous metals within the three dimensional volume being scanned can distort the magnetic fields causing poor quality images.
- The scan room is usually shielded to prevent external electrical interference from swamping the MR signals. All electrical equipment within the scan room must also be fully shielded and electrical conductors entering the room (e.g. monitoring cables) require special radio-frequency filters.

- Rapidly changing magnetic fields cause mechanical vibrations and extremely loud 'knocking' noises, which can potentially damage hearing.

Equipment
Two alternative approaches are feasible:
- specialised 'MRI compatible' equipment within the scan room, or
- conventional equipment outside the scanner's magnetic field in the control room

Standardising on one option keeps anaesthetist, anaesthetic machine, and monitors together. Choice depends upon space, funds, frequency of general anaesthesia, and individual preference. Using conventional equipment at a distance avoids crowding the scanner, is less expensive and allows faulty monitors to be substituted. The anaesthetist can regulate the anaesthetic and monitor the patient without being in the scan room and hazards can be reduced by applying the simple rule that 'nothing enters the scan room except the patient and the trolley'.

A typical set-up is as follows:
- Induction area adjacent to but outside the scan room (beyond the 0.5mT boundary) equipped with a compact conventional anaesthetic machine and monitoring.
- Piped gases, scavenging and suction in both the induction area and the control room.
- Non-magnetic tipping trolley for patient transfer into scanner.
- Compact (e.g. wall mounted) anaesthetic machine and ventilator in the control room with a 10 metre co-axial (Bain) breathing system.
- Respiratory gas/agent side-stream analyser with capnograph display fitted with an extended sampling tube (increases the response time by 5–10 seconds).
- MRI compatible pulse oximeter (fibre-optic patient probe and shielded cable).
- ECG with MRI compatible (carbon fibre) patient leads and electrodes.
- NIBP machine with an extended hose, non-metallic connectors, and a range of cuffs.

Practical considerations and techniques
- Physically and 'magnetically' restricted access makes patient observation and treatment difficult so a secure airway is a priority.
- Neonates and young babies (< 2 months)—will often sleep through a short scan if fed, wrapped up, and placed on their side in scanner.
- Babies and small children (< 15kg), any patient with an intracranial space occupying lesion, suspicion of raised ICP or needing a protected airway—use intubation and IPPV.
- Larger children and adults (if no risk of raised ICP)—use spontaneous ventilation and a standard LMA (NOT a flexible one with a wire spiral).
- If intubating a patient for a head scan use a RAE tube—it keeps the connectors and breathing system clear of the head coil.
- Tape the valve on the pilot tube of a cuffed ETT or LMA outside the aerial coil or the metal of the spring will distort the images.

- Sedation with oral or IV benzodiazepines may be used by radiologists for healthy but claustrophobic adults. Patients with severe back or root compression pain may also require strong analgesia to tolerate positioning for a scan.
- The role of sedation for MRI scanning in children is unclear. Some children's centres have reported successes with structured sedation programmes run by dedicated sedationists. However the safety of having heavily sedated children in the medical imaging department without direct anaesthetic supervision has been questioned.

Tips for IPPV through a 10m breathing system[1]:

- Use a system which functions as a 'T-piece' (Mapleson D or E) so dead space is unaffected by length. Ayre's T-piece and co-axial Bain systems work well and are both suitable for ventilating babies and small children.
- Airway pressures measured near the ventilator may not accurately represent distal pressures at the endotracheal tube.
- Tidal volume delivered to the lungs will be reduced by 'compression losses' of the gas within the system and by expansion of the tubing during inspiration making it difficult to compensate for significant leaks round uncuffed tracheal tubes—change to a slightly larger tube so the leak is minimal.
- As a result of these effects IPPV using a simple pressure generator (e.g. Penlon Nuffield 200 with a Newton valve) may not be effective in children weighing more than 15kg.
- Increased expiratory resistance of some long systems (e.g. Ayres T-piece) generates a positive expiratory pressure which increases with the fresh gas flow.

Intensive care patients:

- Same considerations apply as for CT scanning (see p683) but potential hazards are greater so risk/benefit balance should be assessed carefully.
- Do not scan patients who are haemodynamically or otherwise unstable.
- Electronic pressure transducers, metal containing ICP 'bolts', temporary pacing wires and conventional ECG leads must be removed before the patient enters the scan room.
- Full checks (and if necessary plain radiographs) must be performed to confirm there are no hazardous metallic implants or foreign bodies present.
- Patients who are stable on inotrope infusions can be scanned but the infusion pumps must remain at a safe distance from the magnet—ideally outside the scan room. Prepare duplicate pumps in the control room with extended infusion lines threaded with the breathing system into the scan room. Connect the patient to the running infusions while outside the room, check they are stable and then move into the scanner.

Patient and staff safety

- To avoid accidental injury all patients having an MRI scan must complete a screening/consent form. In case of children or sedated ICU patients these must be completed on their behalf by relatives or staff.
- To prevent injury and property damage all staff must similarly complete a screening questionnaire and leave metallic objects, pagers, credit cards etc outside the room.
- Greatest dangers arise from ferromagnetic implants or foreign bodies—certain types of artificial heart valves, old cerebral aneurysm clips or steel splinters in the eye, where movement could disrupt valve function or precipitate intracranial or vitreous haemorrhage respectively.
- Patients and staff with cardiac pacemakers must remain outside the 0.5mT boundary.
- Anaesthetised and sedated patients should have their ears protected to prevent noise induced auditory damage.
- IV MRI contrast media are paramagnetic but do not contain iodine and have a high therapeutic ratio. Side effects include headache, nausea and vomiting, local burning, and wheals (2.4%). Severe hypotension/anaphylactoid reactions are rare (approximately 1:100 000).
- Commonly used agents are gadopentetate (Magnevist™) at a dose of 0.2–0.4ml/kg and gadodiamide (Omniscan™) at 0.2ml/kg.

Cardiac arrest

- Do not attempt advanced life support in the scan room.
- Do not allow the cardiac arrest team into the scan room.
- Start basic life support with non-metallic self-inflating bag and chest compressions.
- Remove patient from scan room on non-magnetic trolley and continue resuscitation outside 0.5mT boundary.

Further reading

Association of Anaesthetists of Great Britain & Ireland (2002). Provision of anaesthetic services in magnetic resonance units.

Menon DK, Peden, CJ, Hall, AS, Sargentoni J, Whitwam, JG (1992). Magnetic resonance for the anaesthetist Part I: physical principles, applications, safety aspects. *Anaesthesia*, **47**, 240–55.

Peden, CJ, Menon DK, Hall, AS, Sargentoni J, Whitwam, JG (1992). Magnetic resonance for the anaesthetist Part II: anaesthesia and monitoring in MR units. *Anaesthesia*, **47**, 508–17.

Hatch DJ, Sury MRJ (2000). Sedation of children by non-anaesthetists. *British Journal of Anaesthesia*, **84**, 713–4.

Shellock FG (2001). Pocket guide to MR procedures and metallic objects: update 2001. Lippincott Williams & Wilkins Publishers.

---

1 Sweeting CJ, Thomas PW, Sanders DJ (2002). The long Bain breathing system: an investigation into the implications of remote ventilation. *Anaesthesia*, **57**,1183–6.

Chapter 31

Anaesthesia for the elderly

Jeffrey Handel

There is no standard definition of elderly, but it is often arbitrarily taken as >65yr. They have an increased risk of morbidity and mortality associated with anaesthesia and surgery.

Cardiovascular

- Significant cardiovascular disease is present in 50–65% patients.
- Myocardial fibrosis and ventricular wall thickening occur. This reduces ventricular compliance such that small changes in filling may have major effects upon cardiac output and blood pressure.
- Atrial fibrillation is common. Stroke volume is reduced by loss of the atrial boost contribution to ventricular filling.
- Maximal cardiac output with exercise decreases by ~1% per year from the 5th decade.
- Reduced arterial compliance causes systolic hypertension and widened pulse pressure.
- Autonomic responsiveness declines progressively resulting in impairment of cardiovascular responses to hypotension. The hypotensive effect of anaesthetic agents is likely to be more pronounced.
- Capillary permeability is increased leading to a greater risk of pulmonary oedema.

Respiratory

- Ventilatory response to hypoxia and hypercapnia declines and postoperative apnoea is more common. Ventilatory reserve declines.
- O_2 consumption and CO_2 production fall by 10–15% by the 7th decade. Patients are able to tolerate a longer period of apnoea following preoxygenation and minute volume requirement is reduced.
- Loss of elastic recoil increases pulmonary compliance but chest wall compliance falls due to degenerative changes in joints. Therefore total thoracic compliance may fall.
- Loss of septa increases alveolar dead space. Closing volume increases to exceed functional residual capacity in the upright posture at 66yr resulting in venous admixture. Thus normal PaO_2 falls steadily [(13.3−age/30)kPa, or (100−age/4)mmHg].
- Airway protective reflexes decline increasing the risk of postoperative pulmonary aspiration.
- In edentulous patients maintenance of a patent airway and face mask seal may be difficult. Leaving false teeth in situ may help.

Renal

- Renal mass and number of glomeruli fall progressively (by 30% in the 8th decade) resulting in reduced GFR. Creatinine clearance falls comparably although serum creatinine may not rise because of decreased production from a reduced muscle mass (see p124).
- Tubular function deteriorates leading to reduced renin-aldosterone response, ADH sensitivity, and concentrating ability. As a result, all renal homeostatic functions deteriorate so that elderly patients are more susceptible to fluid overload and hypovolaemia. Hypo- and hypernatraemia are more likely to occur.
- Clearance of renally excreted drugs is reduced necessitating dose adjustment. Particular care must be taken with potentially nephrotoxic drugs such as aminoglycosides.

Hepatic

- Hepatic mass and blood flow fall by up to 40% by the 9th decade. Although cellular function is relatively well preserved in healthy patients, the reduction in size reduces clearance and prolongs the effect of drugs that are metabolised and excreted by the liver. These include opioids, propofol, benzodiazepines and non-depolarising muscle relaxants.

CNS

- Brain size and neuronal mass decreases. Average brain weight falls by 18% between the ages of 30 and 80yr. Dementia affects 10% of patients over 65yr of age and 20% over 80yr. However it is important to distinguish between dementia and reversible confusional states due to hypoxia, sepsis, pain, metabolic derangement or depression. The hospital environment may precipitate anxiety and confusion.
- The elderly have lower requirements for opioid analgesics and sedatives and are more susceptible to depression of conscious level and respiration. This is likely to be due to a pharmacodynamic as well as pharmacokinetic effect. Pain threshold may be increased.
- Postoperative cognitive dysfunction is common in the elderly (25% at 1wk, 10% at 2yr post major surgery). It is a complex condition with features of dementia and confusional states which continue after the immediate postoperative period. Disturbance of cerebral perfusion and cellular oxygenation is likely to be a contributory factor. Alterations of central acetylcholine and catecholamine levels as well as central steroid effects from the stress response are thought to play a role.
- The thirst response to reduced ECF volume and increased plasma osmolality is reduced in the elderly, increasing susceptibility to fluid depletion.

Pharmacology

- Total body water is reduced while fat is increased. Volume of distribution of water-soluble drugs is reduced, reducing dose requirements while that of lipid soluble drugs is increased which may prolong clearance. Initial volume of distribution falls because of reduced cardiac output. This reduces dose requirement and is particularly relevant for induction agents. Arm–brain circulation time is prolonged, increasing the time taken for induction agents to take effect.
- Reduced plasma albumin concentration decreases dose requirement of drugs such as barbiturate induction agents, which are bound to albumin.
- MAC of inhaled agents decreases steadily with age (6% reduction per decade) and is reduced by around 40% by the age of 80yr (see p1160). This may be related to a reduction in neuronal mass. Reduction in blood/gas partition coefficient and cardiac output in the elderly result in shorter onset time.
- The risk of gastrointestinal bleeding due to NSAIDs is increased. These agents may also contribute to the development of acute renal failure in the presence of impaired renal perfusion. Angiotensin converting enzyme inhibitors exacerbate this risk. Fluid retention due to NSAIDs may precipitate heart failure in susceptible patients.

Thermoregulation
- Temperature regulation is impaired increasing the risk of hypothermia.
- Postoperative shivering increases skeletal muscle oxygen consumption while vasoconstriction increases myocardial work and oxygen demand.

Endocrine
Glucose loading is increasingly poorly tolerated in elderly patients. The incidence of diabetes rises and may reach 25% in patients above 80yr of age.

Nutrition
Nutritional status is frequently poor in the elderly. Perioperative complications and length of hospital stay may be reduced by nutritional supplementation prior to major surgery.

Haematology and immune system
- Hypercoagulability and deep venous thrombosis become more common with advancing age.
- Disorders causing anaemia are more common and the response of the marrow to anaemia is impaired.
- Immune responses are reduced in the elderly putting them at increased risk of infection. This is due to reduced bone marrow and splenic mass with loss of the thymus.

Anaesthetic management
- Perioperative mortality increases with age. It is influenced by medical fitness, the nature of the surgery, and whether surgery is elective or emergency. Hospital mortality for hip fracture surgery in patients over 70yr of age varies between 5% and 24%. For patients over 80yr undergoing elective bowel surgery for malignancy, hospital mortality is between 0 and 15% for ASA1 patients increasing to 20–30% for ASA3. Mortality is increased if resection is incomplete. Outcome is optimised by thorough preoperative assessment, choice of an anaesthetic technique appropriate to the patient's condition, and meticulous perioperative care to minimise physiological disturbance.

Preoperative assessment and management
- A systematic review is vital. In patients who have sustained a fracture, an underlying medical cause for a fall should be sought.
- Day surgery is particularly appropriate for fit patients undergoing minor surgery as the disorientation associated with a change of environment is minimised.
- The level of physical activity that can be sustained is a useful indicator of cardiovascular and respiratory fitness, but is often limited by joint disease.
- Mental state should be evaluated. The abbreviated mental test or mini mental state examination may be useful in differentiating dementia from acute confusional states.

- Consideration should be given to preoptimisation of medical conditions. This may require cross specialty involvement and high dependency care. The benefits from delaying surgery while this takes place should be balanced against the risks. In patients with lower limb fractures delay in mobilisation may increase the risk of pressure sores, deep venous thrombosis, and pneumonia.
- Regular medications with the exception of oral hypoglycaemics should be continued until the time of surgery. Alcohol should not be withheld the day before surgery and nicotine patches may be helpful in smokers. Sedative premedications should generally be avoided, particularly benzodiazepines, centrally acting anticholinergics and pethidine. Antacid prophylaxis should be considered. Perioperative β-blockade may reduce the risk of myocardial infarction.

Perioperative management

- There is no conclusive evidence that regional or general anaesthetic techniques are superior. Regional anaesthesia may reduce bleeding, risk of DVT, respiratory infection, and cognitive dysfunction. For fractured neck of femur it may reduce mortality at 1 month but has no effect on longer term survival compared with general anaesthesia. The chosen technique should be appropriate for the patient's physiological condition, as with younger patients.
- Careful monitoring is necessary for induction of general anaesthesia and for regional techniques as the hypotensive response to induction agents and to spinal/epidural anaesthesia is likely to be greater in the elderly. Consideration should be given to central venous pressure monitoring as elderly patients are more susceptible to adverse consequences of fluid overload or hypovolaemia. It should be remembered that prolonged arm–brain circulation time delays the onset of IV induction agents—flush drugs with saline. Impatience will lead to inadvertent overdose.
- Temperature should be measured and hypothermia prevented using fluid warmers, active body warming devices, and elevation of ambient temperature.
- Prolonged surgery and periods of hypotension increase the risk of pressure sores. Care should be taken to reduce pressure with soft padding. During long procedures it is advisable to relieve pressure and massage vulnerable areas intermittently.

Postoperative management

- Unless patients are undergoing minor surgery oxygen should be prescribed for at least 24hr. High dependency facilities are ideal after major surgery.
- Fluid balance, vital signs, serum electrolytes, and haematology must be carefully monitored and treated appropriately. Patients with CVS disease may need to have an Hb of 9–10g/dl.
- In postoperative confusion a careful search must be made for reversible organic causes.

- Pain is often poorly managed in patients with confusion and dementia. It is important to realise that these patients also feel pain and poor control may worsen confusion. NSAIDs should be used with caution. IV and SC opioids may be unreliably absorbed and elderly patients may have difficulty using a PCA. Regional techniques or an IV opioid infusion (with appropriate supervision) may be the most appropriate technique of pain relief.
- Early establishment of enteral nutrition by nasogastric tube, if necessary, may improve outcome.
- Early physiotherapy, mobilisation and thromboprophylaxis are extremely important.

When not to operate

- Heroic curative surgery may not be appropriate if the chance of benefiting the patient is felt to be very low. Decisions regarding futility of surgery are difficult and should be taken at consultant level, with involvement of the patient and family. Palliative procedures to improve quality of life should be considered if the patient is adequately prepared. These decisions must be carefully documented.

- Avoid sedative premedications and use regional analgesic techniques where possible to minimise the requirement for opioids.
- Monitor temperature and use active warming devices to prevent hypothermia.
- Maintain a low threshold for invasive monitoring (CVP, Art line).
- In edentulous patients leaving false teeth in place may help to maintain airway patency and face mask seal.
- Drug/MAC requirements are reduced. Use NSAIDs with caution. Consider a COX-2 selective agent or co-administration of a gastroprotective drug.
- Take care with positioning and intermittently relieve pressure during long procedures to reduce the risk of pressure sores.
- In postoperative confusion, search for reversible organic causes in all systems e.g. pain, hypoxaemia, distended bladder, myocardial/cerebral ischaemia, electrolyte disorder, drugs.
- Encourage early mobilisation and consider thromboprophylaxis if mobilisation will not be rapid.

Further reading

The Association of Anaesthetists of Great Britain and Ireland (2001). Anaesthesia and perioperative care of the elderly.

Murray D, Dodds C. Perioperative care of the elderly (2004). *Continuing Education in Anaesthesia, Critical care and Pain*, **4**, 193–196.

Dodds C, Murray D (2001). Pre-operative assessment of the elderly. *BJA CEPD Reviews*, **1**, 181–184.

Jandziol AK, Griffiths R (2001). The anaesthetic management of hip fractures. *BJA CEPD Reviews*, **1**, 52–55.

Chapter 32

Obstetric anaesthesia and analgesia

James Eldridge

Physiology and pharmacology

From early in the first trimester of pregnancy, a woman's physiology changes rapidly, predominantly under the influence of increasing progesterone production by the placenta. The effects are widespread.

- Cardiac output increases by ~50%. Diastolic blood pressure falls in early to mid-trimester and returns to pre-pregnant levels by term. Systolic pressure, although following the same pattern, is less affected. Central venous and pulmonary arterial wedge pressures are not altered.
- Cardiac output increases further in labour, even with effective epidural analgesia, peaking immediately after delivery. It is in this period, when the preload and afterload of the heart are changing rapidly, that women with impaired myocardial function are at greatest risk.
- Uteroplacental blood flow is not autoregulated and so is dependent on uterine blood pressure.
- Aortocaval occlusion occurs when the gravid uterus rests on the aorta or the inferior vena cava. Even in the absence of maternal hypotension, placental blood supply may be compromised in the supine position. After the 20th week of gestation, a left lateral tilt should always be employed. If either mother or fetus is symptomatic, the degree of tilt should be increased.
- Plasma volume increases 50% by term while the red cell mass only increases by 30%, resulting in the physiological anaemia of pregnancy.
- Pregnant women become hypercoagulable early in the first trimester. *Antepartum maternal deaths from pulmonary embolism occur most commonly in the first trimester.* Plasma concentrations of Factors I, VII, VIII, IX, X, and XII are all increased. Anti-thrombin III levels are depressed.
- Arterial CO_2 partial pressure falls to ~4.0kPa (30mmHg). Functional residual capacity is reduced by 20% resulting in airway closure in 50% of supine women at term. This, in combination with a 60% increase in oxygen consumption, renders pregnant women at term vulnerable to hypoxia when supine.
- In labour painful contractions and excessive breathing of Entonox can result in further hyperventilation and marked alkalosis may occur. Arterial pH in excess of 7.5 is common.
- Gastric emptying and acidity are little changed by pregnancy. However, gastric emptying is slowed in established labour and almost halted if systemic opioids are administered for analgesia. Barrier pressure (the difference in pressure between the stomach and lower oesophageal 'sphincter') is reduced, but the incidence of regurgitation into the upper oesophagus during anaesthesia, in otherwise asymptomatic individuals, is not significantly different in the first and second trimesters.
- By 48hr postpartum, intra-abdominal pressure, gastric emptying, volume and acidity are all similar to non-pregnant controls. Although lower oesophageal sphincter tone may take longer to recover, mask anaesthesia is acceptable 48hr after delivery in the absence of other specific indications for intubation.[1]

- Renal blood flow increases by 75% at term and glomerular filtration rate by 50%. Both urea and creatinine plasma concentrations fall.
- Neurological tissue has a greater susceptibility to the action of local anaesthetics during pregnancy—MAC is reduced.
- The volume of distribution increases by 5 litres, affecting predominantly polar (water-soluble) agents. Lipid soluble drugs are more affected by changes in protein binding. The fall in albumin concentration increases the free active portion of acidic agents, while basic drugs are more dominantly bound to α_1 glycoprotein. Some specific binding proteins such as thyroxin binding protein increase in pregnancy.
- Although plasma cholinesterase concentration falls by about 25% in pregnancy, this is counteracted by an increase in volume of distribution, so the actual duration of action of agents such as suxamethonium is little changed.

1 Bogod DG (1994). The postpartum stomach—when is it safe? *Anaesthesia*, **49**, 1–2.

Analgesia for labour

- Most commonly employed 'analgesics' are transcutaneous electrical nerve stimulation (TENS), inhaled nitrous oxide, opioids, and regional techniques.
- Randomised studies show only weak evidence of analgesia for TENS. Opioids in labour act predominantly as sedatives and amnesics—pain scores are minimally changed. Entonox is more efficacious than pethidine, but complete analgesia is never attained. When regional analgesia is contraindicated, a fentanyl PCA may be beneficial. Diamorphine and remifentanil have also been advocated.
- Regional analgesia provides the most effective pain relief. If hypotension is avoided, fetal condition in the first stage of labour may be improved as maternal sympathetic stimulation and hyperventilation are reduced. However a degree of maternal motor block is almost universal, and most randomised studies comparing regional and parenteral analgesia demonstrate an association between epidural analgesia and prolonged labour, together with a higher incidence of instrumental deliveries. Careful obstetric management of labour and appropriate anaesthetic management of analgesia may negate this effect.[1]
- Uterine pain is transmitted in sensory fibres which accompany sympathetic nerves and end in the dorsal horns of T10–L1. Vaginal pain is transmitted via the S2–S4 nerve roots (the pudendal nerve). Spinal, combined spinal/epidural (CSE), and epidural analgesia have largely replaced other regional techniques (paracervical, pudendal, caudal block). In 1997–1998 24% of all parturients in the United Kingdom used regional analgesia. Neuraxial techniques can be expected to provide effective analgesia in over 85% of women.
- Acceptable analgesia must be provided but minimising the incidence of hypotension and motor blockade is important. Reducing the degree of motor block increases maternal satisfaction and may decrease the incidence of assisted delivery. Motor block can be reduced by:
  - Using synergistic agents such as opioids to reduce the dose of local anaesthetic administered.
  - Establishing regional analgesia with low dose epidural local anaesthetic and opioid or low dose intrathecal local anaesthetic and opioid.
  - Using patient controlled epidural analgesia (PCEA) or intermittent top-ups to maintain analgesia. In general, infusions deliver a greater total dose of local anaesthetic than intermittent top-ups, while PCEA delivers the smallest total dose.

The choice of local anaesthetic may also affect motor block. At equimolar doses, ropivacaine produces less motor block than bupivacaine, but it is not as potent as bupivacaine and the relative motor block at equipotent doses remains controversial.

Indications for regional labour analgesia

- Maternal request.
- Expectation of operative delivery (e.g. multiple pregnancy, malpresentation).
- Maternal disease—in particular conditions in which sympathetic stimulation may cause deterioration in maternal or fetal condition.
- Specific cardiovascular disease (e.g. regurgitant valvular lesions).
- Severe respiratory disease (e.g. cystic fibrosis).
- Specific neurological disease (intracranial A–V malformations, space occupying lesions, etc.).
- Obstetric disease (e.g. pre-eclampsia).
- Conditions in which general anaesthesia may be life threatening (e.g. morbid obesity).

Contraindications for regional labour analgesia

- Maternal refusal.
- Allergy (true allergy to amide local anaesthetics is rare so always take a careful history).
- Local infection.
- Uncorrected hypovolaemia.
- Coagulopathy. (Although guidelines suggest that with platelet count >80 × 10^9/l and INR <1.4 neuraxial procedures are safe, clinical judgement for each individual patient remains of paramount importance. The cause of the clotting abnormality and the indication for the procedure have to be considered.)

Relative contraindications for regional labour analgesia

- Expectation of significant haemorrhage.
- Untreated systemic infection (providing systemic infection has been treated with antibiotics, the risk of 'seeding' infection into the epidural space with neuraxial procedures is minimal).
- Specific cardiac disease (e.g. severe valvular stenosis, Eisenmenger's syndrome, peripartum cardiomyopathy). Although regional analgesia has been used for many of these conditions, extreme care must be taken to avoid any rapid changes in blood pressure, preload and afterload of the heart. Intrathecal opioid without local anaesthetic may be advantageous for these patients.
- 'Bad backs' and previous back surgery do not contraindicate regional analgesia/anaesthesia, but scarring of the epidural space may limit the effectiveness of epidural analgesia and increase the risk of inadvertent dural puncture. Intrathecal techniques can be expected to work normally.

Consent

Most anaesthetists do not take written consent before inserting an epidural for labour analgesia, but 'appropriate' explanation must be given. The information offered varies according to local guidelines and with the degree of distress of each individual woman. The explanation and, in particular, the possible hazards discussed must be documented, as many women do not accurately recall information given in labour. Information about labour analgesia should always be available antenatally.

1 Russell R (2000). Editorial—The effect of regional analgesia on the progress of labour and delivery. *British Journal of Anaesthesia*, **84**, 709–712.

Epidural analgesia for labour

- Scrupulous attention to sterile technique is required. Mask and gown should be worn.[1]
- Establish IV access. In the absence of previous haemorrhage or dehydration when low dose local anaesthetic techniques are used, large fluid preloads are unnecessary.
- Position either in a full lateral or sitting position. Finding the midline in the obese may be easier in the sitting position. Accidental dural puncture may be slightly lower in the lateral position.
- Fetal heart rate should be recorded before and during the establishment of analgesia. Whether regional analgesic technique requires routine continuous fetal heart rate monitoring after analgesia has been established is controversial.
- Skin sterilisation with chlorhexidine is more effective than with iodine.
- Locate epidural space (loss of resistance to saline may have slight advantages in both reduced incidence of accidental dural puncture and reduced incidence of 'missed segments' compared with loss of resistance to air).
- Introduce 4–5cm of catheter into the epidural space. (Longer has an increased incidence of unilateral block and shorter increases the chance that the catheter pulls out of the space.) Multihole catheters have a lower incidence of unsatisfactory blocks.
- Check for blood/CSF.
- Give appropriate test dose. An 'appropriate' test remains controversial. Using 0.5% bupivacaine significantly increases motor block. Using 1:200 000 adrenaline to detect IV placement of a catheter has both high false-positive and false-negative rates. Many anaesthetists will use 10–15ml of 0.1% bupivacaine with a dilute opioid (2µg/ml fentanyl) as both the test and main dose. This will exclude intrathecal placement, but may give false negatives if the catheter is IV. The complete absence of a detectable block after such a test dose should therefore warn of possible IV cannulation.
- If required give further local anaesthetic to establish analgesia. There should be no need to use concentrations >0.25% bupivacaine.
- Measure maternal blood pressure every 5min for at least 20min after every bolus dose of local anaesthetic.

Once the epidural is functioning it can be maintained by one of three methods:
- Intermittent top-ups of local anaesthetic administered by midwives (5–10ml 0.25% bupivacaine or 10–15ml 0.1% bupivacaine with 2µg/ml fentanyl).
- A continuous infusion of local anaesthetic (5–12ml/hr of 0.0625–0.1% bupivacaine with 2µg/ml fentanyl).
- Intermittent top-ups of local anaesthetic administered by a patient controlled device (PCEA) (5ml boluses of 0.0625–0.1% bupivacaine with 2µg/ml fentanyl and a 10–15min lockout period).

1 McLure HA Talboys CA et al. (1998). Surgical face masks and downward dispersal of bacteria. Anaesthesia, **53**, 624–626.

Combined spinal epidural analgesia for labour (CSE)

A combination of low dose subarachnoid local anaesthetic and/or opioid together with subsequent top-ups of weak epidural local anaesthetic produces a rapid onset with minimal motor block and effective analgesia. An epidural technique alone can produce a similar degree of analgesia and motor block, but may take 10–15min longer to establish. CSE can be performed as a needle-through-needle technique or as separate injections:

- Locate epidural space at the L3/4 interspace with a Tuohy needle. Pass 25–27 G pencil point needle through the Tuohy needle to locate the subarachnoid space.
- Inject subarachnoid solution (e.g. 0.5–1.0ml of 0.25% bupivacaine with 5–25µg fentanyl). *Do not rotate epidural needle.* Insert epidural catheter.

or

- Perform spinal at L3/4 with a 25–27G pencil point needle.
- Inject subarachnoid solution.
- Perform epidural once analgesia has been established.

Caution: The epidural catheter cannot be effectively tested until the subarachnoid analgesia has receded.

- When the first top-up is required (usually 60–90min after the spinal injection), give the epidural test dose (e.g. 10–15ml of 0.1% bupivacaine with 2µg/ml fentanyl).

Further management of the epidural is the same as for epidural analgesia alone.

Poorly functioning epidural

Look for the pattern of failure. Remember that a full bladder may cause breakthrough pain. Ask the midwife if a full bladder is likely. Carefully assess the spread of the block. It is important to be confident that the epidural could be topped up for a Caesarean section if required. Therefore, if in doubt, re-site the epidural.

Pattern of failure	Remedy
Global failure No detectable block despite at least 10ml 0.25% bupivacaine (or equivalent)	Re-site epidural
Partial failure Unilateral block: feel both feet to assess whether they are symmetrically warm and dry. See if the pattern matches the distribution of pain	Top-up epidural with painful side in a dependent position (Use local anaesthetic and 50–100μg fentanyl) Withdraw catheter 2–3cm and give a further top-up Re-site epidural
Missed segment: true missed segments are rare. Commonly a 'missed segment' felt in the groin is a partial unilateral block	Top-up with opioid (i.e. 50–100μg fentanyl). The intrathecal mode of action will minimise segmental effects Continue as per 'unilateral block'
Back pain: severe back pain is associated with an occipito-posterior position of fetus and may require a dense block to establish analgesia	Top-up with more local anaesthetic and opioid
Perineal pain	Check sacral block and that the bladder is empty Top-up with more local anaesthetic in sitting position Continue as per unilateral block

Complications of epidural analgesia

Hypotension

In the absence of fetal distress, a fall in systolic blood pressure of 20% or to 100mmHg (whichever is higher) is acceptable. However uterine blood flow is not autoregulated and prolonged/severe hypotension will cause fetal compromise. Preload is not routinely required when using low doses of local anaesthetic, but patients should not be hypovolaemic before instituting regional analgesia. When hypotension is detected it should be treated quickly:

● Avoid aortocaval occlusion—make sure that the patient is in the full lateral position.
● Measure the blood pressure on the dependent arm.
● Give an IV fluid bolus of crystalloid solution.
● Give 6mg IV ephedrine and repeat as necessary.

Remember that brachial artery pressure may not reflect uterine artery blood flow. If fetal distress is detected, and is chronologically related to a regional anaesthetic procedure, treat as above even in the absence of overt hypotension.

Subdural block[1]

Subdural block occurs when the epidural catheter is misplaced between the dura mater and arachnoid mater. In obstetric practice, the incidence of clinically recognised subdural block is less than 1:1000 epidurals. However subdural blocks may be clinically indistinguishable from epidural blocks. Definitive diagnosis is radiological. The characteristics of a subdural block are:

● A slow onset (20–30min) of a block that is inappropriately extensive for the volume of local anaesthetic injected. The block may extend to the cervical dermatomes and Horner's syndrome may develop.
● Block is often patchy and asymmetrical. Sparing of motor fibres to the lower limbs may occur.
● A total spinal may occur following a top-up dose. This is likely to be a consequence of the increased volume rupturing the arachnoid mater.
● If a subdural is suspected re-site the epidural catheter.

Total spinal

The incidence of total spinal is variously reported to be 1:5000 to 1:50 000 epidurals. Usually the onset is rapid, although delays of 30min or more have been reported. Delayed onset may be related to a change in maternal position, or a subdural catheter placement. Symptoms are of a rapidly rising block. Initially difficulty in coughing may be noted (commonly seen in regional anaesthesia for Caesarean section), then loss of hand and arm strength, followed by difficulty with talking, breathing and swallowing. Respiratory paralysis, cardiovascular depression, unconsciousness and finally fixed dilated pupils ensue. As expected total spinals are reported more often after epidural anaesthesia rather than analgesia, as larger doses of local anaesthetic are employed.

Management of total spinal is as follows:

- Maintain airway and ventilation, avoid aortocaval compression and provide cardiovascular support.
- Even if consciousness is not lost, intubation may be required to protect the airway.
- Careful maternal and fetal monitoring is essential and, if appropriate, delivery of the fetus. In the absence of fetal distress, Caesarean section is not an immediate requirement. Ventilation is usually necessary for 1–2hr.

Accidental IV injection of local anaesthetic

'Every dose is a test dose.' The maxim is to avoid injecting any single large bolus of local anaesthetic IV. Remember that IV or partial IV positioning of epidural catheters occurs in at least 5% of epidurals. The risk can be minimised by:

- Meticulous attention to technique during placement. Always check for blood in the catheter.
- Always being alert to symptoms of IV injection with every dose of local anaesthetic, even when previous doses have been uncomplicated.
- Divide all large doses of local anaesthetic into aliquots.
- Use appropriate local anaesthetics. Lidocaine and the single enantiomer local anaesthetics are safer than bupivacaine.

1 Reynolds F, Speedy H (1990). The subdural space: the third place to go astray. *Anaesthesia*, **45**, 120–123.

Dural puncture

When loss of CSF is greater than production, as might occur through a dural tear, CSF pressure falls and the brain sinks, stretching the meninges. This stretching is thought to cause headache. Compensatory vasodilation of intracranial vessels may further worsen symptoms.

The incidence of dural puncture should be less than 1% of epidurals. All midwives, as well as obstetric and anaesthetic staff, should be alert to the signs of post dural puncture headache, as symptoms may not develop for several days. If untreated, headaches are not only unpleasant, but very rarely can be life threatening, usually as a result of intracranial haemorrhage or coning of the brain stem.

Management of accidental dural puncture can be divided into immediate and late.

Immediate management

The initial aim is to achieve effective analgesia without causing further complication.

Either:

- If a dural puncture occurs, pass the 'epidural' catheter into the subarachnoid space.
- Label the catheter clearly as an intrathecal catheter and only allow anaesthetist to perform top-ups.
- Give intermittent top-ups through the catheter. (1ml of 0.25% bupivacaine ±5–25µg fentanyl. Tachyphylaxis may occur with prolonged labour.)
- Advantages:
  - The analgesia produced is likely to be excellent.
  - There is no possibility of performing another dural puncture on re-insertion of the epidural.
  - The unpredictable spread of epidural solution through the dural tear is eliminated.
  - The incidence of post dural puncture headache is reduced (but only if the catheter is left in for more than 24hr).
- Disadvantages:
  - The catheter cannot be used to perform an early blood patch.
  - A theoretical risk of introducing infection.
  - The catheter may be mistaken for an epidural catheter.

Or:

- Remove the epidural catheter.
- Reinsert the epidural at a different interspace—usually one interspace higher. If the reason for tap was difficult anatomy, a senior colleague should take over.
- Run the epidural as normal but beware of intrathecal spread of local anaesthetic. The anaesthetist should give all top-ups.

With either technique the patient should be informed at the earliest opportunity that a dural puncture has occurred and of the likely sequelae. Labour itself may be allowed to continue normally. Arrange daily postnatal follow-up.

Late management

Following a dural puncture with a 16–18G Tuohy needle, the incidence of post dural puncture headache is approximately 70%. Not all dural punctures are recognised in labour so be alert to the possibility, even in women who had uncomplicated epidural analgesia. Headaches in the postnatal period are common. The key differentiating factor between a 'normal' postnatal headache and a post dural puncture headache is the positional nature of the latter.

Common features of post dural puncture headache include:

- Typically onset is 24–48hr post dural puncture. Untreated they usually last 7–10d.
- Characteristically worse on standing. Headache is often absent after overnight bed rest, but returns after mobilising.
- Usually in the fronto-occipital regions and radiates to the neck, with associated neck stiffness.
- Photophobia, diplopia, and difficulty in accommodation are common. Hearing loss, tinnitus, and VIth nerve palsy possible.
- Nausea occurs in up to 60%.

Treatment is either to alleviate symptoms while waiting for the dural tear to heal itself, or to seal the puncture. Epidural blood patching is the only commonly used method of sealing dural tears, although neurosurgical closure has been reported.

Prophylactic treatment[1]

- The most effective prophylactic treatment is blood patching. At the end of labour, 20ml blood can be injected through the epidural catheter (having removed the epidural filter). All residual block must have worn off before performing a prophylactic patch as radicular pain is an indication to stop injecting. However, early blood patching has a lower success rate and bacteraemia is common immediately after delivery (7% rising to 80% with uterine manipulation). Blood patching is not without sequelae and the Cochrane database review discourages the use of prophylactic blood patches.
- Bed rest alleviates symptoms, but the incidence of post dural puncture headache after 48hr is the same for those that mobilized throughout. Because of the risk of thromboembolism, bed rest should not be routinely encouraged in asymptomatic women.
- Epidural infusion of saline (1l/24hr) will compress the dural sac and can alleviate symptoms. It may also reduce the flow of CSF through a dural tear. After 24hr of continuous infusion the incidence of post dural puncture headache is marginally reduced. However radicular pain in the lower limbs may occur and patients are immobilised.

1 Sudlow C, Warlow C (2001). Epidural blood patching for preventing and treating postdural puncture headache. *The Cochrane Database of Systematic Reviews 2001*, Issue 2. Art No: CD001791.

Symptomatic treatment

- Simple analgesics (paracetamol, NSAIDs, codeine) are the mainstays of symptomatic treatment. They should always be offered, even though they are unlikely to completely relieve severe post dural puncture headache.
- Adequate fluid intake is to be encouraged although there is no evidence that hydration reduces the incidence of post dural puncture headache.
- Caffeine/theophyllines have become controversial. Concern has been expressed that the incidence of seizures following dural puncture may be increased in the presence of caffeine. These drugs act by reducing intracranial vasodilation, which is partially responsible for the headache. However while symptoms may be improved, they are not cured. Therefore it is probably sensible to avoid using these agents.
- Sumatriptan. Although this cerebral vasoconstrictor is of benefit, it is expensive, is given subcutaneously (6mg) and may cause coronary artery spasm. Its use is best reserved for those in whom blood patching is contraindicated.
- ACTH. Case reports suggest ACTH can effectively alleviate symptoms of post dural puncture headache, probably by increasing the concentration of β-endorphin and intravascular volume.
- Epidural blood patch—see p710.

Epidural blood patch[1,2]

Epidural blood patch performed around 48hr post partum has a 60–90% cure rate at the first attempt (recent studies that have followed women for more than 48hr have found lower success rates). The mechanism of action is twofold:

- Blood injected into the epidural space compresses the dural sac and raises the intracranial pressure. This produces an almost instantaneous improvement in pain.
- The injected blood forms a clot over the site of the dural tear and this seals the CSF leak.

Blood injected into the epidural space predominantly spreads cephalad, so blood patches should be performed at the same or lower interspace as the dural puncture. Suggestions that labour epidurals after blood patching may be less effective, have not been confirmed.

- Consent must be obtained. The patient should be apyrexial and not have a raised white cell count.
- Two operators are required. One should be an experienced 'epiduralist', the other is required to take blood in a sterile manner.
- The patient should have a period of bed rest before performing the patch to reduce the CSF volume in the epidural space.
- Aseptic technique must be meticulous both at the epidural site and the site of blood letting (usually the antecubital fossa).
- An epidural should be performed at the same or a lower vertebral interspace as the dural puncture with the woman in the lateral position to minimise CSF pressure in the lumbar dural sac.
- Once the epidural space has been identified, 20–30ml of blood is obtained.
- Inject the blood slowly through the epidural needle either until a maximum of 20ml has been given or pain develops (commonly in the back or legs). If pain occurs, pause and if the pain resolves, try continuing a slow injection. If the pain does not resolve or recurs then stop.
- To allow the clot to form, maintain bed rest for at least 2hr and then allow slow mobilization.
- As far as possible the patient should avoid straining, lifting or excessive bending for 48hr, although there are obvious limitations when a woman has a new born infant to care for.
- Follow-up is still required. Every woman should have clear instructions to contact the anaesthetists again if symptoms recur even after discharge home.
- Serious complications of blood patching are rare. However backache is common, with 35% of women experiencing some discomfort 48hr post epidural blood patch and 16% of women having prolonged backache (mean duration 27d). Other reported complications include repeated dural puncture, neurological deficits, epileptiform fits and cranial nerve damage.

1 Reynolds F (1993). Dural puncture and headache. Avoid the first but treat the second. *British Medical Journal*, **306**, 874–875.
2 Carrie LE (1993). Post dural puncture headache and extradural blood patch. *British Journal of Anaesthesia*, **71**, 179–180.

Anaesthesia for Caesarean section

With all Caesarean sections, it is vital that the obstetrician clearly communicates the degree of urgency to all staff. A recommended classification is[1]:

Immediate	There is immediate threat to the life of mother or fetus.
Urgent	Maternal or fetal compromise that is not immediately life threatening.
Early	No maternal or fetal compromise, but needs early delivery.
Elective	Delivery timed to suit mother and staff.

For all emergency Caesarean sections, the patient must be transferred to theatre as rapidly as possible. Fetal monitoring should be continued until abdominal skin preparation starts. In most centres, general anaesthesia is used when an 'immediate' Caesarean section is required, but 'urgent' Caesarean sections are usually performed under regional anaesthesia.

There is an expectation that the decision to delivery time should be less than 30min when the indication for Caesarean section is fetal distress. However delivery before this time limit is no guarantee of a successful outcome and delivery after this limit does not necessarily mean disaster. Each case must be individually assessed and the classification of urgency continuously reviewed.

Regional anaesthesia for Caesarean section

Regional anaesthesia for Caesarean section was initially driven by maternal preference. However regional anaesthesia is also more than 16 times safer than general anaesthesia.[2]

Advantages of regional anaesthesia include:

- Improved safety for mother with minimal risk of aspiration and lower risk of anaphylaxis.
- The neonate is more alert promoting early bonding and breastfeeding.
- Fewer drugs are administered, with less 'hangover' than after general anaesthesia.
- Better postoperative analgesia and earlier mobilization.
- Both mother and partner can be present at delivery.

Although regional anaesthesia is safer, maternal refusal remains a contra-indication. Although it is reasonable to give nervous mothers a clear explanation of advantages and disadvantages, mothers should not be forced into accepting regional anaesthesia.

Three techniques are available—epidural, spinal, and combined spinal epidural. Epidural is most commonly used for women who already have epidural analgesia in labour. Spinal is the most popular technique for elective Caesarean section, although in some centres combined spinal epidurals are preferred. Whatever technique is chosen, a careful history and appropriate examination should be performed. This should include checking:

- Blood group and antibody screen. Routine crossmatching of blood is not required unless haemorrhage is expected or if antibodies that interfere with crossmatching are present.
- Ultrasound reports to establish the position of the placenta. A low-lying anterior placenta puts a woman at risk of major haemorrhage, particularly if associated with a scar from a previous Caesarean section.

An explanation of the technique must be offered. Although Caesarean section under regional becomes routine for the anaesthetist, it is rarely routine for the mother. Reassurance and support are important. The possibility of complications must also be mentioned—in particular, the possibility of intra-operative discomfort and its management. Pain during regional anaesthesia is now a leading obstetric anaesthetic cause of maternal litigation. Document all complications that are discussed. Neonates are usually more alert after regional then general anaesthesia. However the speed of onset of sympathectomy that occurs with spinal anaesthesia (as opposed to epidural) results in a greater fall in maternal cardiac output and blood pressure and may be associated with a more acidotic neonate at delivery. In conditions where sudden changes in afterload may be dangerous (i.e. stenotic valvular heart disease) the speed of onset of a spinal block can be slowed by:

- Careful positioning during the onset of the block.
- Using an intrathecal catheter and incrementally topping up the block.
- Using a combined spinal epidural approach and injecting a small dose of intrathecal local anaesthetic. The block can be subsequently extended using the epidural catheter.

While a slow onset of block may be preferable in elective Caesarean section, a rapid onset is necessary for emergency cases. Spinal anaesthesia provides a better quality of analgesia and is quicker in onset than epidural anaesthesia.

1 Lucas DN, Yentis SM, *et al.* (2000). Urgency of Caesarean section: a new classification. *Journal of the Royal Society of Medicine*, **93**, 346–350.
2 Hawkins JL, Koonin LM, *et al.* (1997). Anesthesia-related deaths during obstetric delivery in the United States, 1979–1990. *Anesthesiology*, **86**, 277–284.

Caesarean section: epidural

Advantages	Disadvantages
Easy to top-up labour epidural	Slow onset
Stable BP	Large doses of LA
Intra-operative top-up possible	Poorer quality of block than spinal anaesthesia
Epidural can be used for postop analgesia	

Indications for Caesarean section under epidural anaesthesia:
- Women who already have epidural analgesia established for labour.
- Specific maternal disease (e.g. cardiac disease) where rapid changes in systemic vascular resistance might be problematic.

Technique
- History/examination/explanation and consent.
- Ensure that antacid prophylaxis has been given.
- Establish 16G or larger IV access. Give 10–15ml/kg crystalloid preload.
- Insert epidural catheter at the L2/3 or L3/4 vertebral interspace.
- Test dose then incrementally top-up the epidural with local anaesthetic and opioid:
  - 5–8ml boluses of 2% lidocaine with 1:200 000 adrenaline every 2–3min up to a maximum of 20ml (mix 19ml 2% lidocaine with 1ml 1:10 000 adrenaline rather than using preparatory mixture which contains preservative and has a lower pH).

  or:
  - 5ml 0.5% bupivacaine/levobupivacaine/ropivacaine every 4–5min up to a maximum of 2mg/kg in any 4hr period. (The single enanti-omer local anaesthetics may offer some safety advantage, however lidocaine is still safer than both ropivacaine and levobupivacaine.)
- Opioid (e.g. 100µg fentanyl or 2.5mg diamorphine) improves the quality of the analgesia and a lower level of block may be effective if opioid has been given.
- Establish an S4–T4 block (nipple level) measured by loss of light touch sensation. Always check the sacral dermatomes, as epidural local an-aesthetic occasionally does not spread caudally. Anaesthesia to light touch is more reliable at predicting adequacy of block than loss of cold sensation.[1] Document the level of block obtained and the adequacy of perioperative analgesia.
- Position patient in the supine position with a left lateral tilt or wedge. Give supplemental oxygen by facemask if SaO_2 <96% on air. (This is very important in obese patients who may become hypoxic when supine, and may have benefit for a compromised fetus.)

- Treat hypotension with:
  - Fluid (colloid more effective than crystalloid).
  - 50–100µg phenylephrine IV bolus (expect a reflex bradycardia) or 6mg ephedrine IV. α-agonists may be more effective and be associated with less fetal acidosis than ephedrine.
  - Increasing the left uterine displacement.
- At delivery give 5IU syntocinon IV bolus. If tachycardia must be avoided then a slow IV infusion of 30–50IU syntocinon in 500ml crystalloid is acceptable.
- At the end of the procedure give NSAID unless contraindicated (100mg diclofenac PR).

1 Russell IF (1995). Levels of anaesthesia and intraoperative pain at caesarean section under regional block. *International Journal of Obstetric Anesthesia*, **4**, 71–77.

Caesarean section: spinal

Advantages	Disadvantages
Quick onset	Single shot
Good quality analgesia	Limited duration
Easy to perform	Inadequate analgesia is difficult to correct
	Rapid changes in BP & cardiac output

Spinal anaesthesia is the most commonly used technique for elective Caesarean sections. It is rapid in onset, produces a dense block and with intrathecal opioids can produce long acting postoperative analgesia. However, hypotension is much more common than with epidural anaesthesia.

Technique

- History/examination/explanation and consent.
- Ensure that antacid prophylaxis has been given.
- Establish 16G or larger IV access. Give 10–15ml/kg crystalloid preload.
- Perform spinal anaesthetic at L3/4 interspace using a 25G or smaller pencil point needle. With the orifice pointing cephalad inject the anaesthetic solution e.g. 2.5ml 0.5% hyperbaric bupivacaine with 300µg diamorphine or 15µg fentanyl. (Morphine 100µg is also used, but has little intra-operative benefit. Morphine provides prolonged postoperative analgesia but with a higher incidence of postoperative nausea and vomiting, plus an increased risk of respiratory depression.)
- During the insertion of a spinal anaesthetic, some anaesthetists have patients in a sitting position, while others lie patients on their side. The sitting position usually makes the midline easier to find, and may be associated with a faster onset, although the height of block may be less predictable. A lateral position is associated with a slower onset of block, particularly if a full lateral position is maintained until the block has fully developed. This position also avoids aortocaval compression. With both positions, when 'heavy' local anaesthetic solutions are used, it is important that the cervical spine is kept elevated to prevent local anaesthetic spreading to the cervical dermatomes.
- Continue as for epidural anaesthesia for Caesarean section (p714).

Caesarean section: combined spinal/epidural (CSE)

Advantages	Disadvantages
Quick onset	Rapid change in BP and cardiac output
Good quality analgesia	Technically more difficult with higher failure rate of spinal injection
Intra-operative top-up possible	Untested epidural catheter
Epidural can be used for postop analgesia	

In some centres CSE has become the technique of choice—indications include:
- Prolonged surgery.
- The epidural catheter may be left in situ and used for postoperative analgesia.
- Allows a limited speed of onset of block. A small initial intrathecal dose of local anaesthetic can be supplemented through the epidural catheter as required.

Technique
- History/examination/explanation and consent.
- Ensure that antacid prophylaxis has been given.
- Establish 16G or larger IV access. Give 10–15ml/kg crystalloid preload.

The intrathecal injection may be performed by passing the spinal needle through the epidural needle (needle-through-needle technique) or by performing the intrathecal injection completely separately from the epidural placement either in the same or a different interspace. The needle-through-needle technique is associated with an increased incidence of failure to locate CSF with the spinal needle, but only involves one injection. If a two-injection technique is used, the epidural is usually sited first because of the time delay that may occur in trying to locate the epidural space with a Tuohy needle after the spinal injection. The risk of damaging the epidural catheter with the spinal needle is theoretical.

With either technique, beware of performing the spinal injection above L3/4, as spinal cord damage has been reported.

Needle-through-needle technique
- Position the patient and locate the epidural space with a Tuohy needle. Pass a long 25G or smaller pencil-point needle through the Tuohy needle into the intrathecal space. Inject anaesthetic solution with the needle orifice pointing cephalad (e.g. 2.5ml 0.5% hyperbaric bupivacaine with 300µg diamorphine or 15µg fentanyl).

- Insert epidural catheter. Aspirate the catheter carefully for CSF. Testing the catheter with local anaesthetic before the intrathecal dose has receded may be unreliable. However using the catheter intra-operatively is reasonable, as the anaesthetist is continuously present to deal with the consequences of an intrathecal injection. This may not be true if opioids are given through the catheter for postoperative analgesia at the end of the procedure before the block has receded.

Two needle technique

- Position patient and perform an epidural. After catheter is in position perform a spinal injection at L3/4 or below with a 25G or smaller pencil point needle.
- If the block is inadequate, inject local anaesthetic or 10ml 0.9% saline through the epidural catheter. 0.9% saline works by compressing the dural sac, causing cephalad spread of intrathecal local anaesthetic.
- Continue as for epidural anaesthesia for Caesarean section (p714).

Inadequate anaesthesia

Every patient should be warned of the possibility of intra-operative discomfort and this should be documented. Between 1–5% of attempted regional anaesthetics for Caesarean section are inadequate for surgery. The majority should be identified before operation commences.

Preoperative inadequate block

Epidural

- If no block develops then the catheter is incorrectly positioned. It may be reinserted, or a spinal performed.
- If a partial but inadequate block has developed, the epidural may be resited or withdrawn slightly. Should the toxic limit for the local anaesthetic agent have been reached, elective procedures can be abandoned, but for urgent procedures a general anaesthetic or a spinal anaesthetic will be required. If a spinal is chosen, exceptional care with positioning and observation of the block level is required, as high or total spinal can occur. Use a normal spinal dose of hyperbaric local anaesthetic, as this should ensure adequate anaesthesia, but control the spread with careful positioning.

Spinal

- If no block develops, a repeat spinal may be performed.
- If a partial but inadequate block develops, an epidural may be inserted and slowly topped up.
- Use a GA if required.

Intra-operative inadequate block

In this situation good communication with the mother and surgeon is essential. If possible stop surgery. Identify the likely cause of pain (e.g. inadequately blocked sacral nerve roots, peritoneal pain etc.). Try to give the mother a realistic expectation of continued duration and severity of pain. If the pain has occurred before the delivery of the fetus, it is very likely that a GA is required.

If patient requests GA, in all but exceptional circumstances, comply. If the anaesthetist feels that severity of pain is not acceptable, persuade the patient that GA is required.

Spinal

- Reassure and treat with:
  - Inhaled nitrous oxide.
  - IV opioid (e.g. 25–50µg fentanyl repeated as necessary). Inform the paediatrician that opioid has been given.
  - Surgical administration of local anaesthetic (care with total dose).
  - GA.

Epidural/CSE

- Treat as per spinal anaesthesia but in addition epidural opioid (e.g. 100µg fentanyl) and/or more epidural local anaesthetic can be used.

Preload

A fluid preload is a traditional part of the anaesthetic technique for regional anaesthesia. It has two functions:

- To maintain intravascular volume in a patient who is likely to lose 500–1000ml blood.
- To reduce the incidence of hypotension associated with regional anaesthesia.

However, it is questionable how effectively it prevents hypotension. Volumes as large as 30ml/kg or more of crystalloid solution do not reliably prevent hypotension. In some women, particularly those with severe pre-eclampsia, large preloads are harmful as the rise in filling pressures and the reduced colloid osmotic pressure will predispose to pulmonary oedema. The ineffectiveness of preload may in part be due to the rapid redistribution of fluid into the extravascular space. There is evidence that colloids, such as hetastarch, are more effective.

Preload should be:

- Timely (given immediately before or during the onset of the regional technique to minimise redistribution).
- Limited to 10–15ml/kg crystalloid. Larger volumes should be avoided as they offer little advantage and may be harmful.
- More fluid should only be given as clinically indicated.
- Colloids are preferred by some anaesthetists if excessive fluid load is likely to be harmful.
- Emergency Caesarean section should not be delayed to allow a preload to be administered.

Caesarean section: general anaesthesia

Elective general anaesthesia is now uncommon, limiting opportunities for training. The majority of complications relate to the airway, as failed intubation is much more common in obstetric than non-obstetric anaesthesia (1:250 v. 1:2000 respectively). All obstetric theatres should have equipment to help with the difficult airway and all obstetric anaesthetists should be familiar with a failed intubation drill.

Indications for general anaesthesia include:

- Maternal request.
- Urgent surgery. (In experienced hands and with a team that is familiar with rapid regional anaesthesia, a spinal or epidural top-up can be performed as rapidly as a general anaesthetic.)
- Regional anaesthesia contraindicated (e.g. coagulopathy, maternal hypovolaemia etc.).
- Failed regional anaesthesia.
- Additional surgery planned at the same time as Caesarean section.

Technique

- History and examination. In particular assess the maternal airway—mouth opening, Mallampati score, thyromental distance, neck mobility (see p918).
- Antacid prophylaxis.
- Start appropriate monitoring (see below).
- Position supine with left lateral tilt or wedge.
- Pre-oxygenate for 3–5min or, in an emergency, with four vital capacity breaths with a high flow through the circuit. A seal must be obtained with the face mask. At term, women have a reduced FRC and a higher respiratory rate and oxygen consumption. This reduces the time required for denitrogenation, but also reduces the time from apnoea to arterial oxygen desaturation.
- Perform rapid sequence induction with an adequate dose of induction agent (e.g. 5–7mg/kg thiopental). Isolated forearm techniques suggest that awareness without recall may be common when the dose of induction agent is reduced. A 7.0mm endotracheal tube is adequate for ventilation and may make intubation easier.
- Propofol has also been used for Caesarean section without any major reported complications although at present thiopental probably is still the most commonly used agent in the UK.
- Ventilate with 50% oxygen in nitrous oxide. If severe fetal distress is suspected then 75% oxygen or higher may be appropriate. Maintain $ETCO_2$ at 4.0–4.5kPa (30–34 mmHg).
- Use 'overpressure' of inhalational agent to rapidly increase the end tidal concentration of anaesthetic agent to at least 0.75 of MAC. (e.g. 2% isoflurane for 5min, then reduce to 1.5% for a further 5min).

- At delivery:
  - Give 5IU syntocinon IV bolus. If tachycardia must be avoided then an IV infusion of 30–50IU syntocinon in 500ml crystalloid, infused over 4hr is effective.
  - Administer opioid (e.g. 10–15mg morphine).
  - Ventilate with 35% inspired oxygen concentration in nitrous oxide. Inhalational agent can be reduced to 0.75 MAC to reduce uterine relaxation.
- At end of procedure give an NSAID (e.g. 100mg diclofenac PR). Bilateral ilioinguinal nerve blocks are also effective for postoperative analgesia.
- Extubate awake in the head-down left lateral position.
- Give additional IV analgesia as required.

Effect of general anaesthesia on the fetus

Most anaesthetic agents, except for the muscle relaxants, rapidly cross the placenta. Thiopental can be detected in the fetus within 30s of administration with peak umbilical vein concentration occurring around 1min. Umbilical artery to umbilical vein concentrations approach unity at 8min. Opioids administered before delivery may cause fetal depression. This can be rapidly reversed with naloxone (e.g. 200µg IM). If there is a specific indication for opioids before delivery they should be given, and the paediatrician informed. Hypotension, hypoxia, hypocapnia, and excessive maternal catecholamine secretion may all be harmful to the fetus.

Failed intubation

(For failed intubation drill see pp888, 928)
When intubation fails but mask ventilation succeeds, a decision on whether to continue with the Caesarean section must be made. A suggested grading system is[1]:
Grade 1:   Mother's life dependent on surgery.
Grade 2:   Regional anaesthetic unsuitable (e.g. coagulopathy/ haemorrhage).
Grade 3:   Severe fetal distress (e.g. prolapsed cord).
Grade 4:   Varying severity of fetal distress with recovery.
Grade 5:   Elective procedure.
For Grade 1 cases surgery should continue, and for Grade 5, the mother should be woken. The action between these extremes must take account of additional factors including the ease of maintaining the airway, the likely difficulty of performing a regional anaesthetic and the experience of the anaesthetist. Once a failed intubation has occurred and an airway has been established, reapply fetal monitoring as this may give useful additional information to guide management.

---

1 Harmer M (1997). Difficult and failed intubation in obstetrics. *International Journal of Obstetric Anaesthesia*, **6**, 25–31.

Antacid prophylaxis

Animal data suggests that to minimise the risk from aspiration, the gastric volume should be less than 25ml, non-particulate, and with a pH >2.5. Various strategies are available to achieve this:

Elective surgery

- 150mg ranitidine orally 2hr and 12hr before surgery.
- 10mg metoclopramide orally 2hr before surgery.
- 30ml 0.3M sodium citrate immediately before surgery.
  (pH >2.5 is maintained for only 30min after 30ml 0.3M sodium citrate. If a GA is required after this, a further dose of citrate is required.)

Emergency surgery (if prophylaxis has not already been given)

- 50mg ranitidine by slow IV injection immediately before surgery.
  (Proton pump inhibitors are an alternative.)
- 10mg metoclopramide IV injection immediately before surgery.
- 30ml 0.3M sodium citrate orally immediately before surgery.

Postoperative analgesia

Most post partum women are very well motivated and mobilise quickly. However, effective analgesia does allow earlier mobilization. The mainstays of postoperative analgesia are opioids and NSAIDs. The route that these are given is dependent on the intra-operative anaesthetic technique.

Opioids

- IV patient controlled analgesia or IM opioid can be used although these are not as effective as neuraxial analgesia. A small quantity of opioid may be transferred to the neonate through breast milk, but with a negligible effect.
- Intrathecal/epidural opioid:
  - When given as a bolus at the beginning of surgery, fentanyl lasts little longer than the local anaesthetic and provides almost no post-operative analgesia. Epidural fentanyl may be given as an infusion or as intermittent postoperative boluses (50–100µg up to 2-hourly for 2 or 3 doses) if the epidural catheter is left in situ.
  - Intrathecal diamorphine (300µg) can be expected to provide 6–18hr of analgesia. More than 40% of women will require no other postoperative opioid. Higher doses have been recommended, but are associated with an increased incidence of side effects. Pruritus is very common (60–80%) although only 1–2% have severe pruritus. This can be treated with 200µg naloxone IM or 4mg ondansetron IV/IM.
  - Epidural diamorphine (2.5mg in 10ml saline) provides 6–10hr of analgesia after a single dose. Intermittent doses may be given if the epidural catheter is left in situ.
  - Intrathecal preservative free morphine (100µg) provides long lasting analgesia (12–18hr). Doses above 150µg are associated with increased side effects without improved analgesia. However pruritus and nausea are common. The low lipophilicity of morphine may increase risk of late respiratory depression. Epidural morphine (2–3mg) provides analgesia for 6–24 hr, but pruritus is again common and nausea occurs in 20–40%. Diamorphine is used much more commonly in the UK than morphine. Preservative free pethidine may also be used (10–50mg epidurally).

NSAIDs

NSAIDs are very effective postoperative analgesics, reducing opioid requirements. They should be administered regularly whenever possible.

Retained placenta

- Check IV access with 16G or larger cannula has been obtained.
- Assess total amount and rate of blood loss and cardiovascular stability. Blood loss may be difficult to accurately assess. If rapid blood loss is continuing then urgent crossmatch and evacuation of placenta under general anaesthetic is required.
- Regional anaesthesia is safe provided estimated blood loss is less than 1000ml, but if there are any signs suggesting hypovolaemia, a general anaesthetic may be required.
- Remember antacid prophylaxis.
- For general anaesthesia use a rapid sequence induction technique with cuffed ETT.
- Regional anaesthesia can either be obtained by topping up an existing epidural, or by performing a spinal (e.g. 2ml 0.5% hyperbaric bupivacaine intrathecally). A T7 block reliably ensures analgesia.[1]
- Occasionally uterine relaxation is required. Under general anaesthesia this can be produced by increasing the halogenated vapour concentration. Under regional anaesthesia SL GTN spray or IV aliquots of 100µg glyceryl trinitrate are effective (dilute 1mg in 10ml 0.9% saline and give 1ml bolus repeated as required). With either technique expect transient hypotension.
- On delivery of the placenta give 5IU syntocinon ± syntocinon infusion.
- At the end of the procedure give an NSAID unless contraindicated.

Summary of dosing regimes

Procedure	Technique	Suggested dose
Labour	Epidural loading dose	20ml 0.1% bupivacaine with 2µg/ml fentanyl
	Epidural infusion	10ml/hr 0.1% bupivacaine with 2µg/ml fentanyl
	Top-ups	10–20ml 0.1% bupivacaine with 2µg/ml fentanyl
	CSE	Intrathecal: 1ml 0.25% bupivacaine with 5–25µg/ml fentanyl Epidural: Top-up and infusion as above
	PCEA	5ml boluses of 0.1% bupivacaine with 2µg/ml fentanyl with a 10–15min lockout
LSCS	Spinal	2.5ml 0.5% bupivacaine in 8% dextrose ('heavy') + 250µg diamorphine
	Epidural	15–20ml 2% lidocaine with 1:200 000 adrenaline (1ml of 1:10 000 added to 19ml solution)
	CSE	Normal spinal dose (reduce if slow onset of block is required) If needed, top-up the epidural with 5ml aliquots of 2% lidocaine
Post LSCS analgesia	GA	Bilateral ilioinguinal nerve blocks at end of surgery
		IV aliquots of morphine until comfortable
		Parenteral opioid (IM or PCA as available)
	GA and regional	100mg diclofenac PR at end of surgery, followed by 75mg diclofenac PO 12-hourly
		Simple analgesics as required (i.e. cocodamol, codydramol etc.)
	Regional	Epidural diamorphine (2.5mg) in 10ml 0.9% saline 4-hourly prn

LSCS = lower segment Caesarean section

1 Broadbent CR, Russell R (1999). What height of block is needed for manual removal of placenta under spinal anaesthesia? *International Journal of Obstetric Anesthesia*, **8**, 161–164.

Breast feeding and maternal drug exposure

If a drug is to be transferred from mother to neonate through breast feeding, it must be secreted in the milk, absorbed in the neonatal gastro-intestinal tract and not undergo extensive first pass metabolism in the neonatal liver. In general, for breast fed infants, the neonatal serum concentration of a drug is less than 2% of maternal serum concentration resulting in a sub-therapeutic dose. Most drugs are therefore safe. However there are some exceptions to this rule—either because transfer is much higher or because transfer of even minute quantities of a drug is unacceptable. Drugs with high protein binding may displace bilirubin and precipitate kernicterus in a jaundiced neonate.

Factors that make significant transfer more likely include:
• Low maternal protein binding.
• Lipophilicity or, with hydrophilic drugs, a molecular weight of <200Da.
• Weak bases (which increase the proportion of ionised drug in the weakly acidic breast milk leading to 'trapping').

Transfer to the neonate can be minimised by breast feeding before administering the drug, and if the neonate has a consistent sleep period, administering the drug to mother at the beginning of this.

Although many drugs are excreted in minimal quantities in breast milk with no reports of ill effects manufacturers will often recommend avoiding agents during breast-feeding.

Remember breast feeding constitutes a metabolic and fluid load for the mother, so if surgery is contemplated then keep the mother well hydrated and if the surgery is elective, have the patient first on the list. Try to minimise nausea and vomiting.

The following table gives information on some agents but a full list of drug compatibility with breast-feeding is beyond the scope of this book.

Drug	Comment
Opioids	Minimal amount delivered to neonatal serum. Minor concern about the long duration of action of pethidine's metabolite, nor-pethidine
NSAIDs	Most NSAIDs are considered safe in breast-feeding. Some would advise caution with aspirin because of unsubstantiated concerns about causing Reye syndrome in the neonate
Antibiotics	Penicillins and cephalosporins are safe, although trace amounts may be passed to the neonate
	Tetracycline should be avoided (although absorption is probably minimal because of chelation with calcium in the milk)
	Chloramphenicol may cause bone-marrow suppression in the neonate and should be avoided
	Ciprofloxacin is present in high concentrations in breast milk and should be avoided
Antipsychotics	Generally suggested that these should be avoided although the amount excreted in milk is probably too small to be harmful. Chlorpromazine and clozapine cause neonate drowsiness
Cardiac drugs	Amiodarone is present in milk in significant amounts and breast feeding should be discontinued
	Most β-blockers are secreted in minimal amounts. Sotalol is present in larger amounts. Avoid celiprolol
Anticonvulsants	While carbamazepine does not accumulate in the neonate, phenobarbitone and diazepam may. Neonates should be observed for evidence of sedation

Placenta praevia and accreta

Placenta praevia

Placenta praevia occurs when the placenta implants between the fetus and the cervical os. The incidence is about 1 in 200 pregnancies, but is higher with previous uterine scars and multiparity.

Three questions are used to evaluate the anaesthetic implications of a placenta praevia:

- Is a vaginal delivery possible? (Unlikely if the placenta extends to within 2cm of the os.)
- If not, does the placenta cover the *anterior* lower segment of the uterus. (If it does, the obstetrician will have to divide the placenta to deliver the fetus and blood loss can be expected to be large.)
- Is there a uterine scar from previous surgery? (Placenta accreta is more common if the placenta overlies a uterine scar.)

Diagnosis is usually made by ultrasound, often after a small painless vaginal bleed. Obstetric management is aimed at preserving the pregnancy until the 37th gestational week. Premature labour, excessive bleeding or fetal distress may necessitate delivery. In most circumstances, women with placenta praevia are admitted to hospital and crossmatched blood kept continuously available. If at 37wk gestation a vaginal delivery is not possible, a Caesarean section is performed.

Placenta accreta

Placenta accreta occurs with abnormal implantation of the placenta. Usually the endometrium produces a cleavage plane between the placenta and the myometrium. In placenta accreta vera the placenta grows through the endometrium to the myometrium. In placenta increta the placenta grows into the myometrium, and in placenta percreta the placenta grows through the myometrium to the uterine serosa and on into surrounding structures. Because the normal cleavage plane is absent, following delivery the placenta fails to separate from the uterus, which can result in life threatening haemorrhage.

Incidence is rising, possibly as a result of the increasing numbers of Caesarean sections performed. Placenta accreta is much more common when the placenta implants over a previous scar. A women who has had two previous sections and a placenta that has implanted over the uterine scar has a 50% chance of developing a placenta accreta and two thirds of these will require Caesarean hysterectomy. Diagnosis of percreta is occasionally made with ultrasound or the presence of haematuria, but usually placenta accreta and increta are diagnosed at surgery.

Anaesthetic management

Anaesthetic management is dictated by the likelihood of major haemorrhage, maternal preference and the obstetric/anaesthetic experience levels. Patients with placenta praevia are at risk of haemorrhage because:

- Placenta may have to be divided to facilitate delivery.
- Lower uterine segment does not contract as effectively as the body of the uterus so the placental bed may continue to bleed following delivery.

Further increase in risk occurs sequentially with placenta accreta, increta and percreta. Caesarean hysterectomy is required in 95% of women with placenta percreta with a 7% overall mortality rate.

Although the sympathectomy that occurs with regional anaesthesia may make control of blood pressure more difficult, practical experience shows regional anaesthesia can be safely used for placenta praevia, providing the patient is normovolaemic before the neuraxial technique is performed. Even in Caesarean hysterectomy, the degree of hypotension and blood loss is the same with regional and general anaesthetic techniques. However, if significant haemorrhage does occur, hypotensive and bleeding patients will require reassurance and this may divert the anaesthetist from providing volume resuscitation. Regional anaesthesia should therefore only be undertaken by experienced anaesthetists with additional help available.

Technique

- Experienced obstetricians and anaesthetists are essential.
- All patients admitted with placenta praevia should be seen and assessed by an anaesthetist.
- When Caesarean section is to be performed 2–8U of blood should be crossmatched, depending on the anticipated risk of haemorrhage.
- Obstetric staff experienced in Caesarean hysterectomy should be immediately available.
- Two 14G cannulae should be inserted and equipment for massive haemorrhage must be present.
- If regional anaesthesia is used, a CSE may offer advantages as the surgery may be prolonged.
- For bleeding patients a general anaesthetic is the preferred choice.
- Have a selection of uterotonics to hand (see p734). Even if massive haemorrhage is not encountered, an infusion is advantageous (e.g. syntocinon 30–50IU in 500ml crystalloid over 1–2hr).
- If massive bleeding does occur, hysterectomy may be the only method of controlling bleeding. Excessive delay in making this decision may jeopardise maternal life.
- Do not forget surgical methods of controlling haemorrhage—bimanual compression of the uterus, ligation of internal iliac arteries, temporary compression of the aorta.
- Even if no significant bleeding occurred intra-operatively, continue to observe closely in the postnatal period as haemorrhage may still occur.

Massive obstetric haemorrhage

The gravid uterus receives 12% of the cardiac output and when haemorrhage occurs it can be extremely rapid. In the underdeveloped world, haemorrhage is the leading cause of maternal death. Placental abruption, postpartum haemorrhage and placenta praevia are the principal causes of massive haemorrhage.

The fetus is at greater risk from maternal haemorrhage than the mother. Hypotension reduces uteroplacental blood flow and severe anaemia will further reduce oxygen delivery. In addition abruption may directly compromise blood supply. Fetal mortality may be as high as 35%. Standard protocols for major haemorrhage should be available in every delivery suite.

Aetiology of obstetric haemorrhage

Antenatal

- Placental abruption. Bleeding is often associated with pain. Blood loss may be concealed with retroplacental bleed. Fetal compromise is common. Small bleeds may be treated conservatively.
- Placenta praevia/accreta. Usually a small painless bleed. May be catastrophic.
- Uterine rupture. Fetal distress is most reliable indicator. Classically uterine rupture is said to be painful, but painless dehiscence of a previous uterine scar is not uncommon.

Postnatal

Defined as blood loss of greater than 500ml post delivery. Estimates of 'normal' blood loss after vaginal delivery are of the order of 250–400ml and after Caesarean section around 500–1000ml. Blood loss is usually underestimated.

- Uterine atony. Associated with chorioamnionitis, prolonged labour and an abnormally distended uterus (e.g. polyhydramnios, macrosomia, multiple gestation, etc.).
- Retained placenta. Haemorrhage may be massive, but usually less than 1 litre and occasionally minimal.
- Retained products of conception. This is the leading cause of late haemorrhage, but is rarely massive.
- Genital tract trauma. Vaginal and vulval haematomas are usually self limiting, but retroperitoneal haematomas may be extensive and life threatening.
- Uterine inversion. This is a rare complication in the Western world. It is associated with uterine atony and further relaxation may be required to enable replacement. After replacement uterotonics should be administered.

Diagnosis

Diagnosis of haemorrhage is usually self evident, although be aware that concealed bleeding may occur, especially with placental abruptions. In addition signs of cardiovascular decompensation may be delayed, as women are usually young, fit and start with a pregnancy induced expansion of their intravascular volume. Beware of the woman with cold peripheries—this is abnormal in pregnancy. Hypotension is a late and ominous sign.

Management

In the event of a major haemorrhage requiring surgery, do not delay operation until crossmatched blood is available.

- Call for help.
- Give supplemental oxygen. If laryngeal reflexes are obtunded, intubate and ventilate. In antenatal patients avoid aortocaval compression.
- Insert two 14G cannulae and take blood for crossmatching. Request type specific blood (this can be retrospectively crossmatched).
- Fluid resuscitate with crystalloid and/or colloid.
- If required give Group O Rhesus negative blood (i.e. blood loss of 2–3l and ongoing without the imminent prospect of crossmatched blood being available and/or the presence of ECG abnormalities).
- Start appropriate monitoring of mother and fetus. Urine output and invasive monitoring of central venous and arterial pressures may be indicated depending on rate of blood loss and maternal condition. However early monitoring of CVP is not essential as hypotension is almost always due to hypovolaemia.
- Treat the cause of haemorrhage. If surgery is required:
  - Do not perform a regional technique if the patient is hypovolaemic,
  - Beware of coagulopathies in the presence of concealed abruption.
- With continuing haemorrhage further equipment including warming devices and rapid transfusion devices should be available.
- Correct coagulopathy with platelets, fresh frozen plasma and cryoprecipitate as indicated.
- Once blood loss has been controlled, continue care on a HDU or ICU.

Specific treatment for haemorrhage

Treatment may be with uterotonics or surgery or both depending on the cause:

- Uterotonics can only be used in the postnatal period.
- Most postnatal haemorrhage is due to uterine atony and can be temporarily controlled with firm bimanual pressure while waiting for definitive treatment.

Commonly used uterotonics and doses

Drug	Dose	
Oxytocin (Syntocinon®)	5IU bolus 30–50IU in 500ml crystalloid and titrated as indicated	Synthetically produced hormone causing uterine contraction, peripheral vasodilation and has very mild antidiuretic hormone actions. Early preparations made from animal extracts had significant ADH activity.
Ergometrine	0.5mg IM or 0.125mg by slow IV injection and repeat to a total of 0.5mg	An ergot alkaloid derivative. Produces effective uterine constriction but nausea and vomiting are very common. Systemic vasoconstriction may produce dangerous hypertension in at risk groups (e.g. pre-eclampsia, specific cardiac disease)
Carboprost (Hemabate®) (15-Methyl Prosaglandin $F_{2\alpha}$)	0.25mg intra-myometrially or IM every 10–15min to a max of 2mg	Effective uterine constrictor. Also causes nausea, vomiting, and diarrhoea. May produce severe bronchospasm, alter pulmonary shunt fraction and induce hypoxia (caution in asthmatics)

Amniotic fluid embolism

- Amniotic fluid embolism is the third most common direct cause of maternal death in the UK.
- Incidence: ~1:25,000 live births.
- Effects are probably due to an anaphylactic response to fetal tissue.
- Within the first 30min after amniotic fluid embolism, intense pulmonary vasoconstriction occurs and is associated with right heart failure, hypoxia, hypercarbia and acidosis.
- This is followed by left heart failure and pulmonary oedema.
- Expect a coagulopathy.
- The incidence of amniotic fluid embolism is increased with:
  - Age >25yr.
  - Multiparous women.
  - Obstructed labour, particularly in association with uterine stimulants.
  - Multiple pregnancy.
  - Short labours.
- The clinical features include:
  - Sudden collapse with acute hypotension and fetal distress.
  - Pulmonary oedema (>90%) and cyanosis (80%).
  - Coagulopathy (80%). Haemorrhage may be concealed.
  - Fits (50%).
  - Cardiac arrest (occurs in nearly 90% of women).[1]

Little advance has been made in treating this devastating condition, although care with the use of uterine stimulants and timely diagnosis of obstructed labour may help to reduce the incidence.

Once amniotic fluid embolism has occurred, treatment is purely supportive:

- Airway, breathing, and circulation.
- Senior individuals should be present (obstetric, anaesthetic, paediatric and midwifery).
- Haematology services should be alerted, as large quantities of blood products may be required.
- Early delivery of the fetus is vital for both maternal and fetal survival.
- Pulmonary arterial catheterisation may be useful to guide inotropic support and measure right and left sided filling pressures.
- Measure coagulation profile regularly. Platelets, fresh frozen plasma and cryoprecipitate may all be required.
- Intensive care will be required for those that survive the initial insult.

Early mortality is high (50% within the first hour). Even in those that survive, long term neurological problems are common.

---

1 Clark SL, Hankins GDV, *et al.* (1995). Amniotic Fluid embolism: Analysis of the national registry. *American Journal of Obstetrics and Gynecology*, **172**, 1156–1169.

Cardiac disease and pregnancy

Cardiac disease is the leading cause of indirect maternal death in pregnancy. Although rheumatic disease is now rare, the increasingly elderly maternal population, and the increased survival into child-bearing years of the previous generation of patients with complex congenital cardiac malformations, may increase the frequency with which cardiac disease is encountered. Pregnancy and labour often present a severe stress test to these women. As a generality, if a woman was symptomatic with minimal activity before pregnancy, particularly if symptomatic at rest (New York Heart Association Classification III and IV), the course of pregnancy is likely to be stormy and mortality of the order of 20–30% is to be expected. The period of greatest stress is in the immediate post partum period.

It is beyond the scope of this book to give anything but the broadest plans of how to manage women with cardiac disease during pregnancy:

- Early assessment including echocardiography is vital.
- Plan the delivery—with severe disease, elective Caesarean section offers advantages as appropriate personnel can be guaranteed to be present. A combination of obstetricians, anaesthetists, cardiologists, and paediatricians will need to be involved in decision making.
- Investigations should be performed as indicated. The risk to the fetus from procedures such as chest radiographs is minimal.
- Make sure that the woman is in an appropriate place for delivery (this may be the normal delivery suite or it may be the cardiac theatres in a tertiary centre).
- Remember cardio-prophylactic antibiotics both for labour and delivery.
- Avoid ergometrine.
- Use oxytocin only with extreme caution because of its vasodilating effect, which may decompensate an already compromised individual. If oxytocin must be given, use a slow infusion.
- Expect the period of highest risk to be in the 1–2hr post delivery (cardiac output peaks, auto-transfusion plus blood loss leads to a variable effect on pre- and afterload).
- Continue management on ICU care if appropriate.

General principles

- Conditions associated with pulmonary hypertension have a very high maternal mortality in pregnancy (>70%).
- Extreme caution is required to avoid sudden changes in afterload for patients with fixed cardiac output.
- Cyanotic heart lesions (i.e. right-to-left shunts) will not tolerate reductions in systemic vascular resistance. Nevertheless epidural analgesia is sometimes used to minimise the stress of labour, but onset of analgesia must be slow, and use phenylephrine to maintain afterload. General anaesthesia is probably the technique of choice for Caesarean section.

Aortic stenosis may become symptomatic during pregnancy. Serial echocardiography is often used. Tachycardia and reduction in afterload should be avoided. Loss of sinus rhythm should be treated promptly. General or slow onset regional anaesthesia have both been advocated for Caesarean section. The technique is probably less important than the skill with which it is applied.

- Valvular insufficiencies are usually well tolerated during pregnancy.
- Women with symptomatic Marfan's disease (see p305) particularly if the aortic root is dilated, have a high risk of aortic dissection. They are usually maintained on β-blockers. Unexplained severe chest pain is an indication for a chest X-ray and an echocardiogram.
- Myocardial infarction during pregnancy has a 20% mortality. Infarction occurs most commonly in the third trimester. If possible, delivery should be delayed at least 3wk after infarction. Both elective Caesarean section and vaginal delivery have been advocated. In either case, cardiac stress should be minimised with effective analgesia.

Maternal resuscitation

Maternal cardiac arrest is fortunately rare. The basic algorithms for adult resuscitation (p862) are appropriate for maternal resuscitation with several important differences:

- After 20wk gestation, the mother must be tilted to minimise aortocaval compression. The tilt is ideally provided by a wooden support, but if this is not available an assistant can kneel beside the arrested individual. The hips can then be wedged on to the knees of the assistant.
- After 20wk gestation the fetus should be delivered as soon as possible. This improves the chance of maternal survival (and that of a term fetus) as aortocaval compression severely limits the effectiveness of chest compressions. The fetus is likely to be severely acidotic and hypoxic at delivery.
- Remember that pregnant women have reduced oesophageal sphincter tone and that cricoid pressure and intubation should both be performed as rapidly as possible.
- Normal resuscitation drugs should be used. Adrenaline is the drug of choice despite its effect on uterine circulation.
- Adrenaline is also the drug of choice in major anaphylactic or anaphylactoid reactions. Severe hypotension associated with anaphylaxis results in very poor fetal outcome. Early delivery is vital for the fetus.
- Consideration should be given to the diagnosis and treatment of obstetric causes of maternal arrest.

Common causes of maternal arrest include:
- Haemorrhage
- Pulmonary embolism
- Amniotic fluid embolus
- Cerebral haemorrhage
- Intracranial haemorrhage
- Myocardial infarction
- Iatrogenic events:
  - Hypermagnesaemia—treat with 10ml of 10% calcium chloride.
  - High or total spinal—supportive treatment.
  - Local anaesthetic induced arrhythmia.

Pregnancy induced hypertension, pre-eclampsia, and eclampsia[1]

Pre-eclampsia remains a leading cause of maternal death. It is a systemic disorder and the precise aetiology is complex. Immunological factors, genetic factors, endothelial dysfunction, as well as abnormalities in placental implantation, fatty acid metabolism, coagulation and platelet factors have all been implicated. The earlier in gestation that pre-eclampsia manifests itself, the more severe the disease.

Definitions

- Hypertension: a sustained systolic BP >140mmHg or diastolic BP >90mmHg.
- Chronic hypertension: hypertension that existed before pregnancy.
- Pregnancy induced hypertension: hypertension that develops in pregnancy. In the absence of other signs of pre-eclampsia, this has minimal effect on pregnancy but may be indicative of a tendency to hypertension in later life.
- Pre-eclampsia: pregnancy induced hypertension in association with renal involvement causing proteinuria (>300mg/24hr or 2+ on urine dipstick). Incidence 6–8% of all gestations.
- Severe pre-eclampsia: pre-eclampsia in association with any of the following: a sustained BP >160/110; proteinuria >5g/24hr or 3+ on urine dipstick; urine output <400ml/24hr; pulmonary oedema or evidence of respiratory compromise; epigastric or right upper quadrant pain; hepatic rupture, platelet count <100 × 10^9/l; evidence of cerebral complications. Incidence 0.25–0.5% of all gestations.
- Eclampsia: convulsions occurring in pregnancy or puerperium in the absence of other causes. Almost always occurs in the presence of pre-eclampsia, although signs of pre-eclampsia may not be manifest until after a fit.

Pathophysiology

Cardiorespiratory

- Hypertension and increased sensitivity to catecholamine and exogenous vasopressors.
- Reduced circulating volume, but increased total body water.
- In severe pre-eclampsia systemic vascular resistance is increased and cardiac output reduced. However some women have elevated cardiac output with normal or only marginally increased systemic vascular resistance. Fetal prognosis is improved in this group.
- Poor correlation between central venous and pulmonary capillary wedge pressure.
- Increased capillary permeability which may result in:
  - Pulmonary oedema. In pre-eclampsia the most common mode of maternal death is pulmonary oedema and ARDS. Avoid fluid overload.
  - Laryngeal and pharyngeal oedema. Stridor may result.

Haematological

- Reduced platelet count with increased platelet consumption, hypercoagulability with increased fibrin activation and breakdown. Disseminated intravascular coagulation may result.
- Increased haematocrit resulting from decreased circulating volume.

Renal function
- A reduced glomerular filtration rate.
- Increased permeability to large molecules resulting in proteinuria.
- Decreased urate clearance with rising serum uric acid level.
- Oliguria in severe disease.

Cerebral function
- Headache, visual disturbance and generalised hyper-reflexia.
- Cerebrovascular haemorrhage. Deaths due to intracranial haemorrhage are declining with improved control of blood pressure.
- Eclampsia (resulting from cerebral oedema or cerebrovascular vasoconstriction).

Fetoplacental unit
- Reduced fetal growth with associated oligohydramnios.
- Poor placental perfusion and increased sensitivity to changes in maternal BP.
- Reduction of umbilical arterial diastolic blood flow and particularly reverse diastolic flow are indicative of poor fetal outcome without early intervention.

Management of pre-eclampsia
- There is no effective prophylactic treatment to prevent pre-eclampsia. Some obstetricians may use low dose aspirin in selected high-risk pregnancies, but benefit is unproven.
- In established pre-eclampsia the only definitive treatment is the delivery of the placenta. Symptoms will usually start to resolve within 24–48hr.
- When pre-eclampsia develops at term there is no advantage to delaying delivery. However if pre-eclampsia develops before term, a compromise has to be made between maternal and fetal health. Maternal blood pressure is controlled for as long as possible to allow fetal growth to be optimised. If fetal or maternal condition deteriorates, delivery must be expedited.
- Anti-hypertensive therapy. Blood pressure should be controlled to below 160/110 to prevent maternal morbidity particularly from intracranial haemorrhage, encephalopathy, and myocardial ischaemia/failure.
  - Established oral anti-hypertensive drugs include oral methyldopa/ nifedipine preparations and β-blockers (particularly the combined α- and β-blocker labetalol). Prolonged use of β-blockers may reduce fetal growth.
  - ACE inhibitors are associated with oligohydramnios, still birth, and neonatal renal failure. They should be avoided.

Rapid control of severe hypertension can be achieved with:
- Hydralazine (5mg IV aliquots to a maximum of 20mg).
- Labetalol (5–10mg IV every 10min).
- Oral nifedipine. (SC nifedipine should be avoided because of associated rapid changes in placental circulation which may compromise fetal condition.)

1 Brodie H, Malinow AM (1999). Anaesthetic Management of pre-eclampsia/eclampsia. *International Journal of Obstetric Anaesthesia*, **8**, 110–124.

- In cases resistant to treatment, infusions of sodium nitroprusside or glyceryl trinitrate may be needed. If used, invasive arterial pressure monitoring is required.
- Magnesium prophylaxis in pre-eclampsia effectively reduces the incidence of eclampsia, but increases the frequency with which the side effects of magnesium therapy are seen. Severe pre-eclamptic patients are usually treated with magnesium.
- Fluid management in severe pre-eclampsia is critical. Intravascular volume is depleted but total body water is increased. Excessive fluid load may result in pulmonary oedema, but underfilling may compromise fetal circulation and renal function. General principles are:
  - Individual units are encouraged to develop and follow a fluid management protocol.
  - A named individual should have overall responsibility for fluid therapy in severe pre-eclampsia.
  - Measure hourly urine output.
  - Beware of excessive fluid loads being delivered with drug therapy (i.e. oxytocin or magnesium). Increased concentrations may be required.
  - Be cautious with preload before Caesarean section and avoid preload before regional analgesia.
  - A common approach is to use a small background infusion of crystalloid, and to treat persistent oliguria with 250–500ml of colloid. If oliguria continues, further fluid management is usually guided by central venous pressure.
- Invasive arterial pressure monitoring is indicated in severe pre-eclampsia for:
  - Monitoring the response to laryngoscopy and surgery during general anaesthesia.
  - Taking repeated arterial blood gases.
  - Monitoring rapidly acting hypotensive agents (such as sodium nitroprusside).
- Central venous pressure monitoring is indicated in severe pre-eclampsia:
  - For persistent oliguria (<0.5ml/kg/hr) unresponsive to small fluid challenges.
  - If pulmonary oedema develops.

Beware in severe pre-eclampsia as central venous pressure may not correlate well with pulmonary arterial wedge pressure.

Analgesia for vaginal delivery

- Effective epidural analgesia controls excessive surges in blood pressure during labour and is recommended.
- Check platelet count before performing an epidural. If maternal condition is rapidly deteriorating or if the platelet numbers are falling then a count must be performed immediately before placement. The 'acceptable' level of platelet count is debatable and based on little evidence. However common general guidelines are:
  - If the platelet count is $<100 \times 10^9$/l, a clotting screen is required.
  - If the platelet count is $>80 \times 10^9$/l and the clotting screen is normal then regional techniques are acceptable.

- With a platelet count of $<80 \times 10^9/l$, a very careful assessment from a senior individual is required and the potential risks and benefits should be discussed with the patient.
- Thromboelastography may offer a better method of assessing bleeding potential, but as yet its place is unproven.
- Preload before regional analgesia is not required, but monitor BP and fetus carefully and treat changes in BP promptly with 3mg increments of ephedrine. (The role of phenylephrine in pre-eclamptic patients has still to be established.)

Anaesthesia for Caesarean section

General anaesthesia or regional anaesthesia may be used. General anaesthesia is indicated if significant thrombocytopenia (see above) or coagulopathy has developed.

General anaesthesia

- Assess the airway carefully. Obvious oedema may be apparent. Sometimes partners may be better able to assess the onset of facial oedema. A history of stridor is of major concern. A selection of small tube sizes must be available. Consider awake fibre-optic intubation in severe cases.
- Obtund the hypertensive response to laryngoscopy (e.g. alfentanil 1–2mg, but inform the paediatrician that opioids have been used, or labetalol 10–20mg before induction). In very severe pre-eclampsia, intra-arterial pressure monitoring is needed before induction.
- If magnesium has been used, expect prolongation of action of non-depolarising muscle relaxants. Use a reduced dose and assess muscle function with a nerve stimulator.
- Ensure adequate analgesia before extubation. The hypertensive response to extubation may also need to be controlled with antihypertensive agents (e.g. labetalol 10–20mg).
- Effective postoperative analgesia is required but avoid NSAIDs as these patients are prone to renal impairment and may have impaired platelet count or function. When the proteinuria has resolved, which is often within 48hr, NSAIDs may be introduced.
- Continue care in a high dependency area or ICU.

Regional anaesthesia

Depleted intravascular volume may make severe pre-eclamptic patients more vulnerable to the hypotensive effect of the rapid onset of spinal as opposed to epidural anaesthesia. However recent studies suggest that pre-eclamptic women are actually less prone to hypotension than normal individuals and no difference in fetal outcome could be demonstrated between spinal and epidural anaesthesia. Spinal anaesthesia consistently produces better analgesia.

- As with regional analgesia, platelet count and if necessary clotting screen needs to be assessed (see p744).
- A reduced volume of preload should be used (possibly with colloid).
- Expect ephedrine to have an increased effect. The role of phenylephrine in pre-eclamptic patients has still to be established.
- A slow onset block may be beneficial.
- Effective postoperative analgesia is required but avoid NSAIDs as these patients are prone to renal impairment and may have impaired platelet count or function.
- Care should be continued on an HDU or ICU.

Eclampsia

- Incidence 1:2000 pregnancies in the UK,[1] but there are wide international variations.
- Most fits occur in the third trimester, and nearly one–third occur postpartum, usually within 24hr of delivery.
- Eclampsia is a life-threatening event.
- Management is aimed at immediate control of the fit and secondary prevention of further fits.

Immediate management

- Airway (left lateral position with jaw thrust), breathing (bag and mask ventilation and measure oxygen saturation), circulation (obtain IV access and measure BP when possible, avoid aortocaval compression).
- Control of fits with 4g of magnesium given IV over 5–10min.

Prevention of further fits[2]

- Magnesium infusion at 1g/hr for 24hr. Therapeutic level—2–4mmol/l. Magnesium levels may be monitored clinically (loss of reflexes (>5.0mmol/l), reduced respiratory rate (6.0–7.0mmol/l)) or with laboratory monitoring. Reduce infusion rate with oliguria. (Cardiac arrest may occur at >12.0mmol/l.)
- Patients on calcium channel antagonists are at particular risk of toxicity.
- Toxicity can be treated with IV calcium (e.g. 10ml of 10% calcium chloride).

After the initial fit has been controlled, if eclampsia has developed antenatally a decision has to be made as to when delivery is to be performed. In general the patient should be stabilised on a magnesium infusion and then consideration given to vaginal or operative delivery. Eclampsia is not an indication for emergency Caesarean section. If general anaesthesia is required, expect prolongation of action of non-depolarising muscle relaxants. After delivery patients should be observed on an HDU dependency or ICU.

1 Douglas KA, Redman CWG (1994). Eclampsia in the United Kingdom. *British Medical Journal*, **309**, 1395–1399.
2 The Eclampsia Trial Collaborative Group (1995). Which anticonvulsant for women with eclampsia? Evidence from the Collaborative Eclampsia Trial. *Lancet*, **345**, 1455–1463.

HELLP syndrome

Haemolysis, Elevated Liver enzymes and Low Platelets comprises the HELLP syndrome. It is usually associated with pre-eclampsia or eclampsia, but these are not a prerequisite for diagnosis. Severe HELLP syndrome has a 5% maternal mortality. HELLP rarely presents before the 20th week of gestation, but one sixth present before the third trimester and a further third present postnatally (usually within 48hr of delivery). Symptoms are sometimes of a vague flu-like illness, which may delay diagnosis. Maintain a high index of suspicion.

Features include

- Evidence of haemolysis (a falling Hb concentration without evidence of overt bleeding, haemoglobinuria, elevated bilirubin in serum and urine, elevated LDH).
- Elevated liver function tests—AST (serum aspartate transaminase), ALT (serum alanine aminotransferase), alkaline phosphatase, and γ-glutamyl transferase. Epigastric or right upper quadrant abdominal pain are present in 90% of women with HELLP. Liver failure and hepatic rupture may occur. Extreme elevation in AST is associated with poor maternal prognosis. Most women with right upper quadrant pain and a platelet count of $<20 \times 10^9$/l will have an intrahepatic or subcapsular bleed.
- A falling platelet count. Counts of less than 100×10^9/l are of concern, while a count of less than 50×10^9/l is indicative of severe disease.
- Hypertension and proteinuria are present in 80% of women with HELLP. 50% suffer nausea and vomiting. Convulsions and gastrointestinal haemorrhage are occasional presenting features.

The only definitive treatment is delivery of the placenta, although high dose steroids may delay progress of the disease. If maternal condition is not deteriorating rapidly and the fetus is profoundly premature, delivery may be delayed by 48hr to allow steroids to be administered to promote fetal lung maturity.

- The method of delivery depends on maternal condition and the likelihood of successfully inducing labour. Severe HELLP syndrome will require an urgent Caesarean section.
- The risk of epidural haematoma may preclude the use of regional analgesia/anaesthesia. Consideration must be given to both the absolute platelet number as well as rate of fall in platelet count. All patients require a clotting screen.
- Be prepared for major haemorrhage.
- Further management is supportive, with appropriate replacement of blood products as required.
- Invasive monitoring is dictated entirely by the clinical condition of the patient.
- ARDS, renal failure and disseminated intravascular coagulation may develop.
- After delivery of the placenta, recovery can be expected to start within 24–48hr. These patients should all be on an HDU or ICU.

Incidental surgery during pregnancy

One to two percent of women require incidental surgery during pregnancy.[1] Surgery is associated with increased fetal loss and premature delivery, although this probably reflects the underlying condition that necessitated the surgery rather than the anaesthetic or the surgery itself. The risk of teratogenicity is very small.

General considerations

- When possible delay surgery until the postnatal period or alternatively into the second trimester, when teratogenic risks to the fetus are reduced (the fetus is at greatest risk from teratogenicity in the period of organogenesis, which continues to the 12th gestational week).
- Make sure that the obstetric team are aware that surgery is planned.
- Remember gastric acid prophylaxis.
- Remember DVT prophylaxis. Pregnant women are hypercoagulable.
- Consider regional anaesthesia. The combination of a mother maintaining her own airway together with a minimal fetal drug exposure, is desirable. However data demonstrating that regional anaesthesia is safer than general anaesthesia is lacking.
- Airway management in the first and early second trimester is controversial. In asymptomatic women with no other indication for intubation, it is acceptable not to perform a rapid sequence induction up to 18wk of gestation. However be aware that lower oesophageal sphincter tone is reduced within the first few weeks of pregnancy and intra-abdominal pressure rises in the second trimester. If patients have additional risk factors for regurgitation (e.g. symptomatic reflux, obesity), use a rapid sequence induction.[2]
- Every effort must be made to maintain normal maternal physiological parameters for the gestational age of the fetus throughout the perioperative period.
- Treat haemorrhage aggressively. Avoid hypovolaemia and anaemia as both impact on fetal oxygenation.
- From the 20th week of gestation use left lateral tilt to reduce aortocaval compression. Remember that although upper limb BP may be normal, uterine blood flow may still be compromised in the supine position.
- If general anaesthesia is employed, use adequate doses of inhalational agents. Light anaesthesia is associated with increased catecholamine release, which reduces placental blood flow. The tocolytic effect of inhalational agents is advantageous.
- Fetal monitoring may be beneficial although its value remains unproven. If fetal distress is detected, maternal physiology can be manipulated to optimise uterine blood flow.
- The primary risk to the fetus is premature labour in the postoperative period. Detection and suppression of premature labour is vital. Women should be told to report sensations of uterine contractions so that appropriate tocolytic therapy can be instituted.

- Effective postoperative analgesia is required to reduce maternal catecholamine secretion. Although opioids can be used, they may result in maternal hypercarbia. Regional analgesia with local anaesthetic agents may be preferential. If this would prevent the mother from detecting uterine contractions, consider external uterine pressure transduction—'tocodynamometry'. For minor surgery local anaesthesia and simple analgesics such as paracetamol and codeine may be used. Chronic dosage with NSAIDs should be avoided—in the first trimester because of increased fetal loss and in the third trimester because of the possibility of premature closure of the fetal ductus arteriosus.

Teratogenicity

The fetus is at greatest risk of teratogenesis in the period of major organogenesis. This is predominantly in the first 12wk of gestation, although minor abnormalities may still occur after this. Causes of teratogenicity are diverse and include infection, pyrexia, hypoxia, and acidosis as well as the better-recognised hazards of drugs and radiation. The association of drugs with teratogenicity is often difficult. Epidemiological studies have to be large to establish associations, while animal experiments may not reflect either human dose exposure or human physiology. Although none of the commonly used anaesthetic agents are proven teratogens, specific concerns are addressed below.

Premedication

- Benzodiazepines. Case reports have associated benzodiazepines with cleft lip formation, but this has not been substantiated by more recent studies. A single dose has never been associated with teratogenicity. Long term administration may lead to neonatal withdrawal symptoms following delivery and exposure just before delivery may cause neonatal drowsiness and hypotonia.
- Ranitidine and cimetidine are not known to be harmful but caution is advised with chronic exposure to cimetidine because of known androgenic effects in adults.

Induction agents

- Thiopental. Clinical experience with thiopental suggests that this is a very safe drug to use, although formal studies have not been conducted.
- Propofol is not teratogenic in animal studies. Its use in early human pregnancy has not been formally investigated. Propofol is safe to use during Caesarean section at term.
- Etomidate is also not teratogenic in animal studies. It is a potent inhibitor of cortisol synthesis and when used for Caesarean section, neonates have reduced cortisol concentrations.
- Ketamine should be avoided in early pregnancy as it increases intrauterine pressure, resulting in fetal asphyxia. This increase in intrauterine pressure is not apparent in the third trimester.

1 Mazze RI, Kallen B (1989). Reproductive outcome after anesthesia and operation during pregnancy: A registry study of 5405 cases. *American Journal of Obstetrics & Gynecology*, **161**, 1178–1185.
2 Vanner RG (1992). Gastro-oesophageal reflux and regurgitation during general anaesthesia for termination of pregnancy. *International Journal of Obstetric Anaesthesia*, **1**, 123–128.

Inhalational agents

- Halothane and isoflurane have been used extensively in pregnancy and are safe. At high concentrations, maternal blood pressure and cardiac output fall resulting in a significant reduction in uterine blood flow. The halogenated vapours also cause uterine relaxation, which may be beneficial for surgery during pregnancy.
- Despite early concerns, recent epidemiological studies suggest that nitrous oxide is safe. However nitrous oxide is consistently teratogenic in Sprague Dawley rats if they are exposed to 50–75% concentrations for 24hr during their peak organogenic period. Given that anaesthesia can be safely delivered without nitrous oxide it is sensible to avoid this agent.
- Muscle relaxants: because these agents are not lipophilic, only very small quantities cross the placenta and so fetal exposure is limited. These agents are safe to use.
- Anticholinesterase inhibitors: These agents are highly ionised and so, like muscle relaxants, do not readily cross the placenta and are safe to use. Chronic use of pyridostigmine to treat myasthenia gravis may cause premature labour.

Analgesics

- Opioids readily cross the placenta, but brief exposure is safe. Long-term exposure will cause symptoms of withdrawal when the fetus is delivered. Animal studies suggest possible fetal teratogenicity if prolonged hypercapnia or impaired feeding develop as side effects of opioid exposure.
- Chronic exposure to NSAIDs in early pregnancy may be associated with increased fetal loss and in the third trimester may cause premature closure of the ductus arteriosus and persistent pulmonary hypertension of the newborn. Single doses are unlikely to be harmful. These agents are also used to suppress labour, particularly in the second trimester.
- Bupivacaine and lidocaine are safe. When used near delivery, bupivacaine has no significant neonatal neuro-behavioural effects, while lidocaine may have a mild effect. Cocaine abuse during pregnancy increases fetal loss and may increase the incidence of abnormalities in the genitourinary tract.

Cervical cerclage

Procedure	Surgical treatment of incompetent cervical os
Time	20min
Pain	+
Position	Lithotomy
Blood loss	Nil
Practical techniques	Spinal/epidural
	GA with RSI/cuffed ETT if >18wk
	gestation or reflux

An incompetent cervix may be caused by congenital abnormalities, cervical scarring or hormonal imbalance. Premature dilation of the cervix and fetal loss may result, usually in the second trimester. Cervical cerclage is performed to prevent this premature dilation and is one of the commonest surgical procedures undertaken in pregnancy. Although occasionally inserted before conception, it is usually performed between 14th and 26th week. Emergency cerclage may be required in the face of a dilating cervix and bulging membranes. Not surprisingly emergency treatment is less successful in maintaining a pregnancy than prophylactic cerclage.

Preoperative
- The risks of cerclage include membrane rupture (more common if the membranes are already bulging), infection, haemorrhage and inducing premature labour.
- Careful assessment of airway, gestation, symptoms of reflux, and supine hypotension.
- Remember antacid prophylaxis.
- Explain risks of teratogenicity/spontaneous miscarriage (see p749).

Perioperative
- Both regional and general anaesthesia may be used.
- If general anaesthesia used and uterine relaxation is required to allow bulging membranes to be reduced, the halogenated vapour concentration can be increased.
- For regional anaesthesia, a T8–T10 level is required for intra-operative comfort. If uterine relaxation is required, 100µg aliquots of IV glyceryl trinitrate may be used and repeated as necessary, although transient hypotension is to be expected.

Postoperative
- In the postoperative period women should be observed closely for premature labour.
- Vaginal cervical cerclage sutures are usually removed at the 38th week of gestation.

Special considerations

- Various permutations on cervical cerclage are available. These are broadly divided into transvaginal procedures and trans-abdominal procedures.
- The trans-abdominal procedure requires two operations—one for insertion and a Caesarean section for delivery and removal of the suture. It also carries greater risk of ureteric involvement.
- Transvaginal procedures are much more common. Shirodkar and McDonald procedures are the two commonest methods. They both require anaesthesia for insertion but can be removed without anaesthetic.

Controversies in obstetric anaesthesia

Feeding in labour

In the 1950s the Confidential Enquiries into maternal deaths highlighted aspiration as a major cause of maternal death. As a result a policy of fasting during labour became widespread. Although airway problems continue to be implicated in maternal deaths, aspiration is now rare.

Fasting may adversely affect the progress of labour. Ketosis and hypoglycaemia are common when fasting is combined with the physical effort of labour. This may reduce the likelihood of a spontaneous vaginal delivery. A widely quoted study by Ludka supported this.

Scrutton randomised women to feeding or fasting in labour and found that ketosis and hypoglycaemia were less common when women were fed. However gastric volume was greater in the fed group, and there was no difference in the duration of 1st or 2nd stages of labour, oxytocic requirements or mode of delivery.[1]

Most women do not want to eat when in established labour. However if feeding is to be instituted, suggested recommendations are:

- Only 'low risk' women should be permitted to eat. However identification of 'low risk' women in early labour is notoriously inaccurate.
- Stop all intake of solids if any opioid, epidural, or oxytocic is used.
- Allow only 'low residue' foods that rapidly empty from the stomach (cereals, toast, low fat cheese, and semi-sweet biscuits). Very cold foods such as ice creams are known to delay gastric emptying.
- As particulate matter is known to be especially problematic in the event of aspiration, isotonic sports drinks may offer the ideal solution. These effectively prevent ketosis without increasing gastric volume.

Backache and neurological damage after neuraxial techniques

In the early 1990s two retrospective studies by MacArthur[2] and Russell[3] suggested an association between epidural analgesia in labour and subsequent new backache and headache. Prolonged abnormal posture permitted by effective analgesia was the proposed mechanism. This received widespread media coverage and spurred several prospective studies.

These prospective studies established that previous studies had underestimated the incidence of antenatal backache. No prospective studies have found an increased incidence of 'new' backache at the time of delivery in association with regional anaesthesia. (This excludes a period of short-term backache at the site of needle puncture. The incidence of local tenderness at the site of epidural insertion is roughly 50%, but this usually resolves within a few days.)

Neurological damage does occur after childbirth, but establishing cause and effect is difficult. Neurological sequelae following delivery under general anaesthesia is as common as delivery under regional anaesthesia, suggesting that obstetric causes of neurological problems are probably more common than any effects from the regional technique. Prolonged neurological deficit after epidural anaesthesia occurs in approximately 1:10 000 to 1:15 000.

Epidurals, dystocia and Caesarean section[4]

It has been recognised for many years that epidurals are associated with Caesarean section. However argument continues as to whether this is a *causative* association. Various possible mechanisms have been proposed. These include:

- Reduced maternal expulsive effort resulting from abdominal muscle weakness.
- Change in the way the force of contraction is transferred to the pelvic floor when relaxed by an epidural.
- Change in uterine force of contraction (this is not substantiated by recent studies).
- Interference with the Ferguson reflex (increased oxytocic production between pressure on the pelvic floor in the second stage of labour). This is controversial, as the Ferguson reflex has not been clearly demonstrated in humans.

'Impact studies' (studies of changes in Caesarean section rates when there is a dramatic change in epidural rates) have not found a causative association, and of the many large randomised controlled comparisons of epidural v. opioid analgesia, only two[5] have noted an association. Both of these studies were criticised for methodological problems.

Approximately 50% of the randomised studies did find an association between assisted vaginal deliveries and regional analgesia. This may be minimised by reducing the total dose of local anaesthetic administered.

'Walking' epidurals[6]

Effective analgesia with minimal motor block of the lower limbs can be readily produced with low doses of epidural or intrathecal local anaesthetic, usually in combination with an opioid (e.g. subarachnoid injection of 1ml of 0.25% bupivacaine with 10–25μg fentanyl or an epidural bolus of 15–20ml of 0.1% bupivacaine with 2μg/ml fentanyl. Subsequent epidural top-ups of 15ml of the same solution as required).

In some centres women with minimal motor blockade are encouraged to mobilise. The possible advantages of these techniques include:

- The vertical position, without epidural anaesthesia, is associated with shorter labour, possibly less fetal distress, and greater maternal preference. However the vertical position and mobility do not reduce the need for forceps delivery and the advantages have not been substantiated when walking *with* epidural analgesia.

1 Scrutton MJL, Metcalfe GA, et al. (1999). Eating in labour. A randomised controlled trial assessing the risks and benefits. *Anaesthesia*, **54**, 329–334.

2 MacArthur A, MacArthur C, et al. (1997). Is epidural anesthesia in labor asscoiated with chronic low back pain? A prospective cohort study. *Anesthesia & Analgesia*, **85**, 1066–1070.

3 Russell R, Dundas R, et al. (1996). Long-term backache after childbirth: prospective search for causative factors. *British Medical Journal*, **312**, 1384–1388.

4 Chestnut DH (1997). Epidural analgesia and the incidence of cesarean section. Time for another close look. *Anesthesiology*, **87**, 472–475.

5 Thorp JA, Hu DH, et al. (1993). The effect of intrapartum epidural analgesia on nulliparous labor: a randomised, controlled, prospective study. *American Journal of Obstetrics & Gynecology*, **169**, 851–858.

6 Morgan BM (1995). "Walking" epidurals in labour. *Anaesthesia*, **50**, 839–840.

- Minimal motor block associated with these techniques increases maternal satisfaction scores. Intrathecal, as opposed to epidural, techniques produce a more rapid onset of analgesia, possibly a more rapid cervical dilation and a marginal reduction in assisted delivery.

Mobilization has been criticised because:

- Women usually have adequate leg strength, but it is rarely complete, and is likely to become increasingly compromised with repeat doses of epidural local anaesthetic.
- Impaired proprioception may make walking dangerous even when leg strength has been maintained. Whilst dynamic posturography suggests that following an initial intrathecal dose of 2.5mg bupivacaine and 10µg fentanyl, proprioception is adequate for safe walking, this may no longer be true after repeated epidural top-ups.
- Intrathecal opioid may cause temporary fetal bradycardia, probably by altering uterine blood flow through a change in maternal spinal reflexes.
- Assessing fetal condition is difficult when the mother is mobile.

In practice, when a technique that is likely to permit walking is used, only approximately 50% of women who could walk actually choose to do so. Despite this most women prefer the added sense of control that is engendered by retaining leg strength. If women are to be allowed to walk, always wait at least 30min from the initiation of the block before attempting mobilization. Then:

- Check strength of straight leg raising in bed.
- Ask the woman if she feels able to stand.
- When the woman first stands, have two assistants ready to offer support if required.
- Perform a knee bend.
- Ask the woman if she feels safe.
- Allow full mobilisation.
- After each top-up the same sequence must be repeated.

Chapter 33

Paediatric and neonatal anaesthesia

Simon Berg

Neonatal/infant physiology

Paediatric anaesthesia embraces patients from the premature neonate to the adolescent. Major differences exist between anatomy, physiology, and pharmacological response of children and adults. In anaesthetic terms special considerations apply to the neonate.

> ## Definitions
> Neonate: first 44wk of post-conceptual age (PCA)
> Premature infant: ≤37wk gestational age
> Infant: babies from 1–12 month of age
> SGA: small for gestational age
> Low birth weight (LBW): ≤2.5Kg

Respiratory considerations

- At birth, each terminal bronchiole opens into a single alveolus instead of fully developed alveolar clustering. The alveoli are thick-walled and constitute only 10% of the adult total. Alveolar growth continues by multiplication until 6–8yr.
- Cartilaginous ribs are horizontally aligned so that the 'bucket handle' action of the adult thorax is not possible. Intercostal muscles are poorly developed and the diaphragm has a more horizontal attachment reducing mechanical advantage.
- Ventilation is, therefore, essentially diaphragmatic and rate dependent. Abdominal distension may cause splinting of the diaphragm leading to respiratory failure.
- Closing volume occurs within tidal breathing in the neonate. Minor decreases in functional residual capacity (FRC) increase the pulmonary shunt and lead to lung collapse. The application of continuous positive airway pressure (CPAP) improves oxygenation and reduces the work of breathing.
- Narrow airways result in increased resistance up to the age of 8yr. Nasal resistance represents almost 50% of total airway resistance, accentuating the problem of children with nasal congestion who are obligate nasal breathers.
- Apnoea is a common postoperative problem in preterm neonates. It is significant if the episode exceeds 15s or induces cyanosis or bradycardia. Caffeine (10mg/kg) at induction reduces the incidence by 70%. CPAP may be helpful by the action of distending pressure triggering stretch receptors on the chest wall.
- Due to the higher metabolic rate and alveolar minute volume, volatile agents achieve a more rapid induction and emergence than with adults. They are profound respiratory depressants, and as a consequence most anaesthetised neonates require intubation and controlled ventilation.

Parameter	Neonate	Adult
Tidal volume (spontaneous) (ml/kg)	7	7–10
Tidal volume (IPPV) (ml/kg)	7–10	10
Dead space (ml/kg)	2.2	2.2
VD:VT ratio	0.3	0.3
Respiratory rate	30–40	15
Compliance (ml/cmH$_2$O)	5	100
Resistance (cmH$_2$O/l/s)	25	5
Time constant (s)	0.5	1.1
Oxygen consumption (ml/kg/min)	7	3

Parameters for children over 2yr approximate to adult values.
Estimate respiratory rate from the formula: 24−age/2.

Cardiovascular considerations

- Pulmonary vascular resistance (PVR) falls at birth in response to rises in PaO$_2$/pH and a fall in PaCO$_2$. Subsequent closure of the foramen ovale and ductus arteriosus may reverse with hypoxia and acidosis leading to pulmonary hypertension and right to left shunt (transitional circulation).
- The neonate has small ventricles with reduced contractile mass and poor ventricular compliance. Cardiac output is higher than adults (200ml/kg/min) and rate dependent. Normal systolic pressure is 70–90mmHg with low SVR.
- Heart rates up to 200bpm can be tolerated. Bradycardia occurs in response to hypoxia, and should be treated with oxygen rather than atropine. Neonatal and infant heart rates less than 60bpm require external cardiac compression.
- Autonomic and baroreceptor control is fully functional at term, but vagally mediated parasympathetic tone predominates.
- Incidence of congenital heart disease (CHD) is 7–8 per 1000 live births—10–15% have associated non-cardiac pathology. All neonates with midline defects should be assessed for related cardiac lesions.

Age (yr)	Pulse	Mean systolic blood pressure (mmHg)	Mean diastolic blood pressure (mmHg)
Neonate	80–200	50–90	25–60
1	80–160	85–105	50–65
2	80–130	95–105	50–65
4	80–120	95–110	55–70
6	75–115	95–110	55–70
8	70–110	95–110	55–70
10	70–110	100–120	60–75
12	60–110	110–130	65–80

Mean systolic BP over 1yr = 80 + (age in yr × 2)

Gastrointestinal considerations

- The liver is immature. Enzyme systems have matured by 12wk but some drugs are metabolised more slowly and others by different enzyme pathways from adults. The action of barbiturates and opioids in the neonate is prolonged and enhanced.
- Bilirubin metabolism is affected by a poorly developed glucuronyl transferase system. Rises in unconjugated bilirubin may lead to neonatal jaundice or kernicterus by crossing the blood–brain barrier. Some drugs (e.g. sulphonamides, diazepam, vitamin K) displace bilirubin from plasma proteins and exacerbate jaundice.
- Carbohydrate reserves are low in neonates. The premature baby and stressed neonate are vulnerable to hypoglycaemia.
- Vitamin K-dependent factors are low at term. The routine administration of vitamin K 1mg/kg IV may prevent haemorrhagic disease of the newborn and is mandatory before surgery in the first week of life.

Renal considerations

- Nephron formation is complete at term, but renal function is immature. Renal blood flow is reduced due to high renal vascular resistance. The glomerular filtration rate achieves adult values by 2yr and tubular function by 6–8 months.
- Neonates cannot excrete a large solvent or sodium load. Reduced drug dosages or prolonged frequency intervals may apply.

Haematological considerations

Circulating blood volume is calculated as follows
- Neonate: 90ml/kg
- Infant: 85ml/kg
- Child: 80ml/kg

- Post delivery haemoglobin concentrations range from
  (average 18g/dl) depending on degree of placental tra
  quently haemoglobin concentration falls as the increase
  volume exceeds growth in bone marrow activity, the 'p
  anaemia of infancy' which varies from 10–12g/dl.
- Predominant haemoglobin type at term is HbF (80–90%)
  this has fallen to 10–15% and been replaced by HbA. Hb
  oxygen affinity due to reduced 2,3-diphosphoglycerate (2,
  levels.
- Preoperative haemoglobin less than 10g/dl is abnormal and
  investigated.

Central nervous system

- Neurons are complete at term, but total number of brain ce
  duced. Dendritic proliferation, myelination, and synaptic conn
  develop in the third trimester and first 2yr of life.
- Blood–brain barrier is more permeable in neonates—barbitura
  opioids, antibiotics, and bilirubin all cross more readily.
- Autoregulation of the cerebral circulation is present from birth.
- The brain contains a higher proportion of fat, which may allow v
  agents to reach higher concentrations more rapidly.
- All neonates, however immature, feel pain. The premature neona
  may even be hypersensitive due to a relative increase of transmitt
  mediating nociception with the later development of descending
  inhibitory pathways.
- Dose requirements of volatile agents vary with age. The neonatal M
  is comparable to adult values and decreases with prematurity. MAC
  peaks at one year (approximately 50% greater than adult values), the
  declines to reach adult levels by the onset of puberty (see p1160).

Weight

Approximate weights can be determined from the following formula:

Birth: 3–3.5kg
3–12 month: weight (kg) = [age (month) + 9]/2
1–6yr: weight (kg) = [age (yr) + 4] × 2.

All paediatric patients should be weighed preoperatively.

Thermoregulation

- Poorly developed thermoregulatory mechanism. High surface area to
  volume ratio with minimal SC fat and poor insulation. Vasoconstrictor
  response is limited and the neonate is unable to shiver.
- Non-shivering thermogenesis is achieved by metabolism in brown
  fat found in the back, shoulders, legs, and around major thoracic vessels. This considerably increases oxygen consumption and may worsen
  pre-existing hypoxia. Brown fat is deficient in premature infants.
- Neonates lose heat during surgery by conduction, convection, and
  evaporation but predominantly by radiation. A neutral thermal
  environment is one in which oxygen demand, heat loss, and energy

13–20g/dl
...sfusion. Subse-
...e in circulating
...hysiological

...By 4 months
...r has a higher
...-DPG)

...should be

...ls is re-
...ections

...tes,

...olatile

...te
...ers

...AC

...emperature depends on
...res are 34°C for the
...28°C in the adult.
...egulatory response. Heat is
...al tissues. Prolonged hypo-
...with impaired perfusion.
...g factors are unaffected above
...relaxants is prolonged.

...surgery to warm the walls and raise
...s adequate for larger children but
...e 26°C). In practice this is too hot; a
...an adequate compromise if active
...heat loss and maintain the 'microclimate'
...ould stay closed to avoid draughts.
...; this applies particularly in the anaesthetic
...y large in infants and should be covered
...or even polythene. The rest of the body can
...arm Gamgee.
...device. These include a warming mattress or
...blanket. Overhead radiant heaters may be suitable

...anaesthetic gases. Heated water vapour humidifi-
...ut disposable heat and moisture exchangers are
...y. Use of a circle breathing system also provides
...ning and humidifying anaesthetic gases.
...ve fluids, especially blood, should be warmed.
...s should be kept warm.
...e measurement is essential in neonatal surgery, paediatric
...intermediate to long duration, or where major fluid and
...s is expected.

...ance

neonatal total body weight is water; the value is higher in the
...rm infant and reaches an adult level of 60% by 2yr. Extracellular
...er constitutes 45% of total body water at term (over 50% in the
...eterm) but attains an adult value of 35% by early childhood. Plasma
...olume tends to stay constant at 5% of total body weight independent
of age.
Turnover of water is over double that of the adult. 40% of extracellular
water is lost daily in infants as urine, faeces, sweat, and insensible
losses. A small increase in loss or reduction in intake can rapidly lead
to dehydration.
• Daily fluid maintenance is calculated from calorie requirement;
100kcal/kg for the infant, with older children requiring 75kcal/kg and
adults 35kcal/kg. Each kilocalorie requires 1ml of water for metabolism.

First five days neonatal fluid requirement (ml/kg/d)

	Term	Preterm
Day 1	60	60
Day 2	90	90
Day 3	120	120
Day 4	150	150
Day 5	150	180

Neonatal fluid requirements

- Fluid is initially given cautiously as the kidneys cannot easily excrete a water or sodium load. If under a radiant heater or undergoing photo-therapy, 30ml/kg/day is added to the regime.
- Fluid of choice is 10% dextrose. This is adjusted in increments of 2.5% to achieve normoglycaemia. A blood sugar below 2.6mmol/l is treated with 2ml/kg of 10% dextrose.
- Routinely added electrolytes are sodium 3mmol/kg/d and potassium 2mmol/kg/d. Other electrolytes including calcium are added as indicated.

Paediatric fluid requirements

- Maintenance is calculated using the '4–2–1' regime.
- The fluid of choice is 0.45% saline/5% dextrose:
  - 4ml/kg/hr (100ml/kg/day) for each of the first 10kg
  - 2ml/kg/hr (50ml/kg/day) for each of the second 10kg
  - 1ml/kg/hr (25ml/kg/day) for each subsequent kg

- Maintenance requirement makes no allowance for extra losses from gastroenteritis, intestinal obstruction, and insensible loss from pyrexia. Additional sodium and potassium may also be required.
- Perioperative fluids comprise basic maintenance requirement plus replacement of other observed fluid losses. These are replaced by iso-tonic crystalloid, i.e. 0.9% saline, Hartmann's solution, colloid, or blood according to clinical need. 1% or 2.5% dextrose/Hartmann's (add 10ml or 25ml of 50% dextrose to 500ml Hartmann's) is a useful periopera-tive fluid for infants. Regular blood glucose measurement is essential in neonatal surgery.
- Colloid solutions including albumin, hydroxyethyl starches, and gelatine solutions are all routinely used.
- Transfusion is required after 15% blood loss. Blood volume should be calculated prior to surgery (see p760). Swabs should be carefully weighed and suction recorded.
- Postoperatively use 0.45% saline/5% dextrose (or Hartmann's for older children). 4% dextrose/0.18% saline no longer recommended due to risk of hyponatraemia.

Fluid resuscitation

- Assessment of dehydration and hypovolaemia is made predominantly on clinical grounds. Increased capillary refill time (CRT) ≥ 2s, cold, blue peripheries and an increasing core-peripheral temperature gap with a thready pulse are early signs of hypovolaemia. Rising heart rate is not always helpful and may reflect pain, anxiety, or fever. Oliguria and a reduced level of consciousness are late signs. Hypotension does not occur until over 35% of the blood volume is lost.
- Administer fluid boluses of 20ml/kg crystalloid or 10ml/kg of colloid and then reassess.
- Give blood when 15% of circulating volume lost (p760) and aim for a haemoglobin of 8g/dl or PCV of 25%. Transfused blood should be fresh if possible, warm, filtered, and cytomegalovirus (CMV) negative. It can be rapidly transfused using a syringe and three-way tap.
- 'Swing' of the arterial or pulse oximeter trace is a valuable aid in assessing intravascular loss. CVP may be less sensitive in smaller children because of the greater venous capacitance.

Resuscitation

Clinical assessment of dehydration

Sign	5% dehydration	10% dehydration
Skin	loss of turgor	mottled, poor capillary return
Fontanelle	depressed	deeply depressed
Eyes	sunken	deeply sunken
Peripheral pulses	normal	tachycardia, weak pulse
Mental State	lethargic	Unresponsive

Replacement volume (ml) = wt (kg) x percentage loss
e.g. 10% loss in 5kg infant requires replacement volume of 500ml

Clinical assessment of hypovolaemia

- Shock is the clinical state in which delivery of oxygen and metabolic substrates are inadequate for cellular demand.
- In compensated shock, oxygenation of the vital structures (brain and heart) is maintained by sympathetic reflexes at the expense of non-essential tissues. BP remains normal with an increase in SVR.
- In decompensated shock, hypotension develops and vital organ perfusion is compromised.
- With irreversible shock, there is cyanosis, bradycardia, and gasping respiration. This is a preterminal event.
- Shock may result from loss of fluid (hypovolaemia), pump failure (cardiogenic), or abnormal vessel distribution (distributive).
- The immediate treatment is administration of 100% oxygen and transfusion of 20ml/kg of crystalloid or colloid as often as required. Give blood if no improvement after 40ml/kg.

Sign	Compensated	Uncompensated	Irreversible
Heart rate	↑	↑↑	↑↓
Systolic BP	normal/↑	normal/↓	↑↓
Pulse volume	normal/↓	↓	↓↓
Capillary refill	normal/↑	↑	↑↑
Skin colour	pale	mottled	white/grey
Skin temperature	cool	cold	cold
Mental status	agitated	lethargic	unresponsive
Respiratory rate	normal	↑↑	sighing
Fluid loss	<25%↑	25–40%	>40%

Anaesthetic equipment

Oropharyngeal airway
- Range in size from 000 to 4 (4–10cm in length).
- Rarely useful in neonates who are obligate nasal breathers but may be advantageous in older children or in mask ventilation to prevent gastric distension.
- Estimating the size of the airway is crucial. Incorrect size will worsen airway obstruction. Correct length is equal to the distance from incisors to the angle of the jaw.
- The airway should not be inverted during insertion in infants as this may damage the palate.

Nasopharyngeal airway
- Limited application in paediatric practice. Tolerated at lighter levels of anaesthesia than an oropharyngeal airway and may be of use during induction/recovery of some congenital airway problems or obstructive sleep apnoea.
- Well lubricated prior to insertion; bleeding is possible from mucosal or adenoidal trauma, especially in younger children.
- Appropriate length is equal to the distance from the tip of the nostril to the tragus of the ear.
- If an ET tube is used as a modified nasopharyngeal airway, then the size is calculated by: age/4 + 3.5.

Facemasks
- Clear plastic masks with an inflatable rim provide an excellent seal for spontaneous and assisted ventilation.
- Greater dead space than the traditional black rubber Rendell-Baker masks but less threatening and easier to position.
- Manufactured in a round or tear-drop shape; the round shape is suitable only for neonates and infants. Also available as 'flavoured' masks.
- Transparent design allows for observation of cyanosis/regurgitation and the presence of breathing.
- Size is estimated to fit an area from the bridge of the nose to the cleft of the chin.

Laryngeal mask airway (LMA)[1]
- Indications and insertion techniques are similar to adult use. An alternative method of insertion is to advance the LMA upside down and partially inflated behind the tongue before rotating through 180°.
- Smaller LMA sizes have increased complication rates inversely proportional to the age of the child. The effectiveness of these smaller masks is not established for resuscitation.
- Intubating laryngeal mask airway (ILMA) available in size 3 which is potentially useful for older children.
- ProSeal LMA unavailable in small sizes.

---

1 Bagshaw O (2002). The size 1.5 laryngeal mask (LMA) in paediatric anaesthetic practise. *Paediatric Anaesthesia*, **12**, 420–423.

Size of LMA	Weight (kg)	Cuff volume (ml)
1	0–5	2–5
1.5	5–10	5–7
2	10–20	7–10
2.5	20–30	12–14
3	Large child >30	15–20

Laryngoscopes

- Laryngoscope blades available in different lengths from size 0–3.
- Curved Macintosh blade or straight-bladed Magill for infants (especially ≤6 months—high anterior larynx).
- Polio and McCoy blades are also available.

Tracheal tubes

- Paediatric tracheal tubes should be uncuffed until ~8yr of age.
- Uncuffed tubes are available from 2mm to 7mm. Cuffed tubes start from 5.5mm.
- Paediatric versions of the RAE, armoured, and laser tubes all exist. A north-facing uncuffed preformed tube has been developed for routine paediatric surgery.
- Unlike adults, the paediatric trachea is conical. The narrowest part is at the level of the cricoid ring, the only part of the airway completely surrounded by cartilage. If the tracheal tube is too large, it will compress the tracheal epithelium at this level, leading to ischaemia with consequent scarring and the possibility of subglottic stenosis.
- Correctly sized tube is one in which ventilation is adequate but a small audible leak of air is present when positive pressure is applied at $20cmH_2O$.
- Paediatric 8.5mm connectors can be used in addition to the standard 15mm connector. Catheter mounts should be avoided because of the large dead space involved.

Infant tube sizes	
Weight or age	**Tube size (mm)**
>2 kg	2.5
2–4 kg	3.0
Term neonate	3.5
3 mth–1yr	4.0
Over 2yr	Tube size = age/4 + 4

- Tube length in cm can be calculated as:
  - Age/2 + 12 (or tube size × 3)—oral tube
  - Age/2 + 15—nasal tube.
- Tube size may also approximate to the size of the little finger or diameter of the nostril.
- Tube placement needs to be meticulous to avoid endobronchial intubation or inadvertent extubation.

- To assess the length of tube to be passed below the vocal cords, use the black guide line at the distal end of the tube or the tube size in cm. Ultimately the position must be confirmed clinically.

Anaesthetic breathing systems

Ayre's T-piece with Jackson Rees modification

- Jackson Rees modification of the Ayre's T-piece (Mapleson F) is the most commonly used circuit in paediatric anaesthetic practice. Suitable for all children up to 20kg, beyond which it becomes inefficient. Low-resistance, valveless, lightweight circuit. The expiratory limb exceeds tidal volume to prevent entrainment of room air during spontaneous ventilation. The open-ended 500ml reservoir bag or Jackson–Rees modification allows:
  - Assessment of tidal volume.
  - Ability to partially occlude bag for CPAP or PEEP.
  - Potential for assisted or controlled ventilation.
  - Qualitative appreciation of lung compliance.
  - Reduction in dead space during spontaneous ventilation (FGF washes out expired gas during expiratory pause).
- Scavenging is limited. However, newer versions of the T-piece incorporate a closed bag with an expiratory valve and scavenging attachment. Requirements for fresh gas flow (FGF) are higher in spontaneous than controlled ventilation. Recommendations are 2–3 times alveolar minute volume for spontaneous breathing or 1000ml + 200ml/kg in controlled ventilation. FGF is dependent on the respiratory pattern. A rapid respiratory rate requires a higher FGF. Conversely, an end expiratory pause during controlled ventilation will help reduce FGF.
- Most children require a minimum FGF of 3 litres, which can then be adjusted to achieve normocapnia and an inspired CO_2 concentration of less than 0.6kPa (4.5mmHg). Partial rebreathing allows conservation of heat and humidification.
- End tidal CO_2 concentration may be underestimated in children below 10kg from dilution of expired gases. Sampling should be distal in the circuit.
- A Bain system (co-axial Mapleson D) can be used above 20kg.

Humphrey ADE system

- This hybrid system incorporates the Mapleson A, D, and E circuits in one breathing system.
- Studies indicate that the E mode behaves similarly to the T-piece and that the A mode is efficient in children over 10kg.[1] Both the D and E modes are suitable for controlled ventilation.
- The expiratory valves are of low resistance and do not add appreciably to the work of breathing.

Circle absorption systems

- Low-flow anaesthesia is cost-efficient, reduces atmospheric pollution, and conserves warmth and moisture. The reaction of CO_2 with soda lime is exothermic producing heat and water.

1 Orlikowski, CEP, Ewart MC, Bingham RM (1991). The Humphrey ADE system: evaluation in paediatric use. *British Journal of Anaesthesia*, **66**, 253–257.

- Monitoring of inspiratory and expiratory levels of oxygen, nitrous oxide, CO_2, and volatile agent is mandatory.
- Paediatric circle systems using 15mm lightweight hose are suitable for children over 5kg. The unidirectional valves may increase resistance to breathing and should not be allowed to become damp.
- During controlled ventilation, the leak around the endotracheal tube may require gas flows to be increased.

Bain system

The coaxial Mapleson D system is unsuitable for children under 20kg due to the resistance of the expiratory valve.

Mechanical ventilation

- Standard adult ventilators are suitable down to 20kg.
- Below 20kg, a paediatric ventilator should be able to deliver small tidal volumes, rapid respiratory rates, variable inspiratory flow rates, and different I:E ratios.
- Calculation of tidal volume is meaningless because of compression of gases in the ventilator tubing and a variable leak around the endotracheal tube. More sophisticated ventilators may, however, be capable of measuring expired tidal volume which is of more practical value.
- Some ventilators are designed to work with specific breathing systems. The Newton valve converts the Nuffield Penlon 200 ventilator from time-cycled flow generator to time-cycled pressure generator and can be attached directly to the expiratory limb of the Ayre's T-piece. It is suitable for neonates and children up to 20kg. Many new anaesthetic workstations incorporate integral ventilators attached to circle systems suitable for paediatric practice.
- Pressure controlled ventilation is commonly used and reduces the risk of barotrauma/pneumothorax. This mode will compensate for a leak around the endotracheal tube, but not for changes in lung compliance, partial or complete tube obstruction, or bronchospasm.
- Volume control can make an allowance for changes in lung compliance but at a potential cost of high peak airway pressures.
- Ultimately, setting ventilator parameters is based on clinical observation. Inspiratory flow, pressure, or volume is gradually increased until adequate chest movement is observed. Measurement of capnography and pulse oximetry confirms normocapnia and adequate oxygenation. The peak airway pressure is kept to a minimum. A ventilator alarm is mandatory.
- Most children can be ventilated adequately with inspiratory pressures of $16–20cmH_2O$ and a respiratory rate between 16–24bpm. Normally inspiratory pressure should not exceed $30cmH_2O$. The rate can be adjusted accordingly to achieve normocapnia. A minimum PEEP of $4cmH_2O$ is advisable for infants and neonates to maintain FRC.
- The ability to hand ventilate using the Ayre's T-piece is essential. It should always be available in the event of ventilator failure or unexpected desaturation. Mechanical ventilation may be unsuitable for the small premature neonate. With gastroschisis or exomphalos, hand ventilation can assess changes in lung compliance and determine how much of the abdominal contents can be reduced back into the abdominal cavity. Hand ventilation during repair of a tracheo-oesophageal fistula can be timed to allow the surgeon maximum exposure and time to effect the repair.

Conduct of anaesthesia

Preoperative assessment

The preoperative visit is essential in establishing a rapport with both parents and children and in helping to dissipate anxiety. Communication should be simple, informative, and truthful.

- Avoid wearing a white coat. Involve the parents, but try to question the child directly when appropriate and stay at eye level if possible.
- A preadmission visit reduces parental anxiety and is beneficial to children over 6yr. Play therapists can help provide an informal setting and informatively prepare the child by describing the course of events from the ward to induction of anaesthesia. A collection of photographs or a video may be helpful.

Preoperative investigations

Routine preoperative haemoglobin is indicated for:

- Neonates and ex-premature infants under 1yr.
- Children at risk of sickle-cell disease (see p200).
- Children for whom intra-operative transfusion may be necessary.
- Children with systemic disease.
- A preoperative Hb of less than 10g/dl is abnormal and needs to be investigated. It does not necessarily entail cancellation if the child is haemodynamically stable and otherwise well.

Routine biochemistry is required for:

- Children with metabolic, endocrine, or renal disease.
- Children receiving IV fluids.

The child with a cold

- The preschool child develops 6–8 upper respiratory tract infections (URTI) per yr. Almost 25% of children have a chronic runny nose due to seasonal rhinitis or adenoidal infection.
- Anaesthesia in the presence of an intercurrent URTI is associated with a higher risk of complications in younger children. There is an increased incidence of excess secretions, airway obstruction, laryngospasm, and bronchoconstriction. This risk is increased five-fold using an LMA and by a factor of 10 if the child is intubated.
- Children with moderate to severe chest infections should be postponed. This will include those with productive cough, purulent chest or nasal secretions, pyrexia, and signs of viraemia or constitutional illness, including diarrhoea and vomiting.
- The child with a mild cold is a difficult problem. The history in these cases is crucial. It is important to decide whether the child is at the beginning or end of the URTI. Other members of the family or children at school may have already experienced the same infection, and this can provide useful information.
- A child deemed to be post viral, apyrexial, with no chest signs and constitutionally well is probably fit for surgery even if they have a runny nose.

- URTI requires postponement for 2wk, but this should be 4wk if lower respiratory tract involvement is suspected. Bronchiolitis warrants a delay of at least 6wk.

The child with a murmur

- The majority of pathological murmurs are diagnosed perinatally and these children will already be under the care of a paediatric cardiologist. Antibiotic prophylaxis will apply in certain conditions.
- Previously unreported murmurs are commonly heard at 2–4yr. The majority are functional.
- A pansystolic murmur with normal heart sounds in a child with a normal oxygen saturation and no limitation in exercise tolerance, can be assumed to be innocent and no antibiotic prophylaxis is required. If there are any doubts, surgery should be deferred until a formal assessment has been made.

Premature and ex-premature infants

Account for 13% of births and 47% of neonatal deaths in the UK. Increased incidence of congenital abnormalities, especially SGA babies. Specific problems include asphyxia, hyaline membrane disease (HMD), bronchopulmonary dysplasia (BPD), patent ductus arteriosus (PDA), intraventricular haemorrhage (IVH), retinopathy of prematurity (ROP), hypoglycaemia, anaemia, haemorrhagic disease, increased susceptibility to infection, and impaired thermoregulation.

- Anaesthesia is complicated by difficult vascular access. There is reduced drug metabolism and excretion. Adjust ventilation to minimise barotrauma/high oxygen concentrations. Administer fluids carefully but avoid fluctuations in BP to reduce the possibility of IVH. Increased sensitivity to most anaesthetic agents.
- All neonates feel pain. Adequate pain relief is essential.
- Postoperative apnoea is a common complication. Main predictors are gestational age, postconceptual age, previous apnoeic episodes, and anaemia. Consider caffeine 10mg/kg IV.[1]
- Assessment should identify potential reversible components/degree of chronic infection of BPD, current cardiac status, and underlying neurological disability.
- Inhalational induction is more common because of difficult vascular access and sedative premedication may be necessary.

Consent

- Allow time at the end of preoperative assessment for parents to ask questions. Discuss the options of IV or inhalational induction and obtain consent for a suppository and regional/peripheral nerve block, if indicated, including attendant risks. Discuss the risks associated with general anaesthesia.
- A young person is deemed competent to consent from 16yr. Children under 16yr may have the capacity to decide depending on their ability to understand what is involved (Gillick competence).[2]
- Signed written consent is the preferred option.

1 Welborn LG, Hanallah RS, Fink R, Ruttiman UE, Hicks JM (1989). High-dose caffeine suppresses post-operative apnoea in former preterm infants. *Anesthesiology,* **71**, 347–349.
2 Gillick v West Norfolk and Wisbech AHA (1985), 3 ALL ER 402.

Preoperative fasting (see also p8)

- Fasting instructions are designed to minimise the risk of regurgitation of gastric contents and consequent pulmonary aspiration.
- Fasting reduces gastric volume but does not guarantee an empty stomach. Prolonged fasting does not further reduce the risk of aspiration and in infants can lead to dehydration and hypoglycaemia.
- Infants may be at greater risk of regurgitation. There is reduced lower oesophageal sphincter tone and an increased tendency to distend the stomach during mask ventilation. However, the incidence of pneumonitis following aspiration in children is much less common than in adults.
- Clear fluids can be given safely up to 2hr preoperatively and the intake of fluids (either water or a fruit squash drink) should be encouraged. Children are less irritable at induction and there may be a reduction in postoperative nausea and vomiting.
- The data for milk and solid food are less clear. Breast milk is cleared from the stomach more rapidly than formula milk in infants.
- Every unit should have fasting guidelines. Close liaison with the ward staff ensures that children receive adequate clear fluid preoperatively and that milk feeds for neonates and infants are appropriately timed.

Ingested material	Minimum fast
Clear liquids	2hr
Breast milk	4hr
Light meal, infant formula, and other milk	6hr

Topical anaesthetics

- Topical local anaesthetic preparations reduce the pain of venepuncture and facilitate IV induction.
- Emla® Cream is a eutectic mixture of 5% lidocaine and 5% prilocaine in a 1:1 ratio. It should be applied for at least 45min and can produce vasoconstriction. The duration of action is 30–60min. Emla should be avoided in children <1yr because of the risk of methaemoglobinaemia.
- Ametop® is a 4% gel formulation of amethocaine. There is a shorter onset time (30min) and prolonged duration of action (4hr) after the cream has been removed, compared with Emla. It is licensed from 4wk of age and has vasodilating properties. There may be a higher incidence of allergic reactions. The gel should not be applied for longer than 90min and removed earlier if a rash or itchiness develops.
- It is important to identify the veins to be anaesthetised and not blindly apply the cream to the dorsum of each hand. Keep the area bandaged to prevent removal or licking of cream!
- Ethyl chloride is a cryoanalgesic. It is useful when topical creams are either contra-indicated or forgotten.

Premedication

- Routine sedative premedication is unnecessary.
- Some children will require preoperative sedation. They include the excessively upset child, children with previous unpleasant experiences of anaesthesia and surgery, and certain children with developmental delay. Older children or adolescents may request premedication.
- Infants have not yet developed a fear of strangers and appear relatively undisturbed when separated from their mothers. The preschool child is most at risk. They are vulnerable to separation anxiety in a strange environment but without the ability to reason.
- Even when anaesthesia and surgery are uneventful, there may be a disturbingly high incidence of postoperative psychological problems. Sleep disturbance, nightmares, bed-wetting, eating disorders, and behavioural changes have all been reported. Some authors suggest that sedative premedication especially in the preschool age group may reduce parental anxiety, improve patient compliance, and reduce the incidence of some of these postoperative behavioural changes.
- Oral midazolam (0.5mg/kg) is an ideal premedicant.[1] It acts within 15–30min to reduce anxiety leading to a more cooperative child, but with minimal delay in recovery. The IV formulation is used but is extremely bitter and should be diluted in fruit juice or paracetamol syrup. Midazolam (0.2mg/kg) can also be given intranasally where it has a rapid onset of action within 5–15min but is poorly tolerated because of the burning sensation in the nasal mucosa.
- Ketamine can be given orally (5–6mg/kg) as a sole drug or in combination with midazolam. Its action starts within 15min but it may be associated with excess salivation and emergence delirium. Ketamine 2mg/kg IM may assist in anaesthesia of the uncooperative child who refuses to accept oral premedication.
- Clonidine given orally (4µg/kg) produces good conditions for induction and may reduce postoperative analgesic requirements, but it is associated with hypotension and a delayed recovery.
- Alternative premedicants are trimeprazine (2mg/kg) and promethazine (1mg/kg). They tend to be less predictable and longer lasting. Trimeprazine has both a drying and antiemetic action.
- Modern anaesthetic agents do not require the routine use of anticholinergic agents.
- Antisialogogues are reserved for patients with excessive secretions, e.g. Down's syndrome, cerebral palsy, the suspected difficult airway and co-administration with ketamine. Some anaesthetists still routinely give drying agents for neonates and the smaller child.
- Absorption of orally administered atropine (40µg/kg) is variable. To be certain of efficacy, administer 20µg/kg IM 30min preoperatively or 10µg/kg IV at induction. Glycopyrronium (5µg/kg IM or IV) is a suitable alternative. Atropine should also precede the administration of suxamethonium to protect against possible bradycardia which in children can occur following the first dose. Bradycardias associated

---

1 McCluskey A, Martin GH (1994). Oral administration of midazolam as a premedicant for paediatric day case anaesthesia. *Anaesthesia*, **49**, 782–785.

with gas induction should be treated with IV atropine 10µg/kg and may be prevented by oral atropine preoperatively.
- Children undergoing cardiac surgery are traditionally heavily premedicated. Choices include morphine, which may prevent right ventricular infundibular spasm in uncorrected Fallot's tetralogy, or a combination of drugs, e.g. PethCo®, which comprises a mixture of pethidine, promethazine, and phenergan.

Parents in the anaesthetic room
- In the United Kingdom a parent is routinely allowed into the anaesthetic room while their child is anaesthetised. It is now accepted that enforced separation disempowers the parent and is an emotionally traumatic experience for both parent and child.
- Parents are naturally anxious over loss of control, a strange environment, and the possibility of adverse events. Unfortunately this parental anxiety may communicate itself to the child.
- Parental presence should not be compulsory. It is not always beneficial and may even be counterproductive with a very anxious parent. Evidence of benefit has only been demonstrated for children older than 4yr with a calm parent attending the induction.
- Preschool children are especially at risk of behavioural disturbance, probably because of difficulties in reasoning. In contrast some adolescents may not wish their parents to accompany them.
- Anaesthetic induction appears to be the most distressing event experienced by parents. Separation from the child after induction, watching the child become unconscious, and the degree of stress experienced by the child before induction are all important factors.
- The parent should always be accompanied by a nurse who can comfort them and escort them out of the anaesthetic room once the child is asleep. It is extremely unusual to allow more than one parent into the anaesthetic room. There may rarely be extenuating circumstances, but these should be discussed beforehand with the anaesthetist.

Induction of anaesthesia
- Induction should occur in a child-friendly environment.
- A dedicated paediatric theatre is not always an option. An alternative is a customised paediatric anaesthetic trolley incorporating a comprehensive range of airway and vascular equipment.
- Prepare drugs and equipment before the child arrives. Recheck the weight:

   weight (kg) = (age + 4) × 2

   Precalculate the dose of atropine and suxamethonium in prepared syringes (see p814).
- Pulse oximetry is the minimum monitoring acceptable in the anaesthetic room, although it will not read accurately on the agitated child. Many children will tolerate an ECG and BP cuff prior to induction.

Inhalational induction

- It is important to learn more than one method. Not all children are susceptible to the same technique.
- Sevoflurane is the volatile agent of choice. It is rapidly acting, giving a smooth induction with less cardiovascular depression than halothane. It is not odourless, but is relatively non-irritant. For the suspected difficult airway use sevoflurane in 100% oxygen, otherwise 50% nitrous oxide/oxygen is satisfactory and anecdotally nitrous oxide may obtund the patient's sense of smell, facilitating induction. Emergence delirium is commoner with sevoflurane than halothane. There is a strong association with rapid awakening, particularly in the pre school age group, increased preoperative anxiety and inadequate analgesia.
- Halothane is an alternative, but induction should proceed through incremental increases in concentration. Start with 100% oxygen and add in nitrous oxide once airway is secure. Involve the parent as much as possible. This may involve holding the child or even participating in the induction.
- Position the child either supine on the trolley or across the lap of the parent, so that the parent or anaesthetic assistant can gently restrain the arms if necessary. Warn the parent that the child's head will become floppy and need support.
- For smaller children, a cupped hand method is useful. Occlude the end of the bag to direct all the fresh gas flow towards the patient's mouth and nose.
- A facemask is often tolerated by older children. This can be held by the parent, child, or anaesthetist and the child can be encouraged to blow up the bag 'like a balloon'. A flavoured facemask may be useful initially but the volatile agent rapidly becomes the dominant smell.
- The parent should be warned of abnormal movements when the child is nearly anaesthetised.
- Once anaesthesia is achieved and the eyelash reflex is absent, anaesthesia can be maintained with another volatile agent if desired.

IV induction

- The smaller child sits across the parent's lap and the arm is placed under the parent's axilla, thereby obstructing the child's view. The older child will usually lie on the trolley with the parent on one side holding the child's hand, while the other is cannulated.
- The induction agent of choice is propofol 3–5mg/kg with 1% lidocaine (1ml/10ml propofol) added to reduce pain on injection. It is licensed for use as an induction agent for children over 1 month, but not for infusion below 3yr. The TCI pump is not configured for paediatric use. The dilution of Propofol with an equal volume of saline significantly reduces pain on injection.
- Thiopental at a dose of 4–6mg/kg is a suitable alternative and is licensed for neonates (2mg/kg).
- Ketamine 2mg/kg is reserved for haemodynamically compromised patients or those with severe cardiovascular disease, usually in

conjunction with fentanyl 1–2µg/kg. Emergence phenomena are less common in children, especially in combination with midazolam, but the incidence of PONV and salivation is higher.

Comparison of IV and inhalational induction

- IV induction is simple and safer but is associated with more hypoxia— possibly because children are rarely pre-oxygenated.
- Inhalational induction produces more coughing and laryngospasm.
- Psychological studies suggest that inhalational induction may be more traumatic to the child but the majority of children under 8yr choose this technique if given the choice.
- In practice it seems prudent to opt for IV induction if possible, unless the child actively chooses an inhalational method.

Tips for cannulation

- Securing IV access can be difficult even for paediatric anaesthetists! It is important to realise this, relax and send for help if necessary. Good lighting, competent anaesthetic assistance, and a selection of cannulae with prepared saline-flush syringes are all essential.
- Neonates often have surprisingly good superficial veins on the hand or wrist. Otherwise healthy children between 3 months and 2yr can be notoriously difficult because of the fat pads over hands and feet.
- Compression of a limb by the assistant should be gentle to act as a venous rather than arterial tourniquet. The skin is often mobile and should be gently stretched. In neonates it may be easier for the anaesthetist to flex and squeeze the wrist with the non-cannulating hand.
- Examine the wrists and dorsum of feet for superficial veins. Scalp veins are possible in neonates. Long saphenous and cephalic veins may be palpated.
- In some children, most commonly in the feet, the skin is surprisingly tough and a small nick in the skin with a 21G needle may be necessary. Loosening the cap of the cannula will permit flashback of blood in small veins.
- Transfixion is possible in smaller children. It is potentially useful for all veins but especially in 'blind' long saphenous and femoral vein cannulation. Slowly pull back cannula until in the vein and then gently advance.
- If all else fails, intraosseous access can be an invaluable alternative. Observing aseptic precautions, prepare an area of skin over the antero-medial aspect of the tibia 1cm below and medial to the tibial tuberosity. The intraosseous needle is inserted perpendicularly to the skin and advanced in a twisting pushing movement against the bone until there is a sudden loss of resistance. The position is confirmed if the needle remains upright without support, marrow can be aspirated, and fluid can be administered without SC swelling around the entry site. Children can be successfully anaesthetised via this route although thiopental should be avoided because of its irritant properties. The intraosseous route is particularly useful in fluid resuscitation of the shocked child before definitive IV access can be gained. Routine blood samples including crossmatch can be taken from this site before induction.
- Surgical cut-down is rarely needed, often technically difficult, and should be reserved as a last resort.

Airway management

- Airway complications including coughing, laryngospasm, and upper airways obstruction are more common in children.[1]
- Key to airway management is the triple manoeuvre of head tilt, chin lift, and jaw thrust.
- Hyperextension of the neck in the neonate often occludes the airway and a neutral position is usually more successful. For older children, the adult 'sniffing the morning air' position should be adopted.
- Smaller children do not require a pillow; this may lead to unwanted head flexion.
- The paediatric facemask should be accurately sized and held gently but firmly on the face with the thumb and forefinger. The other fingers should curl around and grip the mandible. It is important to avoid pressing on the floor of the mouth, which will push the tongue forward and obstruct the airway.
- Early use of an oropharyngeal airway may be useful in older children.
- A nasopharyngeal airway may be attempted. This should be well lubricated. It is indicated in cases of micrognathia and can be inserted at lighter levels of anaesthesia.
- The most important technique in management of the airway is judicious use of CPAP. Ensure a good seal with the facemask, and then partially occlude the bag on the Ayre's T-piece.

Laryngospasm (see also p878)

- Laryngospasm is more common in children than adults. Additional risk factors include inhalational induction, asthma, URTI, and chronic lung disease. Children become cyanosed more rapidly than adults because of increased metabolic rate/oxygen consumption and reduced FRC.
- Contrary to the old adage, children do not 'always take a final breath'. Bradycardia is a premorbid event indicating inadequate cardiac output and a significant risk of cerebral hypoxia.

- Partial laryngospasm management
  - 100% oxygen
  - CPAP
  - Gentle assisted ventilation
  - Propofol 1–2mg/kg bolus
- Complete laryngospasm management
  - 100% oxygen
  - CPAP
  - Assisted ventilation may exacerbate the condition by inflating the stomach and forcing the arytenoids and false cords against the true vocal cords
  - Early administration of suxamethonium (1–2mg/kg) and atropine (10µg/kg) may be necessary

---

1 Motoyama EK (1992). Anaesthesia and the upper airway. *International Anaesthesiology Clinics*, **30**, 17–19.

Intubation (for tube sizes see p767)

- Neonatal intubation is not difficult, only different. The neonate has:
  - Proportionately larger head, shorter neck, larger tongue, smaller mandible.
  - Larynx is more anterior/superior (C3–C4 compared with C5–C6).
  - Epiglottis is large, floppy, V-shaped, with obliquely angled vocal cords.
- Awake intubation for neonates is no longer acceptable. In the absence of medical conditions with recognised airway complications, paediatric intubation is usually straightforward. Below 6 months of age, use a straight-bladed laryngoscope. The head should be in a neutral position and the shoulders supported if necessary. Advance the laryngoscope blade past the larynx then withdraw slowly until the larynx becomes visible, i.e. the blade is posterior to the epiglottis. Gentle cricoid pressure is often helpful. If nasal intubation is required use a laryngoscope blade with minimal guttering to allow more room for instrumentation in the oropharynx. Over 6 months of age a curved blade is usually easier. Intubation can be performed in the conventional adult position with the blade resting in the vallecula.
- Most intubated neonates will also require a nasogastric tube (8–10FG).
- Always have a range of endotracheal tubes available including a half size above and below the original estimation.
- Complications are common in children. Oesophageal and endobronchial intubation, extubation, kinking of the tube, and disconnection should all be anticipated. Secretions are far more likely to cause obstruction because of the smaller tube sizes involved, and periodic suction may be necessary.
- Intubation increases the work of breathing. The reduction in cross-sectional area of the neonatal trachea with a size 3.5 tube in situ increases airway resistance by a factor of 16. Most intubated infants should undergo controlled ventilation as part of the anaesthetic technique.

Tube fixation

- Tube fixation is crucial. The neonatal trachea is only 4cm in length. Inadvertent extubation and endobronchial intubation is common.
- Secure with a 'three-point fixation' to prevent movement of the tube in all three planes.
- Two pieces of trouser-shaped Elastoplast may be used with one 'leg' across the upper lip while the other 'leg' is wrapped around the tube. An oropharyngeal airway helps splint the tube.
- There are numerous other methods of fixation, all equally valid. The tube should be secured to the maxilla rather than the more mobile mandible.
- The Portex Polar preformed tracheal tube is a north-facing uncuffed tube which is easy to use, facilitates tube fixation, and reduces the incidence of endobronchial intubation.

Difficult intubation

- The key to difficult intubation is to identify the at-risk patient and plan accordingly with appropriate help, assistance, and equipment. Some conditions are well known to be associated with airway problems (e.g. Pierre–Robin, Treacher–Collins, and Goldenhar syndromes). Other patients can be identified by assessment of the airway preoperatively.
- Premedicate with atropine 20µg/kg IM or glycopyrronium 5µg/kg IM 30min preoperatively to dry secretions or IV at induction. Give ephedrine or pseudoephedrine nose drops. Sedative premedication should be avoided.
- Airway management may be difficult. The traditional method is deep inhalational anaesthesia with CPAP and an IV in situ. Laryngoscopy and intubation are attempted with the patient breathing spontaneously. Halothane is more suitable than sevoflurane at this stage allowing more time for intubation. McCoy and polio blades are both available in paediatric sizes.
- A blind nasal approach to intubation is possible, but experience in the technique is declining.
- LMA will often secure the airway adequately without the need for intubation.
- If intubation is still necessary, it may be possible to pass a bougie through the LMA into the trachea and then railroad an endotracheal tube. A size 3 ILMA is available and may be suitable for a larger child. A fibre-optic bronchoscope can also be used via the LMA.
- Fibre-optic intubation is rarely necessary. Children need to be anaes-thetised but a propofol infusion is an alternative method to volatile anaesthesia. Smaller size neonatal and paediatric bronchoscopes do not all have a suction channel and should be checked to confirm that the selected tracheal tube will fit over them.
- Conventional tubes may present problems in railroading and armoured tubes should be used. Alternatively a guide wire can be inserted into the trachea using the suction channel and the tube passed over it.
- A tracheostomy is rarely required. It is exceedingly difficult as an emergency procedure. Paediatric cricothyroidotomy cannulae are available at 18G and 16G sizes and should be present in the anaes-thetic room.

Rapid sequence induction

- Ranitidine and metoclopramide are not routinely prescribed.
- Preoxygenation does not usually present problems with infants, and older children but may be more difficult in preschool children. Inhalational induction may be necessary.
- Suxamethonium should be preceded by atropine to prevent bradycardia. There is little experience as yet with rocuronium.
- Cricoid pressure often facilitates intubation. If intubation cannot be achieved initially, mask ventilation should gently recommence while cricoid pressure is maintained.

- Nasogastric tube should be routinely used. If already in situ in the neonate it should remain in place rather than being removed. There is no consensus for older children.
- Since the endotracheal tube is uncuffed, a throat pack may help prevent intra-operative aspiration but has no application in the higher-risk periods of induction and reversal.
- Child should be extubated awake in the left lateral position.

Maintenance

- Position the infant and smaller child with both arms raised at the level of the head. Exposure of the hand allows assessment of the pulse, peripheral temperature, colour, and capillary refill. A blocked IV may be more easily cleared and a new cannula may be easier to site.
- Pulse oximeter probe should be sited on the same arm as the IV infusion and contralateral arm to the BP cuff. Avoid oximeter probes on the feet as the trace is usually lost once abdominal surgery commences.
- Check that the endotracheal tube is still in situ, securely fixed and the lungs are ventilating adequately and equally. The connections should all be secure and the tube and breathing circuit supported if necessary.
- Confirm that cannulae are secure, working, and accessible; extension tubing may be necessary. Three-way taps allow administration of drugs and fluid volume when necessary. Neonatal surgery requires a minimum of two cannulae (maintenance and volume). Blood sugar should be checked regularly.
- Even small air bubbles in IV fluids can be potentially harmful to infants, especially in the presence of an ASD or VSD. A bubble trap should be routinely included in the tubing for these patients.
- Theatre temperature should be 21°C and preheated. Child's head should be covered and body exposure reduced to a minimum. It is easier to prevent hypothermia than to treat it. Both IV and cleaning fluid should be warmed.
- Routine monitoring should include ECG, BP (with appropriate size cuff), pulse oximeter, capnography, and full gas monitoring with a ventilator alarm when indicated. Temperature measurement is important and the neonate requires routine use of a precordial or oesophageal stethoscope. The width of the BP cuff should be 20% greater than the diameter of the arm to avoid artefactually raised BP.
- Electronic monitoring is often unreliable with the sick or shocked neonate. It should support but not replace clinical observation. The oesophageal or precordial stethoscope permits a continuous qualitative assessment of heart sounds and ventilation. More importantly, it 'ties' the anaesthetist to the patient.
- Do not let the surgeon start operating until you are ready.
- Anaesthetic complications in paediatric practice are as common during maintenance as at induction or in the postoperative period.

Reversal

- Following surgery, the child should be warm, well saturated, normo-carbic, and pain free. A cold acidotic neonate will not breathe postoperatively.
- LMA can be removed either deep or awake. If an armoured LMA is in situ a bite block will be needed. There is often a stage shortly before waking when the mouth opens slightly to resemble a small yawn; this is an ideal opportunity to deftly remove the LMA.
- Most children should be extubated awake. If warm and with adequate analgesia, this is tolerated well. Exceptions include tonsillectomy and other procedures when coughing is to be avoided. In these cases, deep extubation is preferable.
- Neonates should be extubated awake preceded by an assisted ventilation to preoxygenate the lungs.

Postoperative nausea and vomiting

- Postoperative nausea and vomiting (PONV) is uncommon under the age of 2yr. Predictors of risk include high risk procedures (adenotonsillectomy, squint surgery), travel sickness, and previous PONV. Morphine increases the risk of PONV by 30%. There is no proven benefit of TIVA in children.
- Combinations of antiemetics and the use of 5-HT_3 antagonists with dexamethasone 0.1mg/kg may be more efficacious than simple monotherapy.
- Children considered high risk should receive 0.15mg/kg ondansetron at induction.

Regional anaesthesia

Successful regional blockade provides conditions for light and haemodynamically stable general anaesthesia. The stress response is attenuated and early pain-free emergence is possible leading to a smooth postoperative recovery. Unlike adults, few children tolerate these techniques awake and the majority of regional blocks are performed on anaesthetised patients. Motor blockade is unnecessary and lower concentrations of local anaesthetic can be used. The most widely used solutions are 0.25% bupivacaine/levobupivacaine and 0.2% ropivacaine.

Postoperative pain relief

Similar principles to adult practice (p1028) including the application of multimodal analgesia and specialised pain charts. Assessment can be difficult with infants and neonates.

- Paracetamol and NSAIDs are widely prescribed for minor cases/day surgery and for their morphine-sparing effects. Loading dose of rectal paracetamol is 30–40mg/kg or 20mg/kg for neonates. Drugs are best given regularly.
- Caudal analgesia and peripheral nerve blocks are useful for day cases. Epidural blockade is of proven benefit in abdominal surgery. Below 6 months it is technically easier and possibly safer to insert the catheter via the caudal route.
- Morphine infusions can be administered cautiously to neonates and as nurse-controlled analgesia (NCA) for smaller children. Patient-controlled analgesia (PCA) can be used effectively in children as young as 6yr, although most regimes include a background infusion.
- Liaison with the ward staff is crucial and a standardised pain management approach is the ideal (see below).

Mild to moderate postoperative pain			
Codeine phosphate	1mg/kg	IM, PO, PR	6-hourly
Diclofenac	1mg/kg (over 1yr/10kg)	PO, PR	8-hourly
Ibuprofen	10mg/kg (over 6 month/7kg)	PO	8-hourly
Paracetamol	20mg/kg	PO, PR	6-hourly
	Rectal loading dose		
	Neonate: 20mg/kg	PR	Once
	Child: 30–40mg/kg		
Oramorph	400µg/kg	PO	4-hourly

Severe postoperative pain	
Morphine	50–100µg/kg IV incremental boluses
Morphine infusion	1mg/kg morphine in 50ml saline i.e. 20µg/kg/ml Rate: 1–2ml/hr (20–40µg/kg/hr)
Morphine NCA	1mg/kg morphine in 50ml saline, i.e. 20µg/kg/ml Rate: 1ml/hr. Bolus: 1ml. Lockout: 20min
Morphine PCA	1mg/kg morphine in 50ml saline, i.e. 20µg/kg/ml Rate: 0.2ml/hr. Bolus: 1ml. Lockout: 5min

Caudal block

Caudal extradural analgesia (CEA) has a wide application in children. The technique is easier than with adults with a higher success rate of ~95%. CEA can achieve a higher dermatomal block than adults. Epidural fat is less dense and less tightly packed with the result that local anaesthetic can spread more easily. CEA is used for a range of surgical and orthopaedic procedures below the umbilicus.

Technique

- Position the patient in the left lateral position with the legs flexed at the hip. Aseptic technique is a prerequisite.
- Identify the sacral hiatus as the apex of an equilateral triangle with the base formed by a line joining the posterior superior iliac spines.
- Alternatively with the hips flexed at 90° a line extended from the midline of the femurs will intersect with the sacral hiatus. The natal cleft does not always correspond to bony midline structures.
- Define the boundaries of the sacral hiatus. This is again a triangle with the base formed by a line joining the sacral cornua and the apex representing the lower part of the fourth sacral vertebra. The sacral hiatus is covered by the sacrococcygeal membrane.
- Make a small nick in the skin with a needle to reduce the possibility of a dermoid. Direct a blunt, short-bevel (regional block) needle at 60° to the skin from the midpoint of the line joining the sacral cornua. Alternatively use a 22G or 20G cannula depending on the size of the child. A small 'give' indicates penetration of the sacrococcygeal membrane. Flatten the cannula or needle slightly, then advance. If using a cannula, withdraw the stylet to just behind the cannula before advancing the cannula into the caudal space. Do not advance the needle or cannula any more than is necessary. Advancement of a cannula rather than needle may reduce the incidence of inadvertent dural or vascular puncture. Easy progression of the cannula is a good prognostic indicator of success.
- Test aspiration should be gentle; vessel walls can collapse producing a false negative result. Aspiration should be repeated during injection of the local anaesthetic. The 'whoosh' test using air should be avoided because of the risk of air embolism, but 'Swoosh' test with saline may be helpful. Commonest reason for a failed attempt is positioning the needle too caudally.
- 0.25% bupivacaine is commonly administered—if the planned volume of local anaesthetic is greater than 1ml/kg, use 0.19% bupivacaine (three parts 0.25% bupivacaine to one part saline). Duration of the block averages 4–8hr. Dose—see p787.
- Caudal blockade can be extended with:
  - Clonidine 1µg/kg
  - Diamorphine 30µg/kg
  - Ketamine 0.5mg/kg (preservative-free)
  - Morphine 50µg/kg (preservative-free).
  - Adrenaline has been implicated in cases of spinal ischaemia and should be avoided.

- Clonidine produces postoperative sedation. Morphine and diamorphine increase the incidence of urinary retention and should be reserved for surgery in which catheterisation is required.

Advantages/complications of caudal analgesia
- Simple, safe, successful, with a wide range of indications.
- Motor block, paraesthesia, hypotension, urinary retention, inadvertent dural puncture or intravascular injection can all occur. All these complications are rare using a single-shot caudal technique.

Continuous caudal epidural analgesia
Caudal injection is restricted in its duration of action. A catheter can be introduced into the epidural space via the caudal route. It is a safe and effective method of administering epidural analgesia in infants. The single curve of the back allows the catheter to thread predictably into the epidural space; the tip of the catheter should be close to the level of the dermatomes that need to be blocked.
- Over 2yr of age, the development of a lumbosacral curvature tends to lead to a higher failure rate. However, some authors claim comparable success rates.
- Because of the proximity of the perineum, a caudal catheter should not be left in situ for longer than 36hr.

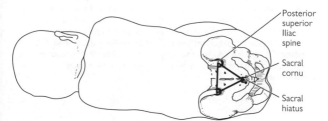

Posterior superior Iliac spine

Sacral cornu

Sacral hiatus

Anatomy for caudal block

Epidural/subarachnoid block

Epidural block (see also p1098)

Epidural blockade is technically more difficult in children and requires experience. The ligamentum flavum is less well developed and the intervertebral spaces are narrower. In infants, the epidural space is rarely located at a depth >15mm and often as superficially as 10mm from the skin. The technique is similar to that used in adults. Either a midline or paramedian approach is acceptable. Severe neurological complications including fatalities have been reported in association with using air to find the epidural space. Reported complications are generally higher in neonates.[1] The caudal route may represent a safer alternative with this group.

- Epidural needle: 18G for infants/children, 19G for neonates/infants (catheter 'end-hole' only).

Subarachnoid block

Spinal anaesthesia is rarely performed in children. One of the few indications is for herniotomy in the high-risk neonate, e.g. the oxygen-dependent premature or ex-premature infant with chronic lung disease.

- Expert assistance is crucial. The infant needs to be firmly gripped in the lateral or sitting position. The technique needs to be precise. The needle should be directed at right angles to the skin in the midline below L3 with L5–S1 reported as the safest approach. Prior infiltration of local anaesthetic into the skin will help prevent patient movement.
- The block has a rapid onset but a duration rarely greater than 40min. If sedation is required during the surgery, the incidence of postoperative apnoea is comparable with a general anaesthetic technique.
- Spinal needle: 5cm 21G.

1 Flandin-Blety C, Barrier G (1995). Accidents following extradural analgesia in children. The results of a retrospective study. *Paediatric Anaesthesia*, **5**, 416–422.

Regional analgesia doses

Caudal extradural blockade required	Sacral: 0.5ml/kg 0.25% bupivacaine Lumbar: 1ml/kg 0.25% bupivacaine Thoracolumbar: 1.25ml/kg 0.19% bupivacaine
Supplements to extend duration of block	Ketamine 0.5mg/kg (preservative-free) Clonidine 1µg/kg Diamorphine 30µg/kg Morphine 50µg/kg (preservative-free)
Lumbar epidural (intra-operative)	0.75ml/kg of 0.25% bupivacaine
Thoracic epidural (intra-operative)	0.5ml/kg of 0.25% bupivacaine
Epidural infusion	60ml of 0.125% bupivacaine + 1mg diamorphine 50ml of 0.125% bupivacaine + fentanyl 2µg/ml Rate: 0.1–0.4ml/kg/hr
Spinal block	0.1ml/kg 0.5% 'heavy' bupivacaine + 0.06ml for needle deadspace
Wound infiltration	1ml/kg 0.25% bupivacaine

Regional nerve blocks

Ilioinguinal and iliohypogastric nerve block

Useful alternative to caudal blockade in herniotomy, hydrocele, and orchidopexy. It should be avoided for neonatal herniotomy as the local anaesthetic may obscure the operating field. The block can be performed under direct vision by the surgeon.

- At a point 1cm medial to the anterior superior iliac spine, direct a regional block needle or blunted 21G needle at right angles to the skin. There is resistance at the aponeurosis of external oblique. At this point 'bounce' the needle until a loss of resistance is encountered.
- Dosage: 0.75ml/kg 0.25% bupivacaine. Retain 1–2ml for an SC fan injection laterally, medially, and inferiorly.
- Advantages: it is an easy block to perform. It decreases the level of anaesthesia and reduces postoperative analgesic requirement.
- Disadvantages: it does not block visceral pain from traction of the spermatic cord or peritoneum and is unsuitable for a high undescended testis. There is a 10% incidence of femoral nerve block.

Dorsal nerve block of penis

This block is indicated for distal surgery to the penis, including circumcision, meatoplasty, and simple hypospadias repair.

- Raise two SC swellings of local anaesthetic either side of the midline, each 5mm from the pubic symphysis at the dorsal base of the penis. Use a 23G or 21G needle.
- Alternatively a simple ring block at the base of the penis can be performed using a 25G needle.
- Dosage: 2–6ml 0.25% of bupivacaine. Avoid adrenaline.
- Advantages: these techniques are safe, simple, and predictable. They avoid the need for injection deep to Buck's fascia close to the corpora cavernosa and penile vessels.
- Disadvantages: does not always block the ventral surface of the penis. Theoretical complications including haematoma and ischaemia are unlikely using the superficial technique.

Axillary block

This block is indicated for hand and lower arm surgery.

- Position the patient supine with the arm abducted to 90° and the elbow flexed.
- Direct a 23G or 25G needle with attached extension tubing just above and parallel to the axillary artery. The needle is advanced until it pulsates or the position can be confirmed with a nerve stimulator. A click or loss of resistance is not always elicited in children.
- Dosage: 0.5ml/kg 0.25% bupivacaine.
- Advantages: safe and effective.
- Disadvantages: upper arm and shoulder surgery cannot be performed. The axillary artery may be difficult to palpate.

Diaphragmatic hernia

Procedure	Repair of defect in diaphragm either by suturing to abdominal wall or with a synthetic graft
Time	1–2hr
Pain	+++
Position	Supine
Blood loss	Usually minimal to moderate
Practical techniques	GA + IPPV, arterial line

Preoperative

- Incidence of 1:3000–4000 deliveries, affecting left side in 85% of cases. Associated with other anomalies.
- Characteristically present in respiratory distress with tachypnoea, cyanosis, and a scaphoid abdomen. The chest radiograph is diagnostic. The diagnosis is usually made antenatally on ultrasound.
- Overall mortality of 50% from lung hypoplasia, abnormal pulmonary vasculature, and pulmonary hypertension.
- Never emergency. Gas exchange should be optimised preferably with FiO_2 <0.5 before surgery. This is not always possible.
- Usually already intubated and ventilated. Ventilatory support can include high-frequency oscillation (HFO) and nitric oxide.
- NG tube essential preoperatively to prevent stomach and small bowel in the chest cavity compressing lung.

Perioperative

- Avoid ventilation via a face mask. Omit nitrous oxide to prevent distension of the gut within the thorax.
- Nasogastric tube, two IV cannulae, arterial line, preferably in the right radial artery for preductal sampling. Oesophageal stethoscope with temperature probe.
- Ventilate with rate, rather than pressure to reduce barotrauma.
- High-dose fentanyl (25µg/kg) to reduce pulmonary vasoconstriction response to surgical stress.
- High risk babies will need the operation on special care baby unit if conventional ventilation not possible.

Postoperative

- Postoperative ventilation for at least 24hr, then attempt to wean.
- Infant may deteriorate within 12hr due to pulmonary hypertensive crises. Pulmonary vasculature is reduced and abnormal. Smooth muscle in the media fails to regress, therefore there is an exaggerated vasoconstrictive response to hypoxaemia and acidosis.
- Rarely, if minimal defect, extubate immediately.

Special considerations

- Pulmonary hypertension is treated by assisted hyperventilation with 100% oxygen and fluid boluses if necessary. Prostacyclin or inhaled nitric oxide can be used for surgery. Extra-corporeal membrane oxygenation (ECMO) is a last resort but has been used.
- To assist weaning a thoracic epidural may be of benefit, inserted either conventionally or via the caudal route.

Gastroschisis/exomphalos

Procedure	Replacement of abdominal contents into the abdominal cavity
Time	2hr
Pain	++/+++
Position	Supine
Blood loss	Moderate
Practical techniques	GA + IPPV

Preoperative

- Obvious neonatal diagnosis from birth, but usually diagnosed in utero. Overall incidence is 1:3000–4000.
- Gastroschisis is a defect in anterior abdominal wall usually on the right, causing herniation of abdominal contents without a covering sac.
- In exomphalos, there is a failure of the gut to return to the abdominal cavity during fetal development resulting in persistent herniation through the extra embryonal part of the umbilical cord, which covers it. This may include other abdominal organs.
- There is an increased incidence of associated anomalies including cardiac disease in exomphalos. A full cardiology assessment should be performed.
- Gastroschisis is associated with low birth weight and thickened bowel wall due to exposure to amniotic fluid.
- Exposed abdominal contents result in large evaporative heat and water losses and predispose to infection. It should initially be covered with cling film or equivalent.

Perioperative

- May already be intubated and ventilated. Otherwise intubate conventionally.
- Nasogastric tube and oesophageal temperature/stethoscope.
- Two IV cannulae for maintenance and volume.
- Arterial monitoring is useful.
- Heat conservation is important. Warm the theatre and use a warming mattress, hot air mattress, or radiant heater. Keep the patient's head covered. Use warmed fluids.
- Fluid losses may be considerable.
- Intra-operative analgesia: fentanyl 5–10µg/kg or epidural if extubation within 48hr is contemplated.

Postoperative
- Postoperative ventilation, especially if the abdomen is tense, should be in the head up position.
- Assiduous attention to fluid balance. There may be large abdominal losses of crystalloid and protein.

Special considerations
- Lines should be sited in the arms as abdominal distension may impair venous return from the lower body.
- Simpler to insert a percutaneous long line or central line at this stage for parenteral feeding. Postoperatively, progressive oedema makes cannulation more difficult.
- Manual ventilation is useful to assess the effect of replacement of abdominal contents on lung compliance to determine the correct degree of abdominal reduction.
- Complete reduction is not always possible. A silo is then created around the extra-abdominal contents to be gradually reduced on the ICU. Fluid loss and infection are major issues.

Tracheo-oesophageal fistula

Procedure	Ligation of fistula + anastomotic repair of oesophageal atresia
Time	2hr
Pain	+++
Position	Left lateral for right thoracotomy
Blood loss	Moderate
Practical techniques	GA + IPPV ± manual ventilation

Preoperative
- Incidence of 1:3500. Commonest type (85%) is oesophageal atresia with a distal fistula. The majority of cases are now diagnosed in utero. It should always be excluded in cases of hydramnios.
- High incidence of prematurity (30%) and cardiac disease (25%).
- Presents clinically with choking and cyanotic episodes on feeding with an inability to pass a nasogastric tube.
- Constant risk of pulmonary aspiration. A double-lumen 'Replogle' tube in the oesophagus allows irrigation and suction.

Perioperative
- Inhalational or IV induction. Gentle mask ventilation to minimise gastric distension via fistula.
- Careful ETT placement. Confirm symmetrical ventilation with the tube distal to the fistula.
- Two IV cannulae for maintenance and volume. Arterial line is useful.
- Intra-operative access will be needed to pass the transanastomotic tube nasally to facilitate oesophageal repair.
- Manual ventilation may be necessary to assess lung compliance after ligation of the fistula, to assist in repair of oesophagus, and to periodically reinflate left lung. Surgical retraction may impede ventilation and blood or secretions can block the tube.
- Intra-operative analgesia: fentanyl (5–10µg/kg) or epidural either by the thoracic or caudal route, if early weaning is anticipated.
- The operation is usually performed via an extrapleural approach.

Postoperative
- The majority of cases are ventilated postoperatively, especially if the oesophageal repair is under tension. It is critical to secure the nasogastric or transanastomotic tube.

Special considerations
- Attention to positioning of the ETT to avoid ventilating the stomach via the fistula. Preoperative bronchoscopy may be useful. The fistula is normally situated on the posterior aspect of the trachea just proximal to the carina. The tube may need to be advanced, withdrawn, or the bevel rotated.

Patent ductus arteriosus

Procedure	Ligation or clipping of ductus arteriosus
Time	1hr
Pain	+
Position	Left thoracotomy
Blood loss	Usually minimal. Occasionally massive if the vessel is torn
Practical techniques	IPPV, fentanyl

Preoperative
- Small premature babies: 25% of premature infants <1.5kg recovering from hyaline membrane disease have a PDA. Associated with other cardiac anomalies.
- Indications are for failure of medical treatment, ventilator dependence, and risk of developing bronchopulmonary dysplasia.

Perioperative
- High-risk group. Operation may be undertaken on the special care baby unit.
- Patient is usually already ventilated with full monitoring.
- Adequate IV access for transfusion. Arterial monitoring.
- IPPV with oxygen, nitrous oxide and fentanyl up to 10µg/kg with a low dose of volatile agent. Replace nitrous oxide with air if frail.
- Active heat conservation.
- Avoid saturations >96% because of retinopathy of prematurity.
- Local infiltration for analgesia, intrapleural block by surgeon, or thoracic epidural if early weaning considered.

Postoperative
Postoperative ventilation until stable, then attempt to wean.

Special considerations
- Sudden ligation of the ductus may precipitate an acute rise in systemic BP and increase the risk of intraventricular haemorrhage. The duct should be clamped gently or alternatively the concentration of the volatile agent can be temporarily increased.
- Older children requiring PDA occlusion tend to be fit, although some present with cardiac failure. Increasingly these procedures are being performed non-invasively as day cases by interventional cardiologists.

Pyloric stenosis

Procedure	Splitting the pylorus muscle longitudinally down to the mucosa
Time	30min
Pain	+
Position	Supine
Blood loss	Minimal
Practical techniques	GA + IPPV, ?RSI

Preoperative
- Incidence of 1:350 births, commoner in first born males. 80% are male, 10% are premature.
- Present with biochemical abnormalities, notably hypochloraemic alkalosis. Operation is never urgent and full resuscitation should occur.
- Electrolytes, particularly chloride, bicarbonate and pH should be within normal limits, with chloride ≥90mmol/l.

Perioperative
- No complete agreement, but there is a risk of pulmonary aspiration from gastric outflow obstruction.
- A nasogastric tube is mandatory and will be in situ. Aspirate, and do not remove. It does not reduce the effect of cricoid pressure and may act as an escape valve if mask ventilation increases intragastric pressure.
- IV is usually in place. Induction may be rapid sequence or non-depolarising relaxant for which some anaesthetists use cricoid pressure. Consider rapid sequence if there is excessive nasogastric loss (>2ml/kg/hr).
- Fentanyl (1μg/kg) + paracetamol suppository (30–40mg/kg) + local infiltration (up to 1ml/kg of 0.25% bupivacaine ± adrenaline). If local given pre-incision, fentanyl can be omitted.
- Extubate awake in the left lateral position.

Postoperative
- Remove the nasogastric tube at the end of the procedure.
- Give paracetamol PO/PR as required.
- Feed within 6hr but maintain IV fluids until feeding is established.
- Use an apnoea alarm overnight.

Special considerations
- Resuscitation: 5% dextrose with 0.45% saline + 20mmol/l KCl. Replace nasogastric loss with 0.9% saline + 20mmol/l KCl. Mild cases may respond to 5% dextrose with 0.45% saline (bicarbonate <32mmol/l), more severe cases will require 0.9% saline. Use colloid initially if hypovolaemia is present.
- May be performed laparoscopically.

Intussusception

Procedure	Reduction of invaginated bowel
Time	1–2hr
Pain	+++
Position	Supine
Blood loss	Moderate, may be large
Practical techniques	RSI + IPPV

Preoperative
- Intussusception is the commonest cause of obstruction in infants over 2 months of age; incidence 2:1000 births.
- Invagination of the bowel into an adjacent lower segment, usually at the terminal ileum or ileocaecal valve. Rarely caused by polyp or Meckel's diverticulum (5% of cases).
- Presents with paroxysmal pain, blood, and mucus in stool (redcurrant jelly stool) and sausage-shaped mass in right abdomen.
- 70% of cases are reduced by air or barium enema.
- Child may be profoundly shocked. Urgent fluid resuscitation with gastric decompression and electrolyte correction will be needed. Colloid and blood may be required. Delay can result in perforated or necrotic bowel. Fluid loss may be greater than expected.

Perioperative
- Rapid sequence induction. Retain the nasogastric tube in situ.
- Fentanyl 2–5µg/kg + volatile agent. Consider an epidural if stable.
- Two secure cannulae of adequate size. CVP line in severe cases.
- Routine monitoring, temperature measurement probe, and urinary catheter.
- Prolonged intussusception with ischaemic gut requiring resection often leads to metabolic acidosis and septic shock. Admission to a paediatric ICU will be required.

Postoperative
Epidural or local wound infiltration and morphine NCA.

Special considerations
No consensus as to whether the child should receive surgery at the base hospital or be transferred to a regional centre. If transferred, this should not delay resuscitation or blood crossmatch, which can be sent with the patient.

Herniotomy

Procedure	Excision of patent processus vaginalis
Time	20min
Pain	++
Position	Supine
Blood loss	Minimal
Practical techniques	SV + LMA, caudal or regional block
	IPPV, caudal or local infiltration
	Spinal or caudal block

Preoperative
- Otherwise fit ASA 1 child. More common in boys.
- 20% of preterm babies present for surgery at ~40wk PCA or when ready to leave the special care baby unit.

Perioperative
- If >5kg inhalational or IV induction with laryngeal mask, then caudal or ilioinguinal block and intra-operative opioids if necessary.
- If <5kg, intubate with controlled ventilation. With neonates, avoid ilioinguinal block as spread of local anaesthetic may obscure the surgical field. Use either caudal or postoperative infiltration.
- Diclofenac suppository (1mg/kg) >1yr or paracetamol suppository (30–40mg/kg) if under 1yr. For neonates, paracetamol suppository (20mg/kg)

Postoperative
- Day case: PRN paracetamol and diclofenac.
- Neonate: PRN paracetamol. Admit overnight.

Special considerations
- The majority of herniotomy repairs are in healthy children and suitable as day cases.
- There is no consensus as to the most appropriate regional block. Caudal blockade is indicated for bilateral herniotomy repair and children up to 20kg. Ilioinguinal block is effective in children over 5kg.
- The ex-premature baby may be small for dates and oxygen-dependent with chronic lung disease. Postoperative apnoea and bradycardia are documented risks associated with general anaesthesia for this group. Hypocarbia and hypothermia should be avoided and an oxygen saturation between 90% and 95% is acceptable. Caffeine (10mg/kg IV) given at induction reduces the risk of apnoea by 70%.
- To avoid general anaesthesia a spinal technique may be used (see p786). This may be technically difficult and complicated by a bloody or dry tap. It is too short acting for bilateral repair. A single-shot caudal is an alternative method. Supplementary sedation results in the same risk of postoperative apnoea as with general anaesthesia.

- Term babies in the first 6wk of life and ex-premature infants up to 60wk' post-conceptual age should be admitted overnight for oxygen saturation and apnoea alarm monitoring.
- A strangulated hernia that does not reduce is an emergency and requires fluid resuscitation and a nasogastric tube. Precautions should be taken against regurgitation and aspiration.

Circumcision

Procedure	Removal of prepuce (foreskin)
Time	20min
Pain	++
Position	Supine
Blood loss	Minimal
Practical techniques	SV, LMA, caudal/penile block/ring block

Preoperative
- Common day case procedure, but move towards more conservative management including simple stretch or preputioplasty.
- Obtain consent for suppository and regional block.

Perioperative
- Inhalational or IV induction. Laryngeal mask.
- Regional block: caudal, penile block, or ring block (see p788).
- Diclofenac suppository (1mg/kg) >1yr or paracetamol suppository (30–40mg/kg) if under 1yr.

Postoperative
- PRN paracetamol 20mg/kg
- Topical lidocaine gel can be applied frequently without exceeding the toxic dose.

Special considerations
- A regional block must be performed prior to the surgery.
- There is no consensus as to the optimal strategy for pain relief. Caudal is technically easier in infants and penile block may be more suitable in children over 10kg. Ring block is technically easier in boys greater than 5kg, producing excellent and consistent analgesia. All methods are effective.
- Circumcision is one of the most painful postoperative day case procedures; parents should be warned and advised to apply topical gel regularly and continue paracetamol for several days.

Orchidopexy

Procedure	Release of undescended testis into scrotum
Time	30min
Pain	++
Position	Supine
Blood loss	Minimal
Practical techniques	SV, LMA + regional block

Preoperative
- Boys, usually over 2yr (2% of population).
- Common day case procedure.
- Obtain consent for suppository and regional block.

Perioperative
- Inhalational or IV induction. Laryngeal mask.
- Regional technique: caudal, ilioinguinal block or local infiltration.
- Diclofenac suppository (1mg/kg) >1yr or paracetamol suppository (30–40mg/kg) if <1yr.
- Give supplementary opioids if indicated.

Postoperative
- PRN diclofenac, paracetamol, codeine phosphate, and anti-emetic.

Special considerations
- Adequate analgesia is difficult if the testis is high. Caudal block should be high volume, low concentration (bupivacaine 0.19%, see pp784, 787). A mid thoracic level is obtained from 1.25ml/kg.
- If ilioinguinal block is used, only the anterior of the scrotum is anaesthetised; use local infiltration for the scrotal incision.
- Testicular traction even with seemingly adequate blockade may lead to intra-operative bradycardia or laryngospasm, especially with an ilioinguinal block. Surgery should be stopped and anaesthesia deepened; supplementary opioids may be required.
- Suspected torsion of the testis is a surgical emergency and the need for a rapid sequence induction will have to be considered. Analgesic techniques are as before.
- A high testis may need surgery in two stages. The first procedure is to identify the testis, and if possible bring it down to the inguinal ring. This is usually performed laparoscopically and will require intubation, controlled ventilation with intra-operative opioids and rectal diclofenac or paracetamol.

Hypospadias

Procedure	Restoration of proximal urethral opening to the tip of the penis
Time	1–3hr
Pain	++
Position	Supine
Blood loss	Minimal
Practical techniques	SV/IPPV + regional block

Preoperative
- Usually an isolated problem, but there may be an association with certain rare dysmorphic syndromes.
- Obtain consent for suppository and regional block.

Perioperative
- Inhalational or IV induction.
- If procedure <1hr use LMA + SV.
- If procedure >1hr use LMA or ETT + IPPV.
- Extended caudal: 1ml/kg 0.25% bupivacaine with ketamine/clonidine/morphine/diamorphine (see pp784, 787).
- Diclofenac suppository (1mg/kg) >1yr or paracetamol suppository (30–40mg/kg) <1yr.
- Employ heat conservation measures.

Postoperative
- Regular NSAIDs/paracetamol. Consider morphine NCA (not always necessary).
- Opioids can be used in the caudal block because the patient will be catheterised, but they must be admitted overnight.

Special considerations
- May be simple procedure, e.g. meatal advancement and glanduloplasty (MAGPI), or extensive involving buccal mucosa graft. The anaesthetic technique can be adjusted accordingly.
- Avoid erection with regional block plus an adequate depth of anaesthesia.

Cleft lip and palate

Procedure	Repair of defect in upper lip and palate
Time	1–2hr
Pain	++
Position	Supine, head ring, shoulder support
Blood loss	Minimal for cleft lip. Moderate for cleft palate
Practical techniques	IPPV. Armoured or RAE tube

Preoperative

- Incidence of 1:300–600 births but can be 1:25 where there is a family history.
- Both lip and palate are involved together in 50% of cases.
- Isolated cleft palate incidence is 1:2000 live births. Increased incidence of congenital abnormalities.
- Associated syndromes often involve a difficult airway, e.g. Pierre–Robin, Treacher–Collins, and Goldenhar syndromes. Therefore make a careful assessment of the airway.
- Discuss risks and complications. Obtain consent for suppository.
- Administer IM atropine 20µg/kg 30min preoperatively if a difficult airway is suspected.

Perioperative

- Inhalational or IV induction. When there is a suspected airway problem, perform inhalational induction with sevoflurane and then maintain with halothane. CPAP will be useful (see pp775, 777). Intubate deep with child breathing spontaneously or following muscle relaxant once a safe
  airway has been established.
- A preformed RAE tube may be obstructed or kinked by the gag, especially the smaller sizes. A reinforced tube will resist compression but needs to be carefully secured at correct length.
- IPPV preferable.
- Use a throat pack and make sure the eyes are protected.
- The surgeon usually places the gag. Encourage local anaesthetic infiltration to improve analgesia and reduce blood loss.
- Fentanyl 2–4µg/kg + paracetamol suppository (30–40mg/kg)<1yr or diclofenac (1mg/kg) >1yr + local infiltration with adrenaline. Clonidine or ketamine can be used as part of an opioid sparing technique. Dexamethasone 0.1mg/kg may prevent postoperative swelling.
- Consider infraorbital nerve block for cleft lip repair[1] and nasopalatine plus palatine block for palatal surgery.
- Codeine phosphate 1mg/kg IM prior to reversal or ketamine 0.5mg/kg IM if infant is floppy or hypotonic.

---

1 Bosenberg AT, Kimble FW (1995). Infraorbital nerve block in neonates for cleft palate repair: anatomical study and clinical application. *British Journal of Anaesthesia*, **74**, 506–508.

Postoperative

- Extubate awake. Suction the pharynx early and carefully to prevent damage to the repair.
- Nasal stents may be inserted to maintain patency of the airway. A tongue stitch is rarely used.
- Routine postoperative analgesia to include regular paracetamol, diclofenac or ibuprofen and codeine phosphate. IV morphine may be required initially.

Special considerations

- Intubation is usually uncomplicated.
- The laryngoscope blade rarely lodges in the cleft. If there is a problem, a roll of gauze can fill the gap.
- Prolonged surgery may cause swollen tongue from pressure of mouth gag.
- Cleft palate repair can produce upper airways obstruction, and extreme care is needed for extubation.
- With airway problems, opioids should be given cautiously. Postoperative monitoring should include pulse oximetry and apnoea alarm.
- Cleft lip is usually repaired at 3 months, cleft palate at 6–9 months. The lip may be repaired at the neonatal stage to improve the scar and assist maternal bonding. There is little evidence to support this.

Congenital talipes equinovarus

Procedure	Correction of club foot abnormality
Time	45min–1hr
Pain	++
Position	Supine, sometimes prone for posterior release
Blood loss	Minimal
Practical techniques	SV, LMA, caudal
	If prone then ETT + IPPV, caudal

Preoperative

- Occurs in 1:1000 births.
- Usually an isolated anomaly but may occur in association with some myopathic diseases, hence increased theoretical risk of Malignant Hyperthermia.
- Obtain consent for suppository and regional block.

Perioperative

- Inhalational or IV induction with LMA. If prone intubate and ventilate. Give additional opioids if indicated.
- Caudal blockade: 1ml/kg 0.25% bupivacaine (see pp784, 787).
- Rectal diclofenac (1mg/kg) >1yr or rectal paracetamol (30–40mg/kg) if <1yr.

Postoperative

Give regular diclofenac, paracetamol plus PRN codeine phosphate + anti-emetic if required for the first day. Oramorph is a useful alternative.

Special considerations

For prolonged pain relief either top-up the caudal at the end of the procedure by using an indwelling 22G or 20G cannula or extend the duration of the block by adding preservative-free ketamine (0.5mg/kg) to the initial dose of bupivacaine. Diamorphine and clonidine will also extend the block. However, the former may lead to urinary retention and the latter increased levels of drowsiness (see also pp784, 787).

Femoral osteotomy

Procedure	Stabilising the hip in congenital dislocation by realigning proximal femur
Time	2hr
Pain	+++
Position	Supine
Blood loss	Moderate/potentially large
Practical techniques	SV + LMA or ETT + IPPV + caudal/epidural

Preoperative
- Usually an isolated defect. Commoner in girls or where there is a family history.
- Obtain consent for a suppository and regional block.

Perioperative
- Inhalational or IV induction. SV + LMA or ETT + IPPV.
- Adequate IV access.
- Caudal block + preservative-free ketamine or clonidine (see pp784, 787). Avoid caudal opioids because of risk of urinary retention. Alternatively lumbar epidural or intra-operative opioids (see pp782, 786).
- Employ heat conservation measures.
- Attention to blood loss.

Postoperative
- Epidural infusion (see pp786, 787).
- Extended caudal or morphine NCA with regular NSAIDs and paracetamol.
- A hip spica provides support and helps with pain relief.

Special considerations
- Blood loss may be extensive if revision surgery.
- A hip spica complicates urinary retention in girls.

Inhaled foreign body

Procedure	Removal of foreign body from bronchial tree
Time	30min
Pain	+
Position	Supine
Blood loss	Nil
Practical techniques	SV or IPPV

Preoperative
- Commonest reason for bronchoscopy in the 1–3yr age group.
- A foreign body in the upper airways may present as an emergency acute airway obstruction.
- Obstruction of the lower airways may follow a history of coughing after several days. Peanut oil is an irritant and leads to mucosal oedema and chemical pneumonitis. A chest radiograph shows characteristic hyperinflation during expiration, but the foreign body is not usually visible.
- Treat symptoms as indicated, e.g. dehydration, pneumonia, wheeze.

Perioperative
- Inhalational induction is usual to avoid displacing the object further. Use 100% oxygen with sevoflurane or halothane.
- Deep inhalational maintenance with halothane (sevoflurane gives too rapid an awakening).
- Apply topical anaesthesia to the vocal cords (10% lidocaine, up to 3mg/kg) and consider a drying agent (atropine 20µg/kg IM 30min preop or 10µg/kg IV at induction, or glycopyrronium 5µg/kg IM or IV).
- Rigid bronchoscopy: the Storz bronchoscope has an attachment for a T-piece.
- If the foreign body is in the lower airway, then use IPPV with a muscle relaxant since the object will be pushed distally by the bronchoscope until it can be grasped by forceps. Give assisted ventilation via a T-piece or high-frequency jet ventilation.
- This may be a difficult procedure.

Postoperative
- If bronchoscopy is traumatic, give dexamethasone 0.25mg/kg IV then 2 doses 8-hourly of 0.125mg/kg.
- Consider physiotherapy, bronchodilators and antibiotics as indicated.

Special considerations
- If tracheal or ball-valve obstruction is suspected, IPPV is contraindicated.
- Intubation may assist lung ventilation and sizing of the bronchoscope if a tracheal foreign body is excluded.

Medical problems

Acute laryngotracheobronchitis (croup)

- Croup occurs predominantly in epidemics in the autumn and early spring. The peak age of incidence is 6 months to 2yr. It is viral in aetiology. The majority of cases are due to parainfluenza, but influenza and respiratory syncitial virus are possible.
- Symptoms are coryzal for the first few days but then progress to a characteristic barking cough/hoarseness with profuse secretions and occasional dysphagia. Pyrexia is mild or absent.
- The larynx, trachea, and bronchi are all involved and become more oedematous leading to the onset of stridor. An anxious child will exacerbate the condition, as the trachea will tend to collapse on inspiration.
- The majority of children respond to conservative measures and reassurance. There is no evidence to support the use of humidified steam tents. In severe cases, steroids (dexamethasone 0.25mg/kg IV followed by two further doses 8-hourly of 0.125mg/kg) and nebulised adrenaline (0.5mg/kg up to a max of 5mg) are required.
- 10% of children are admitted and 1% will require intubation.
- The majority of children have a single isolated episode.

Acute epiglottitis

- This is an acute life-threatening infection caused by *Haemophilus influenzae* Type B (Hib). It most commonly presents at 2–3yr.
- There is a rapid onset of oedema of the epiglottis and aryepiglottic folds. The child has a high temperature, usually greater than 39.5°C and presents sitting or leaning forwards, drooling saliva, unable to swallow, with the tongue pushed forwards. Inspiratory and expiratory stridor is rapidly progressive and a late sign.
- Acute epiglottitis is a medical emergency. The antibiotic of choice is cefotaxime (50mg/kg IV twice daily). Intubation is indicated in 60% of cases; in some centres all children are routinely intubated.
- Following the introduction of the Hib vaccine, this condition is now rare.

Anaesthetic management

- The differential diagnosis between croup and epiglottitis is not always obvious. If epiglottitis is even remotely suspected, there must be liaison with an ENT surgeon at consultant level.
- Induction occurs in the anaesthetic room or operating theatre with the full range of appropriate equipment and monitoring available.
- During anaesthesia, the ENT surgeon should be scrubbed in theatre with the tracheostomy set open.
- Traditionally, IV access has been contraindicated prior to induction because of the risk of acute glottic closure. However, the use of topical cream facilitates atraumatic venepuncture. Unless access is obviously difficult, cannulation should proceed before anaesthesia.
- Inhalational induction is performed in the sitting position with sevoflurane or halothane in 100% oxygen; the choice depends solely on the

operator. Once anaesthetised, the child can be moved to a supine position and maintained with halothane up to concentrations of 5% if needed. Halothane permits a more prolonged attempt at laryngoscopy. CPAP should be routinely applied, but the airway is not usually difficult to maintain.

- In croup laryngoscopy is usually straightforward, but the endotracheal tube required may be surprisingly narrow. Start with one size smaller than normal. Older children may require a tube that has been cut to a longer length. If possible, once the airway is secure, the child should be reintubated nasally since this is better tolerated. Profuse secretions are always a problem and frequent suction is necessary. Intubation is usually required for at least 2–3d and bronchoscopy is indicated if an air leak around the tube fails to develop.

- With epiglottitis intubation may be exceedingly difficult. Laryngoscopy often reveals abnormal anatomy with no obvious glottic opening. Careful inspection may reveal movement of small amounts of mucus indicating tidal flow. The child should be intubated using a stylet so that the tracheal tube can be immediately railroaded if necessary. The tube size will be smaller than predicted.

- Once intubation has been achieved, oedema rapidly settles. Following demonstration of a leak around the tube, extubation is normally possible within 36hr. Dexamethasone is often given prior to extubation to reduce laryngeal oedema.

Sedation

- The expansion of imaging techniques together with new diagnostic and therapeutic interventions has led to a rise in demand for sedation services.
- Compared with general anaesthesia, sedation is neither cheaper nor safer. Safety is paramount and the requirements in terms of personnel and resuscitation equipment are the same.
- With current staff shortages, anaesthetists are not always available to administer sedation and other medical or nursing personnel may be involved.
- Facilities must include sufficient space for a trolley, monitoring, and resuscitation equipment together with all personnel necessary to sedate the child and carry out the specific procedure. All standard anaesthetic equipment should be available for resuscitation.
- Each sedated child must be supervised by an appropriate nurse, or doctor trained in paediatric resuscitation. Experienced medical staff must be immediately available to assist with sedation problems or resuscitation. There must be a contingency for overnight admission if recovery is prolonged.
- The adult concept of sedation where verbal contact is maintained is not practical in children. There may be little difference between deep sedation as defined by the American Academy of Paediatrics and uncontrolled anaesthesia. Ideal conditions achieve depression of the nervous system, allowing the relevant procedures to occur, with preservation of the airway reflexes. In practice this is difficult to achieve.
- It is important not to confuse sedation with analgesia. Painful procedures may require topical anaesthetic cream, infiltration with local anaesthetics, and occasionally systemic opioids.
- Contraindications include children with airway problems, apnoeic episodes, respiratory disease, raised intracranial pressure, risk of pulmonary aspiration, and epilepsy.
- The most frequently used oral sedative drugs are chloral hydrate (50–100mg/kg), triclofos (50–75mg/kg), and to a lesser extent benzodiazepines, trimeprazine, and ketamine. Opioids are also used in combination with other sedatives.
- Midazolam (0.5mg/kg PO) or in incremental bolus doses of 0.05mg/kg IV up to a maximum dose of 0.2mg/kg can produce good conditions for sedation and has the additional property of amnesia. Ketamine (6mg/kg PO or 1–2mg/kg IV) is indicated for short, painful procedures and may be used in combination with midazolam. Emergence delirium is less of a problem with children but a drying agent is often required.
- Propofol can be used alone or in combination with remifentanil for endoscopy sedation, but the use of propofol should be reserved for anaesthetists.[1]

1 Berkenbosch JW, Graft GR, Stort JM, Tobias J (2004). Use of a remifentanil propofol mixture for paediatric flexible fiberoptic bronchoscopy sedation. *Paediatric Anaesthesia*, **14**, 941–946.

- With appropriate planning, organisation, and safety, nurse-led sedation services have been developed at several centres following strict protocols. The children are fasted conventionally but allowed unrestricted clear fluids. A pulse oximeter is mandatory. Surprisingly young children can tolerate scans awake with encouragement, careful explanation, and parental presence.

Further reading

Baum VC, O'Flaherty JE (1999) Anaesthesia for Genetic, Metabolic and Dysmorphic Syndromes of Childhood. Lippincot Williams and Wilkins (pub).

Craven PD, Badawi N, Henderson-Smart DJ, O'Brien M (2003). Regional (spinal, epidural, caudal) versus general anaesthesia in preterm infants undergoing inguinal herniorrhaphy in early infancy. *Cochrane Database Syst Rev.* (3): CD003669

Hatch DJ, Hunter JM (1999). The paediatric patient—Postgraduate educational issue: Update of Paediatric Anaesthesia. *British Journal of Anaesthesia,* **83**, 1–168.

National confidential enquiry into perioperative deaths (1989). Royal College of Surgeons of England and Royal College of Anaesthetists.

Online Mendelian Inheritance in Man. Database of human genes and genetic disorders from Johns Hopkins University with links to Medline and Entrez Pubmed http://www.ncbi.nlm.nih.gov/omim

www.apagbi.org.uk Web site of Association of Paediatric Anaesthetists

www.bnfc.org (BNF for Children 2005)

Paediatric quick reference guide

Age	Approx. weight (kg)	Body surface area (m^2)	% Adult drug dose (approx.)	ETT size (mm)	ETT length (cm)	LMA size	Suxamethonium dose (mg) IV	Atropine dose (μg) IV
Term	3.5	0.23	12.5 (1/8th)	3.5	9	1	7	35
1 month	4.2	0.26	14.5	3.5	10	1	8	40
3 month	6	0.33	15	3.5	10	1.5	12	60
6 month	7.5	0.38	22	3.5/4.0	11	1.5	15	75
1yr	10	0.47	25 (1/4)	4.0	12	1.5/2	20	100
2yr	12	0.53	30	4.5	13	2	24	120
3yr	14	0.61	33	4.5/5	13/14	2	28	140
5yr	18	0.73	40	5.0/5.5	14.5	2.5	36	180
7yr	22	0.86	50 (1/2)	6.0	15.5	2.5	44	220
10yr	30	1.10	60	6.5 cuffed	17	3	60	300
12yr	38	1.30	75 (3/4)	7.0 cuffed	18	3 or 4	75	380

Note : Weights are approximations only. Patients should be weighed accurately.

The critically ill patient

Jerry Nolan

Immediate trauma care

Preparation

Advance warning before the arrival of a severely injured patient in the emergency department enables emergency department staff to alert the trauma team and prepare essential resuscitation drugs, fluid, and equipment before the patient's arrival.

The trauma team

Trauma patient resuscitation is most efficient if undertaken by a team of doctors and nurses; in this way a variety of tasks can be undertaken simultaneously.

Immediate care—ATLS®

The advanced trauma life support (ATLS®)[1] programme provides a framework on which the immediate management of the trauma patient is based. The initial management is considered in four phases:

- Primary survey
- Resuscitation
- Secondary survey
- Definitive care.

The first two phases are undertaken simultaneously. The secondary survey, or head-to-toe examination of the patient, is not started until the patient has been resuscitated adequately.

1 American College of Surgeons Committee on Trauma. Advanced Trauma Life Support® for Doctors. Provider Course Manual. Chicago, American College of Surgeons, 1997.

Primary survey and resuscitation

The primary survey ('ABC principles') looks sequentially for immediately life-threatening injuries:

- Airway with cervical spine control.
- Breathing.
- Circulation and haemorrhage control.
- Disability—a rapid assessment of neurological function.
- Exposure—while considering the environment, and preventing hypothermia.

Airway and cervical spine

The priority during resuscitation of any severely injured patient is to ensure a clear airway and maintain oxygenation. Use basic airway manoeuvres with or without adjuncts such as a Guedel or nasopharyngeal airway. Give the patient high-concentration oxygen; in the unintubated, spontaneously breathing patient this is delivered with a mask and reservoir (non-rebreathing) bag ($FiO_2 = 0.85$).

Assume the presence of a spinal injury in any patient who has sustained significant blunt trauma until clearance procedures have been completed. This implies that the patient has been examined by an experienced clinician and radiological procedures have been completed. A reliable clinical examination cannot be obtained if the patient:

- Has sustained a significant closed head injury
- Is intoxicated
- Has a reduced conscious level from any other cause
- Has significant pain from an injury, which 'distracts' attention from the neck.

Tracheal intubation

Indications for immediate intubation of the severely injured patient include:

- Airway obstruction unrelieved by basic airway manoeuvres
- Impending airway obstruction, e.g. from facial burns and inhalation injury
- GCS <9 (see p825)
- Haemorrhage from maxillofacial injuries compromising the airway
- Respiratory failure secondary to chest or neurological injury
- The need for resuscitative surgery
- Uncooperative patients requiring further investigations

The best technique for emergency intubation of a severely-injured patient with a potential cervical spine injury is:

- Manual in-line stabilisation of the cervical spine by an assistant whose hands grasp the mastoid processes and hold the head down firmly on to the trolley; this reduces neck movement during intubation. Do not apply traction to the neck.
- Preoxygenation.
- IV induction of anaesthesia. All induction drugs have the potential to produce or worsen hypotension and the choice of drug is less important than the way it is used. Extreme caution is essential in patients who may be hypovolaemic; whenever possible, give fluid before anaesthetic induction.

- Paralysis with suxamethonium 1.5mg/kg (though in experienced hands rocuronium 1mg/kg is acceptable).
- Application of cricoid pressure—using one or two hands (there is no strong evidence supporting one technique over the other).
- Direct laryngoscopy and oral intubation.

Placing the patient's head and neck in neutral alignment will tend to make the view at laryngoscopy difficult—expect 20% of patients to have a grade 3 view of the larynx; use of a gum-elastic bougie and McCoy levering laryngoscope is recommended. If intubation is impossible, an LMA will provide a temporary airway, but may not prevent aspiration. The intubating LMA (ILMA) may be easier to insert in the neutral position and provides the opportunity for blind intubation, but consistent success requires ongoing practice. Needle cricothyroidotomy with a 14G cannula followed by jet inflation of oxygen from a high-pressure source (400kPa) will provide satisfactory oxygenation, but the airway is not protected and the cannula is subject to kinking and displacement. Surgical cricothyroidotomy, using a scalpel and a 6.0mm ID tracheostomy or tracheal tube, is a more reliable procedure if the patient cannot be intubated by conventional methods. See also pp890, 934.

Breathing—immediately life-threatening chest injuries

- Tension pneumothorax. Reduced chest movement, reduced breath sounds, and a resonant percussion note on the affected side, along with respiratory distress, hypotension, and tachycardia, indicate a tension pneumothorax. Deviation of the trachea to the opposite side is a late sign, and neck veins may not be distended in the presence of hypovolaemia. Treatment is immediate decompression with a large cannula placed in the second intercostal space, (mid-clavicular line) on the affected side. Once IV access has been obtained, insert a large chest drain (32 FG) in the fifth intercostal space (anterior axillary) line and connect to an underwater seal drain.
- Open pneumothorax. Any open pneumothorax should be covered with an occlusive dressing and sealed on three sides.
- Massive haemothorax (defined as >1500ml blood in a hemithorax) will cause reduced chest movement and a dull percussion note, in the presence of hypoxaemia and hypovolaemia. Start fluid resuscitation and insert a chest drain.

Cardiac tamponade

- Consider cardiac tamponade while examining the chest, particularly if the patient has sustained a penetrating injury to the chest or upper abdomen.
- Distended neck veins in the presence of hypotension are suggestive of cardiac tamponade, although after rapid volume resuscitation myocardial contusion may also present in this way.
- Muffled heart sounds are meaningless in the midst of a busy resuscitation room.
- Sophisticated trauma facilities enable immediate access to ultrasound, which is the most reliable method for diagnosis.

- If cardiac tamponade is diagnosed or suspected after penetrating injury and the patient is deteriorating despite all resuscitative efforts, an urgent thoracotomy and pericardiotomy will be required. If there is time, this is best undertaken in an operating room; however, in extremis, resuscitative thoracotomy should be undertaken in the emergency room.
- In the absence of a suitably experienced surgeon, pericardiocentesis may provide temporary relief from the tamponade while awaiting definitive treatment.

Circulation—management of hypovolaemia

Control external haemorrhage with direct pressure. Hypovolaemic shock is divided into 4 classes according to the percentage of the total blood volume lost, and the associated symptoms and signs. The table provides rough guidance only.

Haemorrhage alone, in the absence of significant tissue injury, causes relatively less tachycardia and may be easily overlooked, particularly in young, fit people who are able to compensate to a remarkable degree. A fall in systolic pressure suggests a loss of >30% of total blood volume (~1500ml in a 70kg adult). A deteriorating conscious level due to hypovolaemia implies at least 40–50% loss of blood volume.

Classification of hypovolaemic shock according to blood loss (adult)

	Class I	Class II	Class III	Class IV
Blood loss (%)	<15	15–30	30–40	>40
Blood loss (ml)	750	800–1500	1500–2000	>2000
Systolic blood pressure	Unchanged	Normal	Reduced	Very low
Diastolic blood pressure	Unchanged	Raised	Reduced	Unrecordable
Pulse (bpm)	Slight tachycardia	100–120	120 (thready)	>120 (very thready)
Capillary refill	Normal	Slow (>2s)	Slow (>2s)	Undetectable
Respiratory rate	Normal	Tachypnoea	Tachypnoea (>20/min)	Tachypnoea (>20/min)
Urine output (ml/hr)	>30	20–30	10–20	0–10
Extremities	Normal	Pale	Pale	Pale, cold, clammy
Complexion	Normal	Pale	Pale	Ashen
Mental state	Alert	Anxious or aggressive	Anxious, aggressive, or drowsy	Drowsy, confused, or unconscious

- Insert 2 short, large-bore IV cannulae (14G or larger); take blood samples for FBC, electrolytes, and crossmatch from the first cannula.
- If peripheral access is difficult, use external jugular vein, femoral vein (avoid in abdominal/pelvic/leg injury), cut-down on a peripheral vein (long saphenous at the ankle), or cannulate a central vein. If the central route is to be used for rapid fluid resuscitation a relatively short, large-bore catheter (e.g. 8.5 Fr introducer sheath) is essential.
- Insert an arterial cannula for blood gas sampling and invasive pressure monitoring. Severely injured patients will have a marked base deficit and its correction by the infusion of appropriate fluid (not bicarbonate) will help to confirm adequate resuscitation.

Fluids

Crystalloid is suitable for the initial fluid resuscitation. Large volumes of 0.9% saline will induce a hyperchloraemic acidosis; however, Hartmann's solution is slightly hypotonic and may increase cerebral oedema in patients with severe brain injury—thus, neither fluid is perfect. The volume status of the patient is best determined by observing the change in vital signs after a reasonably large fluid challenge (e.g., 1 litre of Hartmann's solution). Failure to improve the vital signs implies ongoing haemorrhage, and the need for immediate surgical intervention and blood transfusion. A full crossmatch will take 45min; group-confirmed blood can be issued in 10min and group O blood can be obtained immediately. It is nearly always possible to wait for at least group-confirmed blood; major incompatibility reactions when using group-confirmed blood are extremely rare. The haemoglobin concentration of the severely injured patient should be targeted at greater than 7–8g/dl.

Warm all IV fluids: a high-capacity fluid warmer is necessary to cope with the rapid infusion rates used during resuscitation of trauma patients. Hypothermia (core temperature less than 35°C) is a serious complication and is an independent predictor of mortality. Hypothermia has several adverse effects:

- It causes a gradual decline in heart rate and cardiac output while increasing the propensity for myocardial dysrhythmias and other morbid myocardial events.
- The oxyhaemoglobin dissociation curve is shifted to the left by a decrease in temperature, thus impairing peripheral oxygen delivery in the hypovolaemic patient at a time when it is most needed.
- Shivering may increase oxygen consumption and compound the lactic acidosis that typically accompanies hypovolaemia.
- Even mild hypothermia inhibits coagulation significantly and increases the incidence of wound infection.

In the presence of uncontrolled haemorrhage:

- Aggressive fluid resuscitation may simply accelerate bleeding and increase mortality; however, inadequate fluid resuscitation will cause hypoperfusion of vital organs and may induce life-threatening ischaemia.
- Until surgical control of haemorrhage has been achieved, target fluid resuscitation to a blood pressure that will almost produce adequate vital organ perfusion (permissive hypotension). This target will depend on age and coexisting morbidities: in the normally healthy patient aim

for a pressure around 80mmHg systolic; in the elderly or those with significant co-morbidity a systolic pressure of around 100mmHg may be more appropriate.

• Hypotension increases morbidity and mortality following severe head injury and attempts must be made to maintain an adequate cerebral perfusion as soon as possible. In a patient with even slightly raised intracranial pressure, this implies the need for a mean arterial pressure of at least 90mmHg.

Once haemorrhage control has been achieved, the goals of fluid resuscitation are to optimise oxygen delivery, improve microcirculatory perfusion, and reverse tissue acidosis. Fluid infusion should be targeted at a blood pressure and cardiac output that results in an acceptable urine output, and a falling lactate and base deficit.

Goals for resuscitation of the trauma patient before haemorrhage has been controlled

Parameter	Goal
Blood pressure	Systolic 80mmHg. Mean 50–60mmHg
Heart rate	<120bpm
Oxygenation	SaO_2 >95% (peripheral perfusion allowing Oximeter to work)
Urine output	>0.5ml/kg/hr
Mental state	Following commands accurately
Lactate level	<1.6mmol/l
Base deficit	>−5
Haemoglobin	>8.0g/dl

Disability—rapid neurological assessment

Check the pupils for size and reaction to light and assess the GCS score rapidly (see p825).

If the patient requires urgent induction of anaesthesia and intubation, remember to perform a quick neurological assessment first.

Exposure/environmental control

Undress the patient completely and protect from hypothermia with warm blankets.

Tubes

Insert a urinary catheter; urine output is an excellent indicator of the adequacy of resuscitation. Place a gastric tube; this will enable stomach contents to be drained and reduce the risk of aspiration. If there is any suspicion of a basal skull fracture, use the orogastric route.

Radiographs

Radiographs of the chest and pelvis are required for all patients sustaining significant blunt trauma.

Relatives in the resuscitation room

It is increasingly common for a relative to remain in the resuscitation room while the patient is being resuscitated. Make the trauma team aware of the presence of the relative and assign a member of the emergency department nursing staff to accompany them. Warn relatives before any particularly invasive procedures are undertaken so that they have the option to leave if they wish.

The secondary survey

Do not undertake a detailed head-to-toe survey of the trauma patient until the vital signs are relatively stable. Re-evaluate the patient repeatedly so that ongoing bleeding is detected early. Patients with exsanguinating haemorrhage may need a laparotomy as part of the resuscitation phase.

Head injuries

Most head injury morbidity is caused by a delay in diagnosing and evacuating an intracranial haematoma or the failure to correct hypoxia and hypotension.

- Inspect and palpate the scalp for lacerations, haematomas, or depressed fractures.
- Check for signs of a basal skull fracture: 'racoon' eyes (Battle's sign), bruising over the mastoid process, subhyaloid haemorrhage, scleral haemorrhage without a posterior margin, haemotympanum, cerebrospinal fluid rhinorrhoea, and otorrhoea.
- Brain injury can be divided into primary injury (concussion, contusion, and laceration) and secondary brain injury (hypoxia, hypercarbia, and hypotension). Resuscitation goals include:
  - MAP at least 90mmHg—allows for CPP of 70mmHg in the presence of slightly raised intracranial pressure (e.g. 20mmHg)
  - SaO_2 >95%
  - $PaCO_2$ of 4.5–5.0kPa (34–38mmHg) (if mechanically ventilated)
  - Haemoglobin >10g/dl
- The conscious level is assessed using the GCS. The trend of change in conscious level is more important than one static reading. Record the pupillary response and the presence of any lateralising signs.

Indications for intubation and ventilation after head injury

- GCS <9
- Loss of protective laryngeal reflexes
- Ventilatory insufficiency (PaO_2 <13kPa (100mmHg) on oxygen, $PaCO_2$ >6kP (45mmHg))
- Spontaneous hyperventilation causing $PaCO_2$ <3.5kPa (26mmHg)
- Respiratory arrhythmia
- Copious bleeding into mouth (e.g. skull base fracture)
- Seizures
- To enable CT scanning
- Before transfer to a regional neurosurgical unit:
  - Significantly deteriorating conscious level, even if not in coma
  - Bilateral fractured mandible.

Glasgow Coma Score

	Response	Score
Best motor response	Obeys commands	6
	Localises pain	5
	Normal flexion withdrawal (stimulus to supraorbital notch)	4
	Abnormal flexion to pain	3
	Extension to pain	2
	Nothing	1
Best verbal response	Orientated	5
	Confused	4
	Inappropriate words	3
	Inarticulate sounds	2
	Nothing	1
Eye opening	Eyes open	4
	Eyes open to speech	3
	Eyes open to pain	2
	No eye opening	1

Modification of GCS for children under 5

	Response	Score
Best motor response	Obeys commands (>2yr)	6
	Localises to pain (<2yr)	5
	Normal flexion to pain (>6 months)	4
	Abnormal flexion to pain	3
	Extension to pain	2
	Nothing	1
Best verbal response	Orientated (>5yr)	5
	Words (>1yr)	4
	Vocal sounds (>6 months)	3
	Cries (<6 months)	2
	None	1
Eye opening	Eyes open	4
	Eyes open to speech	3
	Eyes open to pain	2
	No eye opening	1

Using this scoring system the maximum GCS is 9 at 0–6 months, 11 at 6–12 months, 13 at 1–2yr, and 14 at 2–5yr.

Management of intubation in the head-injured patient
- A rapid sequence induction is required with cricoid pressure and manual in-line stabilisation of the head and neck.
- Give thiopental 3–5mg/kg or propofol 1–3mg/kg with suxamethonium 1–2mg/kg and fentanyl 2–5µg/kg or alfentanil 15–30µg/kg.
- Ventilate to a $PaCO_2$ of 4.5–5.0kPa (34–38mmHg).
- Maintain oxygenation (SaO_2 >95%).
- Maintain sedation with a propofol infusion (1–3mg/kg/hr).
- Insert an orogastric tube—nasogastric tubes are contraindicated until a fractured base of skull has been excluded.
- Restore normovolaemia (0.9% saline) and give vasopressors to maintain a mean arterial blood pressure of 90mmHg.

Indications for a CT scan after head injury
Indications for an emergency (immediately after resuscitation) CT scan include:
- GCS 12 or less.
- A deteriorating level of consciousness or progressive focal neurological signs.

Indications for an urgent (within 4hr) CT scan include:
- GCS 13 or 14 followed by failure to improve within 4hr.
- Radiological/clinical evidence of a fracture, whatever the level of consciousness.
- New focal neurological signs which are not getting worse.
- GCS 15 with no fracture but other features, e.g.
  - Severe and persistent headache
  - Nausea and vomiting
  - Irritability or altered behaviour
  - A seizure.

Referral to a neurosurgical unit
Referral to the regional neurosurgical unit is indicated for:
- All patients with an intracranial mass
- Primary brain injury requiring ventilation
- Compound or depressed skull fracture
- Persistent CSF leak
- Penetrating skull injury
- A seizure without full recovery
- Patients deteriorating rapidly with signs of an intracranial mass lesion.

Management of seizures
- Lorazepam 25–30µg/kg IV
- Phenytoin 15mg/kg over 15min
- Thiopental 3mg/kg if required
- Recheck ABC.

Management of increased ICP
- Give mannitol 0.5g/kg (wt [kg] × 2.5 = ml of 20% mannitol).
- Manually hyperventilate the patient's lungs for 30s and reassess pupillary response.

Transfer to a regional neurosurgical unit[1,2]

A doctor with at least 2yr' experience in an appropriate specialty (usually anaesthesia) and an adequately trained assistant should accompany patients with head injuries. The patient should receive the same standard of physiological monitoring during transfer as they would receive in an intensive care unit. All notes (or photocopies), radiographs, blood results, and crossmatched blood should accompany the patient. The transfer team should carry a mobile phone. Head-injured patients must be resuscitated adequately before transfer. Cervical spine protection should be continued and pupillary responses re-assessed every 15min.

Essential equipment for patient transfer includes

- Portable mechanical ventilator, with supply of oxygen
- Portable, battery-powered monitor—ECG, IABP, CVP, SpO_2, $ETCO_2$, Temp
- Suction, defibrillator, battery powered syringe pumps
- Airway and intubation equipment
- Venous access equipment

Essential drugs for the transfer include

- Hypnotics—a propofol infusion is ideal for sedating intubated patients.
- Muscle relaxants and analgesics e.g. fentanyl.
- Mannitol 20%: mannitol (0.5g/kg) may be given after discussion with the neurosurgeon. This may reduce intracranial pressure and will buy time before surgery.
- Vasoactive drugs, e.g. metaraminol, noradrenaline.
- Additional resuscitation drugs.

---

1 The Neuroanaesthesia Society of Great Britain and Ireland and The Association of Anaesthetists of Great Britain and Ireland (1996). *Recommendations for the transfer of patients with acute head injuries to neurosurgical units.* The Association of Anaesthetists of Great Britain and Ireland, London.
2 The Intensive Care Society (2002). *Guidelines for the transport of the critically ill adult.* The Intensive Care Society, London.

Chest injuries

There are six potentially life-threatening injuries (2 contusions and 4 'ruptures'):
• Pulmonary contusion.
• Cardiac contusion.
• Aortic rupture—blunt aortic injury.
• Ruptured diaphragm.
• Oesophageal rupture.
• Rupture of the tracheobronchial tree.

Pulmonary contusion

• Inspection of the chest may reveal signs indicating considerable decelerating forces, such as seat-belt bruising.
• Pulmonary contusion is the commonest potentially lethal chest injury.
• Young adults and children have particularly compliant ribs and considerable energy can be transmitted to the lungs in the absence of rib fractures.
• The earliest indication of pulmonary contusion is hypoxaemia (reduced PaO_2/FiO_2 ratio).
• The chest radiograph shows patchy infiltrates over the affected area, but may be normal initially.
• Increasing the FiO_2 may provide sufficient oxygenation, if not, the patient may require mask CPAP or tracheal intubation and positive pressure ventilation.
• Use small tidal volumes (6–8ml/kg) to minimise volutrauma. Try to keep the peak inspiratory pressure <30cmH$_2$O.
• The patient with chest trauma requires appropriate fluid resuscitation but fluid overload will compound the lung contusion.

Myocardial contusion

• Cardiac contusion must be considered in any patient with severe blunt chest trauma, particularly those with sternal fractures.
• Cardiac arrhythmias, ST changes on the ECG, and elevated CK-MB isoenzymes may indicate contusion but these signs are very non-specific—cardiac troponins are more specific for cardiac contusion.
• Elevated CVP in the presence of hypotension is the earliest indication of myocardial dysfunction secondary to severe cardiac contusion, but cardiac tamponade must be excluded.
• Echocardiography is the best method of confirming a cardiac contusion.
• Patients with severe cardiac contusion tend to have other serious injuries that will mandate their admission to an intensive care unit—the decision to admit a patient to ICU rarely depends on the diagnosis of cardiac contusion alone.
• The severely contused myocardium will require inotropic support (e.g. dobutamine).

Blunt aortic injury

- The thoracic aorta is at risk in any patient sustaining a significant decelerating force (e.g. fall from a height or high-speed road traffic accident). Only 10–15% of these patients will reach hospital alive; without surgery, two thirds of these survivors will die of delayed rupture within 2wk.
- The commonest site for aortic injury is at the aortic isthmus, just distal to the origin of the left subclavian artery at the level of the ligamentum arteriosum. Deceleration produces large shear forces at this site because the relatively mobile aortic arch travels forward relative to the fixed descending aorta.
- The tear in the intima and media may involve either part of or the whole circumference of the aorta, and in survivors the haematoma is contained by an intact aortic adventitia and mediastinal pleura.
- Patients sustaining blunt aortic injury usually have multiple injuries and may be hypotensive at presentation. However, upper extremity hypertension is present in 40% of cases as the haematoma compresses the true lumen causing a 'pseudocoarctation'.
- The supine chest radiograph will show a widened mediastinum in the vast majority of cases. Although this is a sensitive sign of blunt aortic injury, it is not very specific—90% of cases of widened mediastinum are due to venous bleeding. Whenever practical, obtain an erect chest radiograph (providing a clearer view of the thoracic aorta).
- Signs on the chest radiograph suggesting possible blunt aortic injury are: wide mediastinum, pleural capping, left haemothorax, deviation of the trachea to the right, depression of the left mainstem bronchus, loss of the aortic knob, deviation of the nasogastric tube to the right, fractures of the upper three ribs, or fracture of the thoracic spine.
- If the chest radiograph is equivocal, further investigation will be required. Multi-slice spiral CT with contrast has largely replaced aortography as the standard investigation for the diagnosis of blunt aortic injury; a few centres also use trans-oesophageal echocardiography.
- If blunt aortic injury is suspected, the patient's blood pressure should be maintained at 80–100mmHg systolic (using a β-blocker such as esmolol), in an effort to reduce the risk of further dissection or rupture. The use of pure vasodilators, such as sodium nitroprusside (SNP), increases the pulse pressure and will not reduce the shear forces on the aortic wall. Once stable, the patient must be transferred immediately to the nearest cardiothoracic unit (see p340).

Rupture of the diaphragm

- Rupture of the diaphragm occurs in about 5% of patients sustaining severe blunt trauma to the trunk.
- It can be difficult to diagnose initially—the diagnosis is often made late.
- Approximately 75% of ruptures occur on the left side. The stomach or colon commonly herniates into the chest and strangulation of these organs is a significant complication.
- Signs and symptoms may include diminished breath sounds, chest and abdominal pain and respiratory distress.

- Diagnosis can be made on a plain radiograph (elevated hemidiaphragm, gas bubbles above the diaphragm, shift of the mediastinum to the opposite side, nasogastric tube in the chest). The definitive diagnosis is made by instilling contrast media through the nasogastric tube and repeating the radiograph.
- Once the patient has been stabilised, the diaphragm will require surgical repair (see p380).

Oesophageal rupture

- A severe blow to the upper abdomen may tear the lower oesophagus as gastric contents are forcefully ejected.
- The conscious patient will complain of severe chest and abdominal pain, and mediastinal air may be visible on the chest radiograph.
- Gastric contents may appear in the chest drain.
- The diagnosis is confirmed by contrast study of the oesophagus or endoscopy.
- Urgent surgery is essential—mediastinitis carries a high mortality (see p381).

Tracheobronchial injury

- Laryngeal fractures are rare.
- Signs of laryngeal injury include hoarseness, SC emphysema, and palpable fracture crepitus.
- Total airway obstruction or severe respiratory distress is managed by intubation or a surgical airway—tracheostomy is indicated rather than cricothyroidotomy.
- Less severe laryngeal injuries may be assessed by CT before any appropriate surgery.
- Transections of the trachea or bronchi proximal to the pleural reflection cause massive mediastinal and cervical emphysema.
- Injuries distal to the pleural sheath lead to pneumothoraces—these will not resolve after chest drainage, since the bronchopleural fistula allows a large air leak.
- Most bronchial injuries occur within 2.5cm of the carina and the diagnosis is confirmed by bronchoscopy.
- Tracheobronchial injuries require urgent repair through a thoracotomy (see p381).

Abdominal injuries

The priority is to determine quickly the need for laparotomy and not to waste time trying to define precisely which viscus is injured. Inspect the abdomen for bruising, lacerations, and distension. Careful palpation may reveal tenderness. Undertake a rectal examination to assess sphincter tone and to exclude the presence of pelvic fracture or a high prostate (indicative of a ruptured urethra). Abdominal ultrasound, CT or, more rarely nowadays, diagnostic peritoneal lavage, is indicated whenever clinical examination is unreliable:

- In patients with decreased consciousness (head injury, drugs, or alcohol)
- In the presence of lower rib or pelvic fractures
- When prolonged general anaesthesia for other injuries will make reassessment impossible.

Relative merits of diagnostic peritoneal lavage, ultrasound, and CT in blunt abdominal trauma

	Diagnostic peritoneal lavage	Ultrasound	CT scan
Indication	Diagnosis of haemoperitoneum in presence of haemodynamic instability	Screening for free fluid or solid organ injury in all blunt trauma patients	Diagnosis of organ injury in haemodynamically stable patients
Advantages	Fast, 85–98% sensitivity for intra-abdominal bleeding	Fast, sensitivity 83–87%, can detect free fluid and solid organ injury	Most specific for injury (92–98%)
Disadvantages	Invasive, falsely indicates need for laparotomy in some patients who could be managed conservatively, misses injury to diaphragm or retroperitoneum	Operator dependent, misses diaphragm, bowel, and some pancreatic injuries	Takes time to transfer to scanner, misses diaphragm, bowel, and some pancreatic injuries

Pelvic fractures

- Pelvic fractures can cause life-threatening haemorrhage. *In the hypovolaemic, shocked patient the blood is either on the floor, in the chest, in the abdomen, or in the pelvis.*
- Bleeding associated with pelvic fractures arises mainly from the shearing and tearing of large veins lining the posterior pelvis. Bleeding can also arise from the raw, cancellous bony surfaces. Arterial bleeding accounts for major bleeding in less than 10% of cases.
- The two main fracture types responsible for severe haemorrhage are the open book type (or AP-compression) and the vertical shear pattern.
- Suspect pelvic fracture after motor vehicle accidents, especially where the victim has been ejected from the vehicle, pedestrian-vehicle contact, motorcycle accidents, and falls from more than 3m.
- Clinical signs are variable and unpredictable and the diagnosis is made with an AP pelvic radiograph at the end of the primary survey. Widening of the symphysis greater than 2cm or vertical displacement of one side of the pelvis indicates severe disruption and a high likelihood of major haemorrhage.

Treatment

- A widening or diastasis of the symphysis of more than 2cm doubles the pelvic volume. Emergency treatment aims to reduce this volume and tamponade the bleeding vessels. In the emergency room, 'closing the book' using a folded sheet or purpose-made binder wrapped around the pelvis, and tying the legs together can reduce bleeding significantly.
- After stabilisation of the airway and breathing, the next step is rapid, emergency surgical stabilisation of the pelvis with an external fixator. Threaded self-drilling pins are inserted into the wings of the pelvis enabling the 'book' to be closed by clamping both halves of the pelvis together, tamponading the underlying venous bleeding.
- Application of an external fixator takes precedence over laparotomy in the presence of an open book or vertical shear pelvic fracture, otherwise the loss of tamponade associated with the laparotomy incision can lead to catastrophic retroperitoneal bleeding. Once the external fixator is applied, diagnostic peritoneal lavage can be performed (above the umbilicus to avoid pelvic haematoma). Alternatively, emergency focused ultrasound may exclude associated intraperitoneal bleeding. Laparotomy can be undertaken easily with the external fixator in place.
- The external fixator can be applied in the resuscitation room or the operating theatre depending on local policy.

Associated injuries

Bladder injury 20%, urethral injury 14%, liver and splenic injury, spinal fracture, other limb injuries.

Pitfalls

- Open fractures of the pelvis involving perforation of the vagina or rectum may be difficult to diagnose and are associated with a mortality of 30–50%.
- Beware urethral injury; do not attempt to catheterise if there is marked pelvic disruption on the radiograph or marked perineal bruising and urethral bleeding. Call a surgeon to undertake an emergency urethrogram.
- If there is no improvement in vital signs after external fixation, look for other causes of the bleeding, i.e. intraperitoneal (laparotomy), or arterial (angiography). Discuss with a radiologist the possibility of embolising bleeding pelvic vessels.

Anaesthetic considerations

- These patients are usually in Class III shock and need early blood transfusion. Fixators may be applied under LA or GA.
- Patients with a fractured pelvis need analgesia: opioids are the easiest early treatment, but an epidural is effective if not contraindicated.

Spinal injuries (see also p240)

- If a spinal board has been used to transfer the patient to hospital, remove it as soon as possible: spinal boards are designed for extrication, not transport—they are very uncomfortable to lie on and will cause pressure sores quickly. Log roll the patient to enable a thorough inspection and palpation of the whole spine. A safe log roll requires 5 people: 3 to control and turn the patient's body, 1 to maintain the cervical spine in neutral alignment with the rest of the body, and 1 to palpate the spinous processes for tenderness/deformities.

The person controlling the cervical spine should command the team. Thorough clearance of the patient's spine can be complex:

- In the patient who is awake, alert, sober, neurologically normal, and without distracting injuries, the spine may be cleared if there is no pain at rest and, subsequently, on flexion and extension.
- All other patients will require some form of radiological imaging: lateral, AP, and open-mouth radiographs can be used to clear the cervical spine; CT scans may be used to image C1–C2 and/or C7–T1 if these areas are not seen clearly on the radiographs. In the unconscious patient, and those with multiple injuries, it is now common practise to image the entire cervical spine with CT and use 3D reconstruction to rule out significant injury. Some centres require a lateral radiograph as well as the CT scan—this can detect pre-vertebral soft tissue swelling, which may not be seen on a CT scan and which may indicate significant ligamentous injury. Many experts now accept the small possibility of missing a ligamentous injury on the CT scan in unconscious patients and 'clear' the cervical spine to enable optimal treatment and positioning on the ITU.
- The thoracolumbar spine is cleared with lateral and AP radiographs; alternatively, if the patient needs a CT scan of the abdomen and chest, the sagittal images obtained can be used to confirm spinal alignment—these images are often better than can be obtained with radiographs.
- If the patient is expected to regain consciousness within 24–48hr, many clinicians will wait until a clinical examination has been undertaken before clearing the spine formally.

In the conscious patient, a detailed neurological examination should detect any motor or sensory deficits.

Spinal cord injury can be categorised as:

- Incomplete or complete paraplegia
- Incomplete or complete quadriplegia.

Any motor or sensory function below the level of injury indicates an incomplete injury. A cervical or high thoracic injury may cause loss of vasomotor tone, with hypotension and bradycardia; this requires fluid and vasopressor therapy. The principles of resuscitation for the spinal injured patient are much the same as for the head injured patient; the cord perfusion pressure should be maintained and hypoxia avoided. High-dose methylprednisolone therapy is used only rarely in the UK.

Limb injuries (see also p488)

Limb injuries are rarely immediately life-threatening, but should be examined to ensure an adequate circulation and absence of neurological deficit. The priority is to detect injuries that may be limb threatening. Align fractures carefully and splint appropriately, checking for pulses after each intervention. Tibial and forearm fractures are at particularly high risk of causing a compartment syndrome. The signs and symptoms of compartment syndrome are:

- Pain greater than expected and increased by passive stretching of the muscles.
- Paraesthesiae.
- Decreased sensation or functional loss of the nerves traversing the compartment.
- Tense swelling of the involved compartment.
- Loss of pulses is a very late sign—a distal pulse is usually present in a compartment syndrome.

Definitive diagnosis of a compartment syndrome is made by measurement of compartment pressures using a cannula connected to a transducer. In patients with normal blood pressure, compartment pressures in excess of 30–35mmHg are indicative of a compartment syndrome requiring urgent surgical decompression. (See also p490.)

Burns: early management

(See also p515)

General considerations

- Treat immediately life-threatening injuries first.
- Fire is the most common cause of burns in adults; scalding is the most common cause in children. Most injuries occur at home.
- Burns may be associated with alcohol intoxication, epilepsy, or a psychiatric illness. Consider the possibility of non-accidental injury in children.
- Mortality is related to age, total body surface area (TBSA) burnt, and burn depth.

Airway (with cervical spine control)

- Burns to the head and neck may rapidly cause airway obstruction from massive oedema. Inhalation of hot gases usually causes airway injury above the larynx. Signs of potential airway compromise include singed nasal hairs, hoarse voice, productive 'brassy' cough, and soot in the sputum.
- Clinical judgement will determine the need for immediate intubation, particularly if the patient is to be transferred. Maximum wound oedema occurs 12–36hr after injury, although the airway may be compromised much earlier. If in doubt, intubate early using an uncut tracheal tube: the subsequent oedema can be considerable.

Breathing

- Give oxygen 15l/min using a facemask with a reservoir bag.
- Intubation and mechanical ventilation may be required in patients who are:
  - Unconscious from coexisting trauma or from the inhalation of toxic substances such as carbon monoxide (CO).
  - Developing acute respiratory failure due to smoke inhalation or blast injury.
  - In need of extensive resuscitation, sedation, and analgesia following a major burn.

Circulation (with haemorrhage control)

- Burns >25% TBSA produce a marked systemic inflammatory response accompanied by increase in capillary permeability and generalised oedema.
- Insert cannulae through intact skin wherever possible. Start IV fluids for burns:
  - >15% TBSA in adults
  - >10% TBSA in children.
- Hartmann's solution is now the preferred resuscitation fluid for burns; it is cost-effective and readily available.
  - The fluid requirement in the first 24hr in adults is 2ml/kg/% TBSA burn and in children 3ml/kg/% TBSA. Give half the calculated fluid in the first 8hr from the time of injury and give the remainder in the next 16hr.
  - Maintenance fluids are required in addition to the calculated resuscitation fluid.

- These calculated values are merely an estimate—the precise volumes required will be guided by urine output (>0.5–1.0ml/kg) and cardiovascular response.
- Test the urine for haemochromogens (myoglobin/haemoglobin) arising from muscle damage and red cell breakdown. If positive:
  - Increase urine output to 1–2ml/kg/hr.
  - Alkalinise urine: add 25mmol bicarbonate to each litre of Hartmann's solution.
  - Promote diuresis: add 12.5g mannitol to each litre of Hartmann's solution.

Neurological deficit

- Head injury is common in burns associated with road traffic accidents, falls, blasts, or explosions.
- Carbon monoxide (CO) poisoning or alcohol intoxication is a common cause of altered consciousness.

Exposure (with temperature control)

- Remove all clothing to assess the extent of burn injury. If clothing is stuck to the skin, cut around the area leaving the adherent fabric in place. Keep the patient warm.
- Assess % TBSA burnt by reference to an adult or paediatric burn chart. The 'rule of nines' conveniently divides the adult body surface into multiples of 9%; this is inaccurate for small children. The palmar surface of a patient's hand and fingers is ~1% TBSA. Detailed assessment of burn area is made by referring to a Lund and Browder chart (see p841).
- Assess burn depth: burn wounds may be superficial or deep; in practice, most injuries are a mixture of both.
  - Superficial—consist of burns to the epidermis only (sunburn, flashburns) or involving the superficial part of the dermis (producing a blister); these burns are painful and pinprick sensation is preserved. Healing will occur without the need for grafting.
  - Deep—consist of deep dermal burns (no capillary refill beneath the blister since blood vessels are destroyed) or full thickness (involving entire epidermis and dermis, possibly including underlying structures). Burns may have a white, waxy appearance. Pinprick sensation is lost.

Immediate wound care

- Cool the burn wound with cold running water—this helps reduce production of inflammatory mediators and reduces tissue damage. Continue cooling for at least 20min, taking care to prevent hypothermia, especially in the young child. Cooling the burn is an effective analgesic.
- Burn wounds are initially sterile. Cover with 'Clingfilm' to limit evaporation and heat loss, and reduce pain.

Monitoring

- Monitor SaO_2, ECG, urine output, core temperature, and NIBP. The pulse oximeter cannot detect carboxyhaemoglobin (COHb) and will over read the oxygen saturation of haemoglobin: use a co-oximeter to obtain an accurate estimation of the percentage of oxyhaemoglobin.

- Insert an arterial line for unconscious patients and those with major burns and/or inhalational injury.
- Insert a nasogastric tube for large burns (>20% adult, >10% child): gastroparesis is common.
- Check the FBC (including haematocrit), urea/creatinine, electrolytes, glucose, COHb, and crossmatch some blood.

Analgesia

- All burns are painful; although skin sensation is lost over deep burns, the surrounding area is very painful.
- Give morphine IV, titrated to effect, and continue with a morphine infusion or PCA.

Escharotomy

- Eschar is the coagulated dead skin of a full-thickness burn; it cannot expand as tissue oedema progresses. Circumferential burns to limbs may result in limb ischaemia; circumferential burns to the trunk may reduce chest wall compliance and impede ventilation.
- Escharotomy, the release of the burn wound by incision down to SC fat, is performed in the operating room. Incisions are made longitudinally along the medial and lateral sides of limbs; on the trunk, incisions are made along the anterior axillary line down to the upper abdomen. Ensure blood is available; bleeding can be extreme.
- Patients are often already sedated and ventilated. Conscious patients will need additional sedation and analgesia. Full thickness burns are painless, but incisions will extend onto normal skin for a short distance.

Special circumstances

Inhalation of toxic substances

Carbon monoxide poisoning is common: check COHb. The severity of symptoms may not correlate well with the COHb level. Poisoning may mimic alcohol intoxication.

- Carbon monoxide reduces the capacity of blood to carry O_2 and causes tissue hypoxia. The PaO_2 is normal. Carbon monoxide also binds avidly to other haem-containing compounds, especially the cytochrome system. The half-life of COHb is 250min when breathing room air; this is reduced to 40min when breathing 100% O_2. Oxygen therapy should be continued since a secondary peak of COHb occurs after 24hr and is attributed to washout of CO from cytochromes.
- Hyperbaric oxygen therapy reduces the half-life of COHb to just 15–30min; however, the precise role of hyperbaric oxygen is controversial and is highly subject to availability of hyperbaric facilities. Indications for discussion with the nearest hyperbaric facility include:
  - any neurological abnormality or cognitive impairment
  - chest pain, abnormal ECG, or cardiac enzymes
  - pregnancy
  - history of loss of consciousness
  - inability to assess adequately

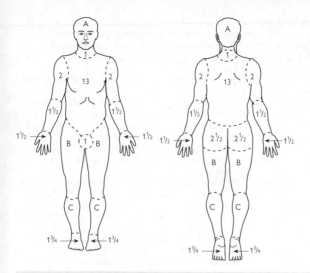

Relative percentage of area affected by growth (age in years)

	0	1	5	10	15	Adult
A: half of head	$9\frac{1}{2}$	$8\frac{1}{2}$	$6\frac{1}{2}$	$5\frac{1}{2}$	$4\frac{1}{2}$	$3\frac{1}{2}$
B: half of thigh	$2\frac{3}{4}$	$3\frac{1}{4}$	4	$4\frac{1}{2}$	$4\frac{1}{2}$	$4\frac{3}{4}$
C: half of leg	$2\frac{1}{2}$	$2\frac{1}{2}$	$2\frac{3}{4}$	3	$3\frac{1}{4}$	$3\frac{1}{2}$

Lund and Browder chart

COHb (%)	Symptoms
0–15	None (smokers)
15–20	Headache, mild confusion
20–40	Nausea and vomiting, disorientation, fatigue
40–60	Hallucinations, ataxia, fits, coma
>60	Death

- Symptoms of COHb poisoning are shown in the table above.
- Other toxic products of combustion may include cyanide, ammonia, phosgene, hydrogen chloride, fluoride or bromide, and complex organic compounds. These toxic substances may produce:
  - A chemical burn to the respiratory tract.
  - Interstitial lung oedema, impaired gas exchange, and ARDS.
  - Systemic acid/base disturbances.
  - Hydrofluoric acid binds serum Ca^{2+} and causes hypocalcaemia.

Chemical burns
- Hands and upper limbs are the most frequently affected areas.
- Staff must protect themselves with gloves, apron, and facemask.
- Remove contaminated clothing as early as possible—store in a secure container for disposal.
- Industrial or household alkalis and acids are commonly used chemicals, e.g. bleach, washing powder, disinfectants, drain cleaner, paint stripper. Immersion in complex hydrocarbons (petrol, diesel) without ignition may cause systemic toxicity. Phosphorus burns may result from fireworks or military applications.
- Tissue damage continues until the chemical is neutralised or diluted by washing with water. Early, continuous, and prolonged (1hr) irrigation with cold water is vital for all burns (except elemental Na, K, or Li).
- Specific treatments include:
  - Hydrofluoric acid, used in the glass industry, is highly toxic. Burns of 2% TBSA can be fatal. Tissue penetration by fluoride ions causes deep chemical burns. Inactivate toxic F^- ions by application of topical calcium gluconate burn gel, 10% gluconate local injections into the burn wound (0.5ml of a 10% solution/cm^2 of surface burn extending 0.5cm beyond the margin of involved tissue; do not use the chloride salt because it is an irritant and may cause tissue damage) and consider intra-arterial (infuse a solution of 10ml of 10% calcium gluconate in 40ml of 5% dextrose over 4hr) or IV (Bier's block—10–15ml of 10% calcium gluconate plus 5000U of heparin diluted up to 40ml in 5% dextrose).
  - Phosphorus: white phosphorus ignites spontaneously when exposed to air; it can be extinguished by water. Apply copper sulphate solution which converts phosphorus to black cupric phosphide.
  - Bitumen: common injury in the United Kingdom from road maintenance. It is liquid at 150°C and causes thermal burns. Cool with water; remove the bitumen with vegetable or paraffin oil.

Electrical burns
- Low voltage (<1000V) causes a local contact burn. The 50Hz A.C. domestic supply is particularly likely to cause cardiac arrest. Muscle spasm may prevent release of the electrical source. There is no associated deep tissue damage.
- High voltage (>1000V) causes flash burn or deep tissue damage due to current transmission. High voltage cables carry 11 000 or 33 000V: electrocution produces an entrance and exit wound, which may require fasciotomy under GA. Haemochromogens released from muscle and damaged red cells may cause renal failure.
- A direct strike by lightning (ultra high voltage, high current) has a very high mortality. Side flash is more common: a nearby lightning strike produces current that flows over the surface of the victim causing superficial burns. Current may flow up one leg and down the other producing an entry and exit wound. Respiratory arrest is common. 'Lichtenberg flowers' is a pathognomonic splashed-on pattern of skin damage resulting from lightning side flash.

The British Burn Association criteria for transfer to a burns centre are

- Burn >10% TBSA adult or >5% TBSA child, and any patient with full thickness burn >5% TBSA.
- Burn to: face, hands, feet, genitalia, perineum, or major joints.
- Electrical or chemical burns.
- Inhalational injury.
- Circumferential burn to the limbs or chest.
- Patients at the extremes of age.
- Patients with poor medical condition, which may complicate treatment.

Analgesia for the injured patient

• Give effective analgesia to the injured patient as soon as practically possible.
• If the patient needs surgery imminently, then immediate induction of general anaesthesia is a logical and very effective solution to the patient's pain; if not, titrate IV opioid (e.g. fentanyl or morphine) to the desired effect.
• Head injured patients require adequate pain relief for any other injuries; careful titration of IV morphine or fentanyl will provide effective pain relief without significant respiratory depression. The popular use of IM codeine in head injured patients is illogical. It is a weak opioid and, in equianalgesic doses, it is a more potent histamine releaser than morphine. It has the same side effects as morphine, including the ability to induce respiratory depression and miosis.
• NSAIDs provide moderate analgesia but are relatively contraindicated in patients with hypovolaemia; these patients depend on renal prostaglandins to maintain renal blood flow.
• Entonox is useful for short procedures such as fracture splintage.
• Local anaesthetic blocks are ideal for the acute trauma patient; unfortunately, relatively few blocks are both simple and effective. Femoral nerve blockade will provide analgesia for a fracture of the femoral shaft. Intercostal nerve blocks will provide analgesia for rib fractures but the duration is relatively short. Continuous thoracic epidural analgesia will provide excellent pain relief for patients with multiple rib fractures.

The multiply injured patient: common dilemmas

- The head injured patient with an abdominal injury—which of a laparotomy or brain CT should be undertaken first? If the patient is haemodynamically unstable the laparotomy has priority. Hypotension will compound any brain injury and bleeding must be controlled rapidly. If the patient is haemodynamically stable, a CT scan of both the brain and the abdomen may be appropriate.
- The head injured patient with lower limb fractures. In general, in the haemodynamically stable patient, limb fractures should be stabilised as soon as possible. In the presence of a significant brain injury, intracranial pressure should be monitored before intramedullary nailing of limb fractures.
- The patient with pulmonary contusion and lower limb fractures. Intramedullary reaming will cause some degree of fat embolism. Whether this results in significant risk to the patient is contentious. In the presence of severe pulmonary contusion, some orthopaedic surgeons would elect to stabilise lower limb fractures temporarily with an external fixator before undertaking definitive nailing at a later date.

Post cardiac arrest resuscitation care

Following cardiac arrest, restoration of a spontaneous circulation (ROSC) is just the first step in what may be a prolonged period of treatment. The anaesthetist may be expected to initiate this treatment in the emergency department, the operating room, the critical care unit, or on the general ward. The aims of post resuscitation care are to:

- Prevent a further cardiac arrest
- Define the underlying pathology
- Limit organ damage
- Predict non-survivors.

Prevention of further cardiac arrest

- Optimise oxygenation—after an immediate return to full consciousness following a short duration cardiac arrest, give oxygen via a facemask.
- Other patients may require assisted ventilation via a tracheal tube. Maintain adequate sedation with a propofol infusion, combined with opioid as required.
- Provide ventilation to maintain normocarbia—excessive ventilation will cause hypocarbia and cerebral ischaemia from cerebral vasoconstriction.
- Correct electrolyte disturbances, particularly K^+, Mg^{2+}, and Ca^{2+}.
- Control the blood glucose tightly: treat the blood glucose with insulin if it exceeds 7mmol/l; maintain in the range 4–7mmol/l.

Define the underlying pathology

- Establish the patient's pre-arrest medical condition.
- Confirm correct placement of tracheal tube and exclude pneumothorax.
- Listen to the heart for evidence of murmurs and seek evidence of ventricular failure.
- Record the GCS.

Limit organ damage

- If there is evidence of ST elevation myocardial infarction (STEMI), consult with a cardiologist: coronary artery reperfusion with thrombolytics or percutaneous coronary intervention (PCI) may be indicated.
- Patients remaining comatose after ROSC, particularly after out-of-hospital cardiac arrest, should be cooled to 32–34°C for 12–24hr and then rewarmed slowly.[1] Cooling can be achieved with ice cold IV saline 20–30ml/kg, application of wet towels to the torso and ice to the groins, axillae, and neck.

Prediction of non-survivors

- Approximately 5% of those sustaining an out-of-hospital cardiac arrest will survive to hospital discharge; the figure for in-hospital cardiac arrest is about 15%.
- Short duration of cardiac arrest/CPR correlates with more rapid ROSC and better neurological outcomes.
- Prognostication in unconscious patients after more protracted CPR remains unreliable for up to 72hr after ROSC.
- Myocardial, neurological and other organ function may all improve slowly, given appropriate support over a period of time: at least 72hr of intensive care should be considered in the comatose patient with ROSC following cardiac arrest.

1 Nolan JP, Morley PT, Vanden Hoek TL, Hickey RW (2003). Therapeutic hypothermia after cardiac arrest. An advisory statement by the Advanced Life Support Task Force of the International Liaison Committee on Resuscitation. *Resuscitation*, **57**, 231–235.

Septic shock

Definitions

- Infection: the inflammatory response to the presence of micro-organisms or the invasion of normally sterile host tissue by those organisms.
- Bacteraemia: the presence of viable bacteria in the blood.
- The Systemic Inflammatory Response Syndrome (SIRS): the patient exhibits two of the following four abnormalities:
  - Temperature >38°C or <36°C.
  - Heart rate >90bpm.
  - Respiratory rate >20 breaths/min or $PaCO_2$ <4.3kPa (32mmHg).
  - White blood cell count >12 000 cells/mm^3 or <4000 cells/mm^3 or >10% immature cells (band forms).
- Sepsis: SIRS resulting from infection.
- Severe sepsis: sepsis associated with organ dysfunction, hypoperfusion or hypotension. Hypoperfusion and perfusion abnormalities include lactic acidosis, oliguria or an acute alteration in mental status.
- Septic shock: sepsis with hypotension (systolic blood pressure <90mmHg or a reduction of >40mmHg from baseline) and perfusion abnormalities or the requirement for vasoactive drugs despite adequate fluid resuscitation in the absence of other causes for hypotension.

Pathology

- The response to sepsis is complex and involves many pro- and anti-inflammatory mediators; the severity of illness is determined more by the nature of the inflammatory response than by the infection.
- Most abdominal sepsis is caused by Gram-negative bacteria which contain endotoxin in their outer membrane. Endotoxin is a lipopoly-saccharide implicated in macrophage and monocyte activation and the release of numerous mediators including tumour necrosis factor (TNF), interleukin 1 (IL-1) and other cytokines, plus prostaglandins, leukotrienes, the complement and fibrinolytic systems, platelet-activating factor, and nitric oxide (NO).
- Pathological effects caused by these mediators include vasodilatation, increased capillary permeability, impaired tissue oxygen utilisation, and myocardial depression.
- Tissues may become hypoxic for several reasons, including hypotension (vasodilatation, hypovolaemia, myocardial depression); microvascular thrombosis (activation of coagulation); tissue oedema acting as a barrier to oxygen diffusion; shunting past some capillary beds. This results in anaerobic metabolism and lactic acidosis. In sepsis, despite adequate oxygen delivery, lactic acidosis may also be caused by mitochondrial dysfunction. Reperfusion of previously hypoxic tissues can cause further release of damaging reactive oxygen species.

Resuscitation

The resuscitation of the septic patient should be started as soon as the condition is recognised; it should not be delayed pending admission to ICU or transfer to the operating room. Induction of anaesthesia in the septic patient is hazardous and every effort should be made to resuscitate the patient adequately preoperatively; whether or not this is achievable will depend on the urgency of the surgery. International guidelines for the treatment of severe sepsis and septic shock have been published recently.[1]

- Anaesthetic induction drugs and volatile agents will compound the vasodilatory and negative inotropic effects of sepsis. Surgery may initially worsen the septic state by further releasing bacteria, endotoxins, and cytokines, and causing haemorrhage and fluid loss.
- Establish vascular access and monitoring as soon as possible and before induction of anaesthesia:
  - 2 functioning, large-bore IV cannulae
  - CVP line
  - Arterial line
  - Urinary catheter
  - In the presence of advanced sepsis consider cardiac output monitoring using the method preferred locally (e.g. pulmonary artery catheter, oesophageal Doppler, etc.); in the absence of a pulmonary artery catheter, measurement of mixed venous oxygen saturation may be valuable
- While establishing monitoring give oxygen and fluid; use crystalloids and/or colloids—there is no good evidence for the benefit of one over the other.
- Resuscitation goals during the first 6hr of resuscitation include:
  - CVP 8–12mmHg
  - Mean arterial pressure (MAP) ≥65mmHg
  - Urine output ≥0.5ml/kg/hr
  - Central venous (superior vena cava) or mixed venous oxygen saturation ≥70%
- Once adequate fluid has been given, start a noradrenaline infusion to maintain MAP ≥65mmHg.
- Ensure crossmatched blood is available—haemoglobin concentration will fall due to haemodilution and there may be excessive blood loss due to a coagulopathy. The haemoglobin concentration should be maintained at >7.0g/dl—a higher target value will be appropriate in the presence of coronary artery disease, acute haemorrhage, or persistent lactic acidosis.
- Ensure that blood cultures are taken before starting antibiotics; give antibiotics at the correct time and in the correct dose. The choice of antibiotics should be guided by local microbiology policies.
- If the patient requires surgery, discuss with critical care staff so that plans can be made for admission to an appropriate unit for Level 2 or Level 3 care.

1 Dellinger RP, Carlet JM, Masur H, et al. (2004). Surviving Sepsis Campaign guidelines for management of severe sepsis and septic shock. Intensive Care Med, 30, 536–555.

Interpretation of investigations in the septic patient

- FBC: expect a high WBC with a neutrophilia (a low WBC is evidence of overwhelming sepsis); a low platelet count is common.
- U&E: urea and sodium raised proportionately more than creatinine indicates dehydration; high creatinine indicates renal impairment.
- Coagulation screen: increased INR indicates septic coagulopathy (unless on warfarin).
- Blood glucose: usually raised, low glucose indicates advanced sepsis or hepatic dysfunction.
- Arterial blood gases: metabolic acidosis is common; there may be compensatory hyperventilation unless the patient is obtunded. Hypoxia is common in severe sepsis.
- Blood lactate: a high blood lactate indicates tissue hypoxia. If there is acidaemia with a normal lactate, check the creatinine and urine output (renal failure is the most likely cause of non-lactic acidosis in the septic patient; another cause is diabetic ketoacidosis).
- The chest radiograph may show evidence of non-cardiogenic pulmonary oedema indicating the development of acute respiratory distress syndrome (ARDS).

Induction and maintenance of anaesthesia

- Rapid sequence induction should be used in any patient with severe sepsis.
- All induction drugs will cause hypotension—use reduced doses. Use of a short acting opioid, such as alfentanil, will enable a significant reduction in the dose of induction drug. Many anaesthetists avoid etomidate in critically ill patients—a single dose suppresses the adrenocortical axis for up to 24hr. Hydrocortisone 50–100mg IV at induction may help prevent problems.
- Ensure that vasopressor drugs are available before inducing anaesthesia: adrenaline drawn up in 2 concentrations (10ml of 1:10 000 and 1:100 000) provides the flexibility to reverse the cardiovascular effects of induction drugs.
- Insert a nasogastric tube if not already in place.
- The use of epidural blockade is controversial in sepsis, although, depending on the precise circumstances, many experienced clinicians still consider the benefits outweigh the risks.
  - A potential bacteraemia may be considered to be a contraindication
  - Coagulopathy may preclude insertion
  - Hypotensive effects are likely to be exaggerated
  - If insertion of an epidural is not contraindicated by other factors, consider inserting a catheter but waiting until the patient is stable before establishing the block.
- Maintain with either a volatile anaesthetic or propofol. A noradrenaline infusion is used to counteract hypotension and maintain a MAP ≥65mmHg.
- The effects and duration of action of opioids other than remifentanil will be increased by impaired hepatic and renal perfusion.
- Avoid NSAIDs in patients who are persistently hypotensive or septic.

Maintaining tissue oxygenation in the operating room
Fluids
- Continue to give fluids aiming for CVP 8–12mmHg.
- Colloid stays in the circulation longer than crystalloid but this difference is probably not as great as was commonly believed.
- Monitor ABG regularly, and give blood to maintain a haemoglobin concentration of 7–9g/dl.

Inotropes/vasoconstrictors
Having ensured adequate fluid resuscitation, use noradrenaline to maintain the MAP $\geq$ 65mmHg—this will counteract the vasodilatation associated with sepsis and also provides some inotropic effect. If cardiac output is thought to be inadequate despite fluid and noradrenaline consider adding dobutamine or adrenaline.

Oxygen and PEEP
- Critically ill patients should be anaesthetised with equipment that can provide positive end expiratory pressure (PEEP) and variable I:E ratios.
- Oxygenation may be impaired by non-cardiogenic pulmonary oedema, which is caused by the increased capillary permeability in sepsis.
- Increase the FiO_2 until SaO_2 is at least 90% and use 5cmH$_2$O PEEP.
- Increase the PEEP to 10cmH$_2$O if the patient is still hypoxic despite FiO_2 0.5. Consider an alveolar recruitment manoeuvre (hold lungs in inspiration at 40cmH$_2$O for up to 40s).
- Modern anaesthetic machines include the facility to give pressure control inverse ratio ventilation and this should be used if the patient remains hypoxic despite FiO_2 >0.6 and PEEP >10cmH$_2$O.

Ventilation
- Increased capillary permeability in sepsis may reduce lung compliance and produce high airway pressures.
- Shear forces caused by ventilation with high tidal volumes or high inspiratory pressures will exacerbate lung injury. In patients with early ARDS, every effort should be made to limit peak airway pressure to 30cmH$_2$O and tidal volume to 6–8ml/kg ideal body weight. These target values can be reconsidered if the resultant minute ventilation fails to achieve a pH >7.15.
- Monitor ABGs regularly: a base deficit or raised lactate indicates inadequate resuscitation, although both of these abnormalities can be associated with an adrenaline infusion.
- A $ScvO_2$ <70% implies inadequate oxygen delivery. Fluids and inotropic treatment may be indicated. An oesophageal Doppler or other technique for measuring cardiac output will assist treatment.
- The trends indicated by these monitors are valuable; single readings taken in isolation are difficult to interpret.

The ICU patient going to theatre

The planning, transfer, and monitoring of a critically ill patient on the ICU needing surgery can be challenging. Physiological instability should be anticipated, detected, and acted upon promptly and effectively. Senior anaesthetists and surgeons must be involved.

Consent

Informed consent is often impossible as the patient may be sedated or comatose. Whilst the family is not able to give consent in law, whenever possible, the reasons for surgery and risks should be discussed with them.

Preoperative assessment

- Routine aspects of the preoperative assessment (e.g. history of previous anaesthetics, chronic medical conditions, allergies, etc.) are just as relevant to the critically ill patient as they are to the elective case.
- Assess the patient's current condition from discussion with critical care and from information on the observation and drug charts.
- Note the current fluid requirements and rate/concentration of inotrope infusions; ensure that there is an adequate supply of inotrope prepared for theatre; consider which vasopressors may be required.
- Note the patient's oxygen requirement, lung compliance, minute volume, and PEEP, etc., to enable prediction of the ventilator settings that will be necessary in theatre. In the absence of a suitable ventilator in the operating room, it will be necessary to use a ventilator from the ICU.
- Check IV access and consider if any additional cannulae may be required. Many ICU patients have had all peripheral access removed.
- Check which antibiotics the patient is receiving and whether any doses will be due in theatre.
- Check the most recent FBC, U&E, and ABG, and ensure that blood has been crossmatched.
- If the patient is being transferred to a more remote facility, such as the X-ray department, ensure adequate anaesthetic assistance. If the patient has very poor lung compliance and is requiring high levels of PEEP, it may be necessary to use an ICU ventilator.
- On rare occasions, it may be necessary to undertake an MRI scan on a critically ill patient—the inability to take ferrometallic objects into the scan room is problematic (see p684).

Transfer to the operating room

- Familiarise yourself with the transport equipment and ensure it is functioning before leaving the ICU.
- If the patient is already ventilated, establish on the transfer ventilator before leaving the ICU to ensure adequate ventilation can be maintained. Modern transfer ventilators have a PEEP facility and the more sophisticated machines can provide pressure control ventilation with variable I:E ratios.

- Consider increasing the patient's sedation for the transfer.
- If the patient is not already sedated and ventilated decide whether to induce in ICU, the anaesthetic room, or theatre: factors influencing the decision will be safety, available assistance, haemodynamic instability, and patient comfort.
- Monitor the patient fully en-route.
- Disentangle all lines, re-establish full monitoring, and check IV access before the start of surgery.

Transfer back to ICU

- Inform the ICU staff when surgery is about to finish; this enables them to prepare to receive the patient and possibly to assist in the transfer.
- Ensure that a full verbal and written handover is given to the ICU medical and nursing staff and communicate the postoperative requirements.

Further reading

Surviving sepsis campaign management guidelines committee (2004). Surviving sepsis campaign guidelines for management of severe sepsis and septic shock. *Critical Care Medicine*, **32**, 858–873. Also at www. survivingsepsis.org

Transferring the critically ill

Safe transfer demands experienced staff and careful preparation. Several studies have demonstrated that patients are often inadequately resuscitated and monitored during transfer. Specialised transport teams improve outcome but are not always available or appropriate. Before transferring any critically ill patient the risks of transfer should be weighed against the potential benefits of treatment at the receiving unit.

Dangers of transfer

- Deranged physiology worsened by movement (acceleration/deceleration leads to cardiovascular instability)—15% of patients develop avoidable hypoxia and hypotension.
- Cramped conditions, isolation, temperature, and pressure changes.
- Vehicular crashes.

Principles of safe transfer

- Staff experienced in intensive care and transfer—specialist transport teams may improve outcome, but may cause delay.
- Use of appropriate equipment and vehicle, extensive monitoring, careful stabilisation, continuing reassessment, direct handover, documentation, and audit.

The transfer vehicle

- Adequate space, light, gases, electricity, and communications.
- Mode: consider urgency, mobilisation time, geography, weather, traffic, and costs.
- Consider air if over 150 miles (remember decreasing PaO_2 at altitude, expanding air spaces requiring naso/orogastric tube, temperature, noise, and vibration).

Aeromedical transfer

- Hazards depend on whether the craft is rotary (helicopter) or fixed wing (aeroplane).
- Helicopters fly at relatively low altitude and therefore avoid some of the problems of aeroplane.
- High altitude decreases the partial pressure of oxygen—at 1500m arterial PaO_2 is about 10kPa (75mmHg). Most aircraft are pressurised to 1500–2000m.
- Decreased barometric pressure leads to expansion of gas-filled cavities (patients should have nasogastric tubes and may need chest drains).
- Pressurising the cabin pressure to sea level can decrease these problems but increases fuel costs!
- Air in the tracheal tube cuff should be replaced by saline.

Problems during transfer

- Vibration leads to failure and inaccuracy of non-invasive BP. Invasive monitoring should be used if at all possible.
- Access to the patient may be limited.
- Acceleration/deceleration may lead to cardiovascular instability.
- Hypothermia, particularly during transfer between vehicles.

Specific considerations for children

- Hypothermia is a greater risk, particularly in the infant. Monitor central temperature and use warming mats, 'bubble wrap', hats, etc., to maintain temperature.
- Secure IV access is paramount before departure.

Calculating oxygen reserves

Operation time (min) for different minute volumes at FiO_2 1.0

Size of oxygen cylinder (volume (litres))	Minute volume 5l/min	Minute volume 7l/min	Minute volume 10l/min
D (340)	56min	42min	30min
E (680)	113min	85min	61min
F (1360)	226min	170min	123min

Battery life

- This can vary greatly, depending on manufacturer, but must be known.
- The charge time is usually considerable.
- Battery life will vary depending on the rate of infusion.

Examples of battery lives for pumps running at 5–10ml/hr

Type	Battery life (estimated) (hr)	Charge time (estimated) (hr)
Graseby 3100	3	14
Alaris IVAC	6	24
Graseby Omnifuse	8	18

Preparation

- Ensure meticulous stabilisation prior to transfer.
- Take a full history and make a thorough examination.
- Full monitoring including invasive BP and CVP where indicated.
- Blood tests, radiographs, and CT prior to transfer.
- Explain procedure to patient and family.

Checklist for preparation

A: airway
- Is the airway safe? If in doubt, intubate.
- Cervical spine control.

B: breathing
- Portable ventilator settings. Check ABG before departure after 15min on the portable ventilator.
- Self-inflating bag-valve-device in the event of a ventilator/oxygen failure.
- Suction.
- Adequate sedation, analgesia, and relaxation.
- Adequate O_2 reserves.
- Insert a chest drain if there is a possibility of a pneumothorax (e.g. fractured ribs).

C: circulation
- Stable circulation with good access. Controlled external bleeding.
- Invasive BP and CVP, when indicated.
- Inotropes—if in doubt have them prepared and ready to run.
- Pumps and batteries.
- Insert a urinary catheter and monitor output.

D: disability
- GCS (mannitol, IPPV), pupillary signs.
- Naso/orogastric tube.

E: exposure
- Temperature loss.
- Splint long bones.

F: forgotten?
- All notes, referral letter, results, radiographs (including CT scans), and blood products.
- Inform the receiving unit that you are leaving the base hospital.
- Inform relatives.
- Take contact numbers.
- Take warm clothing, mobile phone, food, and credit card/money for the team!
- Plan for the return journey.
- Medical indemnity and insurance for death or disability of transfer staff.

Equipment and drug box guidelines

Airway and breathing

Suction equipment	Endotracheal tubes, connectors, and ties
Stethoscope	Tracheostomy tubes (if appropriate)
Face masks, airways, self-inflating bag with reservoir	Laryngoscopes, spare batteries
Gum elastic bougie	

Circulation

Cannulae + IV dressings and tape	IV fluids and giving set
Syringes and needles	Mini sharps receptacle

Resuscitation drugs

Adenosine	Noradrenaline
Hydrocortisone	Diazemuls®
Adrenaline	Salbutamol nebulisers
Lidocaine	Dextrose
Amiodarone	Sodium bicarbonate
Metoprolol	Furosemide
Atropine	Saline ampoules
Naloxone	GTN spray
Calcium chloride	Plain drug labels

Sedation/muscle relaxants

Propofol	Midazolam
Atracurium, vecuronium, or rocuronium	Suxamethonium

Paediatric equipment—extras

Paediatric oxygen mask with reservoir bag	Tracheal tubes
Small cannulae	Paediatric drug doses
Appropriate self-inflating bag with reservoir	Laryngoscope and styles
Intraosseous needle	Magill forceps and suction catheters
Masks and airways	10% dextrose for infusion

Anaesthetic emergencies

Andy McIndoe

Introduction

Anaesthetic emergencies may develop rapidly into life-threatening conditions. Although critical incidents frequently occur in the presence of a theatre team, the anaesthetist is likely to be the person present with the specialist knowledge and skills to deal with the problem. This can give rise to intense pressure. Critical incident protocols and drills have been designed to aid in the management of the more complex or common emergencies, and some are detailed below. However, a protocol driven approach is heavily reliant upon recognition that a serious problem exists.

General considerations to help deal with any unanticipated anaesthetic crisis

Communication

- Declare problems early to the rest of the theatre team before you lose control of the situation. Basic resuscitation measures should be ongoing whilst you figure out the diagnosis.
- No matter whatever or whoever 'caused' the crisis, use objective and non-judgmental comments. Insults tend to provoke an aggressive or withdrawal response from the recipient and inhibit team function.
- To communicate effectively, your messages or commands must be:
  ADDRESSED—Ask specifically named individuals, not 'someone', to perform tasks.
  HEARD—Reduce background noise and distractions by turning off the radio etc.
  UNDERSTOOD—If you make a complex request, ask the recipient to repeat it back to you.
- If the cause of the problem is unknown, say so. Say what you don't know as well as what you do know. Encourage others to contribute.
- Reappraise the situation regularly. Update the rest of the team with new information. If you are still unsure about what to do, send for help—a second person with a fresh approach may pick up on missed clues.

Invoke a team approach

- A team should have one clearly identified leader, who should make effective use of the mixture of skills and resources available within the rest of the team.
- A good team leader is able to step back from the situation to consider the whole picture. This can only be achieved by delegation of responsibility for tasks to other members of the team. It should then be possible to evolve and communicate a plan of action.
- A repeated and systematic ABC approach helps render the patient 'safe', buys thinking time, and increases the likelihood of detecting signs that may lead to a definitive diagnosis.
- Most members of an impromptu emergency team will need to adopt the role of 'team players'. A good team player is adaptable, assumes complete responsibility for delegated problems, and feels comfortable enough to advocate an opinion or feed back information to the rest of the team.

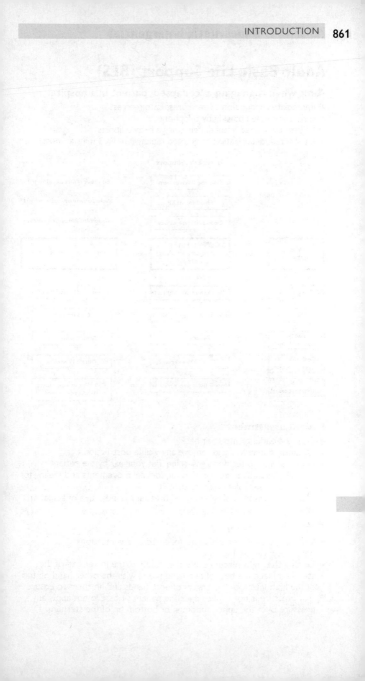

Adult Basic Life Support (BLS)

Aims when managing a 'collapsed' patient in a hospital

- Immediate recognition of cardiorespiratory arrest
- Help summoned quickly by telephone
- CPR to be started immediately using airway adjuncts
- If indicated, defibrillation attempted rapidly (within 3 mins at most).

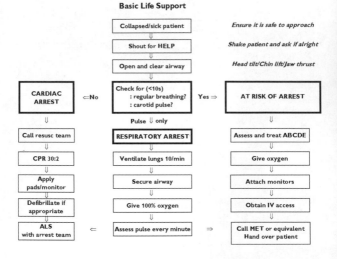

Patient assessment

- Turn the patient onto their back.
- Optimise the airway and remove any visible obstruction.
- Look, listen, and feel for signs of life. Put your ear by the patient's mouth whilst observing for chest/abdominal movements and feeling for a carotid pulse. Take no more than 10s.
- Occasional gasps or slow laboured breathing is indicative of actual or impending cardiac arrest.

Chest compressions

- Give cycles of 30 compressions followed by 2 ventilations.
- Rate of delivery = 100/min.
- **Finding the right place:** Locate the middle of the lower half of the sternum. Place the heel of one hand there, with the other hand on top of the first. Interlock the fingers of both hands and lift them to ensure that pressure is not applied over the patient's ribs. Do not apply any pressure over the upper abdomen or bottom tip of the sternum.

- **Aim to depress the sternum approximately 4-5cm** (or 1/3 of the chest depth) and apply only enough pressure to achieve this.
- The pressure should be firm, controlled, and applied vertically. Erratic or violent action is dangerous.
- About the same time should be spent in the compression phase as in the released phase.

Breathing

- Give 30 chest compressions before giving TWO ventilations.
- Use an inspiratory time of 1s and sufficient volume to make the chest rise.
- Add supplemental oxygen as soon as it is available.
- Once the airway is secured give uninterrupted compressions at 100/min and simultaneously ventilate the lungs at a rate of 10 breaths/min.

Application of defibrillation pads

- Analyse the rhythm using 'quick-look' paddles or self-adhesive pads as soon as is possible.
- Apply self-adhesive defibrillation pads over the sternum and vertically in the mid-axillary line.
- Don't interrupt chest compressions until you are ready to assess the rhythm.
- Defibrillation is indicated for VF/VT.

Suspected cervical spine injury

- Despite the risk of spinal cord damage, untreated cardiorespiratory arrest will kill the patient.
- Potential secondary damage will be minimised by in-line immobilisation of the C-spine.
- Try to use a jaw thrust and/or a Guedel airway to open the airway rather than tilting the neck.
- Avoid placing the patient in the recovery position.

Witnessed monitored VT/VF arrest

- Check the carotid pulse.
- Consider a single precordial thump.
- If a defibrillator is immediately available, give a single 360J shock.
- Start CPR immediately after delivery of the shock without pausing to assess pulse or heart rhythm.

At-risk patients

- Collapsed patients with signs of life (breathing and a pulse) often require urgent medical assessment and intervention to prevent a cardiorespiratory arrest.
- Give 100% oxygen, obtain IV access, and establish ECG, SpO_2, BP, RR, temperature monitoring.
- Look for correctable pathophysiology/biochemistry and establish higher dependency care.

Reference: Resuscitation Council (UK) Guidelines 2005. *http://www.resus.org.uk*

Adult Advanced Life Support (ALS)

2005 Guideline changes

- Shockable rhythms (VF/pulseless VT) should be treated with a SINGLE shock followed by immediate resumption of CPR (**30:2 ratio**) for 2 mins.
- Reassess the rhythm and feel for a pulse AFTER 2 mins of CPR.
- All monophasic shocks are delivered at 360J.
- Biphasic shocks should be 150-200J (1st shock), 150-360J thereafter.
- Treat fine VF as asystole.
- Give adrenaline 1mg urgently for PEA/asystole, then every 3-5 mins.
- Give adrenaline 1mg just before 3rd, 5th, 7th shocks, etc. for VF/VT.
- If VT/VF persists after 3 shocks, give amiodarone 300mg by bolus injection OR lidocaine 1mg/kg.

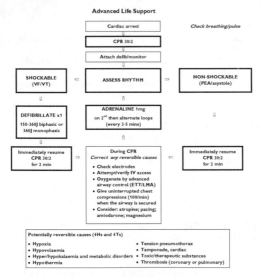

Advanced Life Support

Cardiac arrest — *Check breathing/pulse*

CPR 30:2

Attach defib/monitor

ASSESS RHYTHM

SHOCKABLE (VF/VT)

NON-SHOCKABLE (PEA/asystole)

DEFIBRILLATE x1
150-360J biphasic or
360J monophasic

ADRENALINE 1mg
on 2nd then alternate loops
(every 3-5 mins)

Immediately resume CPR 30:2 for 2 min

Immediately resume CPR 30:2 for 2 min

During CPR
Correct any reversible causes
- Check electrodes
- Attempt/verify IV access
- Oxygenate by advanced airway control (ETT/LMA)
- Give uninterrupted chest compressions (100/min) when the airway is secured
- Consider: atropine; pacing; amiodarone; magnesium

Potentially reversible causes (4Hs and 4Ts)
- Hypoxia
- Hypovolaemia
- Hyper/hypokalaemia and metabolic disorders
- Hypothermia
- Tension pneumothorax
- Tamponade, cardiac
- Toxic/therapeutic substances
- Thrombosis (coronary or pulmonary)

Defibrillation

- For monophasic defibrillators, all shocks should be delivered at 360J.
- For biphasic defibrillators, follow the manufacturer's recommendations. If in any doubt, use 200J initially.
- Electrode polarity is unimportant. Use defibrillation pads to improve electrical contact. One pad is placed to the right of the sternum below the clavicle, the other over the lower left ribs in the mid-axillary line (level with the V6 ECG electrode), avoiding placement over the breast tissue in females. Put the long axis of this pad vertical and make sure it is lateral to the cardiac apex.
- Don't attempt to re-position pads that have already been stuck on the chest—it is more important to deliver the shock quickly.

- Remove transdermal patches to prevent arcing, and place defibrillator pads/paddles 12–15cm away from implanted pacemakers.
- For safety reasons, charge the defibrillator only when the paddles are in contact with the patient. Hold the oxygen mask away from the patient during actual defibrillation, but leave bag connected to ETT.
- Recheck rhythm trace on monitor immediately prior to shock delivery.
- It is the responsibility of the defib operator to visually check that everyone is clear and to state STAND CLEAR prior to delivery of each shock.
- VT and pulseless VT are the commonest causes of reversible cardiac arrest in adults. These are the most 'recoverable' rhythms and it is therefore always worthwhile persisting with CPR whilst they are present. However, successful resuscitation does depend on *early defibrillation*. BLS, IV access, and airway control should not delay delivery of shocks.
- Resume CPR **IMMEDIATELY** after delivering a shock. Delay pulse/rhythm checks for 2mins.

Ventilations

- Once the trachea is intubated, chest compressions should continue uninterrupted (except for pulse checks and defibrillation) at a rate of 100/min whilst ventilations are administered simultaneously at a rate of 10/min.
- A pause in chest compressions allows coronary perfusion pressure to fall substantially and is followed with a delay before the original perfusion pressure is restored after ECM is recommenced.

Adrenaline

- Give adrenaline as soon as IV access is secured for PEA/asystole or after a second shock for VF/VT. Give 1mg every 3–5mins during an arrest.

Atropine

- Give atropine 3mg IV ONCE for slow PEA (rate <60/min)/asystole.
- Consider calcium chloride 10ml 10% slow IV if PEA is thought to be caused by hyperkalaemia, hypocalcaemia, overdose of Ca channel blockers, or magnesium.

Anti-arrhythmics

- Amiodarone should be considered just prior to a 4th shock (300 mg IV bolus followed by 5% dextrose 20ml flush if given peripherally). A further dose of 150mg may be given for recurrent or refractory VF/pulseless VT, followed by an infusion of 900mg over 24h.
- Consider lidocaine 1mg/kg as an ALTERNATIVE treatment.
- Give magnesium sulphate 8mmol (4ml 50% solution) for refractory VF if patient has hypomagnesaemia (e.g. diuretic induced), or torsade de pointes, or digoxin toxicity.
- Bretylium is no longer recommended.

Bicarbonate

- Consider bicarbonate 50mmol in the presence of hyperkalaemia or tricyclic antidepressant overdose.
- Remember that $HCO_3^- + H^+ \Leftrightarrow H_2O + CO_2$, therefore bicarbonate administration requires an increase in minute ventilation. Check ABGs before repeating the dose.

Reference: Resuscitation Council (UK) Guidelines 2005. *http://www.resus.org.uk*

Severe bradycardia

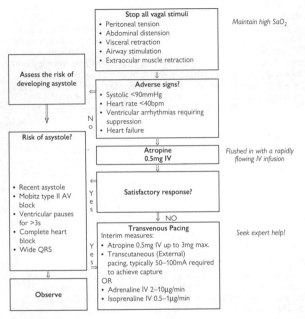

Despite anticholinergic treatment
(see also p86)

Stop all vagal stimuli
- Peritoneal tension
- Abdominal distension
- Visceral retraction
- Airway stimulation
- Extraocular muscle retraction

Maintain high SaO₂

Adverse signs?
- Systolic <90mmHg
- Heart rate <40bpm
- Ventricular arrhythmias requiring suppression
- Heart failure

Assess the risk of developing asystole   ← No

Atropine 0.5mg IV

Flushed in with a rapidly flowing IV infusion

Risk of asystole?   Yes

- Recent asystole
- Mobitz type II AV block
- Ventricular pauses for >3s
- Complete heart block
- Wide QRS

Satisfactory response?   Yes

↓ NO

Transvenous Pacing
Interim measures:
- Atropine 0.5mg IV up to 3mg max.
- Transcutaneous (External) pacing, typically 50–100mA required to achieve capture
OR
- Adrenaline IV 2–10µg/min
- Isoprenaline IV 0.5–1µg/min

Seek expert help!

Observe

Notes

- A transvenous pacing wire can be passed via a Swan Introducer.
- Third degree atrio-ventricular block and second degree Möbitz type II AV block will result in significant bradycardia, haemodynamic instability, and the possibility of asystole. Other significant risk factors for asystole include a recent episode of asystole or ventricular pauses of >3s.
- Indications for referral for preoperative pacing:
  - Second degree AV block—Möbitz type II or 2:1 block
  - Complete heart block
  - Symptomatic sinus node disease
  - Asymptomatic bundle branch block, bifascicular, trifascicular and first degree heart block are not indications for preoperative pacing. Pacing is not usually required for Möbitz type I second degree AV block (Wenckebach) unless the patient is symptomatic.

Atrial fibrillation (See also p82)

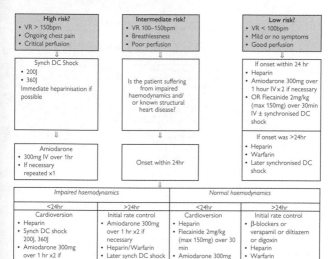

High risk?	Intermediate risk?	Low risk?
• VR > 150bpm • Ongoing chest pain • Critical perfusion	• VR 100–150bpm • Breathlessness • Poor perfusion	• VR < 100bpm • Mild or no symptoms • Good perfusion

High risk →

Synch DC Shock
• 200J
• 360J
Immediate heparinisation if possible

↓

Amiodarone
• 300mg IV over 1hr
• If necessary repeated ×1

Intermediate risk →

Is the patient suffering from impaired haemodynamics and/or known structural heart disease?

↓

Onset within 24hr

Low risk →

If onset within 24 hr
• Heparin
• Amiodarone 300mg over 1 hour IV ×2 if necessary
• OR Flecainide 2mg/kg (max 150mg) over 30min IV ± synchronised DC shock

If onset was >24hr
• Heparin
• Warfarin
• Later synchronised DC shock

↓

Impaired haemodynamics		Normal haemodynamics	
<24hr	>24hr	<24hr	>24hr
Cardioversion • Heparin • Synch DC shock 200J, 360J • Amiodarone 300mg over 1 hr ×2 if necessary	Initial rate control • Amiodarone 300mg over 1 hr ×2 if necessary • Heparin/Warfarin • Later synch DC shock	Cardioversion • Heparin • Flecainide 2mg/kg (max 150mg) over 30 min • Amiodarone 300mg over 1 hr ×2 if necessary • Synch DC shock	Initial rate control • β-blockers or verapamil or diltiazem or digoxin • Heparin • Warfarin • Later synch DC shock

Notes

- At risk patients include those with pre-existing electrolyte disturbance, acidosis, ischaemic heart disease, mitral valve disease, thyrotoxicosis, undergoing cardiothoracic surgery, central line insertion.
- Check CVP line tip and withdraw from right atrium if necessary.
- Check electrolytes and correct if necessary.
- Serum therapeutic range for digoxin = 0.8–2.0µg/l.
- Do not administer verapamil to patients on β-blockers.

UK Resuscitation Council Guidelines 2001. http://www.resus.org.uk
European Resuscitation Council Guidelines 2000. http://www.erc.edu

Narrow complex tachycardia (see also p801)

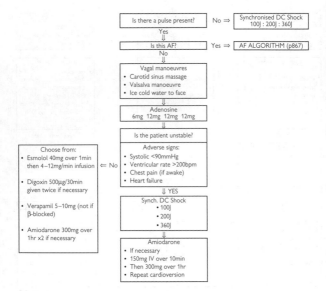

Is there a pulse present? — No ⟹ Synchronised DC Shock 100J : 200J : 360J

⇓ Yes

Is this AF? — Yes ⟹ AF ALGORITHM (p867)

⇓ No

Vagal manoeuvres
- Carotid sinus massage
- Valsalva manoeuvre
- Ice cold water to face

⇓

Adenosine
6mg 12mg 12mg 12mg

⇓

Is the patient unstable?

Adverse signs:
- Systolic <90mmHg
- Ventricular rate >200bpm
- Chest pain (if awake)
- Heart failure

⇐ No

Choose from:
- Esmolol 40mg over 1min then 4–12mg/min infusion
- Digoxin 500µg/30min given twice if necessary
- Verapamil 5–10mg (not if β-blocked)
- Amiodarone 300mg over 1hr x2 if necessary

⇓ YES

Synch. DC Shock
- 100J
- 200J
- 360J

⇓

Amiodarone
- If necessary
- 150mg IV over 10min
- Then 300mg over 1hr
- Repeat cardioversion

Notes
- Exclude light anaesthesia/inadequate analgesia.
- Narrow complex tachycardia with adverse signs (systolic BP <90mmHg; VR >200bpm; ischaemia) requires urgent **synchronised** DC shock.
- Differentiating narrow from broad complex tachycardia can be difficult, especially at high ventricular rates. Vagal manoeuvres or adenosine should slow A-V conduction of an SVT but not a VT.
- Theophylline interacts with adenosine and tends to block its effect.
- Dipyridamole and carbimazole potentiate the effects of adenosine.
- Adenosine should be used with caution in WPW syndrome and should be avoided in asthmatics.
- Atrial fibrillation now has its own algorithm (p867).
- Verapamil should not be administered in the presence of β-blockade.
- Serum therapeutic range for digoxin = 0.8–2.0µg/l.

Broad complex tachycardia

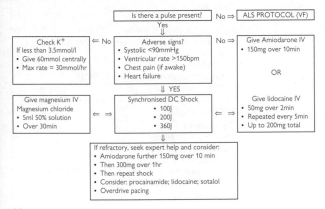

Notes

- Broad complex tachycardia with adverse signs (systolic BP <90mmHg; VR >150bpm; ischaemia) requires urgent synchronised DC shock.
- Secondary treatment is aimed at stabilising sinus rhythm and preventing recurrence (antiarrhythmics and electrolyte correction).
- Torsade de pointes is a polymorphic form of VT characterised by beat-to-beat variation, a constantly changing axis, and a prolonged QT interval. Treat with magnesium 2g IV and correct any electrolyte abnormalities such as hypokalaemia.
- If the patient is not adversely affected by the tachyarrhythmia, correct electrolytes whilst giving antiarrhythmics.

Severe hypotension in theatre

Consider	**Patient:**
	Hypovolaemia
	Obstructed venous return
	Raised intrathoracic pressure including tension pneumothorax
	Anaphylaxis
	Embolus (gas/air/thrombus/cement/fat/ amniotic fluid)
	Primary pump failure/tachyarrhythmia
	Systemic sepsis
	Technique:
	Measurement error
	Excessive depth of anaesthesia
	High regional block (including unexpected central spread from peribulbar/interscalene etc)
	Iatrogenic drug error including LA toxicity, barbiturates + porphyria
Action	100% oxygen; check surgery/blood loss; check ventilation; reduce volatile; lift legs (if feasible); IV fluid challenge; vasoconstrictors/inotropes.
Investigations	ECG; CXR; ABGs; cardiac enzymes.

Risk factors

- Untreated or 'white coat' hypertension preoperatively.
- Preoperative fluid deficit (dehydration, D&V, blood loss).
- Mediastinal/hepatic/renal surgery (blood loss and caval compression).
- Pre-existing myocardial disease/dysrhythmia.
- Multiple trauma.
- Sepsis.
- Carcinoid syndrome (bradykinin).

Differential diagnosis

- Measurement error: palpate the distal pulse manually whilst repeating non-invasive BP; check when pulsation returns against the monitor deflation figure. Invasive BP—check the transducer height.
- Check peripheral perfusion: warm peripheries suggest excessive anaesthesia (GA/regional) or sepsis.
- Suspect tension pneumothorax (particularly following central line insertion) if IPPV and trachea shifted away from a hyper-resonant lung field with diminished breath sounds. Neck veins may be engorged. Treat immediately by decompressing the pleural cavity with an open cannula placed in the 2nd intercostal space in the mid-clavicular line.
- Suspect hypovolaemia if the patient has a HR >100bpm, RR >20bpm, capillary return >2s, cool peripheries, collapsed veins, a narrow and peaked arterial line trace, or marked respiratory swing to either CVP or arterial line trace. Dehydration if the patient is thirsty, has a dry

tongue, is producing dark concentrated urine, and has globally elevated blood cell, urea, creatinine, and electrolyte values.
- Suspect cardiac failure if the patient has HR >100bpm, RR >20bpm, engorged central veins, capillary return >2s, cool peripheries, pulmonary oedema, worsening SaO_2 with fluid challenge.
- Suspect air or gas embolus if the patient had a pre-existing low CVP and open venous bed. Signs are variable but may include sudden ↓$ETCO_2$, ↓SaO_2, loss of palpable pulse, PEA, and rise in CVP.
- Suspect fat embolus or cement reaction in the presence of multiple bony injuries or long bone intramedullary surgery.
- Iatrogenic drug response: histamine release or wrong dilution
- High central neural blockade may be heralded by Horner's syndrome (small pupil, ptosis, stuffy nose, anhydrosis).
- Anaphylaxis—cardiovascular collapse 88%, erythema 45%, bronchospasm 36%, angio-oedema 24%, rash 13%, urticaria 8.5%.

Immediate management
- **ABC** . . . Check what the surgeons are doing (caval compression/blood loss); prevent further losses by clamp or direct pressure. Administer high FiO_2. Maintenance of organ perfusion and oxygenation is more important than achieving blood pressure alone. BP = SVR × CO therefore improvement in cardiac output may help ameliorate low perfusion pressure:
- **'Optimise preload'** (check initial CVP if already sited, change in CVP is more informative than actual CVP). Lifting the legs returns blood into the central venous compartment and also increases afterload.
Fluid challenge of 10ml/kg crystalloid/colloid using a pressure infusor. Assess response (BP/HR/CVP) and repeat if appropriate.
- **Increase contractility:** ephedrine 6mg IV (mixed direct and indirect action); adrenaline 10µg IV ($\beta_{1,2}$ and α activity); consider calcium slowly IV (up to 10ml of 10% calcium chloride).
- **Systemic vasoconstriction** (NB α-agonists increase perfusion pressure but may reduce cardiac output). Metaraminol 1–2mg IV; phenylephrine 0.25–0.5mg IV; adrenaline 10µg IV.

Subsequent management
- Correct acidosis to improve myocardial response to inotropes. Check ABGs and correct respiratory acidosis first. If a severe metabolic acidosis exists (art pH <7.1, base excess <−10) consider using bicarbonate 50mmol (50ml of 8.4% sodium bicarbonate).
- Maintenance infusion of vasoconstrictor (e.g adrenaline or noradrenaline) or inotrope (e.g dobutamine) if required.

Other considerations
- Adrenaline 1:10 000 = 100µg/ml. 1 in 10 dilution results in a 1:100 000 solution (10µg/ml).
- Patients taking β-blockers may not demonstrate a tachycardia despite significant hypovolaemia.

Severe hypertension in theatre

Consider	Inadequate depth of anaesthesia/analgesia
	Measurement error
	Hypoxia/hypercapnia
	Iatrogenic drug error
	Pre-eclampsia
	Raised intracranial pressure
	Thyroid storm
	Phaeochromocytoma
Action	Stop surgery until controlled; confirm readings; increase depth of anaesthesia; analgesia; vasodilators; β-blockade; α-blockade.
Investigations	ECG; cardiac enzymes; TFTs; 24hr urinary catecholamine excretion.

Risk factors

- Untreated or 'white coat' hypertension preoperatively (increased lability).
- Aortic surgery (cross clamp may ↑↑SVR).
- Drugs: MAOIs (+pethidine); ketamine; ergometrine.
- Family history of Multiple Endocrine Neoplasia (type 2) syndrome, medullary thyroid carcinoma, Conn's syndrome.
- Acute head injury.

Differential diagnosis

- Hypoxia/hypercarbia: go through ABC and check for patient colour and SaO_2.
- Inadequate depth of anaesthesia: check volatile agent concentration; sniff test (smell gases); check TIVA pump, line, and IV cannula.
- Inadequate analgesia: if in doubt administer alfentanil 10–20µg/kg and observe effect.
- Measurement error: palpate the distal pulse manually whilst repeating an NIBP; check when pulsation returns against the monitor deflation figure. Invasive BP—check the transducer height.
- Iatrogenic drug response: cocaine, wrong drug such as ephedrine, methoxamine etc. or wrong dilution (remember surgical drugs, e.g. adrenaline with LA, Moffet's solution, phenylephrine).
- Pre-eclampsia: If over 20wk pregnant, check for proteinuria, platelet count ± clotting studies, and LFTs.
- Thyroid storm causing elevated T_4 and T_3 levels.[1]
- Phaeochromocytoma[2] causing elevated plasma noradrenaline levels. Adrenaline will also cause tachydysrhythmias.
- Cushing response = hypertension and reflex bradycardia (baroreceptor mediated). This intracranially mediated response maintains cerebral perfusion in the presence of ↑ICP (see below).

Immediate management

- **ABC** . . . Assuming this is not a physiological response to a correctable cause, the overall aim of symptomatic management is to prevent hypertensive stroke or subendocardial ischaemia/infarct. Apart from increasing the depth of anaesthesia and analgesia (systemic or regional), treatment options at cardiovascular effector/receptor level include:
- **Vasodilators** (may cause tachycardia):
  ↑isoflurane concentration, this is most rapidly achieved by simultaneously increasing fresh gas flow.
  Hydralazine 5mg slow IV every 15min.
  GTN (50mg/50ml start at 3ml/hr and titrate to BP) or SNP.
  Magnesium sulphate 2–4g slow IV (8–16mmol) over 10min, followed by infusion of 1g/hr.
- **β-blockade** (particularly in the presence of ↑HR or dysrhythmias):
  Esmolol 25–100mg then 50–200µg/kg/min. (Note that esmolol is supplied as 10mg/ml and 250mg/ml solutions.)
  Labetalol 5–10mg IV prn (1–2ml increments from a 100mg/20ml ampoule). β:α block ratio = 7:1.
- **α-blockade** (particularly in the presence of normal or ↓HR):
  Phentolamine 1mg IV prn (10mg ampoule made up to 10ml, in 1ml increments).

Subsequent management

- For intense analgesia try remifentanil 0.25–0.5µg/kg/min titrated to BP
- Check for myocardial damage with an ECG, serial cardiac enzymes including CKMB and/or troponins.
- Thyroid function tests, 24hr urine collection for noradrenaline, adrenaline and dopamine excretion.

Other considerations

- Hypertension in the presence of raised intracranial pressure requires CT head and urgent neurosurgical intervention. Maintain MAP >80mmHg, normocarbia, head-up tilt, unobstructed SVC drainage, low airway pressures, and good oxygenation. Consider mannitol 0.5g/kg. Bradycardia can be treated with anticholinergics.

1 Farling PA (2000). Thyroid disease. *British Journal of Anaesthesia*, **85**, 15–28.
2 Prys-Roberts C (2000). Phaeochromocytoma. *British Journal of Anaesthesia*, **85**, 44–57.

Severe hypoxia in theatre

Consider	**Hypoxic gas mixture:** • Incorrect flowmeter settings • Second gas effect (especially on extubation) • Oxygen failure • Anaesthetic machine error **Failure to ventilate:** • Ventilatory depression or narcosis (NB regional block after opioids) • Inadequate IPPV • Disconnection • Misplaced ETT (oesophagus/endobronchial) • Obstruction to the airway, ETT, filter, mount, circuit etc. • ↑airway resistance (laryngospasm, bronchospasm, anaphylaxis) • ↓FRC (pneumothorax, ↑intra-abdominal pressure, morbid obesity) **Shunt:** • Atelectasis • Airway secretions • ↓Hypoxic pulmonary vasoconstriction (vasodilators or β_2 agonists) • CCF with pulmonary oedema • Aspiration of gastric contents • Pre-existing pathology (e.g. VSD, ASD + ↓SVR with reversal of flow) **Poor oxygen delivery:** • Systemic hypoperfusion (hypovolaemia, sepsis) • Embolus gas/air/thrombus/ cement/fat/amniotic fluid) • Local problems (cold limb, Raynaud's, sickle) **Increased oxygen demand:** • Sepsis • Malignant hyperthermia
Action	100% oxygen; check FiO_2; expose patient and check for central cyanosis; check ventilation bilaterally; hand ventilate on a simple system giving 3–4 large breaths initially to recruit alveoli; secure airway; endotracheal suction; initially remove any PEEP; give adrenaline if accompanied by poorly palpable pulses.
Investigations	Capnography; CXR; ABGs; CVP ± PCWP; echocardiography.

Risk factors

- Reduced FRC (obesity, intestinal obstruction, pregnancy) reduces oxygen reserves
- Failure to preoxygenate exacerbates any airway difficulties at induction
- Laryngospasm can result in negative pressure pulmonary oedema
- Head and neck surgery (shared access to the airway) increases the risk of undetected disconnection
- History of congenital heart disease or detection of a heart murmur (left to right communication)
- Chronic lung disease
- Sickle cell disease
- Methaemoglobinaemia (interpreted as deoxyhaemoglobin by pulse oximeters).

Differential diagnosis

- FiO_2: Use an oxygen analyser at all times.
- Ventilation: Cross-check rise and fall of chest with auscultation over stomach and in both axillae, capnograph trace, measured expired tidal volume, and airway pressure.
- Measurement error: does the patient appear cyanosed? Beware in anaemia when 5g/dl deoxyhaemoglobin may not be visible.
- Aspiration/airway secretions: Auscultate and aspirate using tracheal suction catheter ± litmus paper.
- Suspect tension pneumothorax (particularly following central line insertion) if IPPV and trachea shifted away from a hyper-resonant lung field with diminished breath sounds. Neck veins may be engorged. Treat immediately by decompressing the pleural cavity with an *open* cannula placed in the 2nd intercostal space in the mid-clavicular line.
- Suspect hypovolaemia if the patient has a HR>100bpm, RR>20bpm, capillary return >2s, cool peripheries, collapsed veins, a narrow and peaked arterial line trace, or marked respiratory swing to either CVP or arterial line trace.
- Suspect cardiac failure if the patient has HR>100bpm, RR>20bpm, engorged central veins, capillary return >2s, cool peripheries, pulmonary oedema, worsening SaO_2 with fluid challenge.
- Suspect air or gas embolus if the patient had a pre-existing low CVP and open venous bed. Signs are variable but may include sudden ↓$ETCO_2$, ↓SaO_2, loss of palpable pulse, PEA/EMD, and subsequent rise in CVP.
- Suspect fat embolus or cement reaction in the presence of multiple bony injuries or long bone intramedullary surgery.
- Malignant hyperthermia: especially if accompanied by ↑$ETCO_2$, ↑RR, ↑HR, ↑ectopics.
- Anaphylaxis—cardiovascular collapse 88%, erythema 45%, bronchospasm 36%, angio-oedema 24%, rash 13%, urticaria 8.5%.

Immediate management

- **ABC** . . . Expose the chest, all the breathing circuit, and all airway connections. Administer 100% O_2 by manual ventilation—at least 3–4 large breaths initially will help to recruit collapsed alveoli (and gives continuous tactile feedback about the state of the airway). If no improvement:
- **Confirm FiO$_2$:** If there is any doubt about inspired oxygen concentration from the anaesthetic machine, use a separate cylinder supply (as a last resort use room air via a self-inflating bag = 21% O_2).
- **Misplaced ETT**—Cross-check rise and fall of chest with auscultation over stomach and in both axillae and the capnograph trace.
- **Ventilation problem:** Simplify the breathing system until the problem is removed i.e. switch to bag rather than the ventilator, use a Bain circuit instead of the circle system, try a self-inflating bag, + mask rather than ETT etc.
- **Diagnosis of the source of a leak or obstruction:** Is not as important initially as oxygenation of the patient. Make the patient safe first then use a systematic approach. The fastest way to isolate the problem is probably by division. For instance, does breaking the circuit at the ETT connector leave the problem on the patient side or the anaesthetic machine side?
- **Severe right to left shunt:** Severe hypoxia occurs when blood starts flowing through a congenital heart defect in the presence of low SVR, thus bypassing the pulmonary circulation. The resultant hypoxaemia then exacerbates the problem by causing hypoxic pulmonary vasoconstriction which increases PVR and increases the tendency for blood to shunt across the cardiac defect. Treatment is therefore twofold:
  1) Increase SVR—by lifting the legs and giving adrenaline and IV fluid, especially in sepsis
  2) Minimise PVR—by removing PEEP, avoid high intrathoracic pressure, and maximise FiO$_2$
- **Bronchospasm:** Eliminate ETT obstruction by sounding ETT with a gum elastic bougie. Treat by increasing volatile agent concentration, IV salbutamol (250µg)—see Status asthmaticus (p884).

Other considerations

- In chronic bronchitis the bronchial circulation can shunt up to 10% of cardiac output.
- The foramen ovale remains patent in 20–30% of patients but is normally kept closed because left atrial pressure is usually higher than right atrial pressure. IPPV, PEEP, breath holding, CCF, thoracic surgery, or PE can reverse the pressure gradient and result in shunt.

Severe laryngospasm

Condition	Acute glottic closure by the vocal cords
Presentation	Crowing or absent inspiratory sounds and marked tracheal tug
Immediate action	Avoid painful stimuli; 100% oxygen; CPAP; jaw thrust; remove irritants from the airway; deepen anaesthesia, Larsen's manoeuvre
Follow up action	Muscle relaxation if intractable
Also consider	Bronchospasm Laryngeal trauma/airway oedema (especially if no leak with paediatric ETT) Recurrent laryngeal nerve damage Tracheomalacia Inhaled foreign body Epiglottitis; croup

Risk factors
- Barbiturate induction or light anaesthesia especially in anxious patients
- Intense surgical stimulation: anal stretch; cervical dilatation; incision and drainage of abscesses
- Extubation of a soiled airway
- Thyroid surgery
- Hypocalcaemia (neuromuscular irritability)
- Multiple crowns (inhaled foreign body).

Immediate management
- Remove the stimulus that precipitated the laryngospasm.
- Check that the airway is clear of obstruction or potential irritants.
- Give high concentration oxygen with the expiratory valve of the circuit closed and maintain a close seal by mask with two hands if necessary to maintain CPAP. The degree of CPAP can be controlled by intermittently relaxing the airway seal at the level of the mask.
- If the laryngospasm has occurred at induction, it may be relieved by deepening anaesthesia using further increments of propofol (disadvantage = potential ventilatory depression) or by increasing the volatile agent concentration (disadvantage = irritation of the airway, less so with sevoflurane, more with isoflurane). Don't use nitrous oxide, it will decrease oxygen reserves.
- If the laryngospasm fails to improve, remove any airways that may be stimulating the pharynx.
- Suxamethonium 0.25–0.5mg/kg will relieve laryngospasm. If IV access is impossible, consider giving 2–4mg/kg IM or SL.

Subsequent management
- Monitor for evidence of pulmonary oedema.
- CPAP may have inflated the stomach with gas so decompress it with an orogastric tube and recover the patient in the lateral position.

Other considerations
- Risk of laryngospasm may be reduced by co-induction with IV opioids, IV lidocaine, or by topical lidocaine spray prior to laryngoscopy (don't use more than 4mg/kg).
- Unilateral recurrent laryngeal nerve trauma results in paralysis of one vocal cord and causes hoarseness, ineffective cough and potential to aspirate. Bilateral vocal cord paralysis is more serious, leading to stridor on extubation—this may mimic laryngospasm but doesn't get better with standard airway manoeuvres. The patient will require re-intubation and possibly tracheostomy.
- Tracheomalacia is likely to cause more stridor with marked negative inspiratory pressure so treat initially with CPAP. Reconstructive surgery may be necessary.

Air/gas embolism

Condition	Venous gas produces airlock in RV and obstructs pulmonary capillaries
Presentation	↓ETCO$_2$, ↓SaO$_2$, loss of palpable pulse, PEA/EMD, ↑CVP then ↓CVP.
Immediate action	Remove source of embolus; flood wound; compress drainage veins
Follow up action	↑venous pressure; turn off N$_2$O; left lateral head down tilt; CVS support
Investigations	Auscultation; Doppler; ECG; CXR
Also consider	Breathing circuit disconnection (loss of ETCO$_2$ trace and ↓SaO$_2$)
	Pulseless cardiac arrest—other causes of PEA/EMD (4Ts & 4Hs)
	Cement reaction
	Pulmonary embolism of thrombus
	Amniotic fluid embolus

Risk factors
- Patient: spontaneous ventilation (negative central venous pressure); patent foramen ovale (risk of paradoxical emboli).
- Anaesthesia: hypovolaemia; any open vascular access point; operation site higher than heart; pressurised infusions.
- Orthopaedic surgery: multiple trauma; long bone surgery—especially intramedullary nailing; hip surgery.
- General surgery: laparoscopic procedures; hysterectomy; neck surgery; vascular surgery.
- ENT surgery: middle ear procedures.
- Neurosurgery: posterior fossa operations in the sitting position (almost historical).

Diagnosis
- 'At risk' patient, dramatic fall/loss of the ETCO$_2$ trace and fall in SaO$_2$.
- Awake patients complain of severe chest pain.
- Heart rate may rise.
- Sudden rise in CVP due to a fall in cardiac output and rise in PVR.
- Classically a 'millwheel' murmur can supposedly be heard
- Doppler ultrasound is an extremely sensitive (0.25ml air!) but possibly unavailable diagnostic tool.
- PEA/EMD arrest may occur. ECG may show signs of acute ischaemia e.g. ST segment depression >1mm.
- It is claimed that symptoms/signs of air embolus appear following 0.5ml/kg/min of intravascular gas.

Immediate management
- ABC...Eliminate breathing circuit disconnection; give 100% oxygen; check ECG trace and pulse.
- Prevent further gas/air from entering the circulation Get the surgeon to apply compression to major drainage vessels and flood the wound with irrigation fluid or cover with damp pack, stop reaming etc.
- Decompress any gas pressurised system/cavity e.g abdomen during laparoscopy.
- Lower the operation site to below heart level.
- Turn off N_2O (because it will expand any intravascular gas volume).
- Increase venous pressure with rapid IV infusion of fluids ± vasopressors
- If PEA/EMD arrest occurs, start chest compressions and adopt ALS protocol for non VF/VT cardiac arrest.
- Aspirate CV line. Classic teaching is to tip patient head down in left lateral position to keep the bubble in the right atrium or apex of the right ventricle until it dissolves or can be aspirated via a central line advanced into the right atrium. In practice, if there is not already a CVP line in situ aspiration is likely to be difficult.
- Moderate CPAP has been advocated as a means of rapidly increasing intrathoracic and therefore central venous pressure in the event of gas embolus. Whilst this manoeuvre may limit the extent and progress of an air embolus, it must be borne in mind that 10% of patients may have a patent foramen ovale. Sustained rise in right atrial pressure may then lead to a right-to-left shunt and paradoxical air embolism to the cerebral circulation.

Subsequent management
- Ask surgeon to apply bone wax to exposed bone edges.
- Correct any pre-existing hypovolaemia.
- Avoid nitrous oxide for the remainder of the anaesthetic, and maintain a high FiO_2.
- Perform a 12-lead ECG to look for ischaemia. Air in coronary arteries is suggestive of paradoxical air embolism.
- Consider hyperbaric therapy if available. ↑Ambient pressure (3–6 bar) will ↓volume of gas emboli.

Other considerations
Carbon dioxide is the safest gas to use for laparoscopic insufflation. It is non-flammable and more soluble than other agents. Should a gas embolus occur, it will dissolve over time. The priority of management should therefore be to limit the extent and central progress of the gas 'bubble' thereby minimising its systemic cardiovascular effect.

Aspiration

Condition	Chemical pneumonitis; foreign body obstruction and atelectasis
Presentation	Tachypnoea; tachycardia; ↓lung compliance; ↓SaO_2
Immediate action	Minimise further aspiration; secure the airway; suction.
Follow up action	100% oxygen; consider CPAP; empty the stomach.
Investigations	CXR; bronchoscopy
Also consider	Pulmonary oedema
	Embolus
	ARDS

Risk factors

- Full stomach/delayed emptying (many causes)
- Known reflux
- Raised intragastric pressure (intestinal obstruction, pregnancy, laparoscopic surgery)
- Recent trauma
- Perioperative opioids
- Diabetes mellitus
- Topically anaesthetised airway.

Diagnosis

- Clinical: auscultation may reveal wheeze and crepitations; tracheal aspirate may be acidic (but a negative finding does not exclude aspiration).
- CXR: diffuse infiltrative pattern especially in right lower lobe distribution (but often not acutely).

Immediate management

- Avoidance of general anaesthesia in high-risk situations. Use of a rapid sequence technique when appropriate.
- Administer 100% oxygen and minimise the risk of further aspirate contaminating the airway.
- If the patient is awake or nearly awake, suction the oro/nasopharynx and place in the recovery position.
- If the patient is unconscious but breathing spontaneously, apply cricoid pressure. Avoid cricoid pressure if the patient is actively vomiting (risk of oesophageal rupture) and place patient in a left lateral head down position. Intubate if tracheal suction and ventilation indicated.
- If the patient is unconscious and apnoeic intubate immediately and commence ventilation.
- Treat as an inhaled foreign body: minimise positive pressure ventilation until the ETT and airway have been suctioned and all aspirates are clear.

Subsequent management

- Empty the stomach with a large bore nasogastric tube prior to attempting extubation.
- Monitor respiratory function and arrange a CXR. Look for evidence of oedema, collapse, or consolidation.
- If SaO_2 remains 90–95%, atelectasis can be improved with CPAP (10cmH$_2$O) and chest physiotherapy.
- If SaO_2 remains <90% despite 100% oxygen, there may be solid food material obstructing part of the bronchial tree. If the patient is intubated, consider using fibre-optic/rigid bronchoscopy or bronchial lavage using saline to remove any large foreign bodies or semi-solid material from the airway. Refer to ICU postoperatively.

Other considerations

- Corticosteroids may modify the inflammatory response early after aspiration but do not alter the outcome, except by potentially interfering with the normal immune response.
- Prophylactic antibiotics are not generally given routinely (unless infected material aspirated), but may be required to treat subsequent secondary infections.
- If gastric aspirate has been buffered to pH = 7, the resulting aspiration pneumonitis is less severe, volume for volume than if it is highly acidic. However, solid food material can produce prolonged inflammation, even if the overall pH is neutral.
- Blood, although undesirable, is generally well tolerated in the airway.

Status asthmaticus[1]

Condition	Intractable bronchospasm
Presentation	↑ Airway pressure; sloping expiratory capnograph trace
Immediate action	100% oxygen; salbutamol 250µg IV/2.5mg neb; aminophylline 250mg slow IV. Magnesium sulphate 2g IV has been shown to be effective.
Follow up action	Hydrocortisone 200mg
Investigations	CXR; ABGs
Also consider	Breathing circuit obstruction Kinked ETT/cuff herniation Endobronchial intubation/tube migration Foreign body in airway Anaphylaxis Pneumothorax

Risk factors
- Asthma particularly with previous acute admissions, especially to ICU, and/or systemic steroid dependence.
- Intercurrent respiratory tract infection
- Carinal irritation by ETT.

Diagnosis
- Increased airway pressure, prolonged expiratory phase to capnograph trace.
- Central trachea with bilaterally hyperexpanded and resonant lung fields ± expiratory wheeze (absent if severe).
- Severe bronchospasm is a diagnosis of exclusion. The quickest method of ascertaining the source of increased airway resistance is to break the breathing circuit distal to all connectors/filters and to try ventilating directly with a self-inflating bag. If the inflation pressure still feels too high the problem is due to airway/ETT obstruction or reduced compliance.
- Eliminate ETT obstruction by 'sounding' the ETT with a graduated gum elastic bougie (note the distance it can be inserted down the ETT and compare it with the external tube markings).

Immediate management
- ABC . . . 100% oxygen
- Increase volatile agent concentration—sevoflurane is the least irritant and is less likely to precipitate dysrhythmias in the presence of hypercapnia (halothane most likely).
- Salbutamol 250µg IV or 2.5mg by nebuliser up to 5mg every 15min. Alternatively (as an immediate measure) administer 2–6 puffs of β-agonist inhaler into the airway by placing the device in the barrel of

a 50ml syringe. Attach the syringe by Luer lock to a 15cm length of fine bore infusion/capnograph tubing, which can then be fed directly down the ETT. The inhaler can be discharged by pressure applied via the syringe plunger. Use of the fine bore tubing decreases deposition of the drug on the ETT

- Aminophylline 250mg by slow IV injection (up to 5mg/kg)

Subsequent management

- If immediate treatment fails or is unavailable, consider ipratropium bromide (0.25mg neb up to 0.5mg 4–6-hourly), adrenaline IV boluses (10μg = 0.1ml of 1:10 000), ketamine (2mg/kg IV), magnesium (2g slow IV)
- Hydrocortisone 200mg IV
- Check the drug chart and notes for possible drug allergies to agents already administered
- Arrange CXR—check for pneumothorax and ETT tip position (withdraw if carinal)
- Check ABGs and electrolytes (prolonged use of β_2 agonists causes hypokalaemia)
- Refer to ICU.

Other considerations

- Pulsus paradoxus is a systemic blood pressure deficit measured during the spontaneous ventilatory cycle. A paradox of greater than 10mmHg (1.3kPa) indicates severe asthma.
- Gas trapping: Raised mean intrathoracic pressure may result from IPPV in the presence of severe bronchospasm. If pulse pressure falls and neck veins appear distended, consider obstructed venous return and a dependent fall in cardiac output. Intermittently disconnect the ETT from the circuit and observe the (connected) capnograph trace for evidence of prolonged expiration and return of pulse pressure.
- Ventilator setting advice during this phase: 100% oxygen, initially by hand, may need high pressures, slow rate, prolonged expiration, do not worry about CO_2 levels providing SaO_2 is adequate. May be necessary to accept reduced ventilatory rate to allow adequate expiration to occur (permissive hypercapnia).

Further reading

Asthma: a changing perspective on management (1996). *Current Anaesthesia and Critical Care*, **7**, 260–265.

---

[1] British Guideline on the management of asthma. A national clinical guideline. British Thoracic Society. Revised Edition April 2004. www.brit-thoracic.org.uk

Pulmonary oedema

Condition	↑hydrostatic pressure; ↑vascular permeability; ↓plasma colloid osmotic pressure; negative interstitial pressure; obstructed lymphatic drainage.
Presentation	Pink frothy sputum; ↑HR; ↑RR; ↓SaO$_2$; ↑CVP; ↑PCWP.
Immediate action	100% oxygen; ↓PCWP by posture.
Follow up action	Opioids; diuretics; vasodilators.
Investigations	CXR; ECG; ABG; consider PA catheter studies.
Also consider	Asthma MI ARDS Drug reaction Aspiration

Risk factors
- MI or pre-existing myocardial disease (pump failure)
- Drugs/toxins (fluid overload—especially in renal failure and the elderly, drug reaction, myocardial depression)
- Aspiration (chemical pneumonitis)
- Pre-existing lung disease or infection (increased capillary permeability)
- Malnutrition (low oncotic pressure)—rare
- Acute head injury or intracranial pathology (neurogenic)
- Severe laryngospasm or airway obstruction (negative intrathoracic pressure)
- Severe hypertension; LVF; mitral stenosis (high pulmonary vascular hydrostatic pressure)
- Lateral decubitus position (unilateral)
- Impairment of lymphatic drainage (e.g malignancy)
- Rapid lung expansion (e.g re-expansion of a pneumothorax)
- Following pneumonectomy.

Diagnosis
- Clinical: wheeze; pink frothy sputum; fine crackles; quiet bases; gallop rhythm; ↑JVP; liver engorgement.
- Monitors: ↑HR; ↑RR; ↓SaO$_2$; ↑airway pressure; ↑CVP; ↑PCWP (greater than 25–30mmHg).
- CXR: basal shadowing; upper lobe diversion; 'bats wing' or 'stag horn' appearance; hilar haze; bronchial cuffing; Kerley B lines; pleural effusions; septal/interlobar fluid lines.
- ECG: evidence of right heart strain; evidence of MI.

Immediate management

- ABC . . . then management depends upon the current state of the patient.
- If awake and breathing spontaneously: sit up to offload the pulmonary vasculature and improve FRC; high flow 100% oxygen via mask with reservoir bag; furosemide 50mg IV; diamorphine 5mg IV; consider using CPAP 5–10mmHg, and a vasodilator if hypertensive (e.g GTN 0.5–1.5mg SL, or 10mg transcutaneous patch. Beware of IV GTN administration in the absence of invasive BP monitoring).
- If anaesthetised and intubated: commence IPPV with PEEP (5–10cmH$_2$O) in a 15° head up position to reduce atelectasis and improve FRC; aspirate free fluid from the trachea intermittently; drug therapy as above.

Subsequent management

- Optimise fluid therapy and maintain plasma colloid oncotic pressure on the basis of serial CVP measurements. If in doubt, measure PCWP via a PA catheter.
- Consider inotropic support with a β-agonist (e.g. dobutamine) or venesection (500ml) if filling pressures remain high or signs of inadequate circulation persist.

Failed intubation

See also p928.

Condition	Patients die from failure to **oxygenate** NOT failure to intubate
Presentation	1 in 65 patients is likely to present difficulties with intubation
Immediate action	Establish a patent airway with 100% oxygen
Follow up action	Do you need to intubate? Should you continue or wake the patient up?
Investigations	Capnograph; Negative pressure ETT aspiration (bladder syringe); fibre-optic scope,
Also consider	Regional anaesthesia or awake fibre-optic intubation

Diagnosis of misplacement

- Retain a high index of suspicion after difficult intubation.
- Suspect oesophageal placement if you cannot confirm: normal breath sounds in both axillae and absent sounds over the stomach; rise AND fall of chest; normal $ETCO_2$ trace; normal airway pressure cycle.
- The trachea is a rigid structure, the oesophagus is not. If negative pressure is applied to the ETT, failure to aspirate air (e.g. with a bladder syringe directly attached to the ETT) suggests oesophageal placement.
- Confirm ETT placement with fibrescope.
- Remember—if in doubt, pull it out and apply bag and mask ventilation.

Other considerations

- Head down left lateral position used to be advocated as a part of the failed intubation drill. However for the majority of anaesthetists, the ability to manipulate an obstructed airway will be greater with the patient left in the more familiar supine position. In a spontaneously breathing patient who is waking up the airway is often better in the lateral position. Use whichever is most effective, but keep help available to turn the patient if needed.

Immediate management

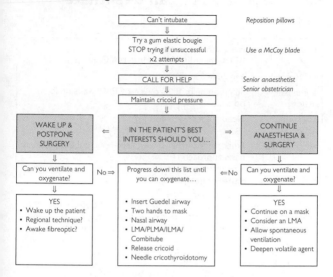

Can't intubate . . . Can't ventilate

See also p934.

Condition	Failure to oxygenate by ETT/facemask/LMA/PLMA/ILMA/Combitube
Presentation	1 in 10 000 anaesthetics
Immediate action	Summon help; 100% oxygen; CPAP; wake up if possible
Follow up action	Needle cricothyroidotomy
Also consider	Emergency tracheostomy; fibre-optic intubation; blind nasal approach

Immediate management

- Call for help, but retain your trained assistant.
- Attempt oxygenation even if it appears futile. Insert both an oral AND nasopharyngeal airway. Emergency oxygen flush. Apply a close fitting facemask with two hands and lift/dislocate the mandible firmly forwards (jaw thrust). Although an assistant may help by bag squeezing, it may be easiest to attempt ventilation by allowing an intermittent leak around the mask.
- Consider using a conventional LMA, Intubating LMA, Proseal LMA, Combitube. No single airway adjunct has clear advantages over others. This is not a time to experiment with unfamiliar devices so stick to whatever you feel comfortable with and abandon them early if they prove to be of no benefit.
- If the patient is making spontaneous effort and respiratory noise, maintain CPAP and 100% oxygen until they awake.

Subsequent management

- **Cricothyroidotomy**: The decision to attempt transtracheal oxygenation is not an easy one to make. However, remember that it is likely to take over a minute to achieve access, and even then, ability to oxygenate will be severely limited. Speed is essential in order to prevent hypoxic cardiac arrest or brain damage.
- Options are surgical cricothyroidotomy or needle cricothyroidotomy.
- Surgical cricothyroidotomy allows insertion of a cuffed tracheostomy tube but is beyond the expertise of most anaesthetists in the emergency situation.
- Extend the neck. You may find access easier if someone else does this for you and simultaneously fixes the skin by applying slight traction bilaterally to the soft tissues of the neck.
- Find the cricothyroid membrane (lies between the superiorly notched thyroid cartilage and the cricoid cartilage).

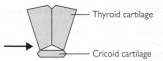

Thyroid cartilage

Cricoid cartilage

- Attach a 20ml syringe containing 10ml of saline to a large bore needle or cannula (14–16G). Advance through the cricothyroid membrane in a slightly caudally inclined direction aspirating until air bubbles freely into the syringe.
- If you have used a needle, hold it firmly in place. If you have used a cannula guard against kinking.
- There are several ways of connecting a needle/cannula to a standard breathing circuit:
  - Connect a 10ml syringe, remove the plunger, and intubate the barrel with a cuffed ETT.
  - Insert an ETT connector from a neonatal 3.5mm ETT to the hub of the needle/cannula.
  - Unscrew the capnograph tubing from the monitor, attach the Luer lock end to the hub of the needle/cannula. Take the other end and attach the sampling end (T-piece) to the common gas outlet. Use your thumb to intermittently occlude the other end of the T-piece.
  - Sanders injector or similar jetting device attached by Luer lock. beware—high pressure oxygen can cause catastrophic surgical emphysema via a misplaced cannula. Check for rise and fall of the chest wall.
- Transtracheal oxygenation by needle/cannula is a temporary emergency measure. Full ventilation is unlikely to be possible. However, there should be flow of oxygen down the bronchial tree to the alveoli.
- If there is significant oxygen leakage upwards, occlude the mouth and nose during the inspiratory phase of ventilation.
- Call urgently for an ENT surgeon to perform an emergency tracheostomy. If possible, improve transtracheal access with a 'Minitrach' or similar device. There are several easy to use commercial kits that exist based around a Seldinger method of insertion. If the patient remains paralysed attempt fibre-optic/blind nasal intubation.
- Consider transtracheal jet ventilation but stop ventilating immediately if surgical emphysema forms in the neck.

Other considerations

- Best treatment is prevention, or at least anticipation of potential airway difficulties. Avoidance of muscle relaxants is prudent until one has determined that ventilation can be achieved manually. Thorough preoxygenation will ensure that the FRC contains approximately 1 litre of oxygen rather than 0.5 litre at induction. Have the kit and personnel required for the creation of a surgical airway close at hand if you anticipate difficulties intubating.
- If the problem is an inability to achieve a seal due to the presence of a beard, quickly apply a large transparent self-adhesive dressing over the whole of the lower face. Make a large hole in it for the mouth and nostrils, and re-apply the mask ± an airway.

- If the problem is an inability to pass a small enough ETT tube down a narrowed trachea (either ETT too short or size unavailable) consider passing an Airway Exchange Catheter. This is a robust guide that resembles a white but hollow gum elastic bougie. It comes with either Luer lock or 15mm connector allowing oxygen to be passed through it into the distal airway whilst a more definitive airway is established either by railroading a larger tube over it or by surgical tracheostomy.
- Commercially available trans-tracheal needles and injectors are now widely available.
- Check that your theatres have a well-stocked difficult/failed intubation trolley available at all times.

Further reading

Benumof JL, Scheller MS (1989). The importance of transtracheal jet ventilation in the management of the difficult airway. *Anesthesiology*, **71**, 769.

Gerig HJ, Schnider T, Heidegger T (2005). Prophylactic percutaneous transtracheal catheterisation in the management of patients with anticipated difficult airways: a case series. *Anaesthesia*, **60**, 801–802.

Padkin A, McIndoe A (2000). Use of the airway exchange catheter for the patient with a partially obstructed airway. *Anaesthesia*, **55**, 87.

Malignant hyperthermia

See also p260.

Condition	Hypermetabolism due to increased skeletal muscle intracellular Ca^{2+}
Presentation	↑$ETCO_2$; ↓SaO_2; ↑HR; CVS instability; dysrhythmias; ↑Core temp
Immediate action	Stop triggers (volatile agents + suxamethonium); hyperventilate with high flow 100% oxygen; dantrolene 1–10mg/kg
Follow up action	Cool; correct DIC, acidosis/↑K^+; promote diuresis (ARF risk)
Investigations	Clotting studies, ABGs, K^+; Urine myoglobin; CK
Also consider	Rebreathing Sepsis Awareness Neuroleptic malignant syndrome Ecstasy Thyroid storm

Risk factors
- Family history.
- Exposure to suxamethonium or volatile agents (even if previous exposures were uneventful).
- Exertional heat stroke. Exercise-induced rhabdomyolysis, central core disease, scoliosis, hernias, strabismus surgery.

Diagnosis
- Sustained jaw rigidity after suxamethonium (masseter spasm).
- Unexplained tachycardia together with an unexpected rise in end-tidal CO_2 (IPPV) or minute volume (SV).
- Falling SaO_2 despite increased FiO_2.
- Cardiovascular instability, dysrhythmias especially multiple ventricular ectopics, peaked T waves on ECG.
- Generalised rigidity.
- Core temperature rise of 2°C per hour.

Immediate management
- Check ABC . . . Turn off all volatile agents, don't administer any further doses of suxamethonium.
- Hyperventilate with 100% oxygen using a high fresh gas flow to flush out volatile agent and expired CO_2.
- Tell the rest of the theatre team what the problem is. Ask for more help and obtain dantrolene immediately.

- Use a fresh breathing circuit ± a 'vapour-free' machine if it is easy to do so, but not if it results in rebreathing of expired CO_2, a low FiO_2, or delays administration of dantrolene.
- When available, give dantrolene 1mg/kg IV (it comes in 20mg ampoules so about 4 are required). Repeat.
  Usually about 2.5mg/kg is required in total, but up to 10mg/kg may be given.
- Stop surgery if feasible, otherwise maintain anaesthesia with TIVA (propofol).
- Reduce core temperature by: evaporation; ice to groins & axillae; cold fluids into IV lines, the bladder via urinary catheter, stomach via NGT, or peritoneal cavity if open.
- Check ABGs and K^+, especially if dysrhythmias occur, and correct acidosis/ hyperkalaemia where appropriate.
- Surgical team—call for senior help to conclude the operation as quickly as is safely possible.

Subsequent management
- Place invasive BP and CVP monitoring lines.
- Send a clotting screen for DIC, and serum CK assay (up to 1000 times normal).
- Send a urine sample for myoglobin estimation secondary to muscle breakdown.
- Monitor for acute renal failure and promote a diuresis with fluids and mannitol.
- Refer to the MH Investigation Unit for *in vitro* muscle contracture tests (IVCTs).

Other considerations
- Dantrolene is formulated with 3g mannitol per ampoule.
- Emptying several ampoules into a sterile dish and adding a large volume of sterile water may help mix dantrolene more rapidly.
- Follow up involves muscle biopsy under LA and *in vitro* halothane, caffeine, ryanodine and chlorocresol contracture tests.
- Beware of using bicarbonate to correct acidosis since the reaction with hydrogen ions produces an increased CO_2 load.

Further reading
Hopkins PM (2000). Malignant hyperthermia: advances in clinical management and diagnosis. *British Journal of Anaesthesia*, **85**, 118–28.

Useful contact—see also p265
UK MH Investigation Unit, Academic Unit of Anaesthesia, Clinical Sciences Building, St James' University Hospital Trust, Leeds LS9 7TF. Emergency hotline bleep 0345 333111.

Anaphylaxis

Condition	IgE mediated type B hypersensitivity reaction to an antigen resulting in histamine and serotonin release from mast cells and basophils
Presentation	Cardiovascular collapse; erythema; bronchospasm; oedema; rash
Immediate action	Remove trigger; 100% oxygen; elevate legs; adrenaline 50µg; fluids
Follow up action	Chlorphenamine 10–20mg; hydrocortisone 100–300mg; ABGs
Investigations	Plasma tryptase; urinary methylhistamine
Also consider	Primary myocardial/cardiovascular problem Latex sensitivity Airway obstruction Asthma Tension pneumothorax

Risk factors
- IV administration of the antigen.
- Note that cross-sensitivities with NSAIDs and muscle relaxants mean that previous exposure is not always necessary.
- True penicillin allergy is a reaction to the basic common structure present in most penicillins (β-lactam ring).

Diagnosis
- Cardiovascular collapse   88%
- Erythema   45%
- Bronchospasm   36%
- Angio-oedema   24%
- Rash   13%
- Urticaria   8.5%

Immediate management
- Check ABC . . . Stop the administration of any potential triggers, particularly IV agents. Muscle relaxants, antibiotics, and NSAIDs are the most frequent triggers.
- Call for help.
- Maintain the airway and give 100% oxygen.
- Lay the patient flat with the legs elevated.
- Give adrenaline in 50µg IV increments (0.5ml 1:10 000 solution) at a rate of 100µg/min until pulse pressure or bronchospasm improves. Alternatively, give adrenaline 0.5–1mg IM (repeated after 10min if necessary).
- Give IV fluid (colloid or suitable crystalloid).

Subsequent management
- Antihistamines: give chlorphenamine (Piriton®) 10–20mg by slow IV.
- Corticosteroids: give hydrocortisone 100–300mg IV.
- Catecholamine infusion as CVS instability may last several hours:
  Adrenaline 0.05–0.1µg/kg/min (= 4ml/hr of 1:10 000 or 5mg/50ml
  saline—70kg adult).
  Noradrenaline 0.05–0.1µg/kg/min (= 4ml/hr of 4mg/40ml
  5% dextrose—70kg adult).
- Check ABGs for acidosis and consider bicarbonate 0.5–1.0mmol/kg
  (8.4% solution = 1mmol/ml).
- Check for the presence of airway oedema by letting down the ETT cuff
  and confirming a leak prior to extubating.
- Consider bronchodilators (see status asthmaticus) for persistent
  bronchospasm (see p884).

Other considerations
- Investigations can wait until the patient has been stabilised. Take a
  10ml clotted blood sample 1hr after the start of the reaction to
  perform a tryptase assay. The specimen needs to be spun down and
  the serum stored at ¯20 °C.
- The anaesthetist should follow up the investigation, report reactions to
  the CSM, and arrange testing with an immunologist (see p954).

Further reading

Anaphylactic reactions associated with anaesthesia 3 (2003). Association of Anaesthetists of Great Britain and Ireland and the British Society of Allergy and Clinical Immunology.

Intra-arterial injection

Condition	Chemical endarteritis characterised by: arterial vasospasm and local release of noradrenaline; crystal deposition within the distal arteries (thiopental); subsequent thrombosis and distal ischaemic necrosis.
Presentation	Intense burning pain on injection; distal blanching; blistering.
Immediate action	Stop injection but leave the cannula *in situ* and administer 1% lidocaine 5ml, and papaverine 40mg, flush with heparinised saline.
Follow up action	Regional sympathetic blockade; anticoagulation.
Investigations	Monitor anticoagulation.
Also consider	Extravasation. Dilution error of drug administered.

Risk factors

- Antecubital lines: inadvertent cannulation of brachial artery or aberrant ulnar artery.
- Radial aspect of wrist: inadvertent cannulation of superficial branch of radial artery.
- Arterial injection is more likely to cause damage with stronger drug concentration (e.g. 5% thiopental).
- Cannula which has been inserted previously and only been flushed with saline (not painful) may present later.

Diagnosis

- Awake patients complain of intense burning pain on injection that may last for several hours.
- Blanching of the skin.
- Blistering.
- Within 2hr: oedema; hyperaesthesia; motor weakness.
- Later: signs of arterial thrombosis ± gangrene.

Immediate management

- Stop injecting!
- Principles of treatment are to dilute the irritant, reverse vasospasm, and prevent thrombosis.
- Keep the cannula in situ—you will need access to reverse local vasoconstriction within the distal arteriolar tree.
- If the drug administered was highly irritant, flush the vessel with isotonic saline or 'Hepsal'.
- Administer LA via the cannula to reduce vasospasm and reduce pain (e.g 5ml 1% lidocaine).
- Administer a vasodilator (e.g papaverine 40mg).
- Once the immediate reaction has subsided, if the hand is well perfused and pink, remove the cannula and apply sufficient pressure to the puncture site to minimise local haematoma formation.

Subsequent management
- Sympathetic blockade and anticoagulation to reduce the risk of thrombosis:
    - Sympathectomy via stellate ganglion or brachial plexus block—probably most easily achieved via the axillary approach, or
    - Guanethidine block: performed like a Bier's block (guanethidine 10–20mg IV + heparin 500U in 25–40ml saline, cuff left inflated for 20min). Guanethidine blocks α-adrenergic neurones and depletes noradrenaline stores. The effects can last for several weeks. Ask for assistance from consultant with a special interest in chronic pain since this block is also used to treat reflex sympathetic dystrophy.
    - Heparinise after achieving sympathetic blockade to minimise the risk of late arterial thrombosis.

Other considerations
Nerve supply to the arm = C_5–T_1. Sympathetic nerve supply to the arm comes from T_1 via the sympathetic chain and the stellate ganglion (fusion of the inferior cervical ganglion and the first thoracic ganglion).

Unsuccessful reversal of neuromuscular blockade

Condition	Competitive antagonism at nicotinic acetylcholine receptor of NMJ
Presentation	Uncoordinated, jerky patient movements during the recovery phase. Inability to maintain an airway OR inadequate spontaneous ventilation
Immediate action	Maintain and protect airway and provide adequate ventilation
Follow up action	Maintain anaesthesia if appropriate; correct the cause
Investigations	Nerve stimulator train-of-four, post-tetanic count; double burst stimulation
Also consider	Non-functional peripheral nerve stimulator (check the battery charge) Volatile agent concentration (maintained by hypoventilation) Hyperventilation (ETCO$_2$ <4kPa) (30mmHg) or CO$_2$ narcosis (over about 9kPa) (68mmHg) Undiagnosed head injury (examine pupils) Cerebrovascular accident

Risk factors
- Recent dose of relaxant/backflow in IVI/drug error.
- Renal and hepatic impairment causing delayed elimination of relaxant in long cases (except atracurium).
- Perioperative administration of magnesium (especially above the therapeutic range 1.25–2.5mmol/l).
- Hypothermia.
- Acidosis and electrolyte imbalance.
- Co-administration of aminoglycoside antibiotics.
- Myasthenia gravis (reduced number of receptors).
- Low levels of plasma cholinesterase (pregnancy, renal & liver disorders, hypothyroidism) or competition with drugs also metabolised by plasma cholinesterase (etomidate, ester LAs, and methotrexate).
- Abnormal plasma cholinesterase (suxamethonium apnoea).
- Ecothiopate eyedrops for glaucoma (historical—now not available on general prescription).

Diagnosis

- Uncoordinated, jerky patient movements are suggestive of inadequate reversal of neuromuscular blockade. Sustained head lift off the pillow for 5s is a good clinical indicator of adequate reversal.
- Train of four is classically measured as adductor pollicis twitches in response to supramaximal stimulation via two electrodes placed over the ulnar nerve—see p994.
- Double burst stimulation is said to be more accurate as a means of quantifying train of four ratio—see p994.
- Post-tetanic count is used to monitor deep relaxation, when the train of four will not show any twitches. Firstly establish that the peripheral nerve stimulator is actually working and has adequate battery charge. A 50Hz tetanic stimulus is applied for 5s followed by single stimuli at 1Hz. Post tetanic facilitation in the presence of non-depolarising blockade allows a number of twitches to be seen. Reversal should be possible with a count of >10.

Immediate management

- ABC . . . then check for signs of awareness, assess anaesthetic depth, and check $ETCO_2$.
- If you have already given a dose of neostigmine ensure it was adequate (0.05mg/kg) and that it did actually enter the circulation (check the IV line for backflow and the site of cannulation for swelling).
- Hypothermia, electrolyte imbalance, and acidosis will impair reversal and should be corrected.
- Aminoglycoside or Mg^{2+} induced poor reversal may improve with calcium gluconate (10ml 10%) titrated IV.

Subsequent management

- Wait patiently—this is not an emergency!
- Suspected myasthenia gravis should be confirmed postoperatively with a 'Tensilon' test.
- If the patient has suffered a period of awareness whilst paralysed, admit it, explain it, apologise, and ensure that the patient has access to professional counselling if required.

Other considerations

- A dual (phase II) blockade occurs when large amounts of suxamethonium are used and the depolarising block is gradually replaced by one of non-depolarising characteristics (fade etc.).

Paediatric Emergencies: Advanced Life Support

Adopt a SAFE approach

- **S**hout for help
- **A**pproach with care
- **F**ree the patient from immediate danger
- **E**valuate the patient's ABC

Assess the airway and breathing first. Give FIVE RESCUE BREATHS (chest seen to rise and fall) before assessing the circulation. Each breath should take about 1-1.5s. Check the carotid pulse in a child but use the brachial pulse in an infant. Feel for no more than 10s.

The most common arrest scenario in children is bradycardia proceeding to asystole—a response to severe hypoxia and acidosis. Basic life support aimed at restoring early oxygenation should therefore be a priority of management. VF is relatively uncommon, but may complicate hypothermia, tricyclic poisoning, and children with pre-existing cardiac disease.

- **All children over 1 yr** should be given basic life support at a ratio of 15:2 (compressions: ventilations) aiming for 100 compressions/min (five cycles).
- Chest compressions should be started if a central pulse cannot be palpated or the child has a pulse rate <60 bpm with poor perfusion.
- Where no vascular access is present, immediate intraosseous access is recommended.
- Once the airway has been secured, chest compressions should be continued at 100/min uninterrupted with breaths administered at a rate of 10/min.
- When circulation has been restored, ventilate the child at 12-20 breaths/min to normalise PCO_2.

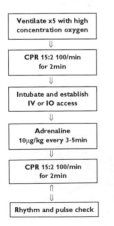

Notes : Consider the following:
- Hypoxia
- Hypovolaemia
- Hyper/hypokalaemia
- Hypothermia
- Tension pneumothorax

- Cardiac tamponade
- Toxin/drug overdose
- Thromboemboli
- Metabolic disturbances

Ventricular fibrillation or pulseless VT

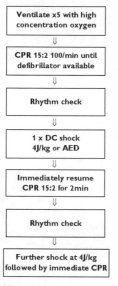

Ventilate x5 with high concentration oxygen

⇓

CPR 15:2 100/min until defibrillator available

⇓

Rhythm check

⇓

1 x DC shock 4J/kg or **AED**

⇓

Immediately resume CPR 15:2 for 2min

⇓

Rhythm check

⇓

Further shock at 4J/kg followed by immediate CPR

*adrenaline 10µg/kg **IV/IO**
every 3-5mins*

*once intubated, give
uninterrupted compressions*

Notes :
- Standard AEDs may be used in children over 8 years.
- Purpose-made paediatric pads are recommended for children aged between 1–8 years, but an unmodified adult AED may be used for children older than 1 year.
- Adrenaline 10 µg/kg = 0.1ml/kg of 1:10 000 solution.
- Consider hypokalaemia, hypothermia, and poisoning.
- Antiarrhythmic agents:
  - 1st line = amiodarone 5mg/kg IV after a third shock
  - 2nd line = lidocaine 1mg/kg IV if amiodarone is not available
  - Torsade de points: magnesium sulphate 25-50 mg/kg
  - Atropine 20mg/kg (minimum dose of 100µg) for bradycardia.

Paediatric doses and equipment[1,2,3]

Weight/BP estimation (1–10yr)
- Child's weight in kg = 2 × (Age in yr + 4)
- Normal systolic BP in mmHg = (Age in yr × 2) + 80

Airway
- ETT internal diameter in mm = (Age in yr ÷ 4) + 4
- ETT length (oral) to lips in cm = (Age in yr ÷ 2) + 12
- ETT length (nose) to lips in cm = (Age in yr ÷ 2) + 15

- LMA#1 (cuff volume 4ml)   <6.5kg
- LMA#2 (cuff volume 10ml)   6.5–20kg
- LMA#2.5 (cuff volume 14ml)   20–30kg
- LMA#3 (cuff volume 20ml)   >30kg

Estimated drug doses (see also p1105)
- Adrenaline   10µg/kg
- Aminophylline   5mg/kg
- Amiodarone   5mg/kg
- Atropine   10–20µg/kg
- Bicarbonate   1mmol/kg
- Calcium Chloride   0.2ml/kg of 10% solution slowly
- Calcium Gluconate   0.6ml/kg of 10% solution
- Cefotaxime   50mg/kg
- Dextrose (10%)   5ml/kg
- Diazepam   0.1mg/kg IV
                      0.5mg/kg PR
- Ketamine   2mg/kg
- Lidocaine   1mg/kg
- Lorazepam   0.1mg/kg recommended for status epilepticus
  (repeatable after 10min)
- Magnesium   25–50mg/kg
- Naloxone   0.1mg/kg
- Neostigmine   50µg/kg
- Paraldehyde   0.1mg/kg
- Phenytoin   20mg/kg
- Salbutamol   2.5mg nebuliser

Circulation
- Blood volume   75ml/kg   (1–10yr)
                      70ml/kg   (>10yr)
- Fluid bolus   20ml/kg

These estimations are not valid for premature infants and are intended as rough guides only.

1 UK Resuscitation Council Guidelines 2005. www.resus.org.uk
2 European Resuscitation Council Guidelines 2000. www.erc.edu
3 Pediatric Advanced Life Support Manual. American Heart Foundation 1997. ISBN 0-87493-621-7.

Paediatric emergencies: neonatal resuscitation

Condition	Acute neonatal asphyxia during the birth process
Presentation	Floppy, blue or pale, heart rate <60bpm, diminished respiratory effort
Immediate action	Open and clear airway, 5 inflation breaths (2–3s at 30cmH$_2$O)
Follow up action	Dry & warm, cardiac compressions (3:1) if <60bpm, review ventilation
Investigations	Record Apgar scores
Also consider	Hypovolaemia, diaphragmatic hernia, pneumothorax

Risk factors

- Known fetal distress; Class 1 emergency Caesarean section; meconium-stained liquor.
- Prolonged delivery; instrumental delivery; shoulder dystocia; multiple births.
- Maternal drugs: opioids, general anaesthesia for Caesarean section.
- Preterm delivery (survival is very poor if gestation <23wk and resuscitation is not recommended).

Diagnosis

- A normal newly delivered baby is pink, breathes spontaneously within 15s, has a heart rate >100bpm, has good muscle tone and is vocal.
- A baby requiring resuscitation is floppy, silent, blue or pale, has a heart rate <100bpm, and gasping, diminished or absent respiratory effort.

Apgar scores			
	0	1	2
Colour	Pale/Blue	Blue extremities	Pink
Heart rate	Absent	<100	>100
Response to stimulation	Nil	Movement	Cry
Muscle tone	Limp	Some flexion	Well flexed
Respiratory effort	Absent	Poor effort/weak cry	Good

Immediate management
- Dry and wrap baby. Keep warm.
- Open and clear airway but keep the neck in a neutral position.
- Give FIVE effective inflation breaths (2–3s at 30cmH$_2$O) of air or oxygen.
- Heart rate should increase, if so continue ventilating until spontaneous effort is adequate.
- If heart rate remains <60bpm commence chest compressions with thumbs around chest at a compression rate of 3:1 breaths.
- Reassess heart rate every 30s.

Subsequent management
- In the neonate that remains unresponsive despite oxygenation, consider intubation and drugs:

Neonate			
	40/40 gestation	**35/40 gestation**	**30/40 gestation**
Weight	3.5kg	2.5kg	1.5kg
ETT internal diameter	3.5mm	3.0mm	2.5mm
ETT length	9.5cm	8.5cm	7.5cm
Adrenaline 1/10 000 (IO/IV)	0.35–1.05ml	0.25–0.75ml	0.15–0.45ml
Sodium bicarbonate 4.2% IV	3.5–7ml	2.5–5ml	1.5–3ml
Dextrose 10% IV	17–35ml	12–25ml	7–15ml
Volume IV (O-Neg/0.9% NaCl)	35–70ml	25–50ml	15–30ml

Other considerations
- If response to resuscitation is prompt (requiring only support breaths) return baby to the parents.
- For ventilatory depression thought to be due to maternal opioids, give naloxone 200µg IM.
- Reasons to transfer to SCBU: ongoing ventilation; major congenital abnormality; prematurity.

Further reading
Newborn Life Support. Resuscitation Council (UK) Guidelines 2005.

Paediatric emergencies: collapsed septic child

Condition	Sepsis with multi-organ failure, capillary leak, and hypoperfusion.
Presentation	Fever >38 °C, ↓BP, ↑HR, ↑RR, oliguria, altered conscious level
Immediate action	100% oxygen, fluid resuscitation, inotropes, antibiotics
Follow up action	Referral to a specialist paediatric critical care unit
Investigations	FBC, Clotting, U&Es, Glucose, blood cultures
Also consider	Hypovolaemia/blood loss, anaphylaxis, poisoning, cardiac abnormality

Risk factors
- Immune deficiency, chronic illness
- Exposure to Gram positive/negative bacteria, *Listeria, Rickettsia*, herpes virus.

Diagnosis
- 'Warm shock' presents early as vasodilatation and often responds to volume resuscitation.
- 'Cold shock' is more serious with lower BP, particularly diastolic hypotension, cold peripheries, capillary refill >2s, and oliguria requiring significant circulatory support.
- Fever >38°C, altered level of consciousness, high white cell count

Immediate management
- ABC . . . 100% oxygen via a non-rebreathing mask ± ventilatory support/intubation.
- Fluid boluses of 20ml/kg crystalloid/colloid up to 100ml/kg to restore normovolaemia.
- Inotropic support with dobutamine (up to 20µg/kg/min) if fluids ineffective
- Correct hypoglycaemia with 10–20% glucose
- If IV fluid and dobutamine is ineffective at maintaining BP, consider:
  - Dopamine (up to 20µg/kg/min)
  - Adrenaline (0.1–1.0µg/kg/min)
  - Noradrenaline (0.1µg/kg/min)
- If pH <7.1 on ABGs and ventilation is adequate, correct acidosis with 8.4% sodium bicarbonate (4.2% in neonates) according to the following formula:
  Sodium bicarbonate required for full correction (mmol) = (weight in kg x 0.3 x base deficit)
  Give 50% correction first then repeat ABGs and re-assess.
- Antibiotics: cefotaxime 50mg/kg IV 6-hourly for older children or ampicillin+gentamicin for neonates (seek microbiologists or PICU advice for up to date guidelines about doses in different ages)

Subsequent management

- Obtain specialist help early. Contact the nearest regional centre/PICU department for advice.
- Consider the possibility of raised intracranial pressure (bulging fontanelle, papilloedema, altered pupils). If suspected catheterise the patient, ventilate to normocapnia, and give mannitol 0.5–1.0g/kg or furosemide 1mg/kg. Avoid LP. CT Head.
- Consider the possibility of meningitis/encephalitis. Look for fever, lethargy, irritability, vomiting, headache, photophobia, convulsions, neck stiffness, raised ICP. Look carefully for purpuric non-blanching spots.
- Consider DIC if mucosal surfaces are bleeding.
- Stabilise for transfer. A retrieval service may be provided by the receiving unit—prepare a handover.

Other considerations

- Significant capillary leakage in severe sepsis may result in pulmonary oedema secondary to fluid resuscitation. This may be reduced by using 4.5% human albumin solution.
- If drugs are required to intubate the child, anticipate an exaggerated fall in blood pressure and adjust the dose accordingly. It is wise to start inotropes and fluid resuscitation before induction.

Paediatric emergencies: major trauma

Condition	Serious injury to chest/abdomen/pelvis/spine/head
Presentation	↑HR, ↓capillary refill, ↑RR, ↓conscious level, bony/visceral injuries
Immediate action	ABCDE, 100% oxygen, 2x IVs or intraosseous access, 20ml/kg IV fluids.
Follow up action	Secondary survey, stabilise for transfer to theatre or critical care
Investigations	CXR, C-spine, ABG, ECG, G&S, blood glucose, CT head, ultrasound abdomen
Also consider	Non-accidental injury, poisoning, fitting

Risk factors
- Pedestrian/cyclist struck by vehicle, unrestrained passenger in RTA.
- Head injuries account for 40% of trauma deaths in children.
- At-risk register.

Diagnosis
- Dependent upon cause and primary mode of injury. Usually involves blood loss with resultant tachycardia and peripheral vasoconstriction. Respiratory rate increased.
- Diminished level of consciousness, respiratory/ventilatory compromise if chest injured.
- Immediately life-threatening conditions include airway obstruction, tension pneumothorax, cardiac tamponade, PEA cardiac arrest.

Immediate management
- *Airway*—100% O_2 (15l/min via non-rebreathing mask). In-line C-spine stabilisation and RSI.
- *Breathing*—Assess for bilateral expansion, breath sounds and evidence of pneumothorax.
- *Circulation*—Assess for tachycardia, capillary refill >2s, two IV cannulae, 20ml/kg crystalloid.
- *Disability*—Pupils & AVPU (**A**lert/Responds to **V**oice/Responds to **P**ain/**U**nresponsive)
- *Exposure* —Remove clothes to assess but **keep warm**. Look for evidence of visceral injuries (CSF leak, blood-stained sputum, blood-stained urine)

Subsequent management

- If repeated fluid boluses of 20ml/kg are required, blood should be given for the third and subsequent bolus. Surgical intervention is likely if an external bleeding point has not been identified and controlled. Likely sites for internal bleeding are abdomen, thorax and pelvis. There may be large blood loss from scalp wounds or into the subdural space in children with head injuries, particularly infants.
- Place a urinary catheter and oro/nasogastric tube.
- Unconscious patients should be ventilated to normocarbia with muscle relaxants but beware of masking seizures.
- Perform a more detailed secondary survey after initial stabilisation.
- Assess the need for surgical intervention.
- Stabilise before transferring out of the department.

Other considerations

- If IV cannulation proves difficult at conventional sites attempt femoral venous access.
- Intraosseous cannulation: useful in all children if IV access is difficult. The most suitable site is the proximal tibia 1–3cm (children) or 0.5–1cm (babies) below and just medial to the tibial tuberosity on the flat, medial aspect of the tibia where the bone lies subcutaneously. The anterior distal femur or humerus is an alternative if the tibia is fractured. Insert an 18G-12G smooth or threaded needle at right angles with the needle directed slightly caudally (away from the growth plate) until loss of resistance is felt and fluid can be injected easily without evidence of extravasation.

Further reading

Advanced Paediatric Life Support: The Practical Approach 3rd Edition 2001.

Paediatric emergencies: acute severe asthma

Condition	Severe bronchospasm
Presentation	Respiratory exhaustion; wheezy/silent chest; ↑RR, ↑HR
Immediate action	100% oxygen, nebulised salbutamol 2.5mg and ipratropium 250µg
Follow up action	Hydrocortisone 4mg/kg, consider adrenaline/aminophylline/$MgSO_4$
Investigations	ABG, CXR, serum theophylline (if already taking this)
Also consider	Anaphylaxis, inhaled FB, pneumonia, epiglottitis, pneumothorax

Risk factors
- History of asthma especially with acute respiratory tract infection.
- Exposure to known triggers (e.g. cold, smoke, allergen, exercise).
- Prematurity and low birth weight.

Diagnosis
- Confused or drowsy from exhaustion, maximal use of accessory muscles, unable to talk.
- Respiratory rate >30 breaths/min (>5yr) or >50 breaths/min (2–5yr) especially with a silent chest.
- PEFR <33% predicted. [Predicted PEFR in litres/min = 5 × (height in cm—80)].
- SaO_2 <92% or PaO_2 <8kPa (60mmHg) in air.
- $PaCO_2$ often normal initially but rises peri-arrest.
- Heart rate >140bpm.

Immediate management
- Check ABC . . . 100% oxygen.
- Nebulised salbutamol 2.5–5mg (10 puffs via inhaler and spacer).
- Nebulised ipratropium bromide 250µg.
- IV hydrocortisone 4mg/kg.
- Review ABC—consider intubation and ventilation (NB gas trapping, so slow respiratory rate preferable).
- If still unresponsive:
  - IM adrenaline 10µg/kg ± IV adrenaline infused at 0.02–0.1µg/kg/min (or consider nebulised adrenaline (2.5–5mg) or IV adrenaline 1µg/kg with ECG monitoring).
  - IV salbutamol titrated to effect up to 15µg/kg IV over 10min, then infused at 1–5µg/kg/min.
  - IV aminophylline 5mg/kg loading dose, then infused at 1mg/kg/hr.
  - IV magnesium sulphate 40mg/kg (max 2g).

Subsequent management
- Rehydrate with 10–20ml/kg crystalloid.
- Oral prednisolone 20mg (2–5yr), 30–40mg (>5yr) for 3d.
- Repeat nebulisers every 20–30min if necessary, otherwise 3–4-hourly.
- CXR to exclude pneumothorax.

Other considerations
- IPPV in severe bronchospasm is difficult and may result in gas trapping and cardiovascular compromise secondary to raised intrathoracic pressure. Consider extending expiratory phase and allowing hypercarbia to occur.
- Volatile agents and ketamine have been used to relieve intractable bronchospasm.
- Avoid the use of known histamine releasing drugs (e.g. thiopental) and NSAIDs.

Further reading
British Guideline on the management of asthma (2003). www.sign.ac.uk

Paediatric emergencies: anaphylaxis

Condition	IgE mediated type B hypersensitivity reaction
Presentation	Stridor, wheeze, cough, ↓SaO₂, CVS collapse, respiratory distress
Immediate action	100% oxygen, Remove trigger, Adrenaline IM, 20ml/kg IV fluid
Follow up action	Chlorphenamine IM/slow IV; Hydrocortisone IM/slow IV
Investigations	ABGs, CXR, Plasma tryptase, urinary methylhistamine
Also consider	Tension pneumothorax, latex allergy, sepsis, acute severe asthma

Risk factors
- Previous allergic reaction.
- History of asthma or atopy.
- Absence of an airway/circuit filter (latex allergy via aerosolised particles).
- Cross sensitivities (e.g. latex and kiwi fruit/bananas; NSAIDs).
- Use of known allergens (nut extracts in ENT, radiographic contrast media, penicillins).

Diagnosis
- Common signs: stridor; wheeze; cough; arterial desaturation; respiratory distress; CVS collapse.
- Less commonly: rash; urticaria; oedema.

Immediate management
- ABC . . . 100% oxygen (NB beware of sudden loss of airway control due to oedema).
- Remove direct contact with all potential triggers (most commonly muscle relaxants/NSAIDs).
- Give IM adrenaline 1:1000 solution: (10µg/kg = 0.01ml/kg 1:1000)

<6months	50µg (0.05ml)
6months–6yr	120µg (0.12ml)
6–12yr	250µg (0.25ml)
>12yr	500µg (0.5ml).

- Give IV fluid volume resuscitation with 20ml/kg crystalloid or colloid and secure more IV access sites.

Age Range	Adrenaline (IM) 1:1000	Chlorphenamine (IV)	Hydrocortisone (IV)
<6 months	50µg (0.05ml)	—	—
6 months–6yr	120µg (0.12ml)	2.5–5mg (>12mths)	50mg (>12mths)
6–12yr	250µg (0.25ml)	5–10mg	100mg
>12yr	500µg (0.5ml)	10–20mg	100–500mg

Subsequent management

- Antihistamine: chlorphenamine IM/slow IV (1–6yr 2.5–5mg; 6–12yr 5–10mg; >12yr = 10–20mg).
- Steroids: hydrocortisone IM/slow IV (1–6yr 50mg; 6–12yr 100mg; >12yr = 100–500mg).
- Frequent and careful review of the unsecured airway.

Other considerations

- Chlorphenamine should not be given to neonates.
- IV adrenaline 1µg/kg (0.01ml/kg of 1:10 000) can be given incrementally titrated to response as an alternative to the IM route, but it must be done with ECG monitoring due to the risk of provoking dysrhythmias.
- Complete a yellow CSM notification and refer to a clinical immunologist for skin-prick testing.

Further reading

Resuscitation Council (UK) guidelines www.resus.org.uk. Anaphylactic reactions associated with anaesthesia 3 (2003). Association of Anaesthetists of Great Britain and Ireland and the British Society of Allergy and Clinical Immunology.

Chapter 36

Airway assessment and management

Jules Cranshaw and Tim Cook

Airway assessment

The difficult airway is the single most important cause of anaesthesia-related morbidity and mortality—up to 30% of deaths attributable to anaesthesia are associated with inadequate airway management.

- Most catastrophes are due to unexpected difficulty.
- Airway assessment has traditionally focussed on detecting difficult direct laryngoscopy and tracheal intubation.
- Prediction of difficult mask ventilation, LMA placement and other rescue techniques is of equal importance.
- Intubation is:
  - Difficult in ~1:50 cases.
  - Impossible in ~1:2000 cases (increasing to ~1:200 for emergencies).
- Facemask ventilation is difficult in ~1:20 cases, impossible in ~1:1500.
- Rescue techniques fail in ~1:20 cases.
- Patients with multiple predictors of difficulty or risk factors for hypox-aemia (e.g. pregnancy, obesity, children) need great care.

History

- Congenital airway difficulties e.g. Pierre Robin, Klippel–Feil, Down's syndromes.
- Acquired airway difficulties e.g. rheumatoid arthritis, Still's disease, ankylosing spondylitis, acromegaly, pregnancy, diabetes.
- Iatrogenic problems e.g. TMJ surgery, cervical fusion, oral/pharyngeal radiotherapy, laryngeal/tracheal surgery.
- Reported previous anaesthetic problems e.g. dental damage or severe sore throat. Check anaesthetic notes, med-alerts, and possibly databases.

Examination

- Adverse anatomical features e.g. small mouth, receding chin, high arched palate, large tongue, bull neck, morbid obesity, large breasts.
- Acquired problems e.g. head/neck burns, tumours, abscesses, radio-therapy injury, restrictive scars.
- Mechanical limitation—reduced mouth opening and anterior temporo-mandibular movement (e.g. TMJ damage, quinsy, post-radiotherapy), poor cervical spine movement.
- Poor dentition e.g. anterior gaps, rotten/sharp/loose teeth, protruding or awkwardly placed teeth.
- Orthopaedic, neurosurgical or orthodontic equipment e.g. halo trac-tion, external fixator, stereotactic locator, surgical collar, dental wiring.
- If using the nasal route check the patency of the nasal passages.
- NB facial hair may hide adverse anatomical features.

Radiology

- A recent CT or MRI scan may help define potentially difficult anatomy and guide management.
- Occipito-atlanto-axial disease is more predictive of difficult laryngo-scopy than disease below C2.
- Plain radiographs are poor predictors of cervical stability but flex-ion/extension views are only indicated for potentially dangerous ligamen-tous (usually atlanto-axial) disruption. In rheumatoid arthritis radiology

correlates poorly with risk. Vertebral settling should be regarded as predictive of difficult intubation and raise the possibility of neck instability.

- Radiographical measures of mandibular length and depth can be used to predict difficult laryngoscopy but are rarely practical.

Predictive tests

Laryngoscopy and tracheal intubation requires creating a clear line of view from the upper teeth to the glottis. This requires mouth opening, extension of the upper cervical spine, and the ability to create a 'sub-mandibular space' (i.e. move the soft tissues within the arch of the mandible out of the way). Most tests of difficult intubation test one or more of these capacities.

Problems with predictive tests of difficult direct laryngoscopy/ intubation:

- Low specificity and positive predictive value. Large numbers of false positives. Generally <10% of patients with features 'predicting' difficult laryngoscopy prove to be difficult to intubate.
- Sensitivity is often less than 50%. Around 50% of difficult cases are not predicted by the tests. Studies that have developed predictive tests often quote higher sensitivity and specificity for the test than is found when it is applied to a general population in routine practice.
- Combining multiple tests increases the specificity (i.e. reduces false positives) but decreases sensitivity (i.e. leads to missing more truly difficult cases).
- Definitions of 'airway difficulty' vary widely. Although the laryngeal view described by Cormack and Lehane is frequently used, it correlates only moderately with measures of difficulty with intubation. Modifications have therefore been proposed.

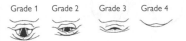

Cormack and Lehane classification of glottic visualisation.

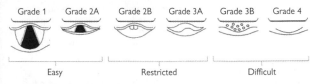

Cook's modified classification of laryngeal view. 1–4 refer to Cormack and Lehane classification. In Cook's classification 'easy' views require no adjuncts, 'restricted' views require a gum elastic bougie, 'difficult' views require advanced techniques to intubate.

Interincisor gap (II gap)

- The distance between the incisors (or alveolar margins) with the mouth open maximally.
- Affected by temporomandibular joint and upper cervical spine mobility.
- <3cm makes intubation difficulty more likely.
- <2.5cm—LMA insertion will be difficult.

Patient protrusion of the mandible

- Class A—able to protrude the lower incisors anterior to the upper incisors.
- Class B—lower incisors can just reach the margin of the upper incisors.
- Class C—lower incisors cannot protrude to the upper incisors.

Classes B and C are associated with increased risk of difficult laryngoscopy.

Mallampati test (with Samsoon and Young's modification)

Examine the patient's oropharynx from opposite the patient's face while the patient opens their mouth maximally and protrudes their tongue without phonating.

- Faucial pillars, soft palate, and uvula visible. (Class 1)
- Faucial pillars and soft palate visible—uvula tip masked by base of tongue. (Class 2)
- Soft palate visible only. (Class 3)
- Soft palate not visible. (Class 4)

Mallampati class 1,2,3,4.

Class 3 and 4 views (i.e. when there is no view of the posterior pharyngeal wall) are associated with an increased risk of difficult laryngoscopy. This test is prone to interobserver variation. Used alone it correctly predicts about 50% of difficult laryngoscopies and has a false positive rate of up to 90%.

Extension of the upper cervical spine

- When limited (<90°) the risk of difficult laryngoscopy is increased.
- Movement may be assessed by:
  - Flexing the head on the neck, immobilising the lower cervical spine with one hand on the neck then fully extending the head. Placing a pointer on the vertex or forehead allows the angle of movement to be estimated.
  - Placing one finger on the patient's chin and one finger on the occipital protuberance and extending the head maximally.

- With normal cervical spine mobility the finger on the chin is higher than the one on the occiput. Level fingers indicate moderate limitation. If the finger on the chin remains lower than the one on the occiput there is severe limitation.

Thyromental distance (Patil test)
The distance from the tip of thyroid cartilage to the tip of mandible, neck fully extended:
- Normal >7cm; <6cm predicts ~75% of difficult laryngoscopies.
- Combined Patil and Mallampati tests (<7cm and class 3–4) increases specificity (97%) but reduces sensitivity (81%).

Sternomental distance (Savva test)
The distance from the upper border of the manubrium to the tip of mandible, neck fully extended and the mouth closed.
- <12.5cm associated with difficulty (positive predictive value 82%).

Wilson score
5 factors—weight; upper cervical spine mobility; jaw movement; receding mandible; buck teeth each scored from 0–2 (subjectively normal to abnormal).
- A total score of ≥2 predicts 75% of difficult intubations; 12% false positives.

Predictors of difficult mask ventilation
Mask ventilation requires the ability to cover the mouth and nose with a facemask, produce a seal, and open the airway.
Predictors of difficulty with facemask ventilation:
- Age >55yr
- Body mass index >26kg/m^2
- History of snoring
- Beards
- Absence of teeth

(The presence of two of the above factors has a >70% sensitivity and specificity.)
- Facial abnormalities
- Receding or markedly prognathic jaw
- Obstructive sleep apnoea

Predictors of problems with back-up techniques
LMA insertion
LMA insertion is likely to form part of a rescue plan when routine airway management fails. The factors associated with difficulty in placing a laryngeal mask are inability to open the mouth more than 2.5cm (impossible if <2.0cm) and intraoral/pharyngeal masses (e.g. lingual tonsils).

Direct tracheal access
If emergency tracheal access is contemplated check:
- The position of the larynx and trachea.
- The accessibility of the cricothyroid membrane and trachea.

Check for gross obesity, goitre or other anterior neck mass, deviated trachea, fixed neck flexion, previous radiotherapy, surgical collar or external fixator preventing access.

Awake techniques including fibre-optic intubation (AFOI)
The most important predictors of AFOI are lack of patient co-operation
and operator inexperience. Use of AFOI for cases of airway obstruction
is controversial.

Further reading

Calder I et al. (2003). Mouth opening. A new angle. Anesthesiology, **99**, 799–801.
Cook TM (2000). A new practical classification of laryngeal view. Anaesthesia, **55**, 274–279.
Cormack RS, Lehane J (1984). Difficult tracheal intubation in obstetrics. Anaesthesia, **39**, 1105–1111.
Langeron O et al.(2000). Prediction of difficult mask ventilation. Anesthesiology, **92**, 1229–1236.
Mallampati SR, Gugino LD, Desai S, Waraksa B, Freiberger D, Lui PL. (1983). Clinical sign to
    predict difficult tracheal intubation. Canadian Anaesthetists Society Journal, **30**, 316–317.
Patil VU, Stehling LC, Zauder HL (1983). Predicting the difficulty of intubation using an intubation
    guage. Anesthesiology Review 1983, **10**, 32–3.
Samsoon G, Young JR (1987). Difficult tracheal intubation: a retrospective study. Anaesthesia, **42**,
    487–90.
Savva D (1994). Prediction of difficult intubation. British Journal of Anaesthesia, **73**, 149–53.
Wilson ME (1993). Predicting difficult intubation. British Journal of Anaesthesia, **71**, 333–334.
Wilson ME, Spiegelhalter D, Robertson JA, Lesser P. (1988). Predicting difficult intubation. British
    Journal of Anaesthesia, **61**, 211–6.
Yentis S (2002). Predicting difficult intubation- worthwhile exercise or pointless ritual? Anaesthe-
    sia, **57**, 105–109.

Unanticipated difficult airway

Despite careful assessment, approximately 50% of airway difficulties arise unexpectedly. Problems may arise from:

- Difficult/failed intubation
- Difficult/failed mask ventilation
- Both

Unexpected difficulty is more likely during emergencies, obstetric cases, and during anaesthesia by inexperienced anaesthetists. When difficulties do occur patients do not die from failure to intubate, but from failure to oxygenate.

Difficult intubation

Management of intubation difficulties can be considered as a four-step process:

A. Primary intubation attempt (includes optimal anaesthesia, optimal position, optimal blade, optimal laryngeal manipulation, use of gum elastic bougie or stylet).

B. Secondary intubation attempt (includes intubation via an LMA or ILMA, use of flexible or rigid fibre-optic systems, lightwands or retrograde intubation).

C. Oxygenation/ventilation via face mask ventilation (but includes use of supraglottic adjuncts).

D. Invasive tracheal techniques (needle or cannula cricothyroidotomy, surgical airway).

The decision to proceed from A-B-C-D depends on failure of each technique. In most cases senior help should be called when plan A fails. Plan D should be reserved for situation of 'can't intubate can't ventilate' (CICV) with progressive desaturation despite optimal attempts at oxygenation.

Difficult intubation with easy ventilation (no aspiration risk)

A calm stepwise approach can be used. If plan A fails plan B will usually succeed. When plans A and B fail, plan C is usually successful. See 'Failed intubation' (p928).

Difficult intubation with difficult/impossible ventilation (can't intubate can't ventilate).

This situation is an emergency and will become life-threatening if not managed correctly. If mask ventilation is difficult, insertion of an LMA (LMA, ILMA or PLMA—choice depends on experience and situation) will rescue the airway in >90% of cases. Where ventilation remains impossible and oxygenation cannot be maintained, invasive techniques (plan D) are lifesaving. All anaesthetists should be equipped and prepared to perform such techniques when the need arises (p934).

Difficult intubation during rapid sequence intubation.

After two attempts at intubation, proceed directly to plan C (omit plan B) and wake the patient up. See 'Rapid Sequence Induction' (pp942–943).

Unanticipated diffult tracheal intubation[1]

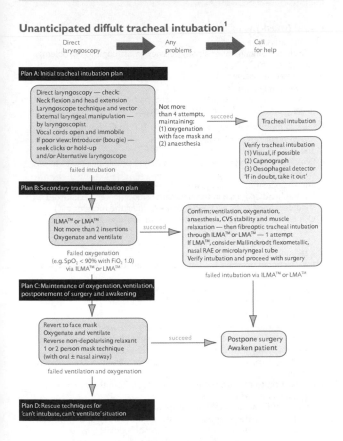

Direct laryngoscopy → Any problems → Call for help

Plan A: Initial tracheal intubation plan

Direct laryngoscopy — check:
Neck flexion and head extension
Laryngoscope technique and vector
External laryngeal manipulation — by laryngoscopist
Vocal cords open and immobile
If poor view: Introducer (bougie) — seek clicks or hold-up
and/or Alternative laryngoscope

→ Not more than 4 attempts, maintaining: (1) oxygenation with face mask and (2) anaesthesia — *succeed* → Tracheal intubation

Verify tracheal intubation
(1) Visual, if possible
(2) Capnograph
(3) Oesophageal detector
'If in doubt, take it out'

failed intubation

Plan B: Secondary tracheal intubation plan

ILMA™ or LMA™
Not more than 2 insertions
Oxygenate and ventilate

succeed →

Confirm: ventilation, oxygenation, anaesthesia, CVS stability and muscle relaxation — then fibreoptic tracheal intubation through ILMA™ or LMA™ — 1 attempt
If LMA™, consider Mallinckrodt flexometallic, nasal RAE or microlaryngeal tube
Verify intubation and proceed with surgery

Failed oxygenation
(e.g. SpO_2 < 90% with FiO_2 1.0) via ILMA™ or LMA™

failed intubation via ILMA™ or LMA™

Plan C: Maintenance of oxygenation, ventilation, postponement of surgery and awakening

Revert to face mask
Oxygenate and ventilate
Reverse non-depolarising relaxant
1 or 2 person mask technique
(with oral ± nasal airway)

succeed → Postpone surgery / Awaken patient

failed ventilation and oxygenation

Plan D: Rescue techniques for 'can't intubate, can't ventilate' situation

[1] With permission of the Difficult Airway Society

Failed (mask) ventilation

This may arise as a result of:
- Failure to maintain upper airway patency (most common problem)
- Laryngospasm
- Laryngeal pathology
- Lower airway pathology

This is always an emergency—an extra pair of hands is helpful. Call for help early but do not let your assistant leave.

Failure to maintain airway patency—(this is Plan C above)
- Pre-oxygenation of all cases prolongs the period before desaturation and reduces risk.
- Switch to 100% oxygen whenever an airway problem appears to be developing.
- Ensure anaesthesia is adequate.
- Put the head and neck in the optimal position (lower neck flexed on shoulders and upper neck extended—'sniffing the morning air').
- Use two-person mask ventilation (one to provide jaw thrust and face-mask seal and one to squeeze the reservoir bag).
- Use an oral or nasal airway (but use care to avoid nasal bleeding).
- If still unable to ventilate by facemask insert an LMA or attempt intubation. If cricoid pressure has been applied reduce or release it but be ready with a sucker.
- If still obstructed with progressive severe desaturation and unable to intubate or awaken the patient, proceed to plan D.

Laryngospasm
May be preceded by stridor or characteristic 'crowing' noise followed by complete airway obstruction. May occur without these signs. Consider in all cases of airway obstruction without obvious supraglottic causes.
- Apply 100% oxygen with the mask held tightly and the expiratory valve closed.
- Use suction to remove secretions and blood from the airway (*if hypoxaemia allows.*)
- Apply CPAP and attempt manual ventilation.
- Forcible jaw thrust or anterior pressure on the body of the mandible just anterior to the mastoid process (Larson's point) may 'break' laryngospasm by a combination of stimulation and airway clearance.
- Deepening anaesthesia with a small dose of propofol (20–50mg) may reduce spasm.
- If oxygenation is falling consider a small dose of suxamethonium (0.1–0.5mg/kg). If laryngospasm is severe a full dose of suxamethonium (1.0mg/kg) should be administered and the trachea intubated. If there is no venous access suxamethonium may be administered IM or into the tongue (3mg/kg).
- As laryngospasm starts to 'break' anaesthesia may be deepened with a volatile agent or further doses of IV agent as appropriate.
- Consider a change in airway management (e.g. exchange a tracheal tube for an LMA), prior to further attempts to wake the patient, to prevent recurrence.

Laryngeal pathology

Unexpected laryngeal pathology causing problems with mask ventilation is a very rare scenario. Cricothyroidotomy may be lifesaving.

Lower airway pathology

Acute severe bronchospasm may present as difficulty in mask ventilation. This may be present in smokers and severe asthmatics or may be part of an adverse drug reaction—see p884. Very rarely lower airway pathology due to diagnosed or undiagnosed mediastinal masses may present as difficulty with ventilation at induction of anaesthesia. Tracheal intubation or use of a rigid bronchoscope to maintain airway patency may be lifesaving.

Paediatric implications

- Tracheal intubation in the absence of structural abnormalities is uncommon.
- Laryngospasm is more common in children.
- Hypoxia occurs rapidly in children if ventilation is inadequate.
- Airway manipulation or use of suxamethonium in the presence of hypoxia may lead to bradycardia and cardiac arrest.

Special considerations

All patients who have airway difficulties should be informed after they have recovered. Inform patient, general practitioner and document fully in notes and databases if appropriate. Complete 'airway alert' if in use.

Failed intubation (see also p888)

Defined as inability to intubate the trachea. The commonest cause is difficulty in viewing the larynx (failed direct laryngoscopy). Remember that patients do not die from failure to intubate but failure to oxygenate.

Optimising primary intubation attempts

Following a few simple rules will eliminate the majority of difficulties with intubation.

- Optimise the position of the head and neck (flexion of the lower cervical spine with extension at the upper cervical spine 'sniffing the morning air'). One pillow.
- Optimal anaesthesia: an unconscious patient with working relaxant.
- Optimal laryngeal position: Optimal External Laryngeal Manipulation (OLEM) by an assistant, or Backwards Upwards and Rightwards Pressure (BURP) during cricoid pressure.
- Use of the correct laryngoscope. Long/polio/straight blade, McCoy laryngoscope.
- Use a gum elastic bougie (or stylet in paediatrics).

Diagnosis of misplacement of the tracheal tube (oesophageal intubation)

- Retain a high index of suspicion after a difficult intubation.
- Capnography is the gold standard for confirmation of tracheal intubation.
- In the absence of capnography suspect oesophageal placement if you cannot confirm: normal breath sounds in both axillae with absent sounds over the stomach; rise and fall of chest; normal airway pressure cycle.
- Use an 'oesophageal detector.' If negative pressure is applied to the ETT the trachea (a rigid structure) does not collapse, while the oesophagus (not rigid) does. Failure to aspirate air with a bladder syringe directly attached to the ETT suggests oesophageal placement.
- Confirm ETT placement with a fibre-optic scope.
- Where there is doubt, pull it out and apply bag and mask ventilation.

Failed elective intubation with difficult ventilation
(see CICV p934)
Proceed directly to plan C

Failed intubation during rapid sequence induction
(see RSI p942)
Proceed directly to plan C

Failed elective intubation with easy ventilation (see p930)

In these cases when the patient has received a full dose of a non-depolarising muscle relaxant and mask ventilation is easy, it may be appropriate to try a full range of secondary intubation techniques (Plan B above)

Techniques for management of elective difficult intubation

Strategies for the 'Can't Intubate, **Can** Ventilate' scenario:

Gum elastic bougie

('Eschmann tracheal tube introducer (reusable)', Sims Portex Ltd, New Portex House, Military Road, Hythe, Kent CT21 5BN, UK. Tel: +44 1303 260551). The gum elastic bougie (GEB) should enable intubation where the laryngeal inlet is partially visible (laryngoscopy grade 2a–3a, p920) and is probably the single most useful piece of difficult intubation equipment. Keep the bougie anterior and in the midline to ensure it does not enter the oesophagus or either piriform fossa. Signs of correct placement are bumps as it passes along the tracheal rings, rotation as it enters the main bronchi and 'hold-up' at approx 40cm. When 'railroading' the ETT keep the laryngoscope in the mouth and rotate the tube 90° counter-clockwise to ensure the bevel is correctly orientated for intubation.

Frova intubating stylet

(Cook Critical Care, Monroe House, Letchworth, SG6 1LN, UK. Tel +44 1462 44 3100) is used similarly to the GEB but is more rigid. It is hollow and has two connectors allowing oxygen insufflation or jet ventilation when required.

Intubation via the classic, ProSeal or intubating LMA

These techniques use an LMA as a 'dedicated airway.' This allows oxygenation and ventilation during intubation and provides a channel through which intubation attempts are made. Intubation via the classic laryngeal mask airway is rarely successful when performed blindly. Alternative techniques include use of a bougie or lightwand to guide intubation. Use of a fibrescope increases success. A suggested technique involves fibre-optic placement of a rigid hollow Aintree catheter (ID 4.7mm, ED 7.0mm, Cook Critical Care), then removal of the LMA and the fibrescope. The Aintree catheter remains in place and has connectors that enable ventilation at this point. A tracheal tube (ID 7.0mm or larger) is then railroaded over the catheter. The same technique is suitable for the ProSeal LMA.

The ILMA (Intavent Orthofix, Maidenhead, UK. Tel +44 1628 594500) is a modification of the classic LMA designed to facilitate blind orotracheal intubation, fibre-optic intubation, or in very co-operative patients awake intubation. It comprises a rigid anatomically curved airway tube terminating in a standard 15mm connector. It is fitted with a rigid metal handle. The mask has a single epiglottic elevating bar replacing the two bars of a classic LMA. As the tracheal tube exits the airway this bar lifts the epiglottis from the route of passage of the tracheal tube. Sizes 3—5 enable intubation in large children and adults. Size 7.0—8.0mm silicone-tipped wire-reinforced tracheal tubes are designed for use with each ILMA and improve successful intubation. Similarly fibre-optic guidance improves success.

Endotracheal tube size fitting through Intavent orthofix LMAs
(if cuffed ETT take off 0.5mm)

LMA	size 1	3.5 id*	distance to bars	108mm
	size 1.5	4.5 id	distance to bars	135mm
	size 2	5.0 id	distance to bars	140mm
	size 2 1/2	6.0 id	distance to bars	170mm
	size 3	6.5 id	distance to bars	200mm
	size 4	6.5 id	distance to bars	205mm
	size 5	7.0 id	distance to bars	230mm
fLMA (flexible LMA)	size 2	3.5 id*	distance to bars	140mm**
	size 2 1/2	3.5 id*	distance to bars	205mm**
	size 3	5.5 id	distance to bars	237mm
	size 4	5.5 id	distance to bars	237mm
	size 5	6.0 id	distance to bars	284mm

* A tube larger than this cannot pass the proximal end of the LMA, at the site of the 15mm connector
** This is longer than an uncut ETT of this size, so not suitable for this technique; fLMA cannot be recommended for this technique!

PLMA	size 3	6.0 id	distance to bowl	190mm
	size 4	6.5 id	distance to bowl	190mm
	size 5	6.5 id	distance to bowl	195mm
ILMA	7.0–8.0mm ILMA tubes			
	distance to epiglottic elevator 160mm			

The combitube

The Combitube™ (Sheridan Catheter Corporation) is an airway device that combines the functions of an oesophageal obturator airway and a conventional endotracheal tube. It has two lumens—an oesophageal lumen with perforations at the pharyngeal level and a tracheal lumen with an open distal end. It has two inflatable cuffs—a large proximal cuff (blue, 85ml) to seal the pharynx and a small distal cuff (white, 10ml) to seal off the proximal oesophagus or trachea. The small size is recommended for general use.

Retrograde intubation

Different methods have been described, all based on the technique of Waters. The airway is anaesthetised (as for awake intubation, see p948). A needle (e.g. a Tuohy needle) is passed through the cricothyroid membrane with the bevel directed cephalad. Correct positioning is confirmed by the aspiration of air. A guidewire (e.g. from a central line kit) is passed via the Tuohy needle and retrieved from the nose or mouth. An introducer is then passed over the guidewire (e.g. a Cook retrograde catheter, a 16G ureteric dilator, or similar). The tracheal tube is passed over the guidewire and introducer into the trachea. The guidewire and introducer are withdrawn from above whilst applying forward pressure on the tube. An alternative technique involves threading the inserted guidewire through the suction port of the fibrescope and using it to guide the scope into the trachea. Cook (Cook Ltd, Letchworth, UK) makes a retrograde intubation kit for use with endotracheal tubes of internal diameter 5mm or larger.

Further reading

Waters DJ (1963). Guided blind endotracheal intubation. *Anaesthesia*, **18**, 158–62.
DAS guidelines. www.DAS.Uk.com

Can't intubate, can't ventilate (see also p890)

Inability to intubate the trachea and ventilate the lungs is always a life-threatening situation. Managed badly it will lead to morbidity or death. It occurs in less than 1:5000 routine anaesthetics. It is more common during emergency anaesthesia, intubation in the emergency department, after multiple attempts at intubation, and with inexperienced anaesthetists. This is plan D of the DAS guidelines (see p924).

Rescue techniques for 'can't intubate, can't ventilate' scenario

Remember insertion of an appropriate LMA will rescue the airway in >90% of cases. It would be rare to attempt any of these procedures without first attempting airway rescue with LMA insertion. Once inserted the LMA should be left in place during tracheal access: it may allow some oxygenation and provides a route of exhalation which is needed if jet ventilation is used.

Cricothyroidotomy

- In the 'can't intubate, can't ventilate' scenario with progressive desaturation, emergency tracheal access is required. Needle cricothyroidotomy is quicker and easier than formal tracheostomy. It is performed at the level of the cricothyroid membrane.
- Appropriate techniques include a cannula over needle technique (e.g. less than 2mm ID, non-kinking cannula such as the Ravussin cannula, VBM GmBH, Sulz, Germany) or larger catheters placed with a Seldinger technique (e.g. Cook Melker Cricothyroidotomy Catheter, 5.0mm cuffed or 4.0/6.0mm uncuffed, Cook, Letchworth, UK).
- Cannulae of less than 4.0mm ID require jet ventilation for adequate ventilation and rely on exhalation via the native upper airway. It is essential to ensure there is no obstruction to expiration otherwise barotrauma may result.
- Catheters of greater than 4.0mm ID permit conventional ventilation and will only provide adequate ventilation if they are cuffed or the upper airway is obstructed. Complications include pneumothorax, surgical emphysema, and bleeding.

IV cannula

- In a critical situation a 14G IV cannula may be used for cricothyroidotomy.
- Position must be confirmed by aspiration of air before ventilating, with the use of an injector or wall oxygen (use of an anaesthetic machine flush is not reliable with modern machines). If using wall oxygen tubing must run from the flowmeter to the patient and there must be a mechanism (e.g. 3 way tap or hole in the tubing) to allow on/off flow to the patient.
- As with all small cannulae exhalation relies on a patent upper airway.
- Complications include misplacement, surgical emphysema, and problems with ventilation and exhalation. There is a high risk of kinking.

Surgical airway

- This technique allows introduction of a size 6.0mm ID tracheal tube into the trachea.
- A scalpel is used to make a horizontal cut in the skin and cricothyroid membrane. The hole in the cricothyroid membrane may be enlarged with the handle of the scalpel blade or a dilator. A cricoid hook allows stabilisation of position while a tracheal tube is passed into the trachea.
- In expert hands this technique establishes a secure airway in 30s. An advantage to the technique, over cricothyroidotomy, is the absence of problems with ventilation once the tube is inserted.
- Complications include bleeding, misplacement, and airway trauma.

Special considerations

- Multiple intubation attempts lead to airway trauma and increase the likelihood of a CICV situation. If one technique has failed twice it is unlikely to work on further attempts. Try something new!
- Difficult and failed intubation is associated with an increased incidence of aspiration. Empty the stomach.
- After rescuing the airway it is necessary to establish a definitive airway as a matter of urgency. ENT assistance is recommended.
- After prolonged obstruction anticipate possible post-obstructive pulmonary oedema.

Can't intubate...can't ventilate[1]

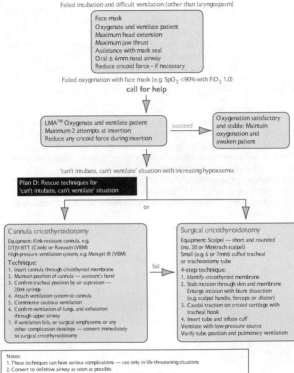

Failed intubation and difficult ventilation (other than laryngospasm)

> Face mask
> Oxygenate and ventilate patient
> Maximum head extension
> Maximum jaw thrust
> Assistance with mask seal
> Oral ± 6mm nasal airway
> Reduce cricoid force - if necessary

Failed oxygenation with face mask (e.g. SpO_2 <90% with FiO_2 1.0)
call for help

LMA™ Oxygenate and ventilate patient
Maximum 2 attempts at insertion
Reduce any cricoid force during insertion

→ succeed →

Oxygenation satisfactory and stable: Maintain oxygenation and awaken patient

'can't intubate, can't ventilate' situation with increasing hypoxaemia

Plan D: Rescue techniques for 'can't intubate, can't ventilate' situation

or

Cannula cricothyroidotomy
Equipment: Kink-resistant cannula, e.g. DTJV-BTT (Cook) or Ravussin (VBM)
High-pressure ventilation system, e.g Manujet III (VBM)
Technique:
1. Insert cannula through cricothyroid membrane
2. Maintain position of cannula — assistant's hand
3. Confirm tracheal position by air aspiration — 20ml syringe
4. Attach ventilation system to cannula
5. Commence cautious ventilation
6. Confirm ventilation of lungs, and exhalation through upper airway
7. If ventilation fails, or surgical emphysema or any other complication develops — convert immediately to surgical cricothyroidotomy

→ fail →

Surgical cricothyroidotomy
Equipment: Scalpel — short and rounded (no. 20 or Minitrach scalpel)
Small (e.g. 6 or 7mm) cuffed tracheal or tracheostomy tube
4-step technique:
1. Identify cricothyroid membrane
2. Stab incision through skin and membrane Enlarge incision with blunt dissection (e.g. scalpel handle, forceps or dilator)
3. Caudal traction on cricoid cartilage with tracheal hook
4. Insert tube and inflate cuff
Ventilate with low-pressure source
Verify tube position and pulmonary ventilation

Notes:
1. These techniques can have serious complications — use only in life-threatening situations
2. Convert to definitive airway as soon as possible
3. Postoperative management — see other difficult airway guidelines and flow-charts
4. 4mm cannula with low-pressure ventilation may be successful in patient breathing spontaneously

---

1 With permission of the Difficult Airway Society

Management of the obstructed airway

The approach to the patient with an obstructed airway differs according to:
- Urgency of intervention
- Level of obstruction
- General condition of the patient.

These cases are always difficult and if managed poorly will develop life-threatening problems. Their management is controversial—airway obstruction is likely to get worse during anaesthesia or airway manipulation due to loss of airway tone, reflex airway responses, trauma or bleeding.

All approaches have potentially life-threatening complications (complete obstruction of the airway on induction, intra-airway haemorrhage, swelling). It is essential to have experienced anaesthetic and surgical involvement. **Have a back-up plan and ensure that all those involved in the case understand what this plan is.**

If time allows obtain appropriate investigations to define the site, extent and severity of obstruction and involvement of related structures.
- Nasendoscopy
- CT/MRI
- Lung function tests with flow-volume loops
- Echocardiography if pulmonary vessel involvement suspected:

Assess the:
- Level—oral; supraglottic; laryngeal; mid tracheal; lower tracheal. Several levels may be affected by one pathology. Inspiratory stridor and voice changes indicate laryngeal obstruction, intrathoracic obstruction may cause expiratory stridor.
- Severity—respiratory distress; accessory muscle use; stridor; hypoxaemia, silent chest, dysphagia and nocturnal panic.
- Lesion—mobility and friability.
- Neck—examine ease of invasive tracheal access.
- Effect of patient position—find the patient's 'best breathing position.' Ask about any tendency to obstruction when lying flat.

Oral, supraglottic and laryngeal lesions

e.g. trauma, burns, tumour, infective causes.
- In semi-elective cases nasendoscopy may help in predicting difficulties but must be performed with great care.
- If emergency access to the trachea is needed (e.g. cricothyroidotomy) this is usually unimpeded by the lesion.
- Consider:
  - Awake fibre-optic intubation.
  - Inhalational induction then direct or fibre-optic laryngoscopy.
  - Elective awake (with local anaesthetic) cricothyroidotomy, tracheostomy or placing a trans-tracheal ventilation catheter (for oxygenation/ventilation in case of obstruction above).
- An experienced surgeon who is scrubbed, equipped, assisted, and ready to perform a cricothyroidotomy or *very* rapid tracheostomy must be available in case complete obstruction occurs during either

awake fibre-optic intubation or inhalational induction. Inserting a rigid bronchoscope may also provide an emergency airway in some cases.
- If unexpected airway obstruction occurs an LMA may assist ventilation during emergency airway access.
- IV induction and attempted laryngoscopy (with or without paralysis) without a backup plan cannot be recommended.

Mid tracheal

e.g. tumour or retrosternal goitre—often present semi-electively but may expand suddenly with haemorrhage. Knowing the site of obstruction is vital. The upper airway is usually normal at laryngoscopy, but difficulties may develop when the tube is inserted into the trachea.
- The site of the lesion may preclude cricothyroidotomy or tracheo-stomy—attempts risk bleeding and complete obstruction.
- Inhalational induction may be very slow and difficult if there is severe narrowing of the airway.
- Awake fibre-optic intubation may be indicated if failure to ventilate under anaesthesia is a significant possibility. However, coughing and distress may lead to increased obstruction and a cycle of decline. Passage of the fibre-optic scope and/or the tube through the narrowing may also hinder spontaneous ventilation and be unpleasant for the patient ('cork in a bottle' phenomenon).
- An endotracheal tube, endobronchial tube or a hollow intubation bougie that also allows jet ventilation (e.g. Cook airway exchange catheter or Frova intubating bougie) may pass the narrowing.
- The obstruction may be high enough in the trachea to allow both the tube cuff and bevel to sit below the obstruction and above the carina.
- IV induction, rapid neuromuscular blockade, (suxamethonium) and early passage of a rigid bronchoscope is also used for marked tracheal obstruction requiring thoracic surgery (e.g. resection, laser or stent insertion). The rigid bronchoscope establishes airway patency and is then used as a dedicated airway for further assessment, oxygenation, ventilation, and surgery.
- Anaesthesia may need to be maintained with an IV technique.

Lower tracheal lesions and bronchial obstruction

e.g. tumours, trauma, large mediastinal masses.
- Best managed by experienced specialists in thoracic centres.
- Cardiopulmonary bypass is sometimes necessary (e.g. pulmonary artery compression).
- IV induction, rapid neuromuscular blockade (suxamethonium), and passage of a rigid bronchoscope may be life-saving.

Further considerations

- A specific tissue diagnosis may allow shrinking of a lesion with antibiotics, steroids, chemotherapy or radiotherapy if time allows.
- Have a management plan for extubation which may need to be delayed. Prolonged instrumentation may cause upper airway oedema.
- Heliox (premixed helium/oxygen containing 21–30% oxygen) may improve flow through a narrowed airway but reduces the FiO_2. Use of a 'Y' connector and oxygen cylinder may be used to increase the FiO_2.

New delivery systems for helium (including ventilators) have recently been marketed (BOC). Heliox may be useful for obstruction at any level but is usually only effective as a temporary measure while organising definitive management.

Further reading

Mason RA, Fielder CP (1999). The obstructed airway in head and neck surgery. *Anaesthesia,* **54,** 625–8.

Ovassapian A, Yelich SJ, Dykes MHM, Brunner EE (1983). Fibre-optic nasotracheal intubation—incidence and causes of failure. *Anesthesia and Analgesia* ,**63,** 692–5.

Rapid sequence induction

Rapid IV induction and muscle relaxation to aid tracheal intubation, combined with cricoid pressure to reduce the risk of pulmonary aspiration. Mask ventilation is relatively contraindicated before tube placement. If airway assessment indicates intubation may be difficult, consider a local/regional technique or awake fibre-optic intubation.

Checks

- Anaesthetic machine, vaporisers, breathing system, ventilator, suction, intubation aids and rescue equipment.
- Two functioning laryngoscopes, and tracheal tube cuff.
- Patient on a tipping trolley or bed.
- Routine monitoring applied.
- Head in the 'sniffing' position—extended on neck, cervical spine flexed on the thorax with a pillow.
- Reliable wide bore IV cannula with fluid running.
- Drawn-up predefined dose of induction agent (thiopental 2–5mg/kg; etomidate 0.2–0.3mg/kg; propofol 1–2.5mg/kg) and suxamethonium (1–1.5mg/kg).
- Emergency drugs.
- Plans for failed intubation and failed ventilation. Difficult intubation may occur in 1 in 20 cases—failure in 1 in 200.

Procedure

- Switch on suction and place in easy reach.
- Preoxygenate through a tight-fitting mask with high flow oxygen for 3min, until ETO_2 is >90% or, in extreme emergency, four vital capacity breaths. (This delays onset of hypoxaemia and buys time for muscle relaxation and intubation. Pregnant, obese, septic, anaemic, paediatric, and patients with respiratory disease desaturate faster. Any entrainment of air undoes the process. Start again. Do not remove the mask until laryngoscopy).
- Cricoid pressure (10N) is applied by a trained assistant.
- Administer induction agent immediately followed by suxamethonium.
- Cricoid pressure is increased to 30N at loss of consciousness.
- Intubate after fasciculations, 45–60 s after suxamethonium.
- Inflate cuff, hand ventilate, and confirm correct tracheal tube placement by capnography and bilateral auscultation of the chest and stomach.
- If the tube is correctly placed, ask the assistant to remove cricoid pressure.

Problems

- Haemodynamic instability. Excessive induction agent produces circulatory collapse especially in the presence of hypovolaemia. Insufficient dosing results in tachycardia and hypertension and risks awareness. Alfentanil (10–30µg/kg) 1min before induction may reduce undesirable haemodynamic responses. In the event of intubation failure this may be reversed with naloxone (400–800µg).

Problems with cricoid pressure

- Correct application is a trained, practised skill.
- The cricoid cartilage is held between the thumb and middle finger and pressure is exerted mainly with the index finger posteriorly.
- Bimanual pressure (other hand behind the neck) is of uncertain benefit.
- Some patients may only tolerate cricoid pressure after induction e.g. distressed children.
- Excessive pressure increases airway obstruction and makes intubation more difficult.
- Backwards Upwards Rightwards Pressure (BURP) may improve laryngeal view but increases the likelihood of airway obstruction. Therefore if intubation fails and ventilation is required return the direction to posterior.
- If a patient vomits after application of cricoid pressure but before induction it should be released. Vomiting does not occur after loss of consciousness.
- A tiring assistant may not be able to maintain cricoid pressure for >5min.

Failed intubation (plan C in DAS guidelines)

- In the event of failed intubation, induction agents/neuromuscular block does not always wear off before the onset of life-threatening hypoxia.
- Oxygenation is essential. Gentle manual ventilation should be part of a failed intubation protocol.
- If ventilation is difficult cricoid pressure should be reduced or released and a 'can't intubate, can't ventilate' protocol adopted (p934). An LMA or ProSeal LMA are suitable rescue devices for this situation.

Paediatric considerations

- Forces required for effective cricoid pressure are not established.
- Young children are unlikely to co-operate with preoxygenation and cricoid pressure. Children desaturate more quickly than adults. RSI may therefore need to be modified with gentle mask ventilation after induction to prevent hypoxaemia before or during laryngoscopy.
- Difficult laryngoscopy and tracheal intubation is fortunately much less common in children.

Further reading

Morris J, Cook TM (2001). National survey of rapid sequence induction. *Anaesthesia*, **56**, 1090–97.
Vanner RG, Asai T (1888). Safe use of cricoid pressure. *Anaesthesia*, **54**, 1–3.

Unanticipated difficult tracheal intubation (rapid sequence induction)[1]

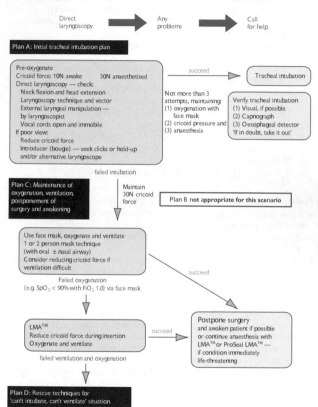

Direct laryngoscopy → Any problems → Call for help

Plan A: Initial tracheal intubation plan

Pre-oxygenate
Cricoid force: 10N awake   30N anaesthetised
Direct laryngoscopy — check:
  Neck flexion and head extension
  Laryngoscopy technique and vector
  External laryngeal manipulation —
    by laryngoscopist
  Vocal cords open and immobile
If poor view:
  Reduce cricoid force
  Introducer (bougie) — seek clicks or hold-up
  and/or alternative laryngoscope

succeed → Tracheal intubation

Not more than 3 attempts, maintaining:
(1) oxygenation with face mask
(2) cricoid pressure and
(3) anaesthesia

Verify tracheal intubation
(1) Visual, if possible
(2) Capnograph
(3) Oesophageal detector
'If in doubt, take it out'

failed intubation

Plan C: Maintenance of oxygenation, ventilation, postponement of surgery and awakening

Maintain 30N cricoid force

Plan B not appropriate for this scenario

Use face mask, oxygenate and ventilate
1 or 2 person mask technique
(with oral ± nasal airway)
Consider reducing cricoid force if
ventilation difficult

succeed

Failed oxygenation
(e.g. SpO_2 < 90% with FiO_2 1.0) via face mask

Postpone surgery
and awaken patient if possible
or continue anaesthesia with
LMA™ or ProSeal LMA™ —
if condition immediately
life-threatening

LMA™
Reduce cricoid force during insertion
Oxygenate and ventilate

succeed

failed ventilation and oxygenation

Plan D: Rescue techniques for 'can't intubate, can't ventilate' situation

[1] With permission of the Difficult Airway Society

Inhalational induction

Indications
- To avoid IV induction—children, needle phobia, difficult IV access
- To maintain airway patency and spontaneous ventilation during induction.
  - Anticipated difficult intubation and/or difficult manual ventilation e.g. acute epiglottitis, perilaryngeal tumours.
  - Inhaled foreign body.
  - Bronchopleural fistula.

Preparation and practice
Explain the process to the patient/parents on the ward. Warn parents about excitation phase. Some anaesthetists prescribe an antisialogogue. Apply routine monitoring whenever possible. A close-fitting facemask speeds induction but in young children a cupped hand around the fresh gas supply may be preferable. When inhalational induction is used for reasons of anticipated airway difficulty, have a back-up plan.
- Inhalational induction is frequently used prior to IV access. In complicated cases have a skilled assistant/second anaesthetist present to secure cannulation.
- Sevoflurane and halothane are the best tolerated agents. Sevoflurane is faster in onset and less arrhythmogenic. Use of a 50:50 nitrous oxide: oxygen mix may improve tolerance and speeds onset of anaesthesia. However, with actual or anticipated airway obstruction 100% oxygen is sensible.
- Halothane may be introduced at 0.5–1% and increased every four breaths or as tolerated. Sevoflurane can be introduced at 8%.
- Single vital capacity breath induction from a four litre reservoir bag containing 5% halothane or 8% sevoflurane in oxygen is suitable for some patients. The patient typically loses consciousness in under a minute.

Difficulties with inhalational induction
- A leak around the mask, low alveolar ventilation (partial/intermittent obstruction; stridor; breath-holding), and a high cardiac output slow induction.
- The correct stage of anaesthesia to cannulate veins, instrument the airway, apply cricoid pressure or intubate is a matter of experience.
- Rapid offset with sevoflurane may cause lightening of anaesthesia during airway intervention. Halothane or sevoflurane induction followed by halothane maintenance may avoid this problem.
- The excitement stage may be long and associated with complications. Induction will only progress past this phase if the airway is patent.
- Application of CPAP may be useful, as may gentle assisted ventilation.
- The traditional view that inhalation induction is safe because if the patient obstructs they will automatically lighten, unobstruct, and start

breathing again is not always reliable: persistent obstruction, laryngospasm, hypoxia and arrhythmias are also possible. Following airway obstruction the patient may not 'lighten', as traditionally described.
- In safe circumstances additional judicious IV induction while maintaining spontaneous breathing may sometimes be appropriate.
- Although inhalational induction may permit direct laryngoscopy and assessment of ease of intubation past an upper airway obstruction, have a back up plan prepared (e.g. equipment for cricothyroidotomy or experienced surgical assistance if an emergency tracheostomy may be necessary).

Paediatric considerations
- Parental explanation and support is essential as their assistance is often useful during induction.
- Optimal positioning will depend on child size. Between the ages of 2–5yr sitting the child on the parent's lap and encouraging them to cuddle/gently restrain them during induction is a useful technique. For older and younger children the trolley may be more appropriate.

Awake fibre-optic intubation

Indications

- Anticipated difficult intubation, laryngoscopy and/or mask ventilation
- Cervical spine instability or cord injury
- To avoid haemodynamic instability during intubation.

Checklist

Decongestant	xylometazoline 0.1% (Otrivine®) or phenylephrine 1% nasal spray—administered in advance if possible
Local anaesthetics	cocaine 5–10% cocaine/lidocaine gel 2% lidocaine spray 10% four syringes of 1.5ml lidocaine 2%
Drugs	midazolam, fentanyl induction agents and neuromuscular blockers
Equipment	6.0/6.5mm nasal endotracheal tube 6/7mm nasopharyngeal airways (cut along length) safety pin Forrester spray warm water in container nasal oxygen catheter
Equipment checks	check scope light functions properly, clean tip and focus check oxygen can be delivered down suction port, and lidocaine injected freely

Preparation

- Full clinical assessment of airway.
- Explanation and consent—co-operation essential.
- Assess nasal passages for patency (on history and unilateral occlusion) and history of epistaxis.
- 1hr pre-procedure: antisialogogue (glycopyrronium 200µg IM—reduces secretions and optimises effect of local anaesthetic) and xylometazoline 0.1% (Otrivine®) nasal spray (or similar).
- IV access.
- Oxygen via nasal catheter.

Technique

- Use mild sedation—midazolam (1–2mg) and fentanyl (50–100µg) or small doses of propofol (10–20mg). Verbal contact must be maintained at all times.
- Determine more patent nostril and spray with cocaine solution (1ml 5%).
- Dilate nasal passage with warmed 6mm then 7mm nasopharyngeal airway lubricated with cocaine or lidocaine gel (cut 7mm along long axis and insert safety pin to aid grip during manipulation of scope).

- Spray oropharynx with lidocaine 10% and use Forrester spray to topically anaesthetise pharynx using lidocaine 2% (2–4 ml) as far back as possible.
- Instil oxygen (2litre/min) through scope to oxygenate patient, clear secretions from the tip, and aid atomisation of injected local anaesthetic.
- Pass *lubricated* fibrescope through the nasopharyngeal airway and having visualised the vocal cords instil 1.5ml lidocaine 2% directly onto the cords. Pass through the cords and repeat for tracheal inlet. The trachea can be identified by rings of cartilage.
- Load warmed, lubricated ET tube onto scope and re-insert through nasal airway into trachea.
- Remove the 'split' 7mm nasopharyngeal airway and advance the endotracheal tube over the scope—be careful not to advance too far or irritation of the carina will cause coughing.
- 90° turn of endotracheal tube anticlockwise allows leading edge of bevel to pass between cords (i.e. bevel facing posterior).
- Remove scope, carefully visualising correct tube placement, and confirm with capnography and bag movement. Do not inflate cuff yet as this may cause panic (increased resistance to respiration).
- Induce anaesthesia, inflate cuff, and fix tube securely.

Complications

Poor compliance/coughing, bleeding in airway (from nasal dilatation), excess secretions, laryngospasm, vomiting, aspiration, airway obstruction.

Special considerations

- Where it is not possible to instil oxygen through the scope, administer oxygen 2–4l/min via nasal cannula.
- Cricothyroid puncture can also be used to anaesthetise glottis: identify the cricothyroid membrane (between thyroid cartilage and cricoid ring) and raise small SC weal with 2% lidocaine. Insert a 20/22G cannula attached to a 5ml syringe containing 2.5ml lidocaine perpendicular to the skin until air can be freely aspirated. This confirms placement within the trachea. The cannula sheath may not easily pass through the membrane in which case a 23/25G needle can be used instead. Inject 2–3ml 2% lidocaine.
- Choice of ET tube. The Portex preformed nasal 'Blue Line' ET tube is extremely pliable when warmed. A 6.5mm tube fits most people although occasionally a 6mm may be needed. Shorten proximally by 3cm to prevent the tube impinging on the nasopharyngeal airway before removal. An alternative would be a 6 or 6.5mm armoured tube. Standard ET tubes will tend to cause nasal bleeding.
- Difficulty in visualising larynx—ask the patient to protrude tongue, swallow or phonate (may improve view) or get assistant to perform gentle jaw thrust.
- 'Red out' indicates too far (oesophagus) or not midline (piriform fossa). Pull back to soft palate and ensure scope is midline. Dimming lights may allow transcutaneous visualisation of the tip.

- 'Tube First' technique. Use 6/7mm nasopharyngeal airways to dilate nasal passage, then insert ET tube 10cm to back of nasal cavity. Pass scope through ET tube and position with good view of laryngeal inlet. If required, spray further 2% lidocaine onto cords at this stage. Advance scope into trachea (view tracheal rings). Use scope as bougie, advancing tube over scope and into trachea (tip of the scope in neutral position).
- Considerations for oral route: use fibrescopic oropharyngeal airway (e.g. Berman Airway®, Vital Signs) which protects fibrescope, holds tongue forward and keeps scope in midline. NB use airway of correct size to ensure tip is just above the laryngeal inlet. Technically much more difficult.
- Contraindications to nasal insertion include coagulopathy, basal skull fracture, CSF leak, and severe nasal disease.
- Positioning depends on preference, either:
  - Patient sitting at least 45° upright facing the operator.
  - Patient supine with operator in normal intubating position.

Further reading

Popat M (2001). Practical Fibre-optic intubation. ISBN 0–7506–4496.6 Butterworth Heinemann.
Ovassapian A, Krejcie TC, Yelich SJ, Dykes MHM (1989). Awake fibreoptic intubation in the presence of a full stomach. *British Journal of Anaesthesia*, **62**, 13–16.
Ovassapian A, Yelich SJ, Dykes MHM, Brunner EE (1983). Fibre-optic nasotracheal intubation—incidence and causes of failure. *Anesthesia and Analgesia*, **63**, 692–5.

Extubation after difficult intubation

Following difficult intubation the airway may occlude when the tracheal tube is removed. Reintubation may then be much more difficult than before due to:

- Airway bruising and swelling.
- Airway contamination with clot, pus or regurgitated material.
- Laryngospasm due to laryngeal or recurrent laryngeal nerve injury.
- New impairments to airway access (e.g. cervical fusion, external fixators, dental wiring).

Extubation must be planned

- Prepare and check the same equipment and personnel as for a difficult intubation.
- Have a plan and a back-up plan.

If an emergency surgical airway could still be required, consider:

- Delaying extubation, ventilating on ICU, and reassessing later.
- Corticosteroid therapy for 24hr before extubation to reduce oedema.
- An elective tracheostomy.
- Positioning a Cook airway exchange catheter (Cook Ltd, Letchworth, UK) in the trachea before extubation. An endotracheal tube may then be rail-roaded into the trachea if required later. These hollow devices also allow apnoeic oxygenation and jet ventilation if needed. Local anaesthetic gel on the catheter improves tolerance. A fibre-optic scope is an alternative but is less well tolerated and does not allow reintubation unless an ETT is already mounted on it. It is therefore far less useful.

Before extubating

- Clear the entire upper airway carefully and suction the trachea.
- Ensure good haemostasis. Can the airway be improved surgically— evacuation of haematoma, relocation of arytenoids, stitches to bring the tongue forward?
- Consider adjuncts the patient will tolerate after extubation e.g. naso-pharyngeal airway, a transtracheal oxygen catheter.
- Empty the stomach if necessary.
- Ensure reversal of neuromuscular blockade.
- Remove any surgical pack(s).
- Perform a leak test. Deflate the cuff (if present) and ventilate to check there is a low pressure leak around the tube. If no leak is present, con-sider delaying extubation.
- Place the patient in their most advantageous position for spontaneous ventilation and airway maintenance. This is often sitting up.
- Preoxygenate, wake patient, and extubate when obeying commands.
- Provide high flow oxygen after extubation.
- Monitor closely in the recovery period for as long as necessary. Consider extended monitoring in a high dependency area.

Practical anaesthesia

Anaphylaxis follow-up

For immediate management of acute anaphylaxis see p896.

Drugs given IV bypass the body's primary defence systems. Potentially noxious chemicals are presented rapidly to sensitive cells such as polymorphs, platelets and mast cells. Degranulation, whether immune or non-immune, releases inflammatory mediators—histamine, prostaglandins, and leukotrienes.

Apparent 'anaesthetic adverse drug reactions' (AADR) may be due to non-drug mechanisms:
- Underlying pathology, e.g. asthma, systemic mastocytosis, malignant hyperthermia.
- Adverse pharmacological effect related to genetic status, e.g. angio-oedema.
- Machine or operator error.
- Vasovagal episode.

Drug involved reactions may be either:
- True allergic reactions: type 1 anaphylaxis (IgE mediated) or type 3 immune complex (IgG mediated).
- Pseudoallergic or anaphylactoid reactions—direct histamine release by active agent or indirect release by complement activation.

Clinically, anaphylactic reactions may be indistinguishable from anaphylactoid responses—the end point in both is mast cell degranulation. Life-threatening reactions are more likely to be immune mediated, implying past exposure.
- Neuromuscular blocking drugs (NMBD) are responsible for 60–70% of serious AADR, frequently on first contact.
- The quarternary ammonium group found in NMBD is widely present in other drugs, foods, cosmetics and hair care products. Previous sensitisation is possible, predominantly in females.

Antibiotic sensitivity
- Penicillin reactions may be IgE mediated but are seldom as severe as AADR.
- If previous penicillin anaphylaxis, neither cephalosporins nor imipenem should be used.
- Incidence of cross-reactivity to newer cephalosporins in patients with penicillin allergy is uncertain as cross-reactivity is often incomplete. Cephalosporins can be given to most patients who declare themselves as 'penicillin allergic'—give slowly and incrementally in case of anaphylactoid (dose related) response.

Incidence
The incidence of AADR is unknown in the United Kingdom. In France, anaphylactic reactions to NMBD have been reported as 1:6500 anaesthetics.

Presentation of anaphylactoid or anaphylactic reactions

- Isolated cutaneous erythema is commonly seen following IV thiopental or atracurium. If there are no further histaminoid manifestations investigation is unwarranted. However, this may be the first clinical feature in severe reactions.
- Timing is important. Onset is usually rapid following IV drug bolus. Slower onset expected if, for example, gelatin infusion, latex sensitivity, or diclofenac suppository responsible.
- Cardiovascular collapse reported in 88%, bronchospasm in 36% and angio-oedema in 24% of AADR with cutaneous signs in ~50%.

Investigation of reactions

Serum tryptase evaluation

Tryptase is a neutral protease released from secretory granules of mast cells during degranulation. *In vivo* half-life is 3hr (compared with 3min for histamine) and it is stable in isolated plasma or serum. Level unaffected by haemolysis, as not present in red or white cells.

- Three venous blood samples preferable—immediately after resuscitation, at 1hr and 6–24hr. Serum separated and stored at minus 20°C for onward transmission to an appropriate laboratory.
- Basal plasma tryptase concentration usually <1ng/ml. Levels up to 15ng/ml seen both in pseudoallergy, i.e. non-specific or anaphylactoid reactions and non-life threatening anaphylaxis. Higher values more likely to indicate IgE mediation.

RAST/CAP tests

- Radioallergosorbent tests (RAST) for antigen-specific IgE antibodies now largely superseded by CAP system (Pharmacia). An antigen coated CAPsule is exposed to the patient`s serum under laboratory conditions. If the serum contains antigen specific IgE a measurable colour change is produced.
- Currently only helpful in confirming penicillin, suxamethonium and latex allergy. Sensitivity low—negative result still requires skin testing.

Skin testing

- Diagnosing AADR depends on skin-prick testing (SPT) or intradermal testing (IDT). In proven NMBD anaphylaxis, no laboratory test has been shown to compare for specificity and sensitivity. Skin testing is probably diagnostic in anaphylaxis, but not in anaphylactoid reactions. Refer patient to a centre experienced in investigating AADR—see below.
- Tests should take place at 4–6wk post-event to allow regeneration of IgE.
- Antihistamines should not have been given within the last 5d.
- SPT used initially. Some drugs, e.g. atracurium and suxamethonium, can produce a false positive result with IDT.
- Testing required to all drugs given before the event. Remember antibiotics, latex, chlorhexidine and lidocaine, if mixed with propofol.

- Suspected local anaesthetic allergy best tested by challenge as recommended by Fisher.[1]
- Negative control is with saline (to exclude dermographia). Positive control is with commercially available histamine solution. The latter demonstrates normal skin response. Weal and flare gives a reference for reactions to test drugs.
- Weal >2mm wider than saline control interpreted as positive. Positive test with undiluted drug is repeated with 1:10 dilution to reduce chance of false positive.
- Following positive result other drugs in the same pharmacological group are tested. In NMBD allergy, up to 60% of people may be sensitive to other relaxants.
- If there is a strong history, but negative SPT—diluted drugs can be tested by IDT.

After testing

- Patient must know the importance and implications of the diagnosis. MedicAlert (12 Bridge Wharf, 156 Caledonian Road, London N1 9UU, UK) can provide a warning bracelet at patient's own expense.
- In the absence of positive skin testing, best advice is given based on the clinical history.
- Ensure hospital notes marked. Inform general practitioner.
- Report reaction to the Medicines and Healthcare Products Regulatory Agency ('yellow card system'). AADR is currently under-reported.

Future anaesthesia

- Avoid all untested drugs related to the original culprit.
- Do not use IV 'test' doses—unsafe if true allergy exists.
- If any doubt about induction agents use inhalational induction. There are no reports of anaphylaxis to inhalational anaesthetics.
- If NMBD reaction, give relaxant-free anaesthetic if possible. In a long-term follow-up of patients with severe reactions to NMBD 3 of 40 subsequent anaesthetics using muscle relaxants produced probable anaphylactic reactions.[2]
- If NMBD must be used, ideally test to your chosen drug by SPT preoperatively.
- In proven NMBD allergy, give chlorphenamine (10mg IV) and hydrocortisone (100mg IV) 1hr pre-induction.

Further reading

Fisher MM, Bowey CJ (1997). Intradermal compared with prick testing in the diagnosis of anaesthetic allergy. *British Journal of Anaesthesia*, **79**, 59–63.
Fisher MM, Merefield D, Baldo B (1999). Failure to prevent an anaphylactic reaction to a second neuromuscular blocking drug during anaesthesia. *British Journal of Anaesthesia*, **82**, 770–773.

1 Fisher MM, Bowey CJ (1997). Alleged allergy to local anaesthetics. *Anaesthesia and Intensive Care*, **25**, 611–614.
2 Thacker MA, Davis FM (1999). Subsequent anaesthesia in patients with a history of previous anaphylactoid/anaphylactic reaction to muscle relaxant.
Anaesthesia and Intensive Care, **27**, 190–193.

Latex allergy

Latex is the sap of *Hevea brasiliensis* (rubber tree). It is a complex mixture of polyisoprene particles in a phospholipoprotein envelope and a serum containing sugars, lipids, nucleic acids, minerals and proteins.

Latex may be found in many of the products used in the operating environment including: gloves, urinary catheters, syringes, drug vial stoppers, IV giving sets, IV cannulae, injection ports, masks, airways, endotracheal tubes, rebreathing bags, bellows and circuits. Many surgical pieces of equipment also contain latex including: drains, bulb irrigation syringes, vascular tags and rubber covered clamps.

Epidemiology

Development of latex sensitivity is dependant on previous exposure. There are certain groups at particular risk of developing latex sensitivity:

- **Health care workers:** estimates have put the risk at between 5–17%, depending on the degree and nature of exposure; the actual figure may well prove to be much higher (up to 50%).
- **Rubber industry workers:** increased incidence of positive skin prick tests to latex, and chronic respiratory symptoms associated with eosinophilia.
- **Neural tube defects (including spina bifida):** reported incidence of latex sensitivity due to recurrent bladder catheterisations is 20–65%.
- **Fruit allergy:** an association between latex and fruit allergy has been described, and cross reactivity demonstrated with certain fruit allergens (banana, avocado, passion fruit, tomato, grape, celery, kiwi fruit, chestnut).

Spectrum

- **Irritant contact dermatitis:** non-allergic irritant contact dermatitis occurs due to damage of skin from irritation of an exogenous substance.
- **Contact dermatitis:** a type IV (delayed) hypersensitivity reaction based on allergic sensitisation. Presents with an eczematous eruption, which can then progress to lichenification and scaling on chronic exposure. Mediated by T lymphocytes.
- **Type I hypersensitivity:** IgE-mediated type I hypersensitivity has been attributed to water-soluble proteins in latex and starch powder-bound proteins. Clinical manifestations may result from exposure to latex via a variety of routes including skin, mucous membranes, inhalation and IV. The three main presentations are:
  - Contact urticaria: particularly in health care workers, typically 10–15min following, and usually at the site of, exposure. This may be the initial step in the progression to more severe reactions.
  - Asthma and rhinitis: characterised by bronchospasm and secretions. Starch powder used as a lubricant for gloves has been implicated.
  - Anaphylaxis, vascular collapse and shock: this is most commonly encountered intra-operatively and although IV and mucous membrane inoculation are the most common triggers, anaphylaxis has been described with donning of gloves and indirect contact with individuals who use latex gloves.

Clinical features of latex anaphylaxis

A careful history with particular reference to risk factors is important preoperatively. Onset is normally 20–60min following exposure and progressively worsens over 5–10min. Presents with hypotension, bronchospasm and commonly rash. It may be difficult to exclude anaphylaxis from anaesthetic drugs since this presents in a similar manner and is treated in the same way (see p896). Subsequent analysis of serum mast cell tryptase confirms anaphylaxis and skin-prick testing will determine the causative factor.

Management of elective surgery

- The prophylactic use of antihistamines and corticosteroids has not been established.
- The patient should be scheduled first on the operating list (latex can remain in the air).
- Items to be particularly careful of include BP cuff, gloves, urinary catheters, anaesthetic reservoir bag/face masks, syringes, elastic in disposable hats/TEDS/underpants, IV giving sets, drug vials with latex stoppers.
- Many companies are now moving towards latex-free equipment, but each theatre suite should have a list detailing which equipment is *guaranteed* latex-free.
- The LMA (Intavent) is latex-free.
- If uncertain about the BP cuff, wrap plastic sheeting around the arm prior to placement.
- Most ETT and airways are latex-free.

Every department should have a latex-free trolley containing the following:

- Non-latex gloves (NB 'hypoallergenic' gloves are non-standardised and often made from latex. Gloves used in latex allergic patients should be made of synthetic rubber such as neoprene or polyvinyl chloride e.g. 'Derma Prene' Ansell Medical or 'Neotech' Biogel).
- Latex-free equipment including masks and airways (plastic), endotracheal tubes (PVC), reservoir bags (neoprene), valves (silicone), IV tubing, bellows and circuits.
- Latex-free (or glass) syringes.
- Latex-free (or Teflon) IV cannulae.
- Barrier protection for placement between latex-containing items and the patients skin (e.g. Webril).
- Drugs for treatment of anaphylaxis and latex-free resuscitation equipment.

Further reading

Kam PC, Lee MS (1997). Latex allergy: an emerging clinical and occupational health problem. *Anaesthesia*, **52**, 570–575.

Woods JA, Lambert S (1997). Natural rubber latex allergy: spectrum, diagnostic approach, and therapy. *Journal of Emergency Medicine*, **15**, 71–85.

Blood exposure incidents

Blood exposure incidents, sometimes referred to as inoculation or needlestick injuries are common in health care settings. These incidents can lead to exposure to blood borne viruses (BBVs), such as hepatitis B (HBV), human immunodeficiency virus (HIV), but the commonest encountered in the UK is Hepatitis C (HCV). Other micro-organisms can also be transmitted leading to local or systemic infection.

Since 1998 there have been four documented cases of UK healthcare workers (HCWs) contracting a blood borne virus in the course of their work. Two doctors and one dentist have contracted Hepatitis C and one nurse has contracted HIV.

Routes of exposure

- Percutaneous injury usually involving a needle (the commonest) or sharp instrument.
- Contact with broken or damaged skin e.g. cuts, abrasions, or eczema.
- Splashes to mucous membranes such as the mouth or eye.

A significant number of these exposures are avoidable by adherence to universal precautions and safe disposal of clinical waste.

Risk of infection following exposure

The risk of infection will depend upon several factors associated with the injury and volume of inoculum. An increased risk is associated with:

- Deep penetrating injury
- Large bore hollow needles
- High viral load of the source patient (donor)
- Injury from a needle that has been in an artery or vein

Risk of seroconversion following needlestick	
HIV	0.3%
HCV	3%
HBV	30%

Prevention (is better than cure)

- Ensure you are immunised against HBV.
- Follow universal precautions, but particularly, do not resheath needles and dispose of your own clinical waste.

First aid

If you are exposed:

- Immediately wash area with soap and water without scrubbing.
- Encourage bleeding of puncture wound.
- If splash to eye or mouth irrigate with water/saline.
- Follow your hospital's policy and procedure for blood exposure incidents.
- Complete incident form—important to record the event in case of health problems developing later.
- Consider whether your injury has led to the patient involved or any-one else being exposed to your blood. This is more likely if your injury has occurred during an interventional procedure.

Post exposure management

- The injury requires rapid assessment. In most hospital settings the Occupational Health Service (OHS) is responsible for this, but different arrangements may be in place out of hours.
- The assessment will consider:
  - The nature of the exposure
  - The likelihood of the source patient being infected with a BBV (see below)
  - The likelihood that the source patient or a third party has been exposed to your blood.
- The OHS will liaise with the source patient's clinical team to obtain consent for testing for BBVs. Most units test routinely for all three BBVs providing consent is given to do so.
- This should be done as a matter of urgency if the source patient is suspected of having HIV infection.
- If consent cannot be obtained a risk assessment of the source patient's status will be required to determine the need for post exposure prophylaxis.
- If consent is withheld or delays are likely post exposure prophylaxis may be commenced based on the risk assessment.

Post exposure prophylaxis (PEP)

- PEP is used following exposure to HBV and HIV. (Antibiotics or antiviral therapy may also be considered after exposures to blood or body fluids of patients suffering from other infectious illnesses.)
- Follow up serology at 6, 12 and 24wk identifies early disease and allows active management. No practice restrictions are required during this period unless seroconversion occurs.
- HBV—depending on immunisation status, victims will receive active immunisation with HBV vaccine alone or in combination with passive protection with HBV immunoglobulin. Treatment should begin within 48hr of injury.
- HIV—ideally PEP should commence within 1hr but may be given up to 1wk following injury. Currently a combination of three antiretroviral agents is recommended for 4wk. The current standard UK starter pack regime is zidovudine 300mg bd, lamivudine 150mg bd and nelfinavir 1250mg bd. The protocol may require alteration if the source patient is not treatment naïve. PEP can produce unpleasant side effects as it is toxic to the liver, kidneys and bone marrow and their function is monitored during treatment. A significant proportion of injured HCWs discontinue treatment because of side effects.
- HCV—No PEP is recommended. Early treatment of acute disease with alpha interferon has been shown to be successful in reducing the risk of long term chronic liver disease.

If occupational health help is not available:

Assess the significance of the injury (see previous page). If exposure has been significant:

- Get colleague to assess the source patient.
- Check to see if testing has been carried out as part of clinical assessment.
- Obtain informed consent for testing for BBVs.
- If consent unavailable obtain clinical/social history to assess risk factors for possible infection (see below).
- If exposure to BBV likely contact on call microbiologist, consultant in communicable disease control or GUM specialist.

Source patient

- Be aware that the injured HCWs blood may have contaminated the source patient as well. Alert senior colleagues that this may have occurred if necessary.
- Co-operate with obtaining consent from source patient for testing for BBVs. This will usually mean ensuring the patient has recovered sufficiently from an anaesthetic to give informed consent.
- In UK there are GMC guidelines concerning testing without informed consent in situations where the patient is anaesthetised, unconscious or has died. Testing can only be supported if there are good reasons to believe the patient is suffering from a condition where prophylaxis for the exposed HCW is available.
- PEP may be started as a result of a risk assessment of the injury whilst awaiting recovery from anaesthesia/sedation etc. However testing without consent may need to be considered if it is unlikely that the patient will be able to give consent within a reasonable timescale, particularly when PEP is associated with significant toxic side effects.
- Consent discussion should cover:
  - Reason for test—injured HCW, possible need for prophylaxis
  - Routine to test for all three BBVs
  - Advantages for source patient—early diagnosis with early treatment and protection for sexual partners
  - Potential disadvantages—distress at serious diagnosis, impact on relationships and difficulty obtaining insurance (but not if negative result)
  - Confidentiality and who will need to know result if positive.
- If consent not available participate in risk assessment of source patient status.
- History consistent with increased risk of infection with BBVs includes:
  - Domicile in a country of high prevalence
  - IV drug abuse
  - Blood/blood product transfusion, especially abroad
  - Male/male sex, sex with prostitutes, casual sex, especially abroad (HBV, HIV)
  - History of jaundice.
- If the decision is made to test source patient without consent ensure patient is informed at the earliest opportunity.

The infected doctor

- Doctors infected with BBVs may represent a risk of infection to patients particularly if they participate in Exposure Prone Procedures (EPPs).
- Occupational health advice must be sought on the range of activities that can be undertaken by infected doctors.
- Currently participation in EPPs is barred for doctors in the UK who are:
  - HBV infected (e-antigen positive or s-antigen positive with a viral load ≥1000 genome copies/ml)
  - HCV infected and HCV polymerase chain reaction (PCR) positive
  - HIV infected.
- Most clinical procedures carried out by anaesthetists do not fall within the definition of EPP. Procedures that may be exposure prone, depending on the technique used, include arterial cutdown or chest drain insertion involving tissue dissection and skin tunnelling.
- Mouth to mouth resuscitation can be undertaken by an EPP restricted worker if no competent non-restricted colleague is available as the benefit to the patient greatly outweighs the small risk of BBV transmission in these circumstances.

Further reading

Department of Health (1998). Guidance for clinical health care workers: protection against infection with blood-borne viruses. Recommendations of the Expert Advisory Group on AIDS and Advisory Group on Hepatitis.
Department of Health (2004). HIV post exposure prophylaxis. Guidance from the UK Chief Medical Officers' Expert Advisory Group on AIDS.
General Medical Council (1997). Serious Communicable Diseases.

Target controlled infusions

Target controlled infusion (TCI) allows the anaesthetist to achieve a target blood concentration of drug for a given patient. The system delivers the required amount of drug (optimised by weight, gender, age) and maintains this calculated target value until changed by the anaesthetist. Propofol has been studied extensively and population pharmacokinetics were incorporated into the *Diprifusor* TCI system in 1996. Recently 'Open' TCI systems have become available offering the advantage of using generic propofol as well as other drugs such as remifentanil e.g. Alaris (Asena Open TCI system) and Fresenius (Base Primea system).

Basic pharmacokinetics

A three-compartment model is used to describe the redistribution and elimination of drugs such as propofol:

- Drug is delivered to the central compartment, V_c, and then distributed throughout the body. The initial bolus is calculated according to the estimated volume of V_c.
- Drug is then distributed to compartments V_2 and V_3. The movement of drug between the compartments is governed by intercompartmental rate constants (e.g. K_{eo} for brain/effect site concentration).

Accuracy

- During infusion measured blood concentrations tend to be higher than predicted.
- Once infusion is stopped this bias is close to zero.
- Because pharmacodynamic variation is much greater than pharmacokinetic variation the target concentration must be titrated to achieve the required effect in any individual patient.

Which numbers to use

With inhalational agents the vaporiser is adjusted to the clinical situation guided by MAC. For propofol, the EC_{50} (effective concentration required to prevent 50% of patients moving in response to a painful stimulus) is 6–7µg/ml with oxygen enriched air and 4–5µg/ml with 67% nitrous oxide in ASA 1–2 patients.

- Inter-individual variations in pharmacokinetics and pharmacodynamics, as well as the interaction between drugs, account for the different responses between patients. The target should be titrated according to the clinical situation. Patients with liver and renal dysfunction show greater pharmacokinetic variability as the drug has altered distribution/elimination.
- In obese patients, the volume of distribution and clearance values are appropriate for body weight and the pharmacokinetics of propofol are unchanged.
- Children require a different set of pharmacokinetic variables for propofol that have not yet been implemented in commercial systems.
- Benzodiazepine premedication, nitrous oxide and opioids all reduce propofol requirements.

Induction of anaesthesia
- Select a target concentration less than anticipated (4–6µg/ml is the requirement in the majority of patients).
- Allow time for the effect site concentration to increase towards the target blood concentration. Oxygen should be administered during the induction phase to ensure an adequate SaO_2.
- Increase the target concentration to achieve the desired level of anaesthesia for the procedure, the individual patient and the balance of other agents such as analgesics.

Rapid induction of anaesthesia using TCI
- Choose a high target such as 6–8µg/ml, but only in young, fit patients.
- Wait to allow for the effect site concentration to rise towards the target concentration.
- Reduce the target value as propofol continues to be redistributed.
- There is no experience in rapid sequence induction of anaesthesia using TCI propofol.

TCI for high risk patients
- Select a low target such as 1µg/ml.
- Wait to allow for the effect site concentration to rise.
- Increase the target in small steps (0.5–1µg/ml) until the desired effect is achieved.

Maintenance of anaesthesia
- 3–6µg/ml is required in the majority of patients but the exact value will depend on the patient, premedication, analgesia and degree of surgical stimulation.
- Titrate to effect.
- The majority of patients will wake at 1–2µg/ml.
- When patients are breathing spontaneously, respiratory rate and $ETCO_2$ are good indicators as to adequacy of anaesthesia.
- The use of moderate doses of opioid analgesics, especially in combination with nitrous oxide, will allow a lower target concentration of propofol to be used—up to one third.

Sedation only
Target concentrations of 0.5–2.5µg/ml are usually required to produce good quality sedation during surgery performed under local/regional anaesthesia. Adding lidocaine to the infusion reduces pain on infusion in the lightly sedated patient.

Effect-site control
The new Open TCI systems offer the possibility of targeting the theoretical effect site concentration rather than blood concentration. A potential advantage would be increased speed of response, but at the risk of increased adverse cardiovascular effects.

IV access

- Requires secure IV access of adequate size to allow the infusion pump to run at its maximum rate of 1200ml/hr (20G or larger). Ideally this access should be visible at all times to ensure the infusion is not disrupted.
- If drug and IV fluids are connected to the same cannula by means of a T-piece or three way tap:
  - Ensure that the fluids are running
  - Prevent reflux by using a one-way valve fitted to the fluid infusion line
  - Minimise the use of extensions to reduce the dead-space.
- Co-administration of drugs by the same giving set is not ideal as a change in the rate of one infusion can affect the other, especially if there is a significant dead-space after the common connection or T-piece.
- The most reliable method is to use a separate, dedicated access site.
- 1–2ml of 1% lignocaine can be injected through the cannula prior to induction, to avoid discomfort from propofol at the start of the infusion.

Benefits of total IV anaesthesia

- Decreases the incidence of PONV.
- Beneficial in laryngoscopy/bronchoscopy where delivery of an inhaled agent may be difficult, and in thoracic surgery, where it does not appear to inhibit the hypoxic vasoconstrictor reflex.
- Safe to use in patients with a history of malignant hyperthermia.
- Recovery with minimal 'hangover'.

Disadvantages

- Increased cost compared with volatile agents.
- Inability to monitor drug concentration.
- Slow recovery following long operations unless the dose of propofol is decreased by combination with remifentanil.
- Interruption to the delivery of propofol may take longer to recognise.

TCI remifentanil

Remifentanil has a rapid onset of action, a short elimination half-life, and a context-sensitive half-time of ~3min, which does not change as the infusion time increases. The pharmacokinetics of remifentanil allow the drug to be easily titrated against patient response using the TCI system. It is often used in combination with propofol TCI and target values of 3–8ng/ml can provide adequate analgesia. Higher values may be required depending on the type of surgery and should be titrated to patient response and dose of hypnotic agent used. The pharmacokinetics of remifentanil have been incorporated into several custom-built TCI systems.

Death on the table

All anaesthetists experience a patient dying on the operating table at some time. In most cases death is expected and the cause is understood. Usually, the patient's relatives and theatre staff will have been informed about the high risk of mortality and are prepared for the event. However, when death is unexpected, the experience can be shattering for all concerned. Added to this is the stress of potential litigation.

Guidelines help to ensure that the legal requirements following a death on the table are fulfilled and may reduce the trauma of the situation. The coroner or equivalent (Procurator Fiscal in Scotland) must be notified of all deaths that occur during anaesthesia, or within 30d of an operation.

- Dealing with the patient. All lines and tubes must be left in place and the patient should be transferred to a quiet area where the relatives can attend.
- Dealing with the relatives. Break the news to the relatives in a sympathetic and considerate way. This should be done by a team of senior staff (surgeon, anaesthetist and nurse). Interpreters, chaplain or social workers may be indicated in specific circumstances. It is highly inadvisable to let the surgeon or any single consultant see the relatives alone, as misunderstandings can occur. The initial interview should convey brief facts about the case to allow the relatives to take in the bad news. A nurse or carer should stay with the family to comfort them and offer practical help as required. After a suitable interval, the team should return and provide further details as appropriate and answer the family's questions. Any queries should be answered as fully and accurately as possible.
- Notifications. The supervising consultant must be contacted, if not already present. The patient's family doctor and the coroner should be informed by telephone at the earliest opportunity.

Unexpected death

When death is unexpected, the cause of death may not be known at the time. The event needs to be accurately documented and in addition to the procedures outlined above, the following must be addressed:

- Equipment—the anaesthetic machine and drug ampoules used should be isolated and checked by a senior colleague, preferably someone unconnected with the original incident. An accurate record of these checks must be kept for future reference. Drug checks should include the identity, doses used, expiry dates, and batch numbers. The drug ampoules and syringes should be kept in case further analysis is required.
- The anaesthetist—the rest of the operating list should be delayed until another anaesthetist and surgeon can take over.
- Documentation—ensure that the medical record is complete and accurate. All entries in the patient's notes should be dated and signed. Details of the case should be clearly documented on an incident form (or equivalent) and copies delivered to the medical director and clinical director. A copy should also be retained by the anaesthetist for the medical defence organization. These should not be filed in the case notes.

- The mentor—a senior colleague should be allocated to act as mentor for the anaesthetist to provide guidance and support. The mentor should help with the notifications, assist in the compilation of reports, liaise with the anaesthetist's family and offer support as necessary.
- The theatre team. A debriefing session should be arranged to help the staff understand the event and come to terms with it. Group counselling may help to reduce post event psychological trauma.

Preparing for legal proceedings

If legal proceedings do ensue, it may be a long time after the event. The medical records will assume utmost importance and form the basis of the case. Anything not recorded in the notes may be assumed not to have been done. The records should be completed within a few hours of the event and must not be altered in any way. An electronically recorded printout alone is insufficient. The record needs to show the reasoning behind the action taken and some indication of the working diagnosis.

The anaesthetist may find it helpful to record a detailed account of the case within a few days of the death, including all the preoperative discussions with the patient and the perioperative events, noting the personnel and times involved. This can be kept in a personal file and used as an aide-mémoire. The anaesthetist's medical defence organization should be consulted for help and further advice. Other healthcare staff should also make statements about the case—normally this is coordinated by the Trust.

Further reading

Association of Anaesthetists of Great Britain and Ireland (2005) Catastrophes in anaesthetic practice. www.aagbi.org

Bacon AK (1989). Death on the table. *Anaesthesia*, **44**, 245–248.

Bacon AK (1990). Major anaesthetic mishaps–handling the aftermath. *Current Anaesthesia and Critical Care*, **1**, 253–257.

Dealing with a complaint

Most doctors receive complaints, the majority of which can be resolved without legal proceedings. Patients are more likely to proceed to a legal claim if there is inadequate information or concern initially. The average acute hospital will investigate 120–160 formal complaints per 1000 doctors annually, but very few are followed by a legal claim and fewer still by a trial. In any service it is recognised that mishaps will occur and mechanisms need to be in place to identify and rectify the causes. There is increasing awareness of the role of 'systems failure' in these cases. Usually a series of mistakes is involved resulting in the adverse incident. The adoption of a 'no blame' culture enables open, honest reporting of failures, which allows appropriate changes to be made thereby improving patient safety.

Background

In the United Kingdom Crown Indemnity was introduced in 1990 and it is the Trust or Health Authority which is sued and is liable, not the individual doctor. The actions of the doctor are considered separately, if required, by the Clinical Director or Medical Director. Crown Indemnity does not cover work performed outside the NHS contract (e.g. private practice, 'Good Samaritan' deeds) and separate medical defence insurance should be arranged to cover any legal claims arising from this work. The defence organization will also provide support for doctors who become the subject of disciplinary proceedings.

Local resolution

Complaints can often be resolved quickly and to the satisfaction of all involved. The aim is to answer the complaint, offer an apology if that is appropriate, amend faulty procedures or practices (for the benefit of others), and to clarify if the complaint is groundless.

Verbal complaints

- Speak to the patient as soon as you hear of any problem. Give the patient a full, clear explanation of the facts and try to resolve any difficulty.
- Speak to a senior colleague for guidance and support. Consider asking a senior consultant or the Clinical Director to see the patient with you as the patient may value their advice and you may value their reassurance.
- Apologise. Saying sorry is not an admission of liability. Patients will appreciate your concern. However, do not apologise for the actions of others, or blame anyone without giving them the opportunity to comment.
- Documentation. Always make a detailed entry in the patient's notes of any dissatisfaction expressed and the action taken in response. Discuss with the Trust complaints manager.

Formal written complaints

Trusts have a legal obligation to comply with national guidelines when dealing with formal complaints. These have to be acknowledged within 2 working days and investigated immediately. The Chief Executive is required to issue a formal response within 20d or provide a letter explaining the delay. Complaints are investigated by copying the correspondence to all the relevant clinical staff and clinical directors for their explanation. The information provided is used to produce a report explaining the course of events and any necessary action taken. When replying:

- Speak to a senior Consultant/Clinical Director. They may have experience of similar events and can help to clarify the issues with you.
- The Trust will have an experienced manager who has responsibility for complaints who should be contacted.
- Inform your medical defence organization who will provide advice and support.
- Record keeping. Keep a full account of the details of the incident.
- Leave a forwarding address if you move. A legal claim may be made many months after the event.

Independent review

Any patient not satisfied with the Trust response, can request an independent review. The review will investigate how the complaint has been handled, not the circumstances of the complaint itself. If this fails to resolve the situation, the case can be referred to the ombudsman (Health Service Commissioner). These procedures do not apply if a legal claim is being pursued.

Legal proceedings

A legal claim can be made up to 3yr after the incident (for children, 3yr after their 18th birthday). Initially, you will be asked for a statement of your involvement in the patient's care. The Trust's legal team will need to work with you and your Clinical Director to produce this.

Preparing a statement

This should include the following:

- Full name and qualifications.
- Grade and position held (including duration).
- Full names and positions of others involved (patients, relatives, staff).
- Date(s) and time(s) of all the relevant matters.
- Brief summary of the background details (e.g. patient's medical history).
- Full and detailed description of the matters involved.
- Date and time that your statement was made, and your signature on every page.
- Copies of any supporting documents referred to in the statement (initialled by you).

The statement should accord with the following points:
- Accuracy. There should be no exaggeration, understatement, or inconsistencies. Check the details with the patient's notes.
- Facts. Keep to the facts, particularly those which determined your decision-making, and avoid value judgments.
- Avoid hearsay. Try to avoid including details which you have not witnessed yourself. If reference has to be made to such information, record the name and position of the person providing it to you, when it was provided and how.
- Be concise. State the essential details in a logical sequence and avoid generalizations.
- Relevance. Include only the details required to understand the situation fully.
- Avoid jargon. Give layman's explanations of any clinical terms used and avoid abbreviations.

Discuss the statement with your Clinical Director and Trust legal department. Make changes as necessary to ensure a clear factual account. Only sign the statement when you are completely happy with the text. Always keep a copy of the final signed version for your own reference. The Trust's legal team should provide advice on the subsequent legal process and discuss the management of the claim with you. Remember good record keeping will help to support your case. Poor records give the impression of poor care. The medical records are the only proof of what occurred and anything not written down may be assumed to have not happened. Any later additions to the notes should be signed and dated with an explanation of the reasons why the entry was not made earlier.

Awareness

Complaints of awareness must be pursued promptly. It is important to confirm what the patient may have heard or felt and document this accurately. If possible, an explanation of the events and causes, if any, should be given. The patient needs reassurance that steps can be taken to reduce the risk of awareness during subsequent anaesthetics. Post-traumatic stress disorder can develop and it is important that these patients are offered counselling.

Further reading

Department of Health (1995). Acting on complaints. *Health Services Circular*
General Medical Council. www.gmc-uk.org
NHS Litigation Authority. www.nhsla.com
National Patient Safety Agency. www.npsa.nhs.uk

Anaesthesia in difficult circumstances

Inhalational anaesthesia

Draw-over anaesthesia is the most suitable inhalational technique for use in the field. The British Military currently use the Penlon Tri-service Apparatus (TSA).[1] The requirements are:

- One-way patient valve and self-inflating bag or Oxford Inflating Bellows.
- Low-resistance drawover vaporiser, e.g. Oxford Miniature Vaporiser (OMV).
- Oxygen by cylinder or concentrator if available.
- Draw-over anaesthesia with isoflurane or halothane in air and supplementary oxygen. Intubation and controlled ventilation, or spontaneous respiration using mask or LMA.
- Supplementary opioid analgesia, usually morphine or nerve blocks.
- Extubate awake.

Advantages of draw-over anaesthesia

- Cheap, practical, simple technique.
- Not reliant on compressed gases.
  - Portability and reliability allowing rapid deployment of anaesthesia equipment to the area of need.
  - Vaporisers (OMV and TEC) are designed for use with different agents and a variety of scales are provided to allow this.

Ketamine

Ketamine is a phencyclidine derivative used as an IV anaesthetic agent and analgesic. It is presented as a colourless liquid, in solutions of 10, 50, or 100mg/ml.

Action

- Non-competitive antagonist at the calcium channel pore of the NMDA receptor.
- Modulates activity at muscarinic and opioid receptors.
- Induces a state of dissociative anaesthesia whereby the patient is in a trance like state with open eyes and laryngeal tone maintained.

Anaesthesia using ketamine

- **IV anaesthesia.** Induction: 1–2mg/kg. The effects of a single dose last for 5–15min. This may be followed by IV maintenance using intermittent boluses (0.25–0.5mg/kg) titrated to response. Alternatively an IV infusion can be used.
- **IV infusion anaesthesia.** Prepare as 1mg/ml in saline. Following IV induction, without muscle relaxation infuse at 0.5–3ml/kg/hr adjusted to response. With relaxants infuse at 0.5–2ml/kg/hr.
- **IM induction** 5–10mg/kg. Onset time usually 5–10min, but slower with smaller doses. The duration of anaesthesia is from 10–75min.
- **Sedation.** For sedation only, or in combination with a regional or local anaesthetic technique 0.25–0.5mg/kg.
- **Analgesia only.** Bolus: 0.25–0.5mg/kg, infusion 0.3–0.6mg/kg/hr.

Uses

- Induction of anaesthesia in shocked/severely ill patients or those with severe asthma.
- Single agent for short repetitive procedures especially in children e.g. plaster changes, radiotherapy, burns dressings.
- Disaster anaesthesia and analgesia for mass casualties.
- Analgesia for positioning prior to a regional block or in combination with a local or regional technique.
- Analgesia in patients with chronic pain.
- ICU sedation in severe unresponsive asthma.
- Extensively used in the third world due to its simplicity and excellent safety record.

Special features of ketamine

- Induction of anaesthesia takes longer with ketamine than with thiopental or propofol.
- Increases sympathetic tone and maintains blood pressure and cardiac output.
- Dysrhythmias are rare.
- Increases cerebral blood flow and cerebral metabolic rate. Contra-indicated in head injury patients.
- Causes an increase in intraocular pressure and is contraindicated in patients with an open eye injury.
- Maintains laryngeal tone but protection of the airway cannot be guaranteed; standard precautions should be taken.
- Stimulates salivation: an antisialogogue premedication is advised, particularly in children.
- Unpleasant dreams/hallucinations and emergence phenomena can be reduced by co-administering a benzodiazepine (e.g. midazolam 1–2mg IV, diazepam 2–5mg IV) or opioid, with minimal interference of recovery. These unpleasant effects occur much less frequently in children and the elderly. (In the UK ketamine is produced as a racemic mixture of R(−) and S(−) isomers. The latter is more potent but less psychoactive. An enantiomer pure product using only the S(-) isomer has been manufactured although is not widely available. It is reported to produce less hallucinations and emergence phenomena.)

Ketamine and midazolam by infusion

- A technique for use with controlled ventilation.
- IV induction: midazolam 0.07mg/kg + ketamine 1mg/kg.
- Maintenance by infusion. Mix ketamine 200mg, midazolam 5mg, and 0.9% saline to a volume of 50ml.
- Infusion rate in ml/h = (patient's body weight in kg)/2.
- The mixture has a shelf life of 72hr.
- Unpleasant dreams or hallucinations are rare.
- Blood pressure and pulse rate tend to be maintained.

1 Houghton IT (1981). The tri-service anaesthetic apparatus. *Anaesthesia*, **36**, 1094–1108.

Other uses of ketamine
- Preservative free ketamine is used to prolong caudal analgesia (see p784).
- Oral administration (1mg/kg) can be used as a sedative and analgesic in children when other drugs are in short supply.

Although ketamine is a useful agent in children, especially in the developing world, it has a variable effect in neonates. They may require a comparatively larger dose to maintain surgical anaesthesia, which can lead to apnoea. Ketamine is difficult to use as a single agent in fit young adults as it often results in repeated, uncontrolled movements. It is also unpredictable in heavy drinkers. Ketamine is probably underused in the UK; its effective use requires experience.

Propofol and alfentanil
- A technique for use with controlled ventilation in patients with an uncompromised circulation.
- IV induction with standard doses of alfentanil and propofol.
- Mix propofol 500mg and alfentanil 2.5mg.
- Initial infusion of ~10mg/kg/hr of propofol.
- Reduce gradually to 5mg/kg/hr according to clinical signs.
- Rapid clear-headed recovery with low incidence of nausea.

Long-term venous access

Cannulae in peripheral veins last for only a few days. For longer-term access several alternatives exist. Before deciding upon which to choose, the following should be considered:
- Indication and duration of proposed therapy for venous access
- Proposed location for administration of therapy (hospital, GP/clinic, home)
- Risk of contamination
- Patient's clinical status (coagulation status, platelet count, sepsis, CVS stability etc.)

The definition of long term central venous access is not standardised e.g. predicted use greater than 6wk or presence of internal anchoring devices.

Indications
- Cancer chemotherapy
- Long-term antibiotics
- Home TPN
- Haemodialysis
- Repeated blood transfusions
- Repeated venesection.

Venous access devices (in ascending duration, costs and complexity)

Short term
- Peripheral cannulae
- Midlines (10–20cm soft catheter) are inserted via the antecubital fossa, with the tip of the device situated in the upper third of the basilic or cephalic vein and short of the great vessels.
- Non-cuffed, non-tunnelled central venous catheters (CVC) are used for resuscitation/central venous monitoring. Non-tunnelled CVCs are rarely used for >10–14d, due to the risk of sepsis. Antimicrobial catheters are available in this type. If only a single lumen catheter is required, avoid multiple channels.
- Tunnelled non-cuffed catheters are used less frequently, as similar cuffed devices offer a more secure fixation and a potential anti-microbial barrier.

Long term
- Peripherally inserted central catheters 'PICC' are long and advanced centrally from the antecubital fossa/upper arm. A PICC can last for several months, if managed correctly.
- Tunnelled, cuffed, central venous catheters ('Hickman type lines') are tunnelled from the insertion site on either the chest or abdominal wall. They can be open ended or contain a two-way valve ('Groshong catheter'). These are used for prolonged therapies and have a Dacron cuff which allows fibrotic tissue ingrowth to provide anchorage and a possible barrier to infection. It takes 3–4wk for fibrous adhesions to develop hence should not be inserted for shorter use.
- SC ports made from either titanium or plastic offer a single or double injection port attached to a central catheter. An SC pocket is formed on the chest or abdominal wall to house the port. They are surgically placed and used for prolonged periods of intermittent therapy e.g. antibiotics for cystic fibrosis. Popular for children.

Device	Normal Duration
Peripheral cannulae	48–72hr
Midlines	14–21d
Non-cuffed, non-tunnelled central venous catheters (CVC)	5–14d
Tunnelled non-cuffed central venous catheters	5–21d
Peripherally Inserted Central Catheters (PICC)	Several months
Tunnelled, cuffed, central venous catheters (Hickman line)	Months/yrs
SC ports	Months/yrs

Site of access

- There is anecdotal evidence to suggest that catheters placed from right side of body have lesser risk of thrombosis than from the left—shorter straighter route to SVC.
- Choose site on basis of patient factors, previous venous access, and clinician experience.
- Look for evidence of thrombosis or stenosis, previous scars from long term access, venous collaterals (suggest great vein stenosis). If doubt exists concerning vessel patency use ultrasound to assess access site. Formal venography is helpful in the difficult case.
- Choose puncture sites and tunnel tract to avoid tight bends, if necessary use multiple puncture sites to avoid >90° bends and catheter kinks.

Site	Advantages	Disadvantages
Arm (cephalic/basilic veins)	Simple to access—veins usually visible and palpable. No vital structures close. Patient comfort	Failure to achieve central position. Higher incidence of thrombosis. Low infusion rates
Right Internal Jugular	Simple to insert. Direct route to central veins. High flow rate—low risk of thrombosis. Lower risk of pneumothorax. Ideal for larger stiff catheters e.g. dialysis	Patient discomfort. Possible higher risk of infection. Tunnelling more difficult to chest wall. Cosmetic considerations
Subclavian	Less patient discomfort. Possibly lower risk of infection	Curved insertion route. Difficult to access. Acute complications—pneumothorax, haemothorax, nerve damage. Catheter may be damaged between clavicle and first rib
Femoral	Easy insertion. Tunnel to mid abdomen	Higher rate of infection/risk of thrombosis. More discomfort

Ultrasound guidance

See NICE guidelines (www.nice.org.uk).
- Appropriate training required.
- Particularly recommended for internal jugular but useful for all sites and ages.
- Useful in context of difficult/repeated long term venous access.
- For subclavian access move lateral to junction of axillary/subclavian vein to allow visualisation with ultrasound.
- Note patent vein at access site does not guarantee central vein patency.

Practical tips for insertion

- Ask patient to take a deep breath on insertion of guidewire/catheter to facilitate central passage.
- Measure catheter length required with correctly positioned guidewire (using fluoroscopy).
- Take care with rigid sheaths and dilators to avoid central vessel damage. Do not insert too deeply (they are generally longer than required).
- Pinch sheath on removal of obturator to avoid bleeding and air embolism.
- Sheaths readily kink—draw back until catheter passes.
- Pass long thin guidewire (70cm+) through soft catheters to increase torque if difficulties passing centrally.
- Screen guidewire, obturator sheath and catheter insertion if any difficulty encountered. Use venography through needle, sheath or catheter if uncertain as to position. 10ml diluted contrast (check allergy) e.g. Ultravist 120®.
- For fixed length catheters (e.g. Groshong) take care to choose correct length for site of access and adequate length of tunnel tract to ensure correct tip position in SVC. Move catheter and cuff along tunnel tract to adjust catheter tip position.
- Flush with saline/heparinised saline before and after use.

Ports

- Ports can be inserted percutaneously under LA ± sedation or under GA. Smaller low profile versions can be sited in the arm.
- Minimise incision and pocket size by placing port anchor sutures within the pocket first and then slide port in over them and tie off (same principle as cardiac valve replacement).
- Access is gained by a specific 'non-coring' needle and advancement through the silicone membrane to the reservoir below. Initial access to a port causes discomfort and EMLA cream can be applied 30min before. There is a distinct clunk as the needle hits the back wall of the port after penetrating the membrane.

Catheter tip position

This is important to reduce risks of thrombosis (with link to infection), catheter perforation into pericardium, pleura or mediastinum, and migration with risk of extravasation injury. Optimal positioning can only be achieved with real time fluoroscopy.

- Tip should ideally lie in SVC, in long axis of vein i.e. not abutting vein at an acute angle.
- It is generally recommended that the tip should lie above the pericardial reflection (to avoid perforation and tamponade). The carina (or right main bronchus) can be used as a radiological landmark to define the approximate upper border of the pericardium.
- It may not be possible to get an adequate catheter tip position above the carina in catheters from the left side (left internal jugular or subclavian) or the right subclavian due to the angulation of the distal catheter segment. Aim to have the last 3–6cm of catheter tip in the long axis of the SVC (this will approximate to the junction of SVC/RA or upper RA in such cases).
- ECG guidance may be used to confirm central position but does not ensure good tip position in SVC (may be angled against vein wall), particularly with left sided catheters.
- Catheter tip may move between lying and sitting/standing. Assess on inspiration and expiration with the patient table flat. It will generally appear much further centrally on supine/head down imaging than on an erect PA film with deep inspiration.

Aftercare

It is essential that staff using such catheters have adequate training in use and use maximum sterile precautions at all times.

- Do not remove anchoring sutures for at least 3wk to allow Dacron cuff to become adherent.
- When used in patients at high risk of thromboembolism, therapeutic doses of warfarin or low molecular weight heparin (LMWH) may reduce the frequency of catheter related thrombosis.
- Beware: some units still lock catheters with strong heparin (e.g. dialysis catheters)—always aspirate catheter and discard before use.
- Thrombosed catheters can be unblocked with urokinase (5000U). Suction all air through 3 way tap to collapse catheter and create vacuum. Then inject urokinase diluted in 2ml saline. Avoid excess pressure that can rupture catheter.

Removing a Hickman line

- Cuffed catheters usually pull out if in situ <3wk—before fibrous adhesions have anchored the cuff.
- Heavily infected catheters usually pull out as the infection breaks down adhesions.
- Push and pull catheter to palpate and visualise cuff shape and tethering. It is difficult to feel cuff if it is just inside the exit site.
- Inject generous LA around cuff site and tunnel tract.

- Cut down (1–2cm incision sufficient) just to the vein side of the cuff. Use forceps to feel catheter as solid structure that rolls under the forceps (incision too small for finger). Free up and remove venous section first; a thin fibrin sheath/capsule will need to be incised to free the catheter. Pull catheter out of vein.
- Then dissect around cuff to free adhesions.
- Try to avoid sharp dissection until the venous section of catheter is removed to reduce risk of embolisation from cut catheter (catheters can pass to RV/PA).

Further reading

Department of Health (2001). Guidelines for preventing infections associated with the insertion and maintenance of central venous catheters. *Journal of Hospital Infection,* **47** (Suppl), 47–67.

Galloway S, Bodenham A (2004). Long-term central venous access. *British Journal of Anaesthesia,* **92**, 722–734.

Galloway S, Bodenham A (2003). Safe removal of long term cuffed Hickman type catheters. *Hospital Medicine,* **64**, 20–23.

Hind D et al. (2003). Ultrasonic devices for central venous cannulation. *British Medical Journal,* **327**, 361–367.

Oesophageal Doppler monitoring

The Oesophageal Doppler monitor (ODM) allows non-invasive cardiac output monitoring. It measures the velocity of blood in the descending aorta and calculates stroke volume and cardiac output, using a nomogram (based on age, weight and height) to estimate aortic diameter. Some models measure aortic diameter using echocardiography. At present most probes are placed in unconscious patients, but with mild sedation/local anaesthesia they can be used in awake patients. Newer non-invasive probes measuring stoke volume and cardiac output from the ascending aorta via the suprasternal notch are also available. The cost of use is low when compared with comparable technologies for cardiac output monitoring.

Method

- The probe is inserted into the oesophagus via the nose or mouth.
- Appropriate entries are made for the age, weight and height of the patient.
- When the transducer is lying 35–40cm from the teeth (~T5/6) a characteristic Doppler signal can be found by manipulating the probe.
- The signal should be a well-defined triangle with a black centre surrounded by red and then some white in the trailing edge of the waveform. This colour spectrum displays the distribution of red blood cell velocities at a given point in time, i.e. a histogram of velocities over time. The brighter (whiter) the colour in the display, the greater the number of RBCs travelling at that given velocity.

Measurements

- **Contractility**—*Peak Velocity (PV)* of blood within the aorta gives a good estimate of contractility. Peak velocity is age dependent.
- **Stoke Volume/Cardiac Output**—*Stroke Distance* is the area under the maximal velocity time curve/waveform and when multiplied by the aortic diameter gives a good estimate of stroke volume.
- **Preload**—blood flow during systole is measured as the *Flow Time*. Flow time is affected by heart rate, limiting its use. When divided by the square root of the heart rate, however, it becomes a useful index of preload and afterload, termed the *Corrected Flow Time (FTc)*. Anything that impedes filling or emptying of the left ventricle will result in a low FTc (<330ms). Most commonly this will be due to hypovolaemia, although obstruction from mitral stenosis or pulmonary embolism will give similar results.
- **Afterload/SVR**—the combination of a low FTc and low PV is strongly suggestive of a high afterload. Conversely vasodilation results in a high FTc (>360ms).

Practical tips

- Lubricate the probe well prior to insertion, as air attenua▮ ultrasound signals.
- Turn the volume up to focus the probe initially. The sharpest ▮ with the best pitch is invariably the right waveform.
- Adjust the following:
  - *Cycle length*. This is essentially a measure of heart rate. Lengthen the 'cycle length' in irregular rhythms to increase accuracy. A cycle length of 5 is a good starting point.
  - *Gain*. This adjusts the contrast between background noise and the Doppler waveform. Aim for a black background to sharply focused signal. A gain of 5 is again a good starting point.
- Always visually check that each waveform is being counted i.e. it has a small white triangle in each corner.
- Be patient when focusing the probe.
- Interference from diathermy is impossible to eliminate but a cycle length of 1 will allow some useful information to be gained.
- Patients having GA and/or epidural may have an FTc approaching 400ms if dilated and well filled.
- It is a dynamic monitor and as such must be refocused prior to each reading.

Normal values		
	Age (yr)	**Velocity (cm/s)**
Peak Velocity	20	90–120
	50	70–100
	70	50–80
FTc	330–360ms	

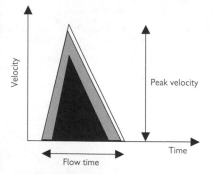

Schematics of a characteristic signal

tic but most commonly is just a starting
y challenge/optimise the cardiovascular

given in boluses e.g. 200ml of colloid to
nat patient. One should look for a
bolus and stop when the Starling curve

represents hypovolaemia and the
d as above to achieve an FTc of
330–360ms. It should be remembered however that there are other
rarer causes for a low FTC, such as pulmonary embolism which will
not correct with fluid alone.

- *Low PV*: consider use of a positive inotrope.
- *Low PV & Low FTc*: Consider agents/manoeuvres to decrease afterload
  e.g. GTN, peripheral warming or reduction of vasoconstrictors.

Indications for use

- Moderate—Major surgery
  - e.g. >2hr + 500ml of blood loss
- High risk patients
  - e.g. extremes of age and co-morbidity
- Haemodynamic instability
  - Fluid flux ± inotropes
  - Critical care.

Cautions and contra-indications for use

- Concurrent intra-aortic balloon pump
- Severe aortic coarctation
- Known pharyngo-oesophageal pathology
- Severe bleeding diatheses.

Further reading

Cholley BP, Singer M. (2003). Esophageal Doppler: Noninvasive cardiac output monitor. *Echocardiography*, **20**, 763–769.

McFall MR, Woods WG, Wakeling HG. (2004). The use of oesophageal Doppler cardiac output measurement to optimize fluid management during colorectal surgery. *Eur J Anaesthesiol*, **21**, 581–583.

McKendry M, μgloin H, Saberi D, Caudwell L, Brady AR, Singer M. (2004). Randomised controlled trial assessing the impact of a nurse delivered, flow monitored protocol for optimisation of circulatory status after cardiac surgery. *British Medical Journal*, **329**, 258.

Depth of anaesthesia monitoring

Awareness is a serious consequence of relaxant anaesthesia with an incidence of around 1:1000. Many incidents are due to errors in anaesthetic administration and can be prevented by careful technique. In an ideal situation anaesthetists could monitor conscious level. Technology to do this reliably has proved difficult to develop and at present depth of anaesthesia is determined in the following ways:

Clinical parameters. Heart rate, BP, pupil size, sweating etc. rely on the sympathetic nervous system and can be affected by factors such as hypovolaemia, arrhythmias, preoperative drug therapy (β blockers, antihypertensive agents) and epidural/subarachnoid block.

Pharmacokinetic modelling. TIVA and TCI systems using pharmacokinetic models to estimate plasma propofol concentration are becoming more common. There is poor correlation between estimated and measured propofol concentrations for individual patients and wide interpatient variability in pharmacodynamic response. There is no equivalent of end-tidal anaesthetic concentration measurement. Secure IV infusion is essential.

Isolated forearm technique. A tourniquet on the upper arm is inflated above systolic BP before muscle relaxation. Spontaneous movements or hand squeezing on command indicates impending or actual awareness. Not all patients who respond have explicit recall postoperatively.

Electroencephalographic monitoring (EEG). A number of methods attempt to measure the effect of anaesthetic agents on the brain. A standard EEG is impractical—time-consuming, electrical interference (mains, diathermy), poor electrode contacts. The use of fewer frontal electrodes and fast-Fourier analysis identifying component waveforms frequencies and corresponding amplitudes has made the interpretation and application of the EEG easier. Techniques include:

- **Compressed Spectral Array.** Fast-Fourier analysis displays amplitudes of component frequencies. As anaesthesia deepens the amplitude of higher frequencies (40–45Hz) decreases with lower frequency amplitudes increasing. Changes are anaesthetic agent dependent, limiting its use as a monitor of depth of anaesthesia.
- **Bispectral Index (BIS).** Combines compressed spectral array information with phase relationships of the EEG's component sine waves and calculates a value between 0 (electrical silence) to 100 (awake) using bifrontal electrodes. 65–85 corresponds to sedation and 40–65 to general anaesthesia. BIS corresponds linearly to the hypnotic state and is agent independent. When using BIS to titrate IV and volatile anaesthesia there is a reduction in anaesthetic usage and faster emergence, however this may encourage 'lighter' anaesthesia. Evidence that BIS reduces awareness is limited. The B-Aware study[1] had two reports of awareness in the BIS-guided group and 11 reports in the routine care group (p = 0.022) of 2463 high risk patients.

Bispectral Index Values	
100	awake
65–85	sedation
45–65	general anaesthesia
<40	burst suppression
0	no electrical activity

- **Auditory Evoked Responses.** Early cortical EEG responses to auditory stimuli administered at 6–10Hz via headphones. Latency of characteristic waveform increases with anaesthesia, with decreasing amplitude as anaesthesia deepens. Correlates with awake to asleep transition but predicts movement poorly. A monitor calculating index of 0–100 developed but wide variability makes it less reliable. Has detected awareness intra-operatively.
- **Patient State Index.** Developed by computer analysis of large numbers of EEGs throughout the anaesthetic process to establish the electrophysiological variability of anaesthetic depth related EEG changes. Calculates an index of hypnosis from patient's EEG and is currently under evaluation.

Minimum alveolar concentration (MAC)[2]. End-tidal anaesthetic agent monitoring provides the most precise estimate of brain anaesthetic agent concentration currently available, provided time is allowed for alveolar/blood/brain equilibration. MAC is the minimum alveolar concentration of anaesthetic at equilibrium producing immobility in 50% of subjects exposed to a standard painful stimulus (skin incision)—the ED_{50}. MAC is normally distributed and has low biological variability. MAC_{awake} refers to the end-tidal concentration producing unconsciousness in 50% of subjects (around 0.5 MAC) and MAC_{bar} the end-tidal concentration inhibiting autonomic reflexes to pain in 50% of subjects.

Variants of MAC

MAC: The minimum alveolar concentration of anaesthetic at 1 atmosphere pressure producing immobility in 50% of subjects exposed to a standard noxious stimulus.

MAC_{awake}: The minimum alveolar concentration of anaesthetic producing unconsciousness in 50% of subjects.

MAC_{bar} : The minimum alveolar concentration of anaesthetic blocking the sympathetic nervous system response to a painful stimulus in 50% of subjects.

MAC is decreased by hypothermia, hypoxia, acidosis, CNS depressant drugs and declines by 6% per decade after 1yr of age. Age-related MAC can be represented by iso-MAC charts, which calculate age-appropriate

1 Myles PS, Leslie K, McNeil J et al. (2004). Bispectral index monitoring to prevent awareness during anaesthesia: the B-Aware randomised controlled trial. *Lancet*, **363**, 1757–1763.
2 White D (2003). Editorial Uses of MAC. *British Journal of Anaesthesia*, **91**, 167–169.

end-tidal volatile concentrations in various nitrous oxide concentrations—see p1160. They may be useful in preventing awareness and also excessive administration of volatile agent in the elderly. Opioids reduce MAC, particularly MAC_{bar}, however are not anaesthetic themselves. It is therefore essential to administer enough volatile agent to prevent awareness, ($>MAC_{awake}$), even when painful surgical stimuli are blocked by high doses of opioids or regional anaesthesia.

Factors increasing MAC	Factors decreasing MAC
Hyperthermia	Increasing age
Hyperthyroidism	Hypothermia
Alcoholism	Hypoxia
	CNS depressants
	N_2O and other volatile agents
	Alpha$_2$ agonists

Lower oesophageal contractility. A balloon in the oesophagus can measure spontaneous and provoked oesophageal contractions. Both reduce in latency and amplitude during general anaesthesia. Its use as a guide to depth of anaesthesia is limited.

Muscle relaxants. If muscle relaxants are not used, patients are free to move if aware. By avoiding total paralysis, a degree of protection may be afforded.

Cardiopulmonary exercise testing

The cardiopulmonary exercise testing (CPX) measurement most commonly used in preoperative testing is the aerobic capacity (or anaerobic threshold—AT). To get a reliable result you need:
- An exercise machine (static bicycle, treadmill, arm crank)
- A computer programmed to increase workload (ramp or step protocol)
- A calibrated pneumotachograph to measure gas volume/composition,
- Continuous 12-lead ECG recording
- Technicians trained to conduct and interpret the test.

The UK's preoperative CPX protocol is available at www.pre-op.org.

The anaerobic threshold is the uptake of oxygen (ml/kg/min) at the point when there is a surge in carbon dioxide production during increasing workload. This is indicated by a steepening of the 'V-slope graph' (i.e. increasing respiratory quotient) and represents the onset of increased anaerobic ATP production. In turn, this reflects the maximum ability of the patient to increase oxygen delivery/consumption, and reflects cardiopulmonary fitness.

CPX results can be used:
- To predict perioperative outcome (death/MI)
- To provide a more precise and complete informed consent
- To plan perioperative management, including ICU/HDU requirement
- To diagnose respiratory or cardiac disease
- To assist in risk reduction.

CPX has been used to categorise patients having major abdominal surgery as 'fit' (AT >11ml/kg/min) or 'unfit' (AT <11ml/kg/min).[1] Postoperative mortality appears to be related both to the presence of ECG ischaemia and AT. When these are both combined the measured positive and negative predictive values increase to 43% and 100% respectively.

Anaerobic Threshold	Mortality rate		
	Test ECG: no ischaemia	Test ECG: ischaemia	Total
>11ml O$_2$/kg/min	0/107 (0%)	1/25 (4%)	1/132 (0.8%)
<11ml O$_2$/kg/min	2/36 (5.5%)	8/19 (43%)	10/55 (18%)
	2/143 (1.4%)	9/44 (20%)	11/187 (6%)

1 Older P, Smith R, Courtney P, Hone R (1993). Preoperative evaluation of cardiac failure and ischaemia in elderly patients by cardiopulmonary exercise testing. *Chest*, **104**, 701–704.

Neuromuscular blockers, reversal, and monitoring

Suxamethonium

- The only depolarising relaxant in clinical use
- Has the most rapid onset of action of all relaxants
- Used if fast onset and brief duration of paralysis are required
- A dose of 1–1.5mg/kg is recommended
- Metabolised by plasma cholinesterase (see below)

Unwanted effects of suxamethonium include:

- Postoperative muscle pains: more common in young muscular adults and most effectively reduced by precurarization—the prior use of a small dose of non-depolarising relaxant, e.g. atracurium (5mg). A larger dose of suxamethonium (1.5mg/kg) is then required.
- Raised intra-ocular pressure: this is of no clinical significance in most patients, but may be important in poorly controlled glaucoma or penetrating eye injuries (p662).
- Hyperkalaemia: serum potassium increases by 0.5mmol/l in normal individuals. This may be significant with pre-existing elevated serum potassium. Patients with burns or certain neurological conditions, e.g. paraplegia, muscular dystrophy, and dystrophia myotonica, may develop severe hyperkalaemia following administration. Patients who have sustained significant burns or spinal cord injuries can be given suxamethonium, if necessary, within the first 48hr following injury. Thereafter there is an increasing risk of life-threatening hyperkalaemia, which reduces over the ensuing months. Avoid suxamethonium until 12 months have elapsed following a burns injury. There may be a permanent risk of hyperkalaemia with upper motor neuron lesions.
- Bradycardias, particularly in children, or if repeated doses of the drug are given. Can be prevented or treated with antimuscarinic agents, e.g. atropine and glycopyrronium.
- Malignant hyperthermia (see p260): suxamethonium is a potent trigger for this condition in predisposed individuals.
- High or repeated doses (probably >8mg/kg) may create dual block which will prolong paralysis.

Cholinesterase

This enzyme occurs in two forms:

- Acetylcholinesterase (true cholinesterase): highly specific for acetylcholine.
- Plasma cholinesterase (pseudocholinesterase or butyrylcholinesterase): capable of hydrolysing a variety of esters. A physiological function for this enzyme has yet to be discovered, but many drugs either interfere with its action, or are metabolised by it.
  - Plasma cholinesterase is synthesised in the liver, has a half-life of 5–12d, and metabolises 70% of a 100mg bolus of suxamethonium within 1min. Genetically, it is encoded on the long arm of

chromosome 3. Several variant genes can occur which result in reduced enzyme activity:

- *The atypical gene.* Heterozygotes will not be sensitive to suxamethonium unless other contributing factors (e.g. concurrent illness, anticholinesterase administration) are present. Homozygotes have a prevalence of ~1:3000 and may remain paralysed for 2–3hr.
- *The fluoride-resistant gene.* Homozygotes are much rarer (1:150 000) and are moderately sensitive to suxamethonium.
- *The silent gene.* Heterozygotes would exhibit a prolongation of the action of suxamethonium, but homozgotes (1:10 000) are very sensitive and develop prolonged apnoea. Usually 3–4hr but may last as long as 24hr.
- Other variants (e.g. H- J- and K-type) also exist. Variant genes thus produce a spectrum of reduced activity of the enzyme, causing mild prolongation of the action of suxamethonium right through to several hours of paralysis.
- The activity of plasma cholinesterase can be measured by adding plasma to benzoylcholine and following the reaction spectrophoto-metrically. Abnormally low values can be further investigated for phenotype by carrying out the reaction in the presence of certain inhibitors, such as dibucaine, sodium fluoride, and a specific inhibitor known as Ro2–0683.

Reduced plasma cholinesterase activity can also occur for acquired reasons. This can occur in the following situations:

- Hepatic disease, renal disease, burns, malignancy, and malnutrition.
- Administration of drugs which share the same metabolic pathway, and therefore compete with suxamethonium for the enzyme, e.g. esmolol, monoamine oxidase inhibitors, methotrexate.
- Presence of anticholinesterases (e.g. edrophonium, neostigmine, ecothiopate eye drops), which inhibit plasma cholinesterase as well as acetyl cholinesterase.
- Pregnancy, where the enzyme activity is reduced by 25%.
- Plasmapheresis and cardiopulmonary bypass.

Many other drugs are metabolised by plasma cholinesterase. Individuals deficient in the enzyme may develop complications with:

- Mivacurium: muscle paralysis will be prolonged
- Cocaine: toxicity is more likely
- Plasma cholinesterase also partially metabolises diamorphine, esmolol and remifentanil. Low enzyme activity does not currently appear to complicate their use.

Further reading

Davis L, Britten JJ, Morgan M (1997). Cholinesterase: its significance in anaesthetic practice. *Anaesthesia*, **52**, 244–260.

Non-depolarising agents

Non-depolarising muscle relaxants (NDMRs) are highly ionised with a relatively small volume of distribution. Structurally, they are either benzylisoquiniliniums (e.g. atracurium and mivacurium) or aminosteroids (e.g. vecuronium and rocuronium). They can also be classified according to their duration of action:

- Short-acting compounds with a duration of action of up to 15min (mivacurium)
- Medium-acting compounds which are effective for ~40min (atracurium, vecuronium, rocuronium, cis-atracurium)
- Long-acting compounds which have a clinical effect for 60min (pancuronium, d-tubocurarine)

Most volatile agents prolong the duration of action of NDMRs. Other drugs may do the same, including aminoglycoside antibiotics, calcium channel blockers, lithium, and magnesium. Neuromuscular block may also be prolonged by acidosis, hypokalaemia, hypocalcaemia, and hypothermia.

Choice of relaxant

Choice is based on individual preference, the length of procedure, and certain patient characteristics:

- Suxamethonium is the drug of choice for rapid sequence induction.
- Many of the benzylisoquiniliniums release histamine, the amount of histamine released being related to the speed of injection. Avoid these drugs in severely atopic or asthmatic individuals. Cis-atracurium, however, does not cause histamine release.
- Like suxamethonium, mivacurium is metabolised by plasma cholinesterase. Patients with reduced levels of this enzyme will exhibit prolonged paralysis.
- Cis-atracurium and atracurium are mainly broken down by Hoffman degradation, a process that is pH and temperature dependent. This metabolism is not affected by the presence of renal failure, so these relaxants are ideal in those with renal impairment.
- Rocuronium, at doses of 0.6mg/kg or greater, gives satisfactory intubating conditions within 60s. Its speed of onset is significantly faster than all other non-depolarising relaxants.
- Mivacurium is useful for short procedures. It does not need to be reversed routinely, providing sufficient time has elapsed (>20min) after a bolus and neuromuscular monitoring is used.

Practical tips when using relaxants

- Calculate dose requirements on lean body mass. NDMRs are highly ionised and do not penetrate well into vessel-poor fat areas.
- Monitor relaxants routinely. This will help you decide when to top-up, when to reverse, and when muscle function has returned.
- Maintenance doses of NDMRs should be approximately a fifth to a quarter of the initial dose.

- Anticipate relaxant drugs wearing off, rather than waiting for patient to cough or move.
- Do not attempt to reverse intermediate-duration NDMRs within 15min of administration.
- Do not wait for suxamethonium to wear off before giving a NDMR. On the very rare occasion that a patient has reduced cholinesterase levels, administering a NDMR will make little difference to the outcome.

Neuromuscular monitoring

Peripheral nerve stimulators allow the degree of neuromuscular block to be assessed. They should apply a supramaximal stimulus (strong enough to depolarise all axons) to a peripheral nerve using a current of 30–80mA. Several peripheral nerves are suitable:

- Ulnar nerve. Electrodes are placed on the medial aspect of the wrist proximal to the hypothenar eminence. Adductor pollicis muscle contraction is assessed.
- Common peroneal nerve. Stimulated immediately below the head of the fibula. Foot dorsiflexion is assessed.
- Facial nerve. Stimulated with electrodes placed in front of the hairline on the temple.

Modes of stimulation

- **Train-of-four (TOF)**. Four supramaximal stimuli are applied over 2s. If non-depolarising muscle relaxant (NDMR) block is profound, no response will be elicited. As neuromuscular function starts to return, the first twitch reappears, followed by the second, third, and finally fourth. Fade is characteristic of partial non-depolarising block. The train-of-four ratio (TOFR) is the ratio of amplitude of the fourth to the first response. Fully reversed patients have no fade and TOFRs of 1. Fade is difficult to assess clinically (visually or by tactile means) once the TOFR has reached 0.4.
- **Double-burst stimulation (DBS)** is a stronger stimulus, where two short bursts of 50Hz tetanus are separated by 750ms. DBS and TOF ratios correlate well, but fade is more accurately assessed with DBS, and an absence of fade is usually good evidence of reversal.
- **Post-tetanic count** can be used to assess deep relaxation when the TOF is zero. A 50Hz tetanic stimulation is applied for 5s followed by 1Hz single twitches. Reversal should be possible at a post-tetanic count of 10 or greater.

These patterns of stimulation are usually assessed by visual or tactile means, but can be assessed more objectively using mechanomyography, electromyography, or accelerometry.

It is sensible to apply the electrodes for nerve stimulation before the induction of anaesthesia, and to assess the effect of stimulation before muscle relaxants are administered, preferably after the patient is unconscious. This enables the anaesthetist to place the electrodes in an optimal position, apply the minimum supramaximal stimulus required, and assess the onset of neuromuscular block once a relaxant has been given.

Muscle groups have differing sensitivities to NDMRs. In general, muscles which are bulkier and closer to the central circulation, e.g. respiratory and anterior abdominal wall muscles, exhibit a block that is less profound and wears off more rapidly. Smaller muscles at a greater distance from the heart, e.g. the muscles of the hand, are more sensitive and remain blocked for longer. Thus, if no residual block is apparent at peripheral muscles, more central muscle will be fully functional. The corollary of this is that patients may start to breathe or cough when there is minimal or no response to peripheral nerve stimulation.

The depth of neuromuscular block required depends on the type of surgery. Certain operations may need profound paralysis, e.g. laparotomies or microsurgery. An adequate non-depolarising block can be maintained at two TOF twitches or one DBS twitch. At this degree of relaxation, patients will be adequately relaxed but also reversible.

Neuromuscular reversal

- Clinical signs of reversal: The ability to breathe is not a good indicator of adequate reversal, as a substantial degree of paralysis may be present with virtually normal tidal volumes. Assessment of sustained muscle contraction is better, e.g. hand grip or head lift for 5s.
- Nerve stimulator: an acceptable recovery from block occurs when the TOF ratio has reached 0.8 or greater. The absence of any detectable fade with double-burst stimulation indicates that the patient has reasonable recovery.
- At the completion of surgery, normal neuromuscular transmission can be facilitated by the use of anticholinesterase drugs (see below).
- Reversal agents should not be given until there is evidence of return of neuromuscular transmission, e.g. at least 2 TOF twitches, 1 DBS twitch or a post-tetanic count greater than 10. Clinically, this might include evidence of breathing or spontaneous muscle movement. Intense neuromuscular block may not be reversible.
- Patients who are inadequately reversed exhibit jerky and uncoordinated muscle movements. If awake, they may appear dyspnoeic and anxious. If residual block is confirmed by TOF or DB stimulation, one further dose of reversal agent may be administered. Agitated patients with reasonable respiratory function and otherwise normal vital signs may be given a small dose of a sedative (e.g. midazolam 1–5mg) whilst awaiting the return of full muscle function. If the block persists, or if the patient is very distressed, anaesthesia, intubation, and artificial ventilation should be undertaken and the cause sought.

Reversal drugs

- These drugs work by blocking acetylcholinesterase, thereby promoting accumulation of acetylcholine. They include:
- Neostigmine. A dose of 0.04mg/kg works within 2min and has a clinical effect for about 30 min.
- Edrophonium. Onset time is faster, but has a duration of action of only a few minutes and is not used in UK except in the 'Tensilon' test.
- Anticholinesterase drugs act at both nicotinic and muscarinic sites, thus producing unwanted side effects which include salivation, bradycardia, bronchospasm and increased gut motility. They are therefore usually administered with antimuscarinic agents (atropine 10–20µg/kg, glycopyrronium 10–15µg/kg).

- Anticholinesterase administration will also result in *plasma* cholinesterase inhibition. Thus if neostigmine is given to reverse a profound block due to mivacurium, block duration may be paradoxically increased (due to inhibition of mivacurium metabolism). Interestingly this effect is less pronounced with edrophonium, which has a lesser effect on plasma cholinesterase.

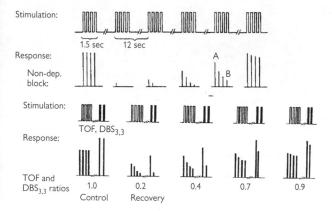

Responses to TOF and DBS stimulations.

Chapter 38

Blood products and fluid therapy

Robert Self, David Walker, and Monty Mythen

Blood products[1]

All donated blood is tested for HIV-1, HIV-2, hepatitis B, hepatitis C and syphilis. Cytomegalovirus (CMV) antibody-negative blood components are available for immunosuppressed patients and neonates. In the UK, white cells are routinely removed from blood components as a precaution against new variant Creutzfeldt–Jacob disease (CJD), leaving a residual leucocyte count of $<5\times10^{6}$/U. This also reduces the risk of CMV transmission.

Whole blood is processed into blood components as follows:
- **Red cells:** most of the plasma is removed, then packed red cells are resuspended in additive solutions—saline, adenine, glucose, and mannitol (SAG-M) or citrate phosphate dextrose adenine (CPDA). Total volume is 190–420ml and haematocrit is 50–70%.
- **Platelets:** pooled buffy coat platelet concentrates are prepared from four donations of whole blood, by a process that includes two centrifugation steps—the 'buffy coat method of preparation'. Platelet concentrates may be produced from a single donor by apheresis. During apheresis, whole blood is sampled from a donor, mixed with anticoagulant and centrifuged. Blood components are separated according to density, the required components (e.g. platelets) are removed and other components (e.g. red cells) are returned to the donor.
- **Fresh frozen plasma and cryoprecipitate:** fresh frozen plasma (FFP) is produced either by centrifugation of whole blood or by apheresis. Plasma is rapidly frozen to maintain activity of labile clotting factors, this produces an average 'unit' of FFP of about 300ml. The Department of Health has recommended that to minimise the risk of CJD transmission, children born after 1996 and patients likely to be exposed to many doses of FFP should receive pathogen-reduced plasma (PRP). This is produced from non-UK sourced plasma by two methods: methylene blue treatment or solvent detergent treatment. Cryoprecipitate is obtained from a single donation of FFP at about 4°C and is rich in factor VIII, von Willebrand factor (VWF), factor XIII, fibronectin and fibrinogen. Each unit of cryoprecipitate is 20–40ml in volume.
- **Plasma derivatives:** albumin, immunoglobulin, and clotting factor concentrates. These products are derived from fractionation of plasma (non-UK sourced).

Other products
- **Artificial oxygen carriers:** these include haemoglobin solutions and perfluorocarbons—use has so far been confined to clinical trials.
- **Recombinant factor VIIa (rVIIa):**[2] originally developed to treat bleeding in patients with haemophilia A or B with inhibitors of factors VIII or IX. Recombinant factor VIIa has also been used in non-haemophiliacs experiencing haemorrhage unresponsive to blood product therapy e.g. trauma, postpartum haemorrhage—this use is unlicensed at present. Average cost of rVIIa therapy for non-approved indications is almost £4000 per patient.

	Red cells	Platelet concentrate	Fresh frozen plasma	Cryo-precipitate
Storage temperature	2–6°C	20–24°C on an agitator rack	–30°C	–30°C
Shelf life	35d	5d	1yr (frozen)	1yr (frozen)
Longest time from leaving controlled storage to completing infusion	Transfuse within 30min of removal from blood fridge. Transfuse unit over maximum of 4hr	Start transfusion as soon as received from blood bank. Transfuse unit within 30min	Once thawed, should be transfused within 4hr	4hr
Unit cost (UK)	£120	£198	£30	£35
Compatibility testing requirement	Must be compatible with recipient ABO and Rh D type	Preferably ABO identical with patient. Rhesus negative females under the age of 45yr should be given Rh D negative platelets	FFP and cryoprecipitate should be ABO compatible to avoid risk of haemolysis caused by donor anti-A or anti-B	
Administration	Infuse through a blood administration set—platelet concentrates should not be infused through giving sets that have been used for blood. Record details of each blood component infusion in the patient's case record.			

1 Handbook of Transfusion Medicine (Edition 3) www.transfusionguidelines.org.uk.
2 Goodnough LT, Lublin DM, Zhang L et al. (2004). Transfusion medicine service policies for recombinant factor VIIa administration. *Transfusion,* **44**, 1325–1331.

Practical uses
Red cells[1]
Transfusion of red cells raises the haemoglobin concentration and thus the oxygen-carrying capacity of blood. Indications for transfusion—see p1006.

Platelets[2]
- Prophylaxis for surgery: A platelet count > 100×10^9/l is recommended before operations in critical sites e.g. brain/eyes. Similar considerations apply to procedures such as epidural anaesthesia (see also pp 699, 1058). For other procedures, a platelet count > 50×10^9/l may be acceptable, however there is limited evidence to guide these decisions.
- Massive transfusion: Maintain count > 50×10^9/l (expected after transfusion of two blood volumes). A higher target of 100×10^9/l is recommended in multiple trauma or central nervous system injury.
- Disseminated intravascular coagulation (DIC): Platelet therapy should be based on frequent platelet counts and clotting tests. In the absence of bleeding, transfusion should not be given to correct a low platelet count.
- Cardiopulmonary bypass (CPB): Platelets should be readily available, but transfusion reserved for patients experiencing excessive postoperative bleeding in whom a surgical cause has been excluded. The decision to transfuse platelets is clinical, based on evidence of microvascular bleeding and excessive blood loss. Near patient testing (e.g. the thromboelastograph, TEG) may aid decision making.
- Liver transplantation: Abnormalities may include reduced coagulation, thrombocytopenia, hyperfibrinolysis, and massive transfusion. Platelet and blood component therapy is guided by the TEG.
- Contraindications to platelet transfusion: Thrombotic thrombocytopenic purpura (TTP) and heparin-induced thrombocytopenia (HIT).

Fresh frozen plasma and cryoprecipitate[3]
- Vitamin K deficiency in the ICU: prolonged prothrombin time (PT) in ICU patients, may be caused by inadequate vitamin K intake. Vitamin K (10mg, 3 times per week) is the treatment of choice.
- Reversal of warfarin: FFP should not be used unless there is evidence of severe bleeding.
- Surgical bleeding and massive transfusion: the decision to use FFP and volume of FFP used should be guided by tests of coagulation, including near-patient tests where available. See section on Massive transfusion on p1012.
- No justification for FFP: FFP should not be used as a simple volume replacement, in plasma exchange (except for thrombotic thrombocytopenic purpura), or to reverse a prolonged INR in the absence of bleeding.

Risks of transfusion

The serious hazards of transfusion (SHOT) scheme is a voluntary scheme for reporting adverse reactions to blood transfusion in the UK and Ireland.

Adverse reactions reported in the 2003 report[4] include:

- **Incorrect blood component transfused (IBCT) 'wrong blood' incidents:** these accounted for 75% of all reports; most errors occurred in clinical areas—the commonest error was failure of the pre-transfusion check.
- **Immune complications:**
  - **Transfusion-related acute lung injury (TRALI)** is caused by antibodies in plasma of a single donor unit reacting with leucocyte antigens in the recipient. Incidence is 1:5–10 000U of products containing plasma transfused—most commonly FFP or whole blood. The risk is greatest with plasma-rich components—more cases are being attributed to FFP and platelets, now that packed red cells are used instead of whole blood. TRALI is probably under-diagnosed and should be considered as a diagnosis in patients developing acute onset pulmonary oedema within 6hr of transfusion. Management is the same as for ARDS/ALI of any cause. In addition the blood bank should be informed. Donors of blood products implicated in TRALI tend to be women immunised against fetal leucocyte antigens in pregnancy.
  - **Acute transfusion reactions (ATR):** defined as occurring up to 24hr following transfusion of blood or components. FFP and platelets are most commonly implicated.
  - **Delayed haemolytic transfusion reactions (DHTR):** defined as occurring more than 24hr after transfusion. Usually a delayed haemolytic reaction related to development of red cell alloantibodies.
- **Transfusion-transmitted infections (TTIs):** 8 reports were probable TTIs—2 hepatitis B virus (HBV), 1 human immunodeficiency virus (HIV), 1 hepatitis A virus (HAV), 1 malaria, and 3 cases of bacterial contamination of platelets. The first possible case of transfusion transmitted CJD was reported in 2003.

1 Murphy MF, Wallington TB et al. (2001). British committee for standards in haematology, blood transfusion task force. Guidelines for the clinical use of red cell transfusions. British Journal of Haematology, **113**, 24–31.
2 British Committee for Standards in Haematology (BCSH), Blood Transfusion Task Force (2003). Guidelines for use of platelet transfusions. British Journal of Haematology, **122**, 10–23.
3 O'Shaughnessy DF, Atterbury C et al. British Committee for Standards in Haematology (BCSH), Blood Transfusion Task Force (2004). Guidelines for the use of fresh-frozen plasma, cryoprecipitate and cryosupernatant. British Journal of Haematology, **126**, 11–28.
4 Serious Hazards of Transfusion (SHOT) Annual Report 2003, www.shotuk.org

Indications and triggers for transfusion

Clinical guidelines for red cell transfusion

- Patients should be given information about the risks and benefits wherever possible, and also be informed about possible alternatives, e.g. autologous transfusion. Patients have the right to refuse blood transfusion.
- Establish the cause of any anaemia. Red cell transfusions should not be given where effective alternatives exist, e.g. treatment of iron deficiency, megaloblastic, and autoimmune haemolytic anaemia.
- There is no absolute level of haemoglobin at which transfusion of red cells is appropriate for all patients (transfusion trigger). Clinical judgement plays a vital role in the decision whether to transfuse or not (see below).
- In acute blood loss, crystalloids or colloids should be used for rapid acute volume replacement. The effects of anaemia need to be considered separately from those of hypovolaemia.
- Local arrangements should provide compatible blood urgently for patients with major bleeding, including emergency O Rh D-negative blood.
- The reason for blood transfusion should be documented in the patient's records.

Indications for blood transfusion

Acute blood loss

First attempt to classify the amount of circulating volume lost (see p820):

- Class I: <15% of circulating blood volume. Do not transfuse unless blood loss is superimposed on a pre-existing anaemia or if the patient is unable to compensate for this level of blood loss because of reduced cardiorespiratory reserve.
- Class II: <30% of circulating blood volume. Will need resuscitation with crystalloids or colloids. Requirement for blood transfusion unlikely unless patient has pre-existing anaemia, reduced cardiorespiratory reserve, or if blood loss continues.
- Class III: <40% of circulating blood volume. Rapid volume replacement is required with crystalloids or colloids; blood transfusion will almost certainly be required.
- Class IV: >40% of circulating blood volume. Rapid volume replacement including blood transfusion.

Next consider the haemoglobin. Plan a target level at which to maintain the patient's haemoglobin:

- Blood transfusion is not indicated when the haemoglobin level is >10g/dl.
- Transfusion is almost always indicated if the haemoglobin level is <7g/dl.
- In patients who may tolerate anaemia poorly, e.g. patients over 65 and those with cardiovascular or respiratory disease, transfusion is indicated if the haemoglobin is <8g/dl.

- It is debateable whether patients whose haemoglobin levels are between 8 and 10g/dl should be transfused. Some will require a transfusion if symptomatic of acute anaemia (fatigue, dizziness, shortness of breath, new or worsening angina).
- Finally consider the risk of further bleeding from disordered haemostasis. Check the platelet count and perform a coagulation screen.

'Group and save' or crossmatch?

- 'Group and save': patient's blood sample is tested to determine ABO and Rh D type and to detect red cell antibodies (in addition to anti-A or anti-B) that could haemolyse transfused red cells. The sample is held in the laboratory for 7d.
- Crossmatch (red cell compatibility testing): as for 'group and save' but in addition the patient's blood is tested to confirm compatibility with each of the units of red cells to be transfused.
- Once 'grouped and saved' (and provided that antibody screening was negative) blood units can be crossmatched against the patient's serum within about 20min.
- There should be a maximum surgical blood ordering schedule (MSBOS) that stipulates which operations require blood to be crossmatched.

Process for red cell or blood product transfusion

Procedures to ensure safe transfusion should include:
- Confirm patient's identity by identification band (and case notes).
- Check blood compatibility label to ensure the blood is correct for patient.
- Check expiry date and unit number.
- Inspect bag to ensure integrity of plastic casing.
- Blood left out of blood fridge for >30min should be transfused within 4hr or discarded.
- Details of the blood unit transfused should be recorded on the anaesthetic chart or clinical notes.
- Volume of blood transfused should be recorded.

Blood conservation techniques

Blood conservation techniques rely upon:
- Increasing the patient's red blood cell mass
- Decreasing perioperative blood losses
- Optimising blood transfusion practices, including both allogeneic (from another human) and autologous (re-infusion of the patient's own blood) transfusion.

Preoperative management
- Optimise preoperative Hb.
- Investigate and treat anaemia. Restrict diagnostic phlebotomy. If possible, stop antiplatelet and anticoagulant medication—this must be balanced against risk of thrombosis.
- Erythropoetin: recombinant human erythropoetin (EPO) stimulates erythropoesis and permits more aggressive preoperative autologous donation. EPO therapy should be started 3–4wk before surgery for maximum effect, and produces the equivalent of 5U of blood. EPO has been considered expensive, this may change with increasing cost of allogeneic blood.
- Preoperative autologous donation (PAD): Patients donate a unit of blood per week in the month prior to their operation. Blood transfusion may be more common in patients undergoing PAD, possibly due to more liberal use of autologous blood. Disadvantages of PAD include: transfusion of the wrong blood due to clerical and laboratory errors, wastage of collected blood, and circulatory overload due to transfusion of whole blood. PAD is not widely used in the United Kingdom, mainly due to organisational difficulties.

Intra-operative management
- **Surgical:** Techniques to minimise blood loss include: less invasive surgery (e.g. endoluminal grafts for abdominal aortic aneurysms), local vasoconstriction with adrenaline, topical haemostatic agents (fibrin glues), tourniquets, and surgical devices, e.g. ultrasonic scalpels/laser techniques.
- **Anaesthetic techniques:** Measures to reduce venous oozing include: avoiding venous congestion (patient positioning), high intra-thoracic pressures, and hypercapnia. Epidural and spinal anaesthesia minimise blood loss by reducing both arterial and venous pressures. Hypotensive anaesthesia has been used in selected patients, however there is a risk of ischaemic cerebral and cardiac complications, especially in the elderly. Hypothermia results in coagulopathy and should be avoided.
- **Pharmacological:** Aprotinin, a serine protease inhibitor, reduces the need for blood transfusion in cardiac and hepatic surgery. Other pharmacological agents that may reduce blood loss include: lysine analogue anti-fibrinolytics (tranexamic acid and epsilon aminocaproic acid), desmospressin (DDAVP), and recombinant factor VIIa. However, further work is needed to examine the efficacy and safety of these agents.[1]

Autologous transfusion[2]

Acute Normovolaemic Haemodilution (ANH)

Perioperative collection of whole blood from the patient, with simultaneous infusion of crystalloid or colloid to maintain normovolaemia. Venesection can be undertaken using a large-bore IV cannula or arterial line into citrated blood bags (available from the blood transfusion department). Once collected, bags should be labelled and stored at room temperature for reinfusion once surgical blood loss has ceased. They must be reinfused to the patient within 6hr. Mathematical models have suggested that significant haemodilution (haematocrit <20%) is required before ANH is efficacious in reducing allogeneic blood transfusion. Risks of significant haemodilution, especially myocardial ischaemia, must be carefully considered.

Indications: current United Kingdom guidelines state that ANH should be considered when the potential surgical blood loss is likely to exceed 20% of the blood volume with a preoperative haemoglobin of >10g/dl.

Advantages of ANH include: no testing required, and reduced risk of incompatible blood transfusion as long as the units are not removed from the operating theatre.

Contraindications: severe myocardial disease, e.g. moderate to severe left ventricular impairment, unstable angina, severe aortic stenosis, or critical left main stem coronary artery disease.

Intra-operative cell salvage

Collection and reinfusion of autologous red cells lost during surgery. Most machines depend on a centrifugal principle using a collection bowl that spins and separates the red cells from plasma, white cells, and platelets. Shed blood is aspirated into a collection reservoir via heparinised tubing. The cells are separated by haemoconcentration and differential centrifugation and finally washed in 1–2 litres of saline. This removes circulating fibrin, debris, plasma, leucocytes, microaggregates, complement, platelets, free haemoglobin, circulating procoagulants, and most of the heparin. Cell salvage produces packed red cells with a haematocrit of 50–60%.

Indications: cell washing devices can provide the equivalent of 10U of bank blood per hour in cases of massive bleeding. The technique is applicable to open heart surgery, vascular surgery, total joint replacements, spinal surgery, liver transplantation, ruptured ectopic pregnancy, and some neurosurgical procedures.

Contraindications: bacterial contamination of the operative field, malignant disease, presence of fat or amniotic fluid in salvaged blood (risk of embolism and disseminated intravascular coagulation (DIC)). Topical clotting agents such as collagen, cellulose, and thrombin and topical antibiotics or cleansing agents used in the operative field should not be aspirated into a cell salvage machine. Complications have been reported in patients with sickle cell disease. However, there is scarce data to support some of these contraindications, and most contraindications are relative rather

1 Kovesi T, Royston D (2003). Pharmacological approaches to reducing allogeneic blood exposure. *Vox Sanguinis*, **84**, 2–10.

2 Napier JA, Bruce M, Chapman J et al. (1997). Guidelines for autologous transfusion II. Perioperative haemodilution and cell salvage. *British Journal of Anaesthesia*, **78**, 768–771.

than absolute.[1] Cell salvage has been used in obstetric haemorrhage, despite contamination of blood with amniotic fluid. In cancer surgery, allogeneic blood transfusion may worsen outcome, possibly by immuno-modulation. Therefore, some centres advocate cell salvage techniques in cancer surgery. The high cost of the machinery and the need for trained operators are drawbacks. Once set up the disposable kits can process limitless units of packed red cells. Current disposable costs are very similar to the cost of one unit of leucodepleted red cells (£120).

Postoperative recovery of blood

Collection of blood from surgical drains followed by reinfusion, with or without processing. The blood recovered is dilute, partially haemolysed/defibrinated and may contain high concentrations of cytokines. Most experience has been gained in cardiac and orthopaedic surgery, especially total knee replacements. The safety and benefit of the use of unwashed blood remains questionable. Some groups have reported considerable savings in the use of bank blood.

1 Waters JH (2004). Indications and contraindications of cell salvage. *Transfusion*, **44**, 40S–44S.

Massive transfusion[1]

Defined as loss of one blood volume in <24hr, 50% blood loss within 3hr, or blood loss of >150ml/min

Goal	Procedure
Restore circulating volume	Two 14G IV cannulae Resuscitation with warmed crystalloid/colloid Warm patient Consider arterial line/central venous access
Contact key personnel	Senior anaesthetist/surgeon/obstetrician Blood bank/haematologist
Arrest bleeding	Early surgical/obstetric intervention Interventional radiology
Request laboratory investigations	FBC, PT, APTT, fibrinogen, X-match—*check patient identity*, biochemistry, arterial blood gas. Repeat clotting, FBC, fibrinogen after products/every 4hr. *May need to give blood products before results available*
Request suitable red cells	Uncrossmatched group O Rh negative in extreme emergency, no more than 2U (Rh positive acceptable if male patient or postmenopausal female). Uncrossmatched ABO group-specific when blood group known (lab will complete X-match after issue). Fully X-match (if time permits or irregular antibodies). Use blood warmer/rapid infusion device. Consider cell salvage if available
Request platelets	Allow for delivery time from blood centre. Anticipate platelet count <50 × 10^9/l after twice blood volume replacement. Target platelet count: 100 × 10^9/l for multiple/CNS trauma, for other situations >50 × 10^9/l
Request FFP (12–15ml/kg body weight)	Aim for PT and APTT <1.5 × control Allow for 30min thawing time
Request cryoprecipitate (1–1.5 packs/10kg body weight)	Replaces fibrinogen and factor VIII Fibrinogen <0.5g/l associated with microvascular bleeding Fibrinogen deficiency develops early when plasma-poor red blood cells used for replacement. Aim for fibrinogen >1.0g/l Allow for delivery time plus 30min thawing time
Suspect DIC	Treat underlying cause if possible

1 Stainsby D, MacLennan S, Hamilton PJ (2000). Management of massive blood loss: a template guideline. *British Journal of Anaesthesia*, **85**, 487–491.

Jehovah's witnesses

The Jehovah's Witness religious movement is 120yr old, with an estimated 6 million members worldwide. Most Jehovah's Witnesses will not accept a transfusion of blood or its primary components, although absolute rules regarding specific blood products do not exist.

Acceptability of blood products and transfusion-related procedures in Jehovah's Witnesses[1] (with permission)

Unacceptable	Whole blood
	Packed red cells
	Plasma
	Autologous pre-donation
Acceptable	Cardiopulmonary bypass
	Renal dialysis
	Acute hypervolaemic haemodilution
	Recombinant erythropoietin
	Recombinant factor VIIa
May be acceptable	Platelets
('matters of conscience')	Clotting factors
	Albumin
	Immunoglobulins
	Epidural blood patch
	Cell salvage

Ethical and legal issues

- Administration of blood or blood products to a competent patient who has refused blood transfusion against their wishes is unlawful and may lead to criminal and/or civil proceedings for assault against the doctor.
- Many Jehovah's Witnesses carry 'Advance Directives', which outline treatments accepted by the individual; family and GP may hold copies.
- Anaesthetists have the right to refuse to anaesthetise Jehovah's Witnesses for elective surgery. However, the anaesthetist is obliged to provide care in emergency cases, and must respect the patient's wishes.[2]
- **Emergencies:** if the patient's Jehovah's Witness status is unknown (e.g. unconscious), the doctor is expected to act in the best interests of the patient—this may include blood transfusion. Opinions of relatives or associates that the patient would not accept a blood transfusion must be verified; evidence of an advance directive should be sought.
- **Children:** the care of children of Jehovah's Witnesses (aged <16yr) may present particular difficulty. For elective procedures, preoperative discussion involving surgeon, anaesthetist, parents, and child should occur. If the parents refuse permission for blood transfusion it may be necessary to apply for a legal 'Specific Issue Order' via the High Court in order to administer a blood transfusion. Two consultants should document that blood transfusion is essential before this serious step is taken.

- In an emergency situation, when a child of Jehovah's Witnesses is likely to die without blood transfusion, blood should be given. Courts are likely to uphold this medical decision.

Preoperative management

- Early communication with the anaesthetic department is essential. Apart from minor surgery a consultant anaesthetist should be available who is prepared to manage the patient.
- Meet the patient as early as possible preoperatively with the results of relevant investigations to ascertain the degree of limitation of normal routine management.
- Involve other specialists, e.g. haematology, intensive care.
- There is a specific consent form for Jehovah's Witnesses. At the preoperative visit establish which treatments are acceptable, including 'Advance Directive' if signed. Make the patient aware of the risks of non-acceptance of blood and blood products.
- Specifically discuss and document whether strategies such as acute normovolaemic haemodilution and perioperative cell salvage may be used.
- Involve the local Jehovah's Witness hospital liaison committee in the discussions. Representatives can help avoid confrontation and assist the understanding of both parties. The address of the local committee may be obtained by contacting hospital information services (Britain): Tel: 0208 906 2211; Fax: 0208 343 0201; E mail: his@wbts.org.uk
- Investigate and treat preoperative anaemia. Oral iron supplements can be used to improve iron stores (ferrous sulphate 200mg twice daily). Recombinant erythropoietin (rEPO) may be used pre-surgery, although the clinical response takes up to a month. Iron supplementation is usually required with rEPO therapy. Discussion of an individual case with a haematologist may be useful.
- Review anticoagulant and antiplatelet drugs, consider stopping.
- Major operations can sometimes be staged to limit acute blood loss.

Intra-operative management

Preoperative assessment must determine which of these techniques are acceptable to the individual patient:

- **Surgical:** consider staged or laparoscopic surgery. Meticulous surgical technique, argon beam diathermy, biological haemostats e.g. Kaltostat and fibrin glues and sealants.
- **Anaesthetic:** reduce venous oozing—avoid venous congestion (patient positioning), high intra-thoracic pressures and hypercarbia. Prevent hypothermia—leads to coagulopathy. Consider the use of invasive monitoring, even when the medical condition of the patient or the nature of the operation would not usually warrant it. The potential benefits and risks of hypotensive anaesthesia and regional anaesthesia should be considered.

1 Milligan LJ, Bellamy MC (2004). Anaesthesia and critical care of Jehovah's Witnesses. *Continuing Education in Anaesthesia, Critical Care & Pain*, **4**, 35–39.
2 The Association of Anaesthetists of Great Britain and Ireland (1999). *Management of anaesthesia for Jehovah's Witnesses.*

- **Drug therapy:** antifibrinolytics e.g. aprotinin, tranexamic acid and epsilon aminocaproic acid (EACA). Desmopressin (DDAVP) increases platelet adherence. Use of these drugs during major surgery may be considered.
- **Acute hypervolaemic haemodilution:** acute normovolaemic haemodilution (ANH) may be unacceptable to Jehovah's Witnesses, as it involves removal and storage of blood from the circulation. However acute hypervolaemic haemodilution (AHH), rapid infusion of fluid to achieve haemodilution without withdrawal of blood, may be acceptable.
- **Intra-operative cell salvage:** acceptable to some Jehovah's Witnesses.
- **Red cell substitutes:** perfluorocarbons and haemoglobin solutions may be acceptable to some Jehovah's Witnesses as an alternative to transfusion. These products are not available in the UK, although there are case reports of 'off licence' use.
- **Alternatives to clotting factors:** there are case reports of the successful use of recombinant factor VIIa in Jehovah's Witnesses undergoing major surgery.

Postoperative management
- Intensive care: low threshold for admission. Treat postoperative oozing aggressively. Remember simple measures such as direct compression. Early re-exploration is mandatory.
- Hyperbaric oxygen therapy: in severe blood loss or anaemia may swiftly reverse hypoxaemia. However, hyperbaric facilities are not readily available and the technique has practical difficulties.

Further reading

Hebert PC, Wells G et al. (1999). A multicenter randomised controlled trial of transfusion requirements in critical care. New England Journal of Medicine, **340**, 409–417.

McGill N, O'Shaughnessy D, Pickering R et al. (2002). Mechanical methods of reducing blood transfusion in cardiac surgery: randomised controlled trial. Brithish Medical Journal 2002, **324**, 1299–1236.

Wallis JP (2003). Transfusion-related acute lung injury (TRALI)— under-diagnosed and under-reported. British Journal of Anaesthesia, **90**, 573–576.

Mahdy AM, Webster NR (2004). Perioperative systemic haemostatic agents. British Journal of Anaesthesia, **93**, 842–858 .

Association of Anaesthetists of Great Britain and Ireland (2001): Blood Transfusion and the Anaesthetist, Red Cell Transfusion.

Association of Anaesthetists of Great Britain and Ireland (2005): Use of Blood Components. www.aagbi.org

Shander A (2003). Surgery without blood. Crit Care Med, **31**, S708–S714.

Fluid and electrolyte therapy

Fluid-compartment equilibrium may be disrupted by illness, anaesthesia, and surgical interventions. These may elicit a combined metabolic, neuroendocrine, immunological, and inflammatory 'stress' response. This response is proportional to the degree of insult and is crudely protective. It normally subsides within several days of surgery, but may be exaggerated and inappropriate.

A short period of fasting in patients undergoing elective minor surgery is well tolerated and does not require fluid replacement. Small volumes of fluid given at the time of minor surgery may be associated with faster recovery and less postoperative nausea and vomiting. At the extremes of age children and elderly patients tolerate dehydration less well and replacement should be considered.

Fluid and electrolyte balance in 70kg man

Water balance

INTAKE (2500ml)	OUTPUT (2500ml)
1500ml oral	1500ml in urine
750ml food	100ml faeces
250ml metabolism	900ml insensible loss

Daily requirements of common electrolytes

	Plasma concentration	Daily requirement
Na^+	135–145mmol/l	1–1.5mmol/kg/d
K^+	3.5–5.0mmol/l	1–1.5mmol/kg/d
Mg^{2+}	0.75–1.05mmol/l	0.1–0.2mmol/kg/d
Ca^{2+}	2.12–2.65mmol/l (total) 1.0mmol/l (ionised)	0.1–0.2mmol/kg/d
Cl^-	95–105mmol/l	0.07–0.22mmol/kg/d
phosphate	0.8–1.45mmol/l	20–40mmol/kg/d

Fluid compartments (70 kg adult)

Total body water 55–60 % (of weight) = 45 litres	Intracellular 30 litres	
	Extracellular 15 litres	Interstitial 12 litres Intravascular 3 litres

Physiological changes during stress response

↑ Anti-diuretic hormone (ADH)	Thirst, water retention, potassium loss
↑ Cortisol (mineralocorticoid effect)	Sodium/ water retention, potassium excretion
↑ Renin–Angiotensin–Aldosterone axis	Sodium reabsorption
↑ Organ osmo/chemoreceptor activity	Endocrine/sympathetic catabolic state
↑ Systemic inflammatory response	Cytokine induced capillary leak

Assessment of dehydration

- This is notoriously inaccurate—most patients are more dehydrated than they look, in-spite of 'adequate' fluid maintenance therapy.
- Every effort should be made to identify and correct perioperative dehydration and hypovolaemia, as it is associated with considerable morbidity.
- This should begin with detailed clinical examination to identify signs and symptoms of dehydration (see table).
- Classical signs and symptoms may be absent, especially in chronic dehydration. Careful examination of fluid balance charts and assessment of periods of fluid restriction, gastro-intestinal losses, blood loss, drugs, bowel preparation, or specific disease states which impact on hydration status is essential.
- In particular, 'third space' losses may account for a significant fluid volume loss, the electrolyte content of which may be large.
- Charting of vital signs over time is useful. Scrutinise trends in BP, pulse, temperature, urine output, and respiratory rate.
- Laboratory indices may be useful. Elevated plasma creatinine/urea/haematocrit/albumin, and low urine acidity/sodium concentration indicate significant dehydration. Plasma lactate/acid base status may highlight metabolic derangement associated with hypovolaemia and hypoperfusion.
- CXR may help identify cardiomegaly/pulmonary oedema due to fluid overload.
- Creatinine clearance is a robust measure of renal function and can be estimated at the bedside (see below).
- CVP monitoring, especially with dynamic fluid challenges, is probably the most reliable method of measuring (and replacing) lost fluid.

Signs and symptoms of dehydration

% body weight loss	Signs and symptoms
5%	Thirst, dry mouth
5–10%	↓ peripheral perfusion, ↓ skin turgor postural dizziness, oliguria, ↓ CVP, lassitude, tachycardia
10–15%	↑ respiratory rate, hypotension, anuria, delirium, coma,
>15%	Life threatening

Estimation of creatinine clearance (Cockcroft and Gault equation)

Approx creatinine clearance = 1.23 × (140–age) × weight (kg)/serum creatinine (µmol/l)

(replace 1.23 with 1.04 for female calculation)

Replacing fluid
- In the fluid replete adult undergoing a significant period of nil by mouth, replace total daily water requirements of 30–40ml/kg/day, plus total daily electrolyte requirements for Na^+, Cl^- and K^+ (see p1018). In pyrexial patients increase fluid by 15% for every 1°C rise in body temperature above normal.
- The perioperative period often proves difficult for assessment of fluid losses. In theatre increased evaporative and 3rd space losses from an open abdomen will not be apparent and may require 10–15ml/kg/hr of crystalloid in addition to calculated basal requirements.
- Most fluids lost are salt-containing and should be replaced with fluids of similar content. Isotonic formulations of crystalloid equilibrate with ECF and are the replacement fluid of choice.
- In the perioperative period Na^+, Cl^-, and K^+ are often replaced routinely. In illness Na^+ stores may be well conserved, whilst obligatory K^+ losses occur and occult total body K^+ deficiency is common. This will not be reflected by plasma concentration.

Daily volume and composition of GI secretions

	Flow (ml/d)	H^+ (nmol/l)	Na^+ (mmol/l)	Cl^- (mmol/l)	HCO_3^- (mmol/l)	K^+ (mmol/l)
Saliva	500–1000	0	30	10–35	0–15	20
Gastric	1500–2000	0–120	60	100–120	0	10
Bile	500	0	140	100	40–70	5–10
Pancreas	750	0	140	70	40–70	5–10
Small/large Intestine	2000–4000	0	110	100	25	5–10

Dynamic fluid challenge
- Use boluses of 100–200ml crystalloid.
- Assess clinical and intravascular endpoints e.g. UOP, HR, SV, BP, and particularly CVP where possible.
- A sustained rise in CVP of >3mmHg suggests patient is well-filled.
- An inadequate response is a failure to sustain clinical/CVS endpoint improvement.
- Repeat boluses with frequent reassessment.
- This should not be considered as treatment for acute blood loss from the vascular compartment.

Crystalloids
Cheap, effective with relatively few adverse effects

Balanced salt solutions (BSS) e.g. Hartmann's (Ringer's lactate) solution
- Physiological solutions
- Osmolality is similar to ECF and thus are useful for restoring extra-cellular volume.
- First line replacement therapy in the perioperative period.

- May reduce iatrogenic hyperchloraemic metabolic acidosis, associated with use of higher chloride containing solutions.
- The addition of K^+ and Ca^{2+} to BSS may limit usefulness in hyperkalaemic states or with citrated blood transfusions.

'Normal' saline 0.9%

- Commonly used for electrolyte replacement
- Contains high sodium and chloride concentrations and may be responsible for hyperchloraemic metabolic acidosis, which is of unknown significance.
- Remains the preferred fluid for hypovolaemic resuscitation in many countries, but intravascular half-life may be limited to 15min. Useful for replacing electrolyte rich GI losses.

Glucose solutions (Dextrose is preferred name in US)

e.g. Glucose 5%, glucose 4%–saline 0.18%

- Glucose 5% is a convenient way of giving free water, used to restore dehydration associated with water loss. Perioperatively hyponatraemia may occur with excessive use.
- Glucose in 10%, 20%, and 50% solutions are available to promote normoglycaemia, but have little role in routine daily fluid management in adults.
- Sugar containing solutions provide 4kcal/g of glucose (Glucose 5% contains 5g/100ml), a considerable energy source, but their potential deleterious osmotic effects limit use, and they have no role as plasma expanders.

Colloids

Colloids are homogenous, non-crystalline substances consisting of large molecules or ultramicroscopic particles, which persist in the vascular compartment to expand the functional plasma volume (lasting several hours to several days). Duration of action is determined by physiochemical properties, integrity of capillary membrane and by metabolic and clearance pharmacokinetics.

Human Albumin Solution (HAS)

- Molecular weight (MW) 69 000.
- Available as a 4.5% solution for the treatment of hypovolaemia, and as a salt-poor 20% solution for the treatment of hypoalbuminaemia.
- Like other blood products is manufactured from fractionation of whole blood. Concern of theoretical transmission of variant Creutzfeld–Jacob (vCJD) has resulted in this product currently being imported from the US and is thus expensive in the UK.

Gelatins

- Succinylated gelatins (MW 30 000) e.g. Gelofusine® 4% is presented in NaCl solution.
- Urea-linked gelatins (MW 35 000) e.g. Haemaccel® 3.5% have been popular, but this product has recently ceased to be manufactured in the UK.
- Manufactured from bovine collagen from BSE-free herds—there have been no reports of vCJD. Succinylated gelatins undergo thermal degradation during manufacture. Succinic anhydride then replaces free amino acid groups with carboxyl groups, resulting in a conformational

change in the molecule size. They have an initially powerful osmotic effect. Administration may rarely lead to histamine release causing bronchospasm, urticarial rash, hypotension, and tachycardia (see below). There is no limit on total volume that may be administered.

Hydroxyethyl starches (HES)

• MW 70 000–450 000.
• Manufactured from hydrolysed amylase resistant maize or sorghum. HES products differ widely and may be characterised by concentration, molar substitution, molecular weight, and degree of substitution (DS), which confers solubility and degree of degradation. Thus there are hetastarches (DS 0.6–0.7), pentastarches (DS 0.5), and tetrastarches (DS 0.4). The greater the DS the greater is the resistance to degradation, which means that plasma expanding activity is prolonged.
• First generation starches were associated with considerable side effects, including, renal impairment, accumulation, pruritus, and clotting derangements and bleeding. Manufacturers recommend a maximum dose which varies with formulation—newly formulated second/third generation HES solutions, with lower molecular weight, may reduce the incidence of unwanted side-effects and may given in volumes of 30 and 50ml/kg respectively.

Dextrans

• Branched polysaccharides derived from bacterial action on sucrose.
• Products are 10% Dextran 40 (MW 40 000), and 6% Dextran 70 (MW 70 000), supplied in 5% dextrose or 0.9% saline solution. Both are plasma expanders, but their use in the UK is less common than other products.
• Interfere with blood crossmatching techniques and reduce factor VIII activity and increase plasminogen activation. Fibrinolysis may also occur resulting in reduced clot strength and impairment of platelet activity causing prolonged bleeding time.
• Manufacturers recommend that initial administration should be limited to 20ml/kg for first 24hr and 10ml/kg thereafter for 5d use only.
• Dextran 40 may be used to promote peripheral blood and microvascular flow, by inhibiting aggregation of red blood cells.

Adverse effects of colloid solutions

There are clinically important differences in safety among colloids. A 2004 systematic review of 113 publications showed that approximately 1.3 cases per million transfusions of albumin result in anaphylactoid reactions. Two fold and four fold increases are seen with dextran and HES solutions respectively, while twelve times the anaphylactoid rate was seen with gelatin products.

An increased incidence of bleeding and coagulopathy is widely reported with artificial colloids, particularly HES solutions. Significant pruritus has also been associated with HES solutions—often occurring some time after administration.

Special considerations in fluid therapy

Colloid vs crystalloid in fluid resuscitation

• No single study has yet been powered for mortality outcome. In rapid major blood loss either type of fluid is suitable to maintain organ perfusion in the short term. For ongoing losses colloids offer faster, longer lasting resuscitation with less volume of infusate. No single colloid solution has been proven to be safest. The aim is to restore adequate organ perfusion, avoiding haemodilution, coagulopathy and hypothermia.

Safety of albumin as a plasma expander

- A recent large RCT comparing albumin and saline for intravascular volume expansion in critical illness concluded a similar outcome using either treatment regime at 28d. This refutes the findings of the 1998 Cochrane Injuries Group who reported adverse outcomes with albumin.

Hypertonic saline in patients undergoing surgery

- Small volume hypertonic saline has theoretical advantages for emergency plasma expansion, but a recent Cochrane review suggests that there is insufficient data available to recommend its use in the perioperative setting.

Fluid and goal-directed therapy

- In emergency surgery there is good evidence that optimal fluid filling, as judged by cardiac stroke volume and cardiac index, reduces perioperative renal failure and reduces length of hospital stay. Only after fluid optimisation and the persistence of organ hypoperfusion (elevated lactate, reduced mixed SvO$_2$, persisting base deficit) should the delivery of oxygen be increased by inotropic support.

Further reading

Conway-D-H, Mayall-R, Abdul-Latif-M-S, Gilligan-S, Tackaberry-C (2002). Randomised controlled trial investigating the influence of intravenous fluid titration using oesophageal Doppler monitoring during bowel surgery. *Anaesthesia*, **57**, 845–849.

Davies SJ, Wilson RJT (2004). Preoptimisation of the high-risk surgical patient. *British Journal of Anaesthesia*, **93**, 121–128.

Gan-Tong-J, Maroof-Mohamed, Moalem-Habib *et al.* (2002). Goal-directed intraoperative fluid administration reduces length of hospital stay after major surgery. *Anesthesiology*, **97**, 820–826.

Sinclair S, James S, Singer M (1997). Intraoperative intravascular volume optimisation and length of hospital stay after repair of proximal femoral fracture: randomised control trial. *British Journal of Anaesthesia*, **315**, 909–912.

The SAFE Study Investigators (2004). A comparison of Albumin and Saline for fluid resuscitation in the intensive care unit. *The New England Journal of Medicine*, **350**, 2247–2256.

Composition of common intravenous fluids

	Na⁺ mmol/l	K⁺ mmol/l	Ca²⁺ mmol/l	Cl⁻ mmol/l	Other	pH	mOsmol/l	Cost £/litre
Normal saline 0.9%	154			154		5	308	1
Glucose 4% saline 0.18%	30			30	Glucose 40g	4	263	1
Glucose 5%					Glucose 50g	4	278	1
Hartmanns solution	131	5	2	111	Lactate 29mmol/l	6.5	278	2
Gelofusine	154	<0.4	<0.4	125	Gelatin 40g	7.4		10
Hydroxyethyl starches (in NaCl)	154			154	Starch 60–100g	5–5.5		25
Albumin 4.5%	<160	<2		136	Albumin 40–50g	7.4		95
Dextran 70 in saline	154			154		4.5		12
Dextran 70 in glucose					Glucose 50g	5		12
Dextran 40 in saline	154			154		4.5		12
Dextran 40 in glucose					Glucose 50g	5		12

Chapter 39

Acute pain

Adrian Dashfield

Introduction

Benefits of acute pain management

Severe postoperative pain and the stress response to surgery cause increased morbidity and mortality.

- CVS—tachycardia, hypertension, and increased peripheral vascular resistance cause increased myocardial oxygen consumption/demand and myocardial ischaemia. Altered regional blood flow (sympathetic stimulation), reduced mobility, venous stasis, and increased clotting cause venous thrombosis.
- RS—abdominal/thoracic pain results in diaphragmatic splinting and weakened cough. Reduction in lung volumes, atelectasis, and sputum retention cause chest infections and hypoxaemia.
- GI—delayed gastric emptying and reduced intestinal motility. This can be a direct effect of pain or as a side-effect of opioids and surgery.
- GU—urinary retention.
- Metabolic/endocrine—release of vasopressin, aldosterone, renin, angiotensin, cortisol, glucagon, growth hormone and catecholamines, and reduction in insulin and testosterone leads to increased protein breakdown, impairment of wound healing/immune function, sodium and water retention, increased fibrinogen and platelet activation and increased metabolic rate.
- Chronic pain—there is some evidence that patients who suffer acute pain are more likely to develop chronic pain.
- Psychological—poor acute pain management can lead to patient anxiety, sleeplessness, fatigue, and distress well into the postoperative period.

Measurement of pain

- Verbal rating scales—stratify pain intensity according to commonly used adjectives such as 'mild', 'moderate', and 'severe'. They are widely applied and easy for patients to use. The semi-quantitative nature makes them less suitable for research purposes.
- Numerical rating scales—take the two extremes of the pain experience and have a numerical scale in-between 'no pain' and 'worst imaginable' for example. These scales are robust and reproducible and easy for patients to understand. A disadvantage is that a digital scale reduces the capacity to detect subtle changes as the digits act as anchoring points.
- Visual analogue scales—similar to numerical rating scales with two extremes of the pain experience on either end of the scale. The patient is asked to mark across the line of standard length (usually 100mm). The distance along this line is used. The continuous data generated make analysis easier than with verbal or numerical rating scales.

Analgesic drugs

Paracetamol

- Action is thought to be inhibition of prostaglandin synthesis within the central nervous system. Analgesic and antipyretic without anti-inflammatory activity.
- Excreted by the kidney after glucuronide and sulphate conjugation in the liver. A hepatotoxic metabolite N-acetyl-p-benzoquinoneimine is normally inactivated by conjugation with hepatic glutathione. In paracetamol overdose, this pathway is overwhelmed leading to hepatic cell necrosis.
- Usually given orally or rectally but available as IV preparation Perfalgan®.
- Recommended dose—4g/d in adults. Most effective when prescribed regularly rather than prn.

Nonsteroidal anti-inflammatory drugs (NSAIDs)

- Analgesic, anti-inflammatory, antiplatelet, and antipyretic action is due to inhibition of the enzyme cyclo-oxygenase (COX) and consequently the synthesis of prostaglandins, prostacyclins, and thromboxane A_2 from arachidonic acid.
- Two types of COX. COX-1 is normally present in the kidney, gastrointestinal mucosa, and platelets where prostaglandin contributes to normal organ function. COX-2 is associated with inflammatory mediators following tissue damage. COX-2 inhibitors may be associated with fewer adverse effects than COX-1 and 2 inhibitors (but see p1029).
- NSAIDs have some central as well as peripheral activity. Absorption from the upper gastrointestinal tract is rapid. Metabolised in the liver, excreted in the kidney.
- Opioid sparing effect of between 20–40%. May be used as the sole analgesic for mild to moderate pain. Side effects with NSAIDs are relatively common.
- The Royal College of Anaesthetists published guidelines[1] for the use of NSAIDs in the postoperative period suggesting a number of precautions and contraindications.
- The VIGOR study,[2] in which patients on low-dose aspirin were excluded, found an increased risk of myocardial infarction for patients given rofecoxib compared to naproxen. Rofecoxib has recently been withdrawn from clinical practice because of further concerns about the risks of cardiovascular events including myocardial infarction and stroke.[3]

Relative contraindications	Absolute contraindications
Impaired hepatic function, diabetes, bleeding or coagulation disorders, vascular disease	History of gastrointestinal bleeding or ulceration
	Known hypersensitivity to NSAIDs
Operations where there is a high risk of intra-operative haemorrhage (e.g. cardiac, major vascular, and hepatobiliary surgery)	Severe liver dysfunction
	Cardiac failure (NSAIDs cause sodium, potassium and water retention)
Operations where an absence of bleeding is important (eye surgery, neurosurgery)	Dehydration, hypovolaemia, or hypotension
	Hyperkalaemia
Non aspirin-induced asthma	Pre-existing renal impairment
Concurrent use of ACE inhibitors, potassium-sparing diuretics, anticoagulants, methotrexate, ciclosporin, and potentially nephrotoxic antibiotics such as gentamicin	Uncontrolled hypertension
	Aspirin-induced asthma
Pregnant and lactating women. Age >65yr (renal impairment is more common)	

1 Royal College of Surgeons and College of Anaesthetists (1990): Report of the Working Party on Pain after Surgery.
2 Bombardier C, Laine L, Reicin A, et al. (2000). Comparison of upper gastrointestinal toxicity of rofecoxib and naproxen in patients with rheumatoid arthritis. VIGOR Study Group. New Engl J Med, 343, 1520–1528.
3 FDA (2004). FDA Public Health Advisory: Safety of Vioxx. US Food and Drug Administration. www.fda.gov/cder/drug/infopage/vioxx/PHA_ioxx.htm

Comparison of NSAIDs and COX-2

	NSAIDs	COX-2
Efficacy for moderate to severe acute pain management (Numbers Needed to Treat—NNT)	Diclofenac 50mg (2.3) Ibuprofen 400mg (2.4) Ketorolac 10mg (2.6)	Celecoxib 200mg (4.5) Parecoxib 20mg (3.0) Valdecoxib 20mg (1.7)
Renal function	Can affect renal function in the immediate postoperative period	Similar adverse effects on renal function
Gastrointestinal	Acute gastro-duodenal damage and bleeding can occur with short-term use. Risk increased with higher doses, history of peptic ulceration, long-term use, and the elderly	Less clinically significant peptic ulceration than NSAIDs (VIGOR and CLASS studies)
Platelet function	Inhibit platelet function but do not significantly increase surgical blood loss in normal patients. Associated with higher incidence of post-tonsillectomy haemorrhage	Do not impair platelet function
Aspirin-exacerbated respiratory disease	10–15% of asthmatics affected when given aspirin. Cross-sensitivity with NSAIDs	Do not produce bronchospasm
Bone healing	Impaired in animal models. No good evidence that this is clinically important	Similar to NSAIDs

Inhalational analgesia

- Entonox (50% nitrous oxide, 50% oxygen) is a quick acting, potent analgesic of short duration which relies on patient self-administration.
- Isonox (isoflurane 0.2–0.75% in Entonox). Lower concentrations of isoflurane produce less drowsiness.[1]
- It is ideal for procedures of short duration such as dressing changes, removal of drains, catheterisation, labour pain, and application of traction etc.
- Side-effects of Entonox include drowsiness, nausea, excitability, and augmentation of respiratory depressant drugs.
- Entonox diffuses rapidly into and increases gas-containing cavities. Contraindications thus include pneumothorax, decompression sickness, intoxication, bowel obstruction, bullous emphysema, and head injury.

Opioids

Opioid drugs act as agonists at opioid receptors found mainly in the brain and spinal cord but also peripherally. There are three principal classes of opioid receptor:

- μ—analgesia, nausea and vomiting, bradycardia, respiratory depression, miosis, inhibition of gut motility, pruritus. Endogenous agonists are β-endorphins.
- κ—analgesia, sedation, dysphoria, diuresis. Endogenous agonists are dynorphins.
- δ—analgesia. Endogenous agonists are enkephalins.

Morphine—remains the 'gold' standard against which all new analgesics are compared. It is the least lipid-soluble opioid in common use. Metabolised in the liver, with only 10% excreted unchanged by the kidney. Metabolite morphine 6-glucuronide is more potent than morphine. Other main metabolite is morphine 3-glucuronide which has no analgesic activity. Both metabolites are excreted in the kidney. Accumulation can occur after prolonged use in patients with impaired renal function. Dose ranges and dose intervals vary according to route of administration.

Diamorphine—a prodrug (diacetylmorphine) rapidly hydrolysed to 6-monoacetylmorphine and then morphine. Diamorphine is much more lipid soluble than morphine and thus has a more rapid onset of action than morphine when given by epidural or IV route.

Fentanyl—highly lipid-soluble synthetic opioid with a short duration of action because of rapid tissue uptake. The high lipid solubility makes it suitable for trans-dermal administration. Metabolites of fentanyl are inactive. Fentanyl is commonly administered IV, epidurally or intrathecally.

Pethidine—analgesic with anticholinergic and some local anaesthetic activity. Primarily metabolised in the liver with metabolites excreted in the kidney. One of the main metabolites is norpethidine with a half-life of 15–20hr. Norpethidine is a potent analgesic. High blood concentrations can lead to central nervous system excitation. Patients with impaired renal function are at risk. Pethidine can be used to treat postoperative

---

1 Ross JAS (2000). Isoflurane Entonox mixtures for pain relief during labour. *Anaesthesia*, **55**, 711–712.

shivering associated with volatile anaesthetic agents, epidural and spinal anaesthesia.

Codeine is a prodrug for morphine. Usually administered for the treatment of mild to moderate pain. About 10% of the dose is converted to morphine. Metabolism to morphine requires an enzyme (CYP2D6) which is part of the cytochrome P450 system. 8–10% of Caucasians lack this enzyme, obtaining little or no benefit.

Tramadol—synthetic centrally-acting opioid-like drug. Less than half of its analgesic activity is at the µ-opioid receptor. It inhibits noradrenaline and serotonin uptake at nerve terminals. Lower tolerance and abuse potential, less respiratory depression, and constipation compared to other opioids reported. Metabolised in the liver and excreted in the kidney. Main metabolite of tramadol is O-desmethyltramadol (M1) which is more potent. Formation of M1 also depends on the presence of CYP2D6 within the cytochrome P450 system (see codeine).

All opioids are equianalgesic if adjustments are made for dose and route of administration. Allowance should be made for long-term opioid therapy, incomplete cross-tolerance between opioids, differing half-lives and inter-patient variability.

Equianalgesic dosages		
Opioid	**IM/IV (mg)**	**Oral (mg)**
Morphine	10	25
Diamorphine	5	—
Fentanyl	0.15–0.2	—
Pethidine	100	250
Codeine	—	175
Tramadol	100	100

Opioids have a similar spectrum of side-effects. There is considerable inter-patient variability and some patients may suffer more side effects with one particular drug compared to another.

Side-effects include respiratory depression (decreased respiratory rate, tidal volume, and irregular respiratory rhythm), sedation, euphoria, dysphoria, nausea and vomiting, muscle rigidity, miosis, bradycardia, myocardial depression, vasodilatation, delayed gastric emptying, constipation, and pruritus.

Opioid antagonists act at all opioid receptors. Naloxone (Narcan®) is the most commonly used. By titrating the dose of naloxone administered, it is possible to reverse side-effects such as respiratory depression, nausea and vomiting, and sedation without antagonising the analgesic effects. It must be remembered that naloxone is effective for about 60min.

Opioids—routes of administration

- *Oral*. Oral bioavailability of most opioids is limited due to first-pass metabolism. The slower onset and longer duration of controlled-release formulations make rapid titration impossible. Immediate-release oral opioids (e.g. morphine syrup, oxycodone) are preferred for early management of acute pain.
- *Intermittent SC or IM opioids*. Traditional route of administration ordered 4-hourly PRN. A reluctance to give opioids more frequently than 4-hourly often leads to failure of regimens. Blood levels of an opioid need to reach minimum effective analgesic concentration (MEAC) before any relief of pain is perceived. This requires an adequate initial dose. The only way to achieve good pain relief is to titrate the dose of opioid for each patient.
- *Intermittent IV opioids*. To achieve sustained pain relief without excessive drowsiness and respiratory depression, small doses of opioids should be given often. This technique of opioid administration is suitable for recovery wards but not for routine maintenance of analgesia by untrained staff. Commonly used regimens are 1–3mg of morphine or 20–60µg fentanyl every 5min until the patient is comfortable. Morphine can take up to 15min to exhibit its full effect.
- *Continuous IV infusion*. To avoid 'peaks and troughs' in blood opioid concentrations associated with intermittent administration, continuous opioid infusions are sometimes used. Close observation and monitoring of the patient is essential. Patients are best made comfortable with IV boluses to 'load' the patient.
- *Intra-nasal diamorphine*. Very effective in children (>1yr) needing acute analgesia. A suitable dosing regime is 0.1mg/kg in 0.2ml saline (0.1ml to each nostril). To prepare solution, add 10mg diamorphine to 20/weight (kg) of saline (ml) and draw up 0.2ml.
- *Transmucosal administration*. Fentanyl lollipops (oral transmucosal fentanyl citrate) allows absorption from the oral mucosa. More frequently used for anaesthetic premedication in children. Can be used for 'breakthrough' analgesia in opioid-tolerant patients with cancer.
- *Transdermal administration*. Very lipid-soluble opioids are absorbed through skin. Fentanyl patches are available in 4 sizes (25–100µg/hr) and patches are replaced every 72hr. Although not suitable for acute pain management, in chronic pain the recommended dose based on daily parenteral morphine dose is:

Daily parenteral morphine dose (mg)	Transdermal fentanyl dose (µg/hr)
8–22	25
23–37	50
38–52	75
53–67	100
68–82	125
83–97	150

The Oxford league table of analgesic efficacy (Courtesy of Pain Research Unit, Oxford—www.ebandolier.com)

Analgesic	Number of patients in comparison	At least 50% pain relief (%)	NNT	Lower confidence interval	Higher confidence interval
Valdecoxib 40mg	473	73	1.6	1.4	1.8
Valdecoxib 20mg	204	68	1.7	1.4	2.0
Diclofenac 100mg	411	67	1.9	1.6	2.2
Rofecoxib 50mg	1900	63	1.9	1.8	2.1
Paracetamol 1000mg + codeine 60mg	197	57	2.2	1.7	2.9
Parecoxib 40mg (IV)	349	63	2.2	1.8	2.7
Diclofenac 50mg	738	63	2.3	2.0	2.7
Ibuprofen 600mg	203	79	2.4	2.0	4.2
Ibuprofen 400mg	4703	56	2.4	2.3	2.6
Ketorolac 10mg	790	50	2.6	2.3	3.1
Paracetamol 650mg + tramadol 75mg	679	43	2.6	2.3	3.0
Ibuprofen 200mg	1414	45	2.7	2.5	3.1
Diclofenac 25mg	204	54	2.8	2.1	4.3
Pethidine 100mg (IM)	364	54	2.9	2.3	3.9
Morphine 10mg (IM)	946	50	2.9	2.6	3.6
Parecoxib 20mg (IV)	346	50	3.0	2.3	4.1
Ketorolac 30mg (IM)	359	53	3.4	2.5	4.9
Paracetamol 500mg	561	61	3.5	2.2	13.3
Paracetamol 1000mg	2759	46	3.8	3.4	4.4
Paracetamol 600/650mg + codeine 60mg	1123	42	4.2	3.4	5.3
Aspirin 600/650mg	5061	38	4.4	4.0	4.9
Tramadol 100mg	882	30	4.8	3.8	6.1
Tramadol 75mg	563	32	5.3	3.9	8.2
Paracetamol 300mg + codeine 30mg	379	26	5.7	4.0	9.8
Tramadol 50mg	770	19	8.3	6.0	13.0
Codeine 60mg	1305	15	16.7	11.0	48.0

Patient-controlled analgesia

Patient-controlled analgesia (PCA) refers to self-administration of IV opioids and helps overcome the marked variability in response to post-operative opioids. Patients titrate their plasma opioid concentration to remain in the analgesic window (above the minimum effective analgesic concentration (MEAC) and below the minimum toxic concentration (MTC)). The inherent safety of PCA lies in the fact that excessive doses of opioid will not be delivered should the patient become sedated. No-one but the patient is allowed to operate the PCA demand button.

PCA regimens

- The most commonly used opioid is morphine. Fentanyl, pethidine, tramadol, and other opioids have also been used. No opioid is noticeably superior to any other although a greater incidence of pruritus may be seen with morphine; on an individual basis one opioid may be better tolerated than another.
- The optimal bolus dose consistently results in analgesia without side-effects. Initial values for PCA variables are given below.
- For paediatric use of PCA see p782.

PCA variable	Drug and dose	Comments
Loading dose	0mg	Patients should be comfortable before starting PCA
Bolus dose	Morphine 1mg Pethidine 10mg Fentanyl 20µg Diamorphine 0.5mg Tramadol 10mg	Patients over the age of 70yr may require half this amount
Concentration	Varies depending on pumps used and hospital protocols	Should be standardised in hospital protocols for each drug
Lock-out interval	5min is usual	
Background infusion	0mg/hr	If used, the background infusion rate (mg/hr) usually should not exceed the bolus dose (mg)
Dose limit	30mg morphine or equivalent in 4hr	No clear opinion on how this facility should be used. Often no dose limit is set

Complications

- Equipment malfunction is rare. Interference in pump operation has been reported following current surges or static electricity. Modern PCA pumps have a number of 'fail-safe' design features where the program defaults to the lowest setting possible for a bolus dose. Most machines have a battery back-up lasting up to 8hr. Failure of anti-reflux valves has led to cases of respiratory depression.
- Operator error is much more common. Programming errors, the use of the wrong drug or incorrect drug concentrations, and incorrect background infusions have all been reported and have led to fatalities due to respiratory depression.
- Side-effects related to opioid use such as nausea and vomiting, pruritus, sedation, respiratory depression, urinary retention, confusion, constipation, and hypotension.

Troubleshooting

- Nausea and vomiting—consider:
  - Adding anti-emetic to the PCA (ondansetron 4mg, cyclizine 50–100mg, haloperidol 2mg)
  - Prescribe anti-emetic on a regular basis
  - Change opioid.
- Breakthrough pain: Add regular NSAID and paracetamol if not contraindicated. Increase bolus dose or consider background infusion if severe.
- Respiratory depression: This is caused by direct action of opioids on the respiratory centre. All opioids, given in equianalgesic doses, have the same potential for respiratory depression. This is a relatively uncommon side-effect and if doses are properly titrated, the risk is small. The best early clinical indicator of respiratory depression is increasing sedation. Opioid doses are adjusted so that the sedation score remains below 2. Respiratory depression (respiratory rate <8/min) is reversed with IV naloxone (100–400µg).

Sedation score	
0	Patient wide awake
1	Easy to rouse. Mild drowsiness
2	Moderate drowsiness. Easy to rouse
3	Severe drowsiness. Difficult to rouse
S	Asleep, but easy to rouse

Epidural analgesia

Epidural analgesia is considered by many to be the 'gold standard' analgesic technique for major surgery. It can provide complete analgesia for up to 3d. Patients can mobilise and resume normal activities more quickly with epidural analgesia compared to parenteral opioids. Beneficial effects of epidural analgesia result from attenuation of the 'stress response' following surgery:

- The efficacy of epidural analgesia, regardless of agent used, location of catheter, type of surgery, time or type of pain assessment has recently been demonstrated.[1]
- The incidence of postoperative atelectasis and pulmonary infection is reduced, improving postoperative oxygenation.[2] Effective pain relief allows the patient to cough, breathe deeply, and cooperate with physio.
- The incidence of postoperative myocardial infarction is reduced. The myocardial oxygen supply:demand ratio is improved by the reduction of sympathetic activity, improved pulmonary function, and reduced thrombotic tendency.
- The hypercoagulable response to surgery is attenuated and fibrinolytic function is improved by attenuation of the stress response. This has been shown to be of benefit for graft survival in patients undergoing lower limb revascularisation.
- Increased postoperative mobility reduces the incidence of DVT.
- Epidural analgesia improves intestinal motility by blocking nociceptive and sympathetic reflexes as well as limiting systemic opioid use. The duration of postoperative ileus is reduced so permitting earlier feeding.
- Intra-operative neuraxial block reduces postoperative blood transfusion requirements.
- There is however no survival benefit in high risk patients despite being beneficial in terms of pain relief and respiratory function.[3]

Contraindications

- Patient refusal—a full explanation of the risks and benefits of the technique must be given to every patient.
- Untrained staff—staff must have a good understanding of the techniques used and be able to recognise and treat complications.
- Contraindications to catheter or needle placement include local or general sepsis, hypovolaemia, coagulation disorders, concurrent treatment with anticoagulant drugs, and some central neurological diseases (see pp696, 1054, 1098).

Troubleshooting

- Breakthrough pain—consider:
  - Adding regular PO/PR/IV NSAID and paracetamol if not contraindicated
  - Bolus dose (3–5ml) followed by increased infusion rate
  - Check all connections and insertion site
  - Check block level (with ice or touch). If block patchy or unilateral, withdraw catheter to 2cm in space
  - Bolus dose of opioid only (fentanyl 50–100µg, diamorphine 2–3mg).

- Pruritus—give naloxone (50–100µg) and consider adding 300µg to infusion fluids, or removing opioid from epidural infusion. Antihistamines may give some relief.
- Hypotension—check fluid status of patient, probably relatively hypovolaemic. Check block height. Consider reducing infusion rate. If acute/severe raise legs, give fluid bolus ± ephedrine (6mg boluses).
- Motor block—reduce infusion rate. Consider reducing local anaesthetic concentration.

Complications of epidural anaesthesia

Complication	Incidence (%)	Management
Dural puncture	0.16–1.3	Bed rest, analgesia, hydration, blood patch (see pp702, 706)
Headache	16–86	Bed rest, analgesia, hydration, suspect dural puncture
Nerve or spinal cord injury	0.016–0.56	Immediate neurological assessment
Catheter migration	0.15–0.18	Remove catheter and re-site if appropriate
Epidural haematoma	0.0004–0.03	MRI or CT scan. Immediate neurosurgical assessment. Antibiotics (see also p21)
Epidural abscess	0.01–0.05	
Respiratory depression	0.13–0.4	Decrease in opioid concentration may be required
Hypotension	3–30	IV fluids ± vasopressors. Temporarily reduce or stop infusion
Pruritus	10	Naloxone IV (50–100µg) ± antihistamine
Urinary retention	10–30 (in males)	Catheterisation
Motor block	3	Check for catheter migration. Temporarily cease infusion. Consider epidural haematoma (p21)
Other		Possible increased risk of anastomotic leakage after bowel surgery. No evidence to support this

1 Block BM, Liu SS, Rowlingson AJ, et al. (2003). Efficacy of postoperative epidural analgesia: A meta-analysis. *JAMA*, **290**, 2455–2463.
2 Ballantyne JC, Carr DB, deFerranti S, et al. (1998). The comparative effects of postoperative analgesic therapies on pulmonary outcome: cumulative meta-analyses of randomized, controlled trials. *Anesth Analg*, **86**, 598–612.
3 Rigg JRA, Jamrozik K, Myles PS, et al. (2002). Epidural anaesthesia and analgesia and outcome of major surgery: a randomised trial. *Lancet*, **359**, 1276–1282.

Drugs used for epidural analgesia

To minimise the side effects of each class of drug and provide optimal analgesia a combination of an opioid and a low concentration of local anaesthetic solution is given by continuous infusion. Commonly used mixtures are:

- 0.125% bupivacaine with 5µg/ml fentanyl or 100–125µg/ml diamorphine
- 0.1% bupivacaine with 5µg/ml fentanyl or 100µg/ml diamorphine
- 0.0625% bupivacaine and 2µg/ml fentanyl or 50µg/ml diamorphine

There is no universally accepted optimal combination of drugs. Infusion rates vary according to the concentration, surgical site, and dermatomal level of epidural catheter placement. Usual infusion rates for the above solutions are 8–15ml/hr for adult patients and reduced rates of 4–8ml/hr in patients over 70yr of age. Some anaesthetists reduce or avoid epidural opioids in the very elderly and use local anaesthetic solutions only.

Intrathecal opioids

Opioids can be administered intrathecally in combination with local anaesthetic during spinal anaesthesia. The opioid is delivered directly into CSF so avoiding distribution into epidural fat and blood vessels. Consequently the doses used are much smaller compared to epidural or parenteral routes.

Opioid	Intrathecal dose	Onset (min)	Duration (hr)	Epidural dose
Morphine (preservative free)	0.1–0.2mg	15–30	8–24	2–3mg
Pethidine (preservative free)	10–25mg	<5	1–2	10–50mg
Fentanyl	10–25µg	<10	1–4	50–100µg
Diamorphine	0.25–0.5mg	<10	10–20	2.5–5mg

- The more lipid soluble the drug, the more rapid the onset and the shorter the duration of action.
- Pethidine has local anaesthetic as well as opioid properties. It can be used as the sole drug for spinal anaesthesia (requires higher doses).
- Delayed or late respiratory depression can occur with the less lipid soluble drugs (particularly morphine). Increasing patient age, high doses of opioid administered intrathecally, concurrent use of sedatives or systemic opioids are associated with increased risk of respiratory depression.
- Diamorphine (if available) offers the best combination of duration of analgesia with fewest side-effects.

Stimulation-produced analgesia: TENS and acupuncture

- Stimulation techniques activate the body's pain-modulation systems. The gate control theory of pain by Melzack and Wall in 1965 provided a model to explain this phenomenon.
- Incoming noxious pain signals are reduced by presynaptic and postsynaptic inhibition in laminae 1–5 in the dorsal horn of the spinal cord. Modulatory input arrives via descending pathways and lateral branches from myelinated afferent A-fibres. A-fibres arise in low-threshold mechanoreceptors activated by transcutaneous electrical nerve stimulation (TENS) and in high-threshold mechanoreceptors responsive to low-frequency needle manipulation (acupuncture).
- A-fibres are recruited at 50–200Hz and respond to low intensity stimulation. Pain relief occurs immediately but lasts only as long as stimulation continues. A stimulation increases levels of inhibitory neurotransmitters dynorphin A and B in the dorsal horn.
- A-fibres are recruited at 2–4Hz and respond to high intensity stimulation. Pain relief takes 20–30min but lasts hours or days. A stimulation also increases inhibitory neurotransmitter metenkephalin levels in the dorsal horn.

The opioid-dependent patient

The principles of acute pain management in the opioid dependent patient are similar to those previously described. The aim is to bring acute pain under control. Involvement of a multidisciplinary team will often be necessary to manage behavioural, psychological, psychiatric, and medical problems encountered in this group of patients.

- **Tolerance, dependence, addiction, and pseudoaddiction**—tolerance is a decrease in sensitivity to opioids resulting in less effect from the same dose. Physical dependence is a physiological phenomenon characterised by a withdrawal reaction when the drug is withdrawn or an antagonist is administered. Addiction is a pattern of drug abuse characterised by compulsive use to experience a psychological effect and to avoid withdrawal reaction. Pseudoaddiction is iatrogenic drug-seeking behaviour normally due to under-treatment of acute pain by the physician.

- Symptoms and signs of withdrawal include yawning, sweating, anxiety, rhinorrhoea, lacrimation, tachycardia, hypertension, diarrhoea, nausea, vomiting, abdominal pain, and cramps. On average, these symptoms peak at 36–72hr after the last dose. Aims of treatment must be provision of analgesia, prevention of opioid withdrawal, and management of abnormal drug-taking behaviour. Non-opioid analgesics such as paracetamol and NSAIDs should be prescribed regularly if possible.

- Opioid-dependent patients normally fall into one of three groups; opioid addicts, chronic non-cancer pain, and cancer pain. The principles of management are the same for each group.

Opioid requirements will in general be much higher than in non opioid-dependent patients. The initial dose prescribed should take the patient's current opioid requirement into account. It may be difficult to judge current opioid use when illicit drugs have been taken. The GP, local pharmacist, or drug rehabilitation centre may provide helpful information.

- Opioid-tolerant patients report higher pain scores and have lower incidence of opioid-induced nausea and vomiting.

- Opioid-tolerant patients are at risk of opioid withdrawal if non-opioid analgesic regimens or tramadol are used.

- PCA settings may need to include a background infusion to replace the usual opioid dose and a higher bolus dose.

- Total dose should be increased until acceptable analgesia is achieved or until side-effects prohibit any further dose increases. PCA with larger than average bolus doses is the preferred means of administrating opioids.[1,2] Opioid rotation may be of use particularly with an agent of higher intrinsic opioid agonist activity.[3]

- The aim is to eventually discharge the patient on no more opioid than was used before admission. Normally dose reductions of 20–25% every day towards the pre-admission opioid intake will avoid symptoms of withdrawal.

- Oral or SC clonidine (50µg tds) can be used to treat symptoms of opioid withdrawal.

- An objective assessment of function, i.e. ability to cough, may be a better guide to opioid requirements than pain scores. Patients with an addiction to opioids tend to exaggerate pain in the hope of receiving increased dosages.
- Whenever possible, regional analgesic techniques should be used (e.g. continuous lumbar plexus, brachial plexus, or epidural infusions).
- Liaise with all clinicians involved in the treatment of these patients.

1 Macintyre PE, Ready LB (2001). Acute Pain Management-A Practical Guide. 2nd edition. Harcourt Publishers Limited, London.
2 Mitra S, Sinatra RS (2004). Perioperative management of acute pain in the opioid-dependent patient. *Anesthesiology*, **101**, 212–227.
3 De Leon-Casasola OA, Lema MJ (1994). Epidural bupivacaine/sufentanil therapy for postoperative pain control in patients tolerant to opioid and unresponsive to epidural bupivacaine/morphine. *Anesthesiology*, **80**, 303–309.

The patient with a substance abuse disorder

A substance abuse disorder (SAD) exists when the extent and pattern of substance use interferes with the psychological and sociocultural integrity of the person.[1] (American Psychiatric Association 1994).

Effective management of acute pain in patients with SAD may be complicated by:
• Psychological and behavioural characteristics
• Presence of the drug of abuse
• Presence of tolerance, physical dependence, and the risk of withdrawal
• Medications used to assist with drug withdrawal or rehabilitation
• Complications related to drug abuse including organ impairment.

Ethical dilemmas can arise as a result of the need to balance concerns of undermedication against anxieties about safety and possible abuse or diversion of the drugs.

Management of pain in patients with SAD should focus on:
• Prevention of withdrawal
• Effective analgesia
• Symptomatic treatment of affective and behavioural problems.

Patients with SAD may be abusing CNS depressant drugs (alcohol, benzodiazepines, opioids) or CNS stimulant drugs (cocaine, amphetamines, ecstasy, cannabinoids).

Drugs used in the treatment of SAD include:
• Methadone—long-acting pure opioid agonist. In the acute pain setting methadone should be continued at the same dose. If the patient is unable to take methadone orally, substitution with parenteral methadone or other opioids may be required in the short term.
• Naltrexone—pure opioid antagonist administered orally. Binds to opioid receptors for 24hr following a single dose. May create difficulties in the acute pain setting. It is recommended that naltrexone is stopped 24hr before surgery. Usual maintenance dose is 25–50mg daily.
• Buprenorphine—partial opioid agonist used in the treatment of opioid addiction. Commonly prescribed doses of 8–32mg. Continuation of buprenorphine pre-surgery has been suggested although it may be difficult to obtain good analgesia with full agonist opioids. Multimodal analgesic strategies should be used.

Patients in drug-free recovery may be concerned about the risk of relapse into active SAD if given opioids for acute pain management. Use of multimodal analgesic strategies, reassurance that the risk of reversion is small, and information that ineffective analgesia can paradoxically lead to relapses in recovering patients, help avoid undertreatment.

---

1 American Psychiatric Association (1994). Diagnostic and Statistical Manual of Mental Disorders. 4th edition, Washington DC.

Acute neuropathic pain following surgery

The occurrence of persistent pain following surgery is becoming increasingly recognised. Acute postoperative neuropathic pain does not usually occur in isolation, there will also be nociceptive pain as a result of tissue damage/inflammation.

- Approximately 14% of patients presenting to the pain clinic attribute their pain to surgery, with the pain beginning acutely.
- Patients may complain of an unusual type of pain different from the usual postoperative nociceptive pain. Patients often describe the pain as burning or shooting in nature. Pain may extend beyond the territory of a single peripheral nerve.
- The pain is often poorly responsive to opioid analgesia despite high doses being administered.
- Allodynia (pain following a normal innocuous stimulation), hyperalgesia (pain disproportionate to a noxious stimulus), and dysaesthesias (spontaneous unpleasant abnormal sensations) are often seen.
- The presence of a neurological deficit such as brachial plexus avulsion or spinal cord injury make the presence of acute neuropathic pain more likely.

Treatment

There is currently no published evidence to guide treatment of acute neuropathic pain.

Mechanisms of neuropathic pain involve central nervous system changes and increased peripheral nerve excitability. Drug therapy focuses on reducing neuronal hyperexcitability and reducing activity of the NMDA receptor in an attempt to reverse neuronal changes.

- Parenteral ketamine (NMDA receptor antagonist, 5mg/hr) and lidocaine (neuronal membrane stabilisation, 5mg/kg over 30–40min followed by 0.5–1.5mg/kg/hr) can be given in the acute phase to alter both peripheral and central neuronal plasticity. Treatment may take up to a week or more. This should be supervised by a suitably qualified pain specialist.
- Tricyclic antidepressants or anticonvulsant drugs (carbamazepine, gabapentin, or pregabalin) can be used to supplement treatment. These drugs are commonly used in established chronic pain conditions. Common side-effects are drowsiness, dizziness, and gait disturbance.
- Acute neuropathic pain after surgery is well recognised but poorly studied. Clinical trials are required to confirm the efficacy of treatments.

Chapter 40

Postoperative nausea and vomiting

Gordon Yuill and Carl Gwinnutt

General principles

Definitions
- Nausea is the subjective sensation of the need to vomit.
- Vomiting is the forced expulsion of stomach and gastrointestinal contents through the mouth.

Incidence
- 20–30% after general anaesthesia (GA) with volatile anaesthetics.
- Up to 70% in high risk patients.

Associated morbidity
- Decreased patient satisfaction, delayed hospital discharge, unexpected hospital admission.
- Wound dehiscence, bleeding, pulmonary aspiration, oesophageal rupture
- Fluid and electrolyte disturbances.

Anatomy and physiology
Chemoreceptor trigger zone (CTZ)
- Major impact on the vomiting centre – area postrema, floor of fourth ventricle.
- Poorly developed blood-brain barrier, activated by systemic stimuli.

Vomiting centre
- Lateral reticular formation of the medulla, close to fourth ventricle. Responsible for controlling and coordinating nausea and vomiting.
- Afferents—CTZ, vestibular apparatus, cerebellum, higher cortical and brain stem centres, solitary tract nucleus.
- Efferents—cranial nerves V, VII, IX, X, XII and spinal nerves to GI tract, diaphragm and abdominal muscles.
- Receptors—Dopaminergic (D_2), muscarinic, serotoninergic (5-HT_3), histaminic (H_1), opioid, neurokinin (NK_1).

Risk factors contributing to PONV
- Patient
  - Age—children > adults, decreased incidence after 50yr of age
  - Females (3x risk)
  - Previous PONV or motion sickness (2–3x risk)
  - Smokers (0.6x risk).
- Surgical
  - Breast, ophthalmic (strabismus repair), ENT, gynaecological, laparoscopic, laparotomy, craniotomy (posterior fossa), genitourinary, orthopaedic (shoulder procedures).
- Anaesthetic
  - Premedication—decreased risk after benzodiazepines and clonidine, increased risk after opioids.
  - Type of anaesthesia—GA 11x risk of regional technique, propofol TIVA less than volatile.

- Intra-operative drugs—opioids, nitrous oxide, inhalational agents (ether and cyclopropane > modern agents), IV agents (thiopental, etomidate and ketamine are emetogenic, propofol is possibly anti-emetic), neuromuscular blocker antagonists (including PONV due to muscarinic effects on GI tract).
- Adequate hydration decreases risk. Avoid too early resumption of food/fluids.

Management of PONV

Multi-factorial, multiple pathways and neurotransmitters, therefore a multi-modal approach is required.

Pharmacologic methods

- Prophylaxis vs treatment remains controversial.
- Prophylaxis with ondansetron is reported to be cost-effective in high-risk patients where PONV >30–33%.
- Combination therapy—combining two or more agents with different modes of action is believed to be more effective, e.g. ondansetron and dexamethasone.

Non-pharmacologic methods

Ginger root extract, acupuncture—pericardium (P6) point on palmer aspect of wrist (NNT = 5), hypnosis, suggestion, homeopathy.

Current research and other agents

- Neurokinin receptors are found in the medulla and are believed to play a role in the final nausea and vomiting pathway. Current research is beginning to show NK_1 antagonists to be more effective than ondansetron.
- Propofol (20mg IV), benzodiazepines, clonidine (0.15–0.3mg IV at induction) and the cannabinoid nabilone (1–2mg PO 12-hourly) have all been used in the prophylaxis and treatment of PONV.
- Persistent nausea and vomiting in palliative care is often treated with continuous SC infusions. Drugs used include cyclizine (150mg/24hr), dexamethasone (4mg/24hr), haloperidol (2.5–10mg/24hr) and levomepromazine (2.5–25mg/24hr).

The vomiting patient

- Reassurance
- Correct vital signs appropriately
- Ensure adequate analgesia and hydration
- Look for surgical cause (e.g. distended abdomen—site or aspirate NG tube)
- Anti-emetics:
  - Check if a prophylactic anti-emetic was given
  - Choose a different class for each subsequent administration
  - 1st line—anticholinergic, antihistamine, antidopaminergic
  - 2nd line—5-HT_3 antagonist
  - Combination anti-emetic therapy—5-HT_3 antagonist and dexamethasone
  - Consider other agents (see above).

Drugs available for the prophylaxis and treatment of PONV

Drug	Action	Dose, route & frequency	Number needed to treat	Side effects	Other points
Hyoscine hydrobromide	Anticholinergic	0.2–0.4mg SC or IM 6-hourly	3.8	Dry mouth, blurred vision, dizziness	Useful for motion sickness, labyrinth disorders, posterior fossa surgery, opioid related nausea
Cyclizine	Antihistamine	50mg PO, IM or IV 8-hourly		Sedation, dry mouth, blurred vision. Tachycardia and hypotension when given IV	Useful for motion sickness, labyrinth disorders, opioid related nausea
Prochlorperazine	D_2 antagonist	12.5mg IM 3mg buccal 6-hourly		Extrapyramidal, sedation	Useful for opioid related nausea
Metoclopramide	D_2 antagonist	10mg IM or IV	10	Extrapyramidal, sedation, abdominal cramping, dizziness	Promotes gastric emptying, ↑ lower oesophageal sphincter barrier pressure. Useful for opioid related nausea
Droperidol	D_2 antagonist	0.5–1.25mg IV 2.5–5mg PO 8-hourly	5	Extrapyramidal, sedation, neurolepsis, GI disturbances, abnormal LFTs	Used in technique of neurolept analgesia. Withdrawn from British National Formulary—QT prolongation

Drug	Class	Dose		Side effects	Notes
Haloperidol	D_2 antagonist	1–2mg 12-hourly		Extrapyramidal sedation, neurolepsis, neuroleptic malignant syndrome, GI+ LFT disturbance	Useful for treatment of delirium in the critically ill
Ondansetron	5-HT$_3$ antagonist	1–8mg PO IM or IV 8-hourly	5	Hypersensitivity reactions, headache, dizziness, transient elevated liver enzymes	Paediatrics—drug of first choice due to its lesser side effect profile (0.1mg/kg)
Dolasetron	5-HT$_3$ antagonist	12.5mg IV 24-hourly	5	Hypersensitivity reactions, abdo pain, ECG changes	
Granisetron	5-HT$_3$ antagonist	1mg IV 12-hourly		Hypersensitivity reactions, transient elevated liver enzymes	
Tropisetron	5-HT$_3$ antagonist	2mg IV 24-hourly	6.7 (nausea) 5 (vomiting)	Hypersensitivity reactions, headache, dizziness, abdo pain	
Dexamethasone	Steroid	6–10mg IV Single prophylactic dose	4	Wound infection, adrenal suppression	Better in combination with other drugs

PONV avoidance strategy

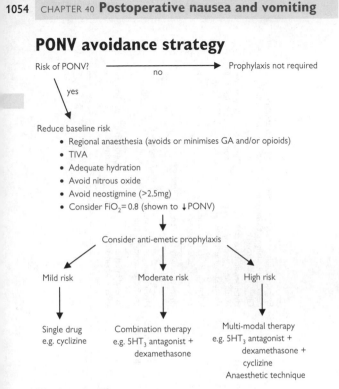

Risk of PONV? ──────── no ──────────► Prophylaxis not required

↓ yes

Reduce baseline risk

- Regional anaesthesia (avoids or minimises GA and/or opioids)
- TIVA
- Adequate hydration
- Avoid nitrous oxide
- Avoid neostigmine (>2.5mg)
- Consider FiO_2= 0.8 (shown to ↓PONV)

Consider anti-emetic prophylaxis

Mild risk	Moderate risk	High risk
Single drug e.g. cyclizine	Combination therapy e.g. $5HT_3$ antagonist + dexamethasone	Multi-modal therapy e.g. $5HT_3$ antagonist + dexamethasone + cyclizine Anaesthetic technique

Further reading

Habib AS, Gan TJ (2004). Evidence based management of postoperative nausea and vomiting: a review. *Canadian Journal of Anesthesia,* **51**, 326–341.

Ku CM, Ong BC (2003). Postoperative nausea and vomiting: a review of current literature. *Singapore Medical Journal,* **44**, 366–374.

Tramer MR (2001). A rational approach to the control of postoperative nausea and vomiting: evidence from systematic reviews. Part 1. Efficacy and harm of anti-emetic interventions and methodological issues. *Acta Anaesthesiologica Scandinavica,* **45**, 4–13.

Tramer MR (2001). A rational approach to the control of postoperative nausea and vomiting: evidence from systematic reviews. Part 2. Recommendations for prevention and treatment, and research agenda. *Acta Anaesthesiologica Scandinavica,* **45**, 14–19.

Regional anaesthesia

David Conn and Barry Nicholls

General principles
Used correctly, regional anaesthesia can provide prolonged postoperative analgesia or a safer alternative to general anaesthesia. Detailed knowledge of anatomy, technique, and possible complications is important for correct placement. Experience avoids 'two frightened people either end of a needle'!

Patient selection
Patient refusal and local sepsis are the only absolute contraindications to regional anaesthesia; therapeutic anticoagulation (prosthetic valves, etc.) needs to be assessed on an individual basis.
- All procedures should be discussed with the patient before arriving in the anaesthetic room.
- Informed verbal and/or written consent, documented in the notes, should be obtained.
- Any potential complications that are likely to influence the decision to proceed should be discussed with the patient and recorded in the notes/anaesthetic record.
- Consider the appropriateness of the technique. Supraclavicular or infraclavicular blocks in a compromised respiratory patient or sciatic/femoral nerve block with bupivacaine for day case knee arthroscopy are rarely acceptable.
- Avoid bilateral blocks—double the complication rate.
- Beware using blocks in forearm or tibial fractures as they may mask compartment syndromes.

Complications following regional anaesthesia
See pp30, 1070.

Regional anaesthesia awake or asleep?
- Anaesthetised or heavily sedated patients are unable to respond to paraesthesia/intraneural injection, which may precede neurological trauma and damage. However, regional analgesia performed in such patients has never been demonstrated to produce an increased incidence of neurological sequelae.
- Paediatric regional anaesthesia is almost exclusively performed under a general anaesthetic. Of over 24 000 central and peripheral blocks in paediatric patients, the complication rate was 1.5:1000 (all associated with central blocks) with no permanent neurological damage.
- The majority of regional techniques can be performed on awake or lightly sedated adult patients with minimal discomfort.
- Continuing verbal contact with patients has distinct advantages in the likelihood of inadvertent paraesthesia, IV, intrathecal, or intraneural injection, both for recognition and management.
- In a case of neurological damage following operation, clarification of the cause (anaesthetic/surgical) is facilitated if documentation of no paraesthesia, pain, or bleeding was present when performing the block.
- On balance therefore, perform blocks on awake patients whenever possible. Judicious doses of analgesics/sedatives (fentanyl 50–100µg with midazolam 1–2mg) will improve patient tolerance.

Anticoagulation and regional anaesthesia

Bleeding and compression neurapraxia is a potential complication of regional anaesthesia in anticoagulated patients or those with clotting abnormalities. Peripheral nerve blockade may still be used where compression can be achieved or bleeding is unlikely (superficial nerves). More proximal/perivascular techniques are best avoided. Central neuraxial blocks require particular consideration.

Anticoagulation and central neuraxial blocks

- Full anticoagulation with warfarin or standard heparin (SH) is an absolute contraindication to central neuraxial blockade, and a relative contraindication to peripheral nerve blockade.
- Partial anticoagulation with low molecular weight heparin (LMWH) or low-dose warfarin (INR <1.5) is a relative contraindication to central neural blockade and each patient should be assessed individually, with respect to risk/benefit.
- Half life of heparin is ~90min. Hence need to wait for 4hr following IV infusion of heparin.
- The table opposite is based upon the ASRA Consensus Conference recommendations.[1]
- These are guidelines only and a balance of risks and benefits should be sought before embarking on any regional technique.
- The risks following plexus and peripheral techniques remain undefined. It is not unreasonable to apply the same criteria to such blocks although this may be more restrictive than necessary especially in areas with compressible vasculature.
- Other useful techniques to reduce haematoma rates include: use the smallest needle possible—use a spinal technique rather than epidural, do not thread an epidural catheter further than 4cm, minimise recurrent passes, abort technique if unduly difficult, use weak LA solutions with opioid, and have a high index of suspicion.
- An epidural haematoma should be suspected in any patient who complains of severe back pain a few hours/days following any central neuraxial block or with any prolonged or abnormal neurological deficit. An immediate MRI scan and neurosurgical referral are indicated. (see p36)

Recommendations for neuraxial blockade and anticoagulants

Drug	Type	Recommendations	Notes
Thrombolytic Therapy	rt-PA, streptokinase etc	Avoid administration for 10d following block	Very high risk. Fibrinogen level may be a useful indicator
		Avoid block after thrombolytic therapy—time period unknown	
Unfractionated heparin	Minidose SC 5000U BD	No contraindication to neuraxial block. If possible delay dose until after block	Check platelet count after 4d of therapy
	IV Intra-operative administration	Give heparin >1hr after block	If bloody/traumatic tap discuss need for heparin with surgeon
		Do not remove catheter until 2–4hr after dosage and repeat APTR ideally	
	Full IV anti-coagulation (cardiac surgery)	Unknown risk if undertaken after neuraxial block	
LMWH	Preop dose	Wait at least 10–12hr after dose	Anti-Xa levels not helpful
	High dose treatment	Perform block more than 24hr after last dose	
	2hr before surgery	Avoid neuraxial block	
	Postop OD dosing	First dose more than 6–8hr postop	If bloody/traumatic tap delay postop dose for 24hr
		Epidural catheter removed more than 10–12hr after last dose and more than 2hr before next dose	

1 Horlocker TT, et al. (2003). Regional anesthesia in the anticoagulated patient: Defining the risks (the second ASRA Consensus Conference on neuraxial anesthesia and anticoagulation. *Reg Anesth Pain Med*, **28**, 172–197.

Table contd.

Drug	Type	Recommendations	Notes
Warfarin	Postop BD dosing	Increased risk of haematoma. Give first dose more than 24hr postoperatively. Remove catheter more than 2hr before *first* dose	
	Long term	Stop 4–5d preop. INR <1.5 (<1.2 ideal)	Monitor INR
	Preop	Check INR if first dose more than 24hr pre-block, or more than one dose administered	
Anti-platelets	NSAIDs	No increased risk	No useful test of function
	Clopidogrel	Stop for 7d pre-block	
	Ticlopidine	Stop for 14d pre-block	
	Abciximab	Stop for 24–48hr pre-block	Avoid for 28d post-block
	Eptifibatide, Tirofiban	Stop for 4–8hr pre-block	Avoid for 28d post-block
Thrombocytopenia	Various causes	Epidural relatively contraindicated below 100 × 10⁹/l. Spinal/epidural contraindicated below 50 × 10⁹/l	
Synthetic pentasaccharide	Fondaparinux (Arixtra®) 2.5mg OD	First dose more than 6hr postop. Epidural catheter removed more than 36hr after last dose, and 12hr before next dose (omit one treatment)	
Oral direct thrombin inhibitor	Ximelagatran (Exanta®) 24mg bd	First dose 12–24hr postop. Epidural catheter removed more than 8hr after last dose and 2–4hr before next dose	

Nerve identification

Location of a nerve or plexus can be achieved by:
- Loss of resistance (epidural, paravertebral)
- Measured advancement of the needle (peribulbar, intercostal)
- Relation to arterial pulsation/transfixion (femoral, brachial plexus)
- Paraesthesia
- Percutaneous electrical stimulation
- Ultrasound.

Peripheral nerve stimulation

- This is the commonest method used to identify nerves percutaneously.
- Indicates motor supply of the nerve. Sensory stimulation can be achieved with some peripheral nerve stimulators.
- Patient cooperation is desirable but not essential—sedation or GA are possible, but the patient should not have received neuromuscular blocking drugs.
- Possible reduced potential for nerve damage, as there is no need for direct physical contact with the nerve cf paraesthesia.
- Usually comfortable for the patient.

Using a peripheral nerve stimulator (PNS)

- Connect the stimulating needle to the negative lead (black) and ground electrode or ECG pad to positive lead (red).
  - 'Negative to needle, positive to patient'.
- Keep the ECG pad at least 20cm from the site of injection. Start with current of 1.5mA and 1–2Hz. This causes stimulation of Type A motor fibres in mixed nerves, without sensory stimulation.
- Insert the insulated needle. At all times move the needle slowly and gently, watching for signs of stimulation. Aim for movement in 1–2mm steps.
- When stimulation is achieved try to optimise position of the needle to obtain good motor response without paraesthesia, with a stimulating current of 0.2–0.5mA.
- Inject 1ml solution; the motor response should disappear (nerve is displaced by solution). Inject the full volume after careful aspiration, fractionating the dose if it is greater than 5ml.
- If the motor response does not disappear with the initial 1ml, suspect needle may be within the nerve sheath. Reposition before further injection.
- If there is any pain or increased resistance to injection, stop immediately, and reposition the needle—possible intraneural positioning.

Needle design

- Long bevelled (10–14°) needles are easier to pass through tissues, but have less feel. Intraneurally they will cut a small number of fibres.
- Short bevelled (18–45°) needles have more resistance and may give more feedback to the operator. Intraneurally they may damage (not cut) fibres.
- Pencil-point needles split fibres if used intraneurally and have side injection ports to minimise intraneural injection.

- There is no compelling evidence to support decreased nerve damage with any particular needle design.
- Insulated needles concentrate current density at the tip of the needle improving accuracy, but they are not essential for nerve localisation.
- Uninsulated needles are adequate for superficial nerves/plexuses. With deeper nerves and plexuses excessive superficial muscle contraction may confuse identification.

Motor response elicited with peripheral nerve stimulation

Nerve stimulated	Response
Median*	Finger and wrist flexion and pronation of the wrist. Thumb opposition
Ulnar*	Adduction of thumb, flexion ring and little finger, supination. Ulnar deviation
Radial*	Wrist and finger extension. Thumb abduction
Musculo-cutaneous	Elbow flexion (biceps, brachialis)
Femoral	Quadriceps contraction—patellar twitch
Sciatic-tibial	Plantar flexion of foot and inversion—flexion of toes
Sciatic-peroneal	Dorsiflexion of foot and eversion—extension of the toes
Cervical roots	Contraction of scalenus medius C3, scalenus anterior C4, deltoid C5
Cervical trunks	Shoulder surgery: (C5–C6)—deltoid and biceps contraction
	Humerus and forearm surgery—forearm or hand movement, especially extension
Cervical cords	Lateral cord: elbow flexion (1° musculocutaneous). Medial cord: finger and wrist flexion. (1° ulnar nerve) Posterior cord: wrist, fingers, and thumb extension (1° radial nerve)
Lumbar plexus	Quadriceps contraction L2–L3

* Pure ulnar/radial/median nerve stimulation can only be achieved at the axilla or below. Cords/trunk stimulation gives a less defined motor response.

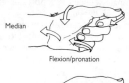

Median

Flexion/pronation

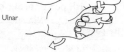

Ulnar

Ulnar deviation/thumb adduction

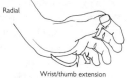

Radial

Wrist/thumb extension

Motor response of medial/ulnar/radial nerves to stimulation.

Characteristics of different local anaesthetic agents

- Potency is directly related to lipid solubility.
- Duration of action is related to protein binding at the site of action and factors which affect removal of drug from the site, e.g. blood supply.
- Speed of onset/latency depends on the local availability of unionised free base. This can be improved by increasing the concentration of local anaesthetic or increasing the pH of the local anaesthetic/tissues. It is also dependent on the pKa of drug and the pH of the solution (a high pKa is associated with slow onset in normal pH settings, e.g. bupivacaine).

	pKa	Relative lipid solubility	Relative potency	Protein binding (%)	Onset	Duration
Procaine	8.9	1	1	6	Slow	Short
Amethocaine	8.5	200	8	75	Slow	Long
Lidocaine	7.7	150	2	65	Fast	Medium
Prilocaine	7.7	50	2	55	Fast	Medium
Etidocaine	7.7	5000	6	96	Fast	Long
Mepivacaine	7.6	50	2	78	Fast	Medium
Ropivacaine	8.1	400	6	94	Medium	Long
Bupivacaine	8.1	1000	8	95	Medium	Long
Levobupivacaine	8.1	1000	8	95	Medium	Long

Choice of agent

- If rapid onset peripheral blockade for surgery is needed use lidocaine or prilocaine 1–2%. These agents diffuse more readily than bupivacaine (high protein binding capacity).
- If postoperative analgesia only is required use bupivacaine 0.25–0.5%, for its extended duration of action.
- In high-volume plexus anaesthesia or multiple blocks consider the use of levobupivacaine or ropivacaine (reduced toxicity).
- Continuous infusion—consider the use of less toxic drugs, i.e. ropivacaine and levobupivacaine. The addition of fentanyl or clonidine may augment blockade.

Mixtures of local anaesthetics

- A mixture of short acting LA (lidocaine/prilocaine) with long acting LA (bupivacaine/levobupivacaine) is commonly used—caution, side effects and toxicity are cumulative.

Drug	Characteristics
Lidocaine	Short-acting amide. Moderate vasodilatation. Cerebral irritation before cardiac depression. Duration enhanced and peak plasma levels reduced by adrenaline
Prilocaine	Short-acting amide. No vasodilatation. Rapid metabolism and low toxicity. Metabolised to o-toluidine causing methaemoglobinaemia (care in obstetrics/anaemia)
Bupivacaine	Long-acting amide. Racemic mixture of R and S enantiomers. Profound cardiotoxicity in higher doses
L-bupivacaine (levobupivacaine)	S-enantiomer of bupivacaine. Enhanced vasoconstriction. Reduced intensity and duration of motor block with less cardiotoxicity than bupivacaine
Ropivacaine	Long-acting amide. Reduced intensity and duration of motor block. Less cardiotoxic than bupivacaine or levobupivacaine
Amethocaine	Long-acting ester. Rapid absorption from mucous membranes or transdermal route. Relatively toxic
Benzocaine	Short-acting ester. Low potency. Used as lozenges
Cocaine	Short-acting ester. Slow onset, profound vasoconstriction. Limited local anaesthetic use, toxic

Topical local anaesthetics

EMLA (eutectic mixture of local anaesthetic)
• Contains lidocaine 2.5% + prilocaine 2.5%, Arlatone (emulsifier), Carbopol (thickener), distilled water and sodium hydroxide.
• Application 1–5hr before venepuncture.
• Side effects are blanching and vasoconstriction.
• Avoid on broken skin/mucous membranes and in infants under 1yr.

Ametop (topical amethocaine gel)
• Contains amethocaine 4%, xanthan gum, methyl and propyl-p-hydroxy-benzoate, water, and saline.
• Application 30min before venepuncture, and 45min before cannulation.
• Side effects are erythema, oedema, and pruritus.
• Remove gel after 1hr.
• Not recommended in babies under 1 month.
• Lasts for 4–6hr after removal of cream.

Adjuvant drugs and additives

Bicarbonate	Added to increase the pH of a solution—increases unionised LA
	May increase the speed of onset
	Add 1ml 8.4% to 10ml lidocaine/prilocaine or to 20ml bupivacaine
Adrenaline	Decreases vascular reabsorption, increasing the duration by making more drug available
	Reduces peak plasma levels (lidocaine, mepivacaine)
	Is of reduced benefit with a long-acting LA
	Less effective in epidurals
	The total dose of adrenaline should not exceed 200µg. This should be reduced by 50% during halothane anaesthesia
	Avoid the use of adrenaline in digital nerve, penile blocks and around the sciatic nerve
	Effective concentration 5µg/ml adrenaline. Add 0.1mg of adrenaline (1ml of 1:10 000) to 20ml of LA
Clonidine	Prolongs the duration of sensory and motor block
	Induces post block analgesia
	Acts on α_2 adrenergic receptors
	Effective in epidural/caudal/spinal anaesthesia (see p784)
	Use is limited by hypotension and sedation
	Dose: for caudal blocks 1–2µg/kg
	For peripheral blocks 1µg/kg
Ketamine	An NMDA receptor agonist with weak local anaesthetic properties
	All opioids have been used. Of debatable benefit in peripheral blocks
	Intra-articular morphine 2–5mg in knee surgery is used in combination with LA by some surgeons. Evidence is weak
Opioids	Proven synergism with epidural/intrathecal LA
	All opioids have been used. Of debatable benefit in peripheral blocks
	Intra-articular morphine 2–5mg in knee surgery is used in combination with LA by some surgeons. Evidence is weak
Dextrose	Used to increase baricity of LA for intrathecal use. Heavy bupivacaine contains 80mg/ml
Hyaluronidase	Used in peribulbar and retrobulbar blocks of the eye to enhance LA spread. Dose 5–30U/ml

Local anaesthetic toxicity

High plasma levels of local anaesthetic can be found in:
- Drug overdose
- Direct intravascular injection
- Rapid absorption/injection into a highly vascular area
- Cumulative effect of multiple injections or continuous infusion.

Recommended maximum doses as quoted by manufacturers' data sheets are a guide only. Equally important are:
- The site of injection with relation to vascularity and absorption.
- Metabolic status: acidosis, hypoxia, and hypercarbia all potentiate the negative inotropic/chronotropic effects of local anaesthetics.
- Whenever possible, keep within the maximum dosing recommendations, aspirate carefully before injection, and divide large-volume injections into smaller aliquots. Inject slowly.

Maximum recommended doses of common agents (BNF)		
Agent	**Maximum recommended doses**	**Maximum recommended doses with vasoconstrictor**
Bupivacaine	2mg/kg	2mg/kg
Levobupivacaine	2mg/kg	2mg/kg
Ropivacaine	3mg/kg	3mg/kg
Lidocaine	3mg/kg	6mg/kg
Prilocaine	6mg/kg	8mg/kg
Cocaine	1.5–3mg/kg	

Treatment of toxicity
- Stop injection or infusion as appropriate.
- ABC: 'airway, breathing, circulation'.
- Mild symptoms may be best treated by oxygen, plus small doses of midazolam (1–4mg) to increase the convulsant threshold. Beware of hypoventilation/acidosis from sedation, which will exacerbate the toxicity.
- For moderate to severe toxicity, cardiovascular collapse is normally preceded by convulsions and is worsened by hypoxia and acidosis.
- Prevent/treat convulsions and maintain oxygenation. Use thiopental, propofol or midazolam. Paralyse and intubate if convulsions recur and ventilate with 100% oxygen.
- If cardiovascular collapse ensues, begin CPR (p864).
- Early intervention leads to better outcome.
- Bretylium is no longer available and amiodarone is the antiarrhythmic of choice.

- Vasopressors such as adrenaline or vasopressin should be used in the event of cardiovascular collapse.
- Propofol *may* decrease cardiac toxicity, suppress bupivacaine induced seizures, reduce the effective tissue level of bupivacaine and act as an antioxidant to improve recovery from tissue hypoxia.[1]

Symptoms and signs of toxicity	
Potentially fatal toxicity	Respiratory arrest
	Cardiac arrhythmias
	Cardiovascular collapse
Moderate toxicity	Altered conscious state
	Convulsions
	Coma
Mild toxicity	Perioral tingling
	Metallic taste
	Tinnitus
	Visual disturbance
	Slurred speech

Methaemoglobinaemia (prilocaine toxicity)

- Oxidation of haemoglobin to methaemoglobin by o-toluidine. Methaemoglobin has a reduced oxygen carrying capacity resulting in cyanosis. O-toluidine is formed by metabolism of prilocaine in the liver.
- Methaemoglobinaemia occurs with high doses of prilocaine (>600mg).
- Avoid prilocaine in pregnancy and anaemia.
- Treatment: methylthioninium chloride (methylene blue) 1mg/kg IV.

1 Weinberg GL (2002). Current concepts in resuscitation of patients with local anesthetic cardiac toxicity. *Reg Anesth Pain Med,* **27**, 568–575.

Head and neck blocks

- Depending on the site, most surgery on the face and scalp relies upon infiltration rather than blockade of specific nerves.
- Formal blockade of nerves such as the maxillary and mandibular have all but vanished.
- Local anaesthetic techniques of the face and scalp relate more to the type of surgery i.e. ear, nose, and dental.

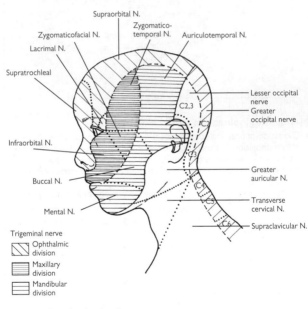

Nerve supply to head and neck.

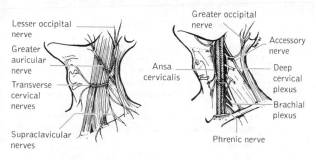

Superficial and deep cervical plexus.

Cervical plexus anatomy

- C1 has no cutaneous sensory branch.
- C1–C3 gives meningeal branches to the posterior cranial fossa.
- C1–C4 anterior primary rami form the cervical plexus, anterior to the scalenus medius but deep to the sternomastoid and the internal jugular vein.
- Supplies the ear, anterior neck, and 'cape area' (anterior and posterior aspect of shoulder and upper chest wall).
- Complete sensory analgesia of the anterior neck can be achieved with blockade of superficial branches of the cervical plexus (lesser occipital, greater auricular, transverse cervical, and supraclavicular nerves).
- Deep cervical plexus segmentally supplies the deep muscles of the neck and diaphragm.
- Motor and sensory connection to the diaphragm (phrenic nerve).

Greater/lesser occipital nerve blockade

Greater/lesser occipital nerve blockade is indicated for operations on the occipital scalp.

- Landmarks: greater occipital protuberance, mastoid process, posterior occipital artery.
- Technique:
  - Draw a line joining the occipital protuberance to the mastoid process.
  - Palpate the posterior occipital artery; the greater occipital nerve accompanies the artery.
  - Inject 5ml of solution.
  - Infiltrate from this point along the line to the mastoid process with 5ml solution to block the lesser occipital nerve.

Superficial cervical plexus block

Superficial cervical plexus block is indicated for carotid endarterectomy (with or without a deep cervical plexus block), neck and thyroid surgery, and ear and mastoid procedures (including a greater occipital nerve block).

- Landmarks: posterior border of sternomastoid, cricoid cartilage.
- Technique:
  - Position the patient with their head turned slightly to the opposite side
  - Draw a line from the cricoid to the posterior border of the sternomastoid and mark it (ask the patient to lift their head off the pillow to find the posterior border of the sternomastoid).
  - Insert a 22G needle perpendicular to the skin.
  - A click or pop is felt as the needle passes through the cervical fascia.
  - Inject 10ml local anaesthetic solution at this point or fan the injection cranially and caudally along the posterior border of the muscle.

Deep cervical plexus block

Indications are as for superficial cervical plexus block.

- Landmarks: mastoid process, Chassaignac's tubercle (transverse process C6).
- Technique:
  - Draw a line connecting the tip of the mastoid process and the Chassaignac tubercle; draw a second line parallel but 1cm posterior to the first.
  - The C2 transverse process lies 1–2cm (one finger's breadth) caudad to the mastoid process, C3/4 transverse processes lie at 1.5cm intervals along the second line.
  - After raising a skin weal a 22G 50mm needle is inserted perpendicular to the skin, with a slight caudad angulation to contact the bone (the transverse process).
  - Either paraesthesiae (nerve root) or bony contact is acceptable as there is free communication between paravertebral spaces. 4ml of solution is injected at each level.
  - Paraesthesiae can be elicited by 'walking' in an anteroposterior direction off the anterior tubercle of the transverse process.
  - Alternatively: single injection at C4 level using a peripheral nerve stimulator (Winnie). The junction of the interscalene groove and the superior border of thyroid cartilage is at C4 level. Stimulate the scalenus anterior C4, scalenus medius C3 and inject 10–15ml.
- Complications:
  - Inadvertent injection into the dural cuff (epidural/intrathecal).
  - Injection into the vertebral artery.
  - Phrenic nerve block, brachial plexus block.
- Clinical tips:
  - Avoid in patients with contralateral phrenic nerve palsy.
  - Do not perform bilateral deep cervical plexus blocks; there is the danger of bilateral recurrent laryngeal or phrenic nerve palsy.

Upper limb blocks

Brachial plexus anatomy

Formed from anterior primary rami of C5–C8 and T1 nerves which emerge from the intervertebral foramina and form:

- Roots: between scalene muscles.
- Trunks: (C5–6) upper, (C7) middle, (C8, T1) lower, beneath the floor of the posterior triangle, between the sternomastoid and trapezius muscles above the middle third of the clavicle, posterior to the sub-clavian artery.
- Divisions: each trunk divides into anterior and posterior divisions behind the clavicle.
- Cords: formed at the outer border of the first rib; they enter the axilla with the axillary artery, lying in their true anatomical relationship medial, lateral, and posterior to the second part of the artery behind pectoralis minor.
- Branches of the cords are formed around the third part of the axillary artery within the axilla. A fascial sheath accompanies the brachial plexus from the scalene muscles down to the mid point of the upper arm, although the musculocutaneous and radial nerves leave the sheath before then.
- The site of injection within the fascial sheath affects the spread of local anaesthetic.
  - An interscalene block commonly misses the lower roots C8, T1 (ulnar sparing).
  - Supraclavicular/infraclavicular: at this level the divisions become the cords. The narrow shape of the perivascular sheath allows predict-able spread of LA and rapid onset of block.
  - Axillary injection (single shot) commonly misses the radial nerve and the musculocutaneous nerve.

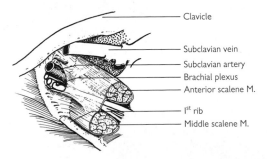

Clavicle

Subclavian vein
Subclavian artery
Brachial plexus
Anterior scalene M.

1st rib
Middle scalene M.

Brachial plexus passing over the first rib.

Interscalene brachial plexus block (classical Winnie)

Indications for this block are shoulder, humerus, or elbow surgery.

- Landmarks: cricoid cartilage, posterior border of sternomastoid, external jugular vein, interscalene groove.
- Technique:
  - The patient should be supine, with one small pillow under their head and neck.
  - The head should be turned comfortably to the opposite side.
  - At the level of the cricoid cartilage draw a line laterally to intersect the posterior border of the sternomastoid; this usually corresponds to where the external jugular vein crosses.
  - Palpate the scalenus anterior underneath the lateral border of the sternomastoid. Moving the fingers laterally, palpate the interscalene groove, between scalenus anterior and medius.
  - To aid palpation ask the patient to their lift head gently off the pillow (contracting the sternomastoid) or sniff (contracting scalene muscles).
  - Stand to the side of patient or at their head, raise a weal and insert a 22G 25–50mm needle perpendicular to the skin in all directions with a slight caudal direction. Aim at the contralateral elbow.
  - On entering the fascial sheath a 'pop' may be elicited; advance until motor stimulation is achieved (C5 deltoid C6 biceps)
  - After careful aspiration inject 10–20ml for postoperative analgesia or 20–40ml for complete brachial plexus block.
- Complications:
  - Phrenic nerve block in all cases (100%).
  - Horner's syndrome if the stellate ganglion is affected (10–25%).
  - Vessel puncture (external/internal jugular, common carotid, vertebral).
  - Intrathecal/epidural injection.
  - Recurrent laryngeal nerve palsy causing a hoarse voice (5–10%).
- Clinical tips:
  - Take care in patients with COPD, and do not use in patients with contralateral phrenic nerve palsy.
  - In view of potential complications always perform this block on awake or lightly sedated patients.
  - The plexus is very superficial in thin people (1–2cm deep). In all patients, the plexus should be identifiable within 25mm.
  - Avoid in obese patients with short necks, as landmarks can be impossible to locate.
  - If unable to find the interscalene groove, consider a higher approach at the level of the thyroid cartilage, or a lower approach (subclavian perivascular).
  - Digital compression above the injection site whilst injecting will aid caudal spread.
  - Look for fullness in the posterior triangle on injection—if there is no swelling the injection is too deep, if there is cutaneous swelling it is too superficial.
  - Use a short bevelled needle to aid 'feel'.
  - *Phrenic nerve* stimulation indicates that the needle is too anterior (on scalenus anterior); *levator scapulae* stimulation indicates that the needle is too posterior (dorsal scapular nerve).

- Best used for surgery of the shoulder as this is the only brachial plexus block that anaesthetises the suprascapular nerve.
- Catheter insertion: after entering the interscalene sheath bring the hub of the needle towards the neck. Advance slightly, maintaining stimulation, and insert the catheter after distending the space with local anaesthetic.

Subclavian perivascular (supraclavicular) block (SPV)

This block is indicated for humerus, elbow, or hand surgery.
- Landmarks: interscalene groove, subclavian artery.
- Technique:
  - Position the patient lying flat, with their head turned 30° to the opposite side.
  - Palpate the interscalene groove (as described for the interscalene approach).
  - Follow the interscalene groove caudally until the subclavian artery is felt above the clavicle (50% of patients), or until the neck 'flattens out'.
  - With a finger on the subclavian artery insert a 22G 50mm needle into the posterior part of the groove, posterior to the subclavian artery.
  - Keeping the hub of the needle against the neck (this ensures needle direction is parallel to the long axis of the interscalene groove), direct the needle directly caudad; aim for the ipsilateral nipple or great toe.
  - As the needle enters the fascial sheath a distinct 'pop' will be felt; advance slowly until specific motor response is elicited (flexion/extension of the wrist or fingers).
  - The first rib may be encountered. If so 'walk' the needle anteroposteriorly on the rib until the plexus is encountered.
  - Inject 0.5ml/kg up to 40ml of LA in increments.
- Complications:
  - Subclavian artery puncture (20%).
  - Pneumothorax (0.1%).
- Clinical tips:
  - Best avoided if the subclavian artery cannot be palpated.
  - Can use a Doppler probe to locate the artery.
  - There should be absolutely no medial direction to the needle (risk of pneumothorax). Keep the hub of the needle against the side of the neck.
  - If the artery is punctured change to a more posterior direction.
  - If using a peripheral nerve stimulator aim for muscle contractions below the elbow (flexion/extension of the wrist or fingers).
  - May miss the ulnar component: this is not the best block for hand surgery.

Vertical infraclavicular block (VIB)

This block is indicated for humerus, elbow, or hand surgery.
- Landmarks: suprasternal notch, anterior prominence of the acromion.

- Technique:

Brachial plexus

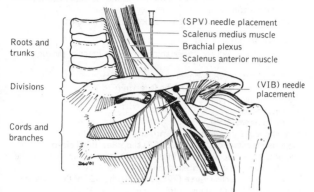

Subclavian perivascular (SPV) and vertical infraclavicular (VIB) approaches to the brachial plexus.

- Position the patient supine without a pillow, with the arm to be blocked resting on the upper abdomen.
- Palpate the spine of the scapula moving anteriorly to locate the anterior prominence of the acromion.
- Mark a point midway on a line joining the anterior prominence of the acromion and the suprasternal notch, below the clavicle.
- Palpate the subclavian artery above the clavicle; your mark should be just lateral to this.
- Using a 22G 50mm insulated needle insert below (but not touching) the clavicle, and advance vertically at right angles to the bed.
- Insert slowly until stimulation of the posterior cord (extension of wrist and fingers) is elicited.
- Depth 20–50mm.
- After careful aspiration inject 0.5ml/kg up to 50ml of LA in increments.
- Complications:
  - Vessel puncture—subclavian artery, subclavian/cephalic vein (15%).
  - Pneumothorax (<0.5%).
  - Horner's syndrome (<5%).
- Clinical tips:
  - No response—move the needle medially 5–10mm. Keep an absolutely vertical approach
  - Confirm the lateral landmark by externally rotating the humerus—if you are on the acromion there will be no movement.
  - Flexion of the elbow or forearm motor responses (musculocutaneous) indicate the lateral cord and may result in inadequate block.
  - Ensure an absolutely vertical direction of injection to avoid pneumothorax.

1079

- there is subclavian puncture the position is too medial—move laterally.
- If there is pectoral muscle contraction at the expected depth the position is too medial.
- This block is contraindicated in anticoagulated patients.

Axillary brachial plexus

Accompanying the axillary artery and vein in the brachial plexus sheath are:
- The medial cutaneous nerve of the arm (C8, T1).
- The medial cutaneous nerve of the forearm (C8, T1).
- The median nerve (C5–C8, T1).
- The ulnar nerve (C7–C8, T1).
- The radial nerve (C5–C8, T1).

Outside the axillary perivascular sheath are:
- The musculocutaneous nerve (C5–C7) supplying 'BBC' biceps, brachialis and coracobrachialis (motor) and sensory to the skin on the radial border of the forearm from the elbow to the wrist.
- The intercostobrachial nerve (T2), supplying the skin of the axilla and the medial side of the upper arm.

Axillary plexus block

This block is indicated for elbow, forearm, and hand surgery.
- Landmark: axillary artery, insertion of pectoralis major muscle.
- Technique:
  - The patient should be supine with their arm abducted to 90° and elbow flexed to 90°.
  - Palpate the axillary artery and mark its position.

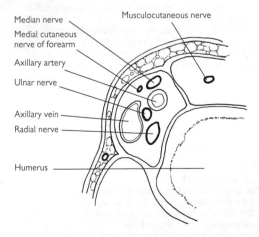

Relationship of the axillary artery and nerves in the axilla.

- Draw a line down from the anterior axillary crease (insertion of the pectoralis major) crossing the axillary artery.
- At this point raise a weal and, fixing the artery between the index and middle fingers, insert a 22G 50mm needle angled slightly proximally to pass either above or below the artery to stimulate either median or ulnar nerve respectively.
- A perceptible click or pop is felt on entering the fascial sheath, and specific motor responses can be elicited (median, radial or ulnar nerve).
- Inject 40–50ml of LA in increments.
- **Four** different techniques can be employed:
  1. Transarterial—injecting 20ml of solution both anterior and posterior to the artery;
  2. Multiple injections—finding each of the four nerves separately, the success of the block being increased when each successive nerve is identified;
  3. Single loss of resistance using a short bevelled needle—fascial click, injecting either through the needle or after insertion of a cannula;
  4. Infiltration—fanwise injection of 15ml of solution each side of the artery.
- Complications: vessel puncture—axillary artery or veins.
- Clinical tips:
  - The fascial sheath may be multicompartmental causing unreliable spread.
  - Remember 'M&M are tops'—musculocutaneous and median nerves are above the artery (ulnar below, radial behind).
  - The musculocutaneous nerve lies outside the sheath and needs to be blocked separately by injection of 10ml into the body of coraco-brachialis (using a peripheral nerve stimulator, direct the needle towards the head of the humerus: the motor response is flexion of the elbow 'hitching a ride').
  - To reduce tourniquet pain infiltrate LA subcutaneously across the base of the axilla.
  - Decide on the area of operation and target the primary nerve if using a single injection technique.

Mid humeral block

All four peripheral nerves can be separately identified and blocked from the same point of entry. This block is indicated for elbow, forearm, and hand surgery.
- Landmarks: brachial artery, humeral canal.
- Technique:
  - The patient should be supine with their arm abducted and forearm supinated.
  - The brachial artery is palpated and marked at the junction of the upper and middle third of the humerus (humeral canal).
  - Draw a line from the insertion of deltoid to cross the brachial artery at this point. This is about 4 finger breadths below the axilla. Mark and raise a weal.

- Insert a 22G 50mm insulated needle above, and parallel to, the artery in a proximal direction to elicit a motor response from the median nerve—flexion of the fingers.
- Return to the skin, and then angle the needle 25° above the artery aiming at the superior border of the humerus to pass between coracobrachialis and biceps to elicit a response from the musculo-cutaneous nerve—flexion of the elbow.
- Return to the skin, redirect the needle inferior and superficial to the artery to elicit an ulnar motor response—thumb adduction, wrist flexion.
- Return to the skin, move the insertion point inferiorly (skin traction) and direct the needle passing under the humerus, to elicit a radial motor response—extension of finger and thumb.
- Inject 6–10ml on each nerve.
- The medial cutaneous nerve of the arm and forearm can be blocked by SC infiltration over the brachial artery at this level (5ml).
- Complications: vessel puncture of the brachial artery.
- Clinical tip: depending on site of the operation, different concentrations of solution can be used for each nerve, allowing varying durations of anaesthesia and postoperative analgesia.

Elbow blocks
Indicated for surgery on the forearm and hand, or supplementing partially effective proximal blocks.
- Landmarks: flexion crease of the elbow, brachial artery, biceps tendon, medial, and lateral epicondyles.
- In all cases the arm should be slightly abducted with the elbow slightly flexed, the forearm supinated.

Median nerve technique
- The median nerve is medial and deep to the brachial artery, partially covered by the biceps muscle tendon.
- The brachial artery is palpated and a 22G 50mm needle is inserted medial to it.
- A click may be felt as the needle pierces the deep fascia, and a motor response elicited (finger flexion and thumb opposition).
- 5–8ml of solution is slowly injected.
- On withdrawal of needle another 5–8ml of solution is deposited subcutaneously along the medial border of the biceps tendon to block the medial cutaneous nerve of the forearm.

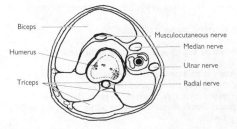

Biceps

Humerus

Triceps

Musculocutaneous nerve

Median nerve

Ulnar nerve

Radial nerve

Mid humeral block.

Radial nerve

- Palpate the intermuscular groove between the biceps and brachioradialis.
- Insert a 22G 50mm needle 2cm above the flexion crease in this groove, towards the lateral epicondyle. Elicit a specific motor response—thumb extension.
- 5–8ml of solution is slowly injected.
- On withdrawal of the needle, inject 5–8ml of solution subcutaneously along the lateral border of the biceps tendon to block the lateral cutaneous nerve of the forearm.

Ulnar nerve

- The patient should be supine with the arm across their body and elbow flexed to 90°.
- The ulnar groove is palpated and a 22G 50mm needle is inserted 1–2 cm proximal to the medial epicondyle in line with the ulnar groove, at 45° to the skin, directed proximally.
- Paraesthesia or a specific motor response is elicited and 5ml of solution injected.
- Caution—do not block the nerve in the ulnar groove as there is a risk of pressure neurapraxia.
- SC infiltration of 5ml between the olecranon and lateral epicondyle of the humerus will block the posterior cutaneous nerve of the forearm.

Clinical tips

- Elbow blocks can be useful for augmenting patchy axillary or supra/infraclavicular techniques.
- If surgery is limited to cutaneous distribution of one nerve, individual nerves can be targeted.

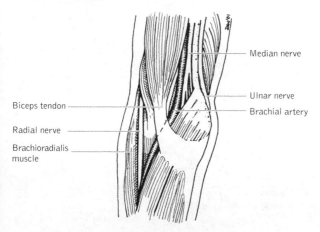

Biceps tendon

Radial nerve

Brachioradialis muscle

Median nerve

Ulnar nerve

Brachial artery

Elbow block (medial, radial, and ulnar) (ante-cubital fossa right arm).

Wrist blocks

The arm is abducted and the forearm supinated. This block is indicated for hand surgery:

- If surgery is limited to cutaneous distribution of one nerve, individual nerves can be targeted.
- Wrist blocks can be used in conjunction with wrist tourniquets for hand surgery.
- Wrist blocks give minimal motor block.

Median nerve

- Insert a 25G 25mm needle between the tendons of the palmaris longus and flexor carpi radialis (FCR) at the level of the proximal palmar crease. If there is no palmaris longus, insert the needle about 5mm medial to FCR.
- Resistance is felt as the needle passes through the flexor retinaculum. Inject 3–5ml of solution.
- On withdrawal of the needle, subcutaneously infiltrate 2–3ml to block the palmar cutaneous branch.
- Alternatively, an injection can be made 3 finger breadths proximal to the skin crease to block the palmar cutaneous branch and the median nerve together.

Ulnar nerve

- Insert a 25G 25mm needle medial to the ulnar artery, lateral to the tendon of the flexor carpi ulnaris at the level of the wrist crease, directed towards the ulnar styloid.

or

- On the medial aspect of the wrist, insert a 25G 25mm needle underneath the tendon of the flexor carpi ulnaris, directed laterally.
- At a depth of approximately 1cm slowly inject 3ml of solution.
- SC infiltration around the ulnar aspect of the wrist will block the dorsal cutaneous branch.

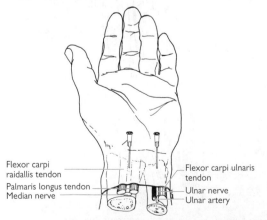

Flexor carpi raidallis tendon
Palmaris longus tendon
Median nerve

Flexor carpi ulnaris tendon
Ulnar nerve
Ulnar artery

Wrist block (median and ulnar nerves).

Radial nerve
- The arm is abducted and the forearm slightly pronated.
- The radial nerve is entirely sensory and cutaneous at this level. A field block of the terminal branches is achieved by infiltration of 5–8ml of LA over the radial aspect of the wrist, 2 finger breadths proximal to the metacarpal base.

Digital nerve block
- Technique:
  - Palpate the metacarpophalangeal (MCP) joint and insert a 25G 25mm needle perpendicular to the skin just distal to the joint. Advance the needle towards the palmar surface, slowly injecting 2–3ml on each side of the phalanx.
  - Insert a 25G 25mm needle into the web space to a point just proximal to the head of the MCP joint, injecting 5ml of solution into each space. Massage the space to aid spread.
  - Avoid adrenaline-containing solutions.

IV regional anaesthesia (IVRA)—Bier's block
- Technique:
  - Apply a double cuff tourniquet (or single cuff) to either the wrist or the upper arm.
  - Select a suitable vein and insert a 20G IV cannula, distal to the cuff.
  - Insert a 20G IV cannula into the other hand (safety needle).
  - Elevate or use an Eschmark bandage to exsanguinate the arm. Inflate the distal and then the proximal cuff, to 100mmHg above systolic pressure, checking for absence of radial pulse. Deflate the distal cuff.
  - Inject a dilute solution of local anaesthetic, e.g. prilocaine 0.5%, 40ml for a small arm, 50ml for a medium arm, or 60ml for a large arm. (Lidocaine 0.5% maximum dose 250mg is a possible alternative if prilocaine is unavailable).
  - Wait 5–10min for the block to take effect.
  - The minimum time to cuff deflation is 15min with prilocaine or 20min with lidocaine.
- Complications: accidental deflation of the cuff causes IV injection of a large volume of local anaesthetic solution.
- Clinical tips:
  - Useful for cutaneous anaesthesia but often inadequate for bony surgery.
  - Use only for short procedures—<30min.
  - Use only lidocaine or prilocaine
  - Bupivacaine and ropivacaine are contraindicated.
  - If tourniquet pain is a problem, inflate the distal cuff, then deflate the proximal cuff
- Anaesthesia and analgesia with this technique is a mixture of LA blockade and possibly cuff induced ischaemia/neurapraxia.

Lower limb blocks

Anatomy of the lumbar plexus

The lumbar plexus lies within the psoas muscle, formed from the ventral rami of L1–L3 and the major part of L4. It gives rise to:

- Iliohypogastric nerve (L1)
- Ilioinguinal nerve (L1)
- Genitofemoral nerve (L1–L2)
- Lateral femoral cutaneous nerve (L2–L3)
- Femoral nerve (L2–L4)
- Obturator nerve (L2–L4).

Lumbar plexus block (posterior approach or 'psoas compartment' block)

This block is indicated for hip, knee, and femoral shaft surgery. In combination with sciatic nerve block it can be used for all operations on the knee, ankle, and foot including the use of a tourniquet.

- Landmarks: posterior superior iliac spine (PSIS), line joining the iliac crests (Tuffier's line—intercristine line).
- Technique:
  - Position the patient laterally, operative side uppermost, and draw a line parallel to the spinous processes, passing through the PSIS (approximately 3 finger breadths from the midline).
  - Mark where it crosses the intercristine line.
  - Insert a 22G 100mm insulated needle perpendicular to the skin with a slight caudad angle. Insert until a transverse process is encountered (probably L4) then redirect the needle to pass either superior or inferior to it. Advance 2–4cm looking for quadriceps stimulation.
  - Inject 30–40ml of solution.
- Complications:
  - Vascular injection—inject slowly, with repeated aspiration.
  - Epidural/intrathecal injection or spread.
- Clinical tips:
  - Avoid medial angulation as epidural/intrathecal injection may occur.
  - Useful for intra/postoperative analgesia in surgery for a fractured femoral neck.
  - Of little value for total hip replacement because the hip joint is also innervated by the sciatic nerve and the cutaneous innervation will include the subcostal nerve.

Femoral nerve block (anterior approach to lumbar plexus)

This block is indicated for surgery to the anterior thigh, knee, or femur.

- Technique:
  - Palpate the femoral artery at the level of the inguinal ligament.
  - Mark a point 1cm lateral to the pulsation and 1–2cm distal to the ligament.

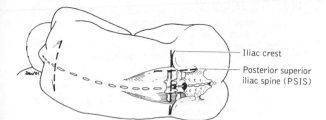

Posterior approach to the lumbar plexus (psoas compartment block).

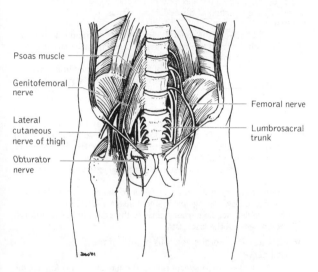

Lumbar plexus.

- Insert a 22G 50cm needle at 45° to the skin in a cephalad direction. Two distinct 'pops' may be felt as the needle passes through fascia lata and iliopectineal fascia.
- Stimulation of rectus femoris ('dancing patella') indicates correct location of the needle. Inject 10–30ml of solution.
- Complications: vascular injection.

- Clinical tips:
  - Sartorius stimulation (medial thigh twitching) is either from direct muscle contact or anterior division of the nerve—not acceptable for a good effect. Move needle laterally.
  - Commonly called a 3:1 block (femoral, lateral cutaneous nerve of thigh, obturator) when using high volume and distal pressure to aid cephalad spread. This is an unreliable method for obturator nerve block.

Obturator nerve block

This block is indicated for adductor spasm and knee surgery (optional).
- Landmarks: insertion of adductor tendons.
- Technique:
  - Position the patient supine with the leg placed in a 'figure of four' position. Hip abducted and externally rotated—knee flexed.
  - Identify the insertion of the adductor magnus and brevis into the pubis.
  - At a point between the tendons, 1cm inferior to the pubis, insert a 22G 80mm insulated needle in the horizontal plane aiming at the ipsilateral anterior superior iliac spine.
  - At a depth of 5–6cm resistance of the obturator membrane may be felt. Following a 'pop' a motor response (adductor stimulation) may be elicited. Inject 5–15ml of LA.

Lateral cutaneous nerve of the thigh

Block of this nerve is indicated for analgesia of lateral femoral incisions (hip surgery, surgery for fractured neck of femur, or skin graft donation). It is commonly blocked by a femoral nerve block or femoral 3:1 block, and psoas compartment block.
- Landmarks: anterior superior iliac spine, inguinal ligament.
- Technique:
  - At a point 2cm medial and 2cm inferior to the anterior superior iliac spine, below the inguinal ligament insert a 22G 25–50cm short-bevelled needle perpendicular to the skin. 10ml of solution is injected beneath the fascia lata.

Subcostal nerve (lateral cutaneous branch of the T12 intercostal nerve)

This nerve is blocked in conjunction with the lumbar plexus for hip surgery (posterior approach).
- Landmarks: anterior superior iliac spine, iliac crest
- Technique: using 22G 80mm needle make an SC infiltration backwards from the anterior superior iliac spine along the iliac crest using 8–10ml of solution.

Anatomy of the sacral plexus

The sacral plexus is formed from the lumbosacral trunk (L4–L5), the ventral rami of S1–S3 and part of S4. The plexus lies on piriformis on the anterior surface of the sacrum, covered by the parietal pelvic fascia. It gives several branches to the pelvis but only two nerves emerge to supply the leg:
- the posterior cutaneous nerve of the thigh (S1–S3)
- the sciatic nerve (L4–L5, S1–S3).

Sciatic nerve block (posterior approach–Labat)

This block is indicated for ankle and foot surgery. In combination with femoral nerve block it can be used for all surgery on the knee and lower leg.

- Technique:
  - Put the patient in Sim's position (recovery position with operative side uppermost) and arrange the knee, greater trochanter, and posterior superior iliac spine (PSIS) in a line.
  - Draw a line connecting the PSIS and greater trochanter. At its mid point, drop a perpendicular line (5cm) to intersect another line joining the greater trochanter and the sacral hiatus.
  - Insert a 22G 100mm needle perpendicular to the skin to a depth of 8–10cm, and elicit motor stimulation—foot eversion (peroneal) or plantar flexion (tibial). Inject 15–20ml of solution.
  - Three other approaches to the sciatic nerve have been described: the inferior approach (Raj), the lateral approach (Ichiangi), and the anterior approach (Beck).
- Clinical tips:
  - Only the classical posterior approach guarantees block of the posterior cutaneous nerve of the thigh.
  - If the nerve cannot be immediately identified, 'walk' the needle along the perpendicular line (the sciatic nerve must cross this line at some point).
  - The onset of block is slow and may take up to 60min.
  - The tibial and peroneal components may divide anywhere from the sciatic notch to the popliteal fossa. Peroneal nerve stimulation alone (dorsiflexion and eversion of the foot) doesn't ensure tibial anaesthesia. Aim for foot inversion and plantar flexion.
  - In ~25% of patients it is impossible or difficult to block the sciatic nerve by the alternative anterior approach. The nerve lies underneath the femur (external rotation of femur may help).
  - Avoid adrenaline containing solutions as the nerve has a poor blood supply.

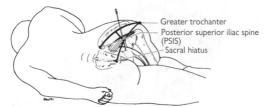

Greater trochanter
Posterior superior iliac spine (PSIS)
Sacral hiatus

Posterior (Labat) approach to the sciatic nerve.

Anatomy of the nerve supply of the lower leg and foot

Below the knee the sciatic nerve supplies all motor and sensory innervation except for a cutaneous strip following the long saphenous vein to the medial border of the foot (saphenous nerve—terminal branch of the femoral nerve). The sciatic nerve divides at the upper angle of the popliteal fossa into:

- The tibial nerve (L4–S3), branching into the sural and tibial nerves.
- The common peroneal nerve (L4–S2), dividing into the superficial peroneal and deep peroneal nerves.

Popliteal block posterior approach

The popliteal fossa is a diamond-shaped area bounded inferiorly by the medial and lateral heads of the gastrocnemius and superiorly by the long head of biceps femoris (laterally) and the superimposed heads of semimembranosus and semitendinosus (medially). The posterior skin crease marks the widest point of the fossa, and with the knee slightly flexed, the muscular boundaries of the fossa can be identified. This block is indicated for ankle and foot surgery.

- Landmarks: popliteal skin crease, biceps femoris, vastus lateralis, semimembranosus, and semitendinosus.
- Techniques:

Posterior approach

- With the patient prone, flex the knee, identify and mark the muscular borders of the fossa and then straighten the leg.
- Mark a point 10cm proximal to the popliteal skin crease, in the midline between biceps femoris (laterally) and semitendinosus and semimembranosus (medially).
- Insert a 22G 50/100mm needle (depending on the size of the patient) at this point, directing the needle proximally at an angle of 45°.
- At a depth of 4–8cm the sciatic nerve or components will be found (tibial—plantar flexion, common peroneal—dorsiflexion)
- Inject 20–30ml of local anaesthetic.

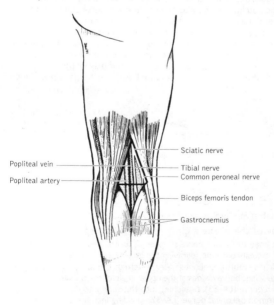

Popliteal vein

Popliteal artery

Sciatic nerve

Tibial nerve
Common peroneal nerve

Biceps femoris tendon

Gastrocnemius

Popliteal fossa block (right leg).

Lateral approach
- Supine, with the knee slightly flexed, mark the groove between vastus lateralis (above) and biceps femoris (below)
- Draw a line down from the superior border of the patella, where it crosses this groove
- Insert a 22G 50mm needle, directed posteriorly 25–30° and slightly caudally
- The needle passes through biceps femoris into the popliteal fossa— initially passing the common peroneal nerve, then the tibial nerve.
- Inject 10ml of local anaesthetic around each nerve.
- Clinical tips
  - The sciatic nerve is two nerves loosely bound together; commonly dividing into the tibial and peroneal nerves 5–12cm above the popliteal crease. In a small proportion of people, it is separated for its entire course.
  - High volume popliteal techniques—often block both nerves, but individual localisation of both nerves may improve success rate.

Intra-articular block

This block is indicated for knee arthroscopy.
- Landmarks: medial border of the patella.
- Technique:
  - Fully extend the knee.
  - Identify the gap between the medial border of the patella and the femur.
  - Insert a 22G 50mm needle into the knee joint.
  - Inject 30ml of local anaesthetic—0.5% L-bupivacaine with adrenaline onset 40min duration 3–5hr.
  - Inject portal sites with 1% lidocaine by surgeon.
- Clinical tips:
  - Sterile technique is of the utmost importance when injecting into a major joint.
  - Addition of morphine 2–5mg may improve postoperative analgesia.
  - Adrenaline-containing solutions have the advantage of minimising bleeding into the joint.

Saphenous nerve block

This is indicated in combination with sciatic nerve block for ankle and foot surgery.
- Landmarks: tibial tuberosity, medial tibial condyle.
- Technique:
  - The patient should be supine, with their leg externally rotated.
  - Identify the tibial tuberosity and inject 10–15ml subcutaneously from the tibial tuberosity towards the medial tibial condyle.

Ankle and foot blocks

To ensure anaesthesia of the forefoot all of the following nerves need to be blocked: deep and superficial peroneal, tibial and sural nerves.

Deep peroneal nerve
- Technique:
  - 3cm distal to the inter-malleolar line palpate the extensor hallucis longus tendon (dorsiflexion of the big toe); lateral to this is the dorsalis pedis artery.
  - Insert a 23G 25mm needle just lateral to the artery, until bony contact is made; withdraw slightly injecting 2ml.

Superficial peroneal nerves
- Landmarks: injection point is the same as for the deep peroneal nerve.
- Technique: after performing blockade of the deep peroneal nerve infiltrate subcutaneously laterally and medially to the plantar junction of the foot with 10ml of local anaesthetic. This blocks the medial and lateral cutaneous branches.

Tibial nerve
- Technique:
  - Draw a line from the medial malleolus to the posterior inferior calcaneum.
  - Palpate the posterior tibial artery.
  - Insert a 22G 50mm needle just behind the artery, advancing until stimulation is elicited (plantar flexion of the toes). If bone is encountered, withdraw slightly injecting 6–10ml.

Sural nerve
- Landmarks: lateral malleolus, Achilles tendon.
- Technique: using a 22G 50mm needle, inject 5ml subcutaneously between the lateral malleolus and the lateral border of the Achilles tendon.

Digital nerve blocks
- Metatarsal approach: 22G 50mm needle at mid metatarsal level, 6ml.

or
- Digital approach: a 22G 50mm needle distal to the metatarso-phalangeal joint, 3–6ml.

or
- Web space: a 23G 25mm needle in the web space, 6ml.
- Avoid adrenaline-containing solutions.

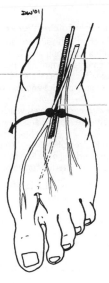

Superficial peroneal nerve

Dorsalis pedis artery

Deep peroneal nerve

Ankle block I.

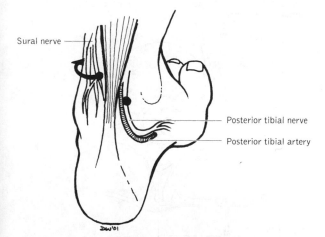

Sural nerve

Posterior tibial nerve

Posterior tibial artery

Ankle block II.

Trunk blocks

Anatomy of the nerve supply to the thorax and abdomen

- The muscles and skin of the chest and abdomen are supplied by the spinal nerves of T2–T12 with a contribution of L1 in the inguinal region. These mixed spinal nerves emerge from the intervertebral foramen into the paravertebral space dividing into dorsal and ventral rami.
- The dorsal rami supply the deep muscles and skin over the dorsum of the trunk.
- The ventral rami form the intercostal nerves, which pass into the neurovascular plane between the internal and innermost intercostal muscles.
- A lateral cutaneous branch is given off before the costal angle, piercing the intercostal muscles and overlying muscles in the mid-axillary line.
- The intercostal nerves end as an anterior cutaneous nerve.

Thoracic paravertebral block (see also p354)

- This block is indicated for pain relief after:
  - thoracic surgery
  - breast surgery
  - fractured ribs
  - open cholecystectomy
  - renal surgery.
- Landmarks: spinous processes of the thoracic vertebrae.
- Technique:
  - The patient should be sitting or lying with the operative side up.
  - Palpate the cephalad aspect of the spinous process and make a mark 2.5–3cm laterally.

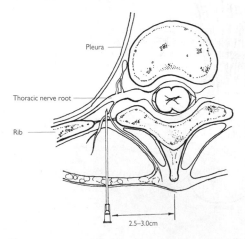

Pleura

Thoracic nerve root

Rib

2.5–3.0cm

Thoracic paravertebral block.

- Insert a 22G 80mm needle perpendicular to the skin to contact the transverse process of the vertebra below.
- Withdraw the needle, reinserting it to pass cephalad to the transverse process, advancing until you feel a change in resistance/loss of resistance or paraesthesia is elicited (usually 1–1.5cm). Inject 5ml per level or 15ml to obtain spread in 3–5 segments.
- To insert a catheter use a 16G Tuohy needle using loss of resistance to air/saline.
- Complications:
  - Intravascular injection of local anaesthetic.
  - Epidural or intrathecal injection.
  - Pneumothorax. Frequency is operator dependent.

Intercostal nerve block

Indications as for thoracic paravertebral block.
- Technique:
  - The patient should be prone or lateral with the operative side up.
  - Feel for the angle of the rib at the posterior axillary line; place the index and middle fingers either side of the rib.
  - Insert a 22G 50mm needle perpendicular to the skin, to touch the lower border of the rib.
  - Pass the needle beneath the rib, insert 3–4mm. A click or loss of resistance or paraesthesia may be felt—inject 3–5ml.
  - For catheter insertion use 16G Tuohy needle with an oblique angulation parallel to the rib until there is loss of resistance to air/saline.
- Complications:
  - Intravascular injection.
  - Bleeding.
  - Pneumothorax.
  - Local anaesthetic drug toxicity.
- Clinical tips:
  - It is important to be able to feel the rib.
  - Multiple levels increase the risk of pneumothorax.
  - Bilateral block best achieved with the patient prone but risks bilateral pneumothorax and rapid absorption of local anaesthetic drug.

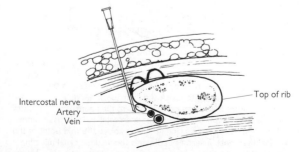

Intercostal nerve block.

Interpleural block

- This block is indicated for:
  - Fractured ribs
  - Breast surgery
  - Unilateral upper abdominal surgery—open cholecystectomy
  - Chronic pancreatic pain.
- Landmarks: posterior angle of the sixth rib.
- Technique:
  - Position the patient laterally with the operative side uppermost.
  - Use a 16G Tuohy needle with a one-way or self-sealing valve connected to a bag of IV saline.
  - Introduce the needle at 45° to the sixth rib to touch upper border.
  - Connect the infusion to the side arm of the sheath adaptor and turn on.
  - Advance the needle over the top of the rib (avoiding the neurovascular compartment) until there is free flow of saline (the space between parietal and visceral pleura is entered).
  - Thread an epidural catheter through the self-sealing valve of the adaptor, 8–10cm into the space, and secure.
  - Inject 20ml solution.
- Complications: pneumothorax.
- Clinical tips:
  - Using a closed system ensures that no air is introduced into the space from outside.
  - Effect is due to spread into the paravertebral gutter, blocking sympathetic as well as somatic nerves.
  - Keep the saline infusion no more than 10cm above the height of the needle hub to avoid false loss of resistance.
  - Go above the rib to avoid intercostal artery—potential for massive haematoma.

Inguinal field block

Iliohypogastric, ilioinguinal and genitofemoral nerves, plus branches from overlapping intercostal nerves, supply the inguinal region.
Indicated for inguinal hernia surgery.

- Technique:
  - At a point 2cm (two fingers' breadth) medial to the anterior superior iliac spine insert a 22G 50mm short bevelled needle perpendicular to the skin.
  - A pop is felt as the needle passes through the aponeurosis of the external oblique muscle. Inject 8ml blocking the iliohypogastric nerve.
  - Redirect the needle deeper to pass through the internal oblique muscle, injecting 8ml between the internal oblique and the transversus abdominis to block the ilioinguinal nerve.
  - Further fan-wise SC infiltration superficial to the aponeurosis will block the cutaneous supply from the lower intercostal and subcostal nerves.
  - Palpate the deep inguinal ring (1–1.5cm above the mid point of the inguinal ligament). Insert a needle into the inguinal canal injecting 5ml to block the genital branch of the genitofemoral nerve. This can only reliably be done at the time of surgery.

- SC infiltration at the medial end of incision or fan-wise from the pubic tubercle will block contralateral innervation.
- All the above (with the exception of the genitofemoral block) are best done before surgery as they rely on the spread of LA between the fascial layers. This can be done either by surgeon or anaesthetist.
- Complications:
  - Intravascular injection.
  - Intraperitoneal injection.
  - Femoral nerve block—ipsilateral leg weakness.

Penile block

This is indicated for circumcision:
- Anatomy: The nerve supply to the penis and scrotum is primarily via the dorsal nerve of the penis and posterior scrotal branches of the pudendal nerve (S2–S4), with additional branches from the ilioinguinal, genitofemoral, and posterior cutaneous nerve of the thigh.
- Landmarks: symphysis pubis.
- Technique:
  - Palpate the symphysis pubis above the root of the penis.
  - Insert a 22G 25–50mm needle to touch the inferior border of the pubis and advance 1–2cm until loss of resistance is felt.
  - The needle will be deep to the superficial fascia of the penis (Buck's fascia), Inject 5–10ml blocking both dorsal nerves. Need to direct angle 5 degrees from the midline in each side
  - Complete the block by injecting subcutaneously around the root of the penis onto the scrotum to block input from ilioinguinal and genitofemoral nerves.
  - Never use adrenaline-containing solutions.
- Complications: intravascular injection, bleeding.

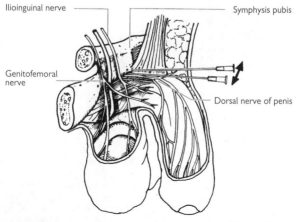

Penile block.

Central neuraxial blocks (see also p699 and p786)

Spinal and epidural anatomy

- The spinal cord terminates at L1–L2 adults, L3 infants.
- The line joining the iliac crests (intercristine or Tuffier's line) is at the L3/4 interspace.
- The subarachnoid space ends at S2 in adults and lower in children (care with paediatric caudal block, use cannula rather than needle).
- The subarachnoid space extends laterally along the nerve roots to the dorsal root ganglia.
- There is a capillary interval (potential space) between the dura and the arachnoid mater (subdural space). This space is widest and most easily accessible in the cervical region.
- The epidural (extradural) space lies between the walls of the vertebral canal and the spinal dura mater. It is a potential low-pressure space, occupied by areolar tissue, loose fat, and the internal vertebral venous plexus.
- The ligamentum flavum is thin in the cervical region reaching maximal thickness in the lumbar region (2–5mm).

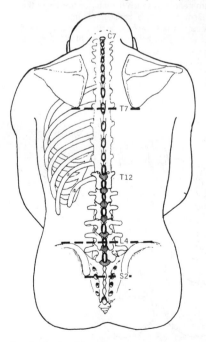

Bony landmarks of the spine.

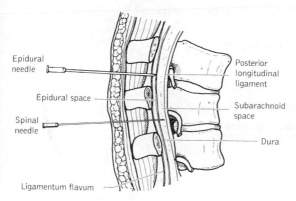

Subarachnoid and epidural spaces.

Spinal block

- Indications for spinal block are:
  - Lower abdominal surgery (Caesarean section, inguinal hernia).
  - Lower limb surgery.
  - Perineal surgery.
- Landmarks: spinous processes of the lumbar vertebrae and the line joining the iliac crests (Tuffier's line).
- Technique:
  - The patient should be sitting or lying on their side.
  - Mark a line joining the iliac crests.
  - Identify the spinous processes at the level of this line.
  - The nearest interspace at this level is L3/4 (there is significant variation).
  - Spinal blocks should always be carried out caudal to this space.
- After raising an SC weal, insert a 22–29G needle of your choice:
  - Midline: at the level of the interspace, insert a needle in the midline (coronal plane). With 15° cephalad angulation, advance until a click or pop is felt, at an approximate depth of 4–6cm.
  - Paramedian: 1–2cm lateral to the upper border of the spinous process. Insert a needle perpendicular to the skin to contact the lamina of the vertebra. Withdraw slightly, reinserting the needle 15° medially and 30° cephalad to pass over the lamina through the interlaminar space. Advance until a click or pop is felt (the dura is pierced).
- After free flow of CSF inject the desired volume. Check for free flow of CSF after injection.

Needle design

- Quincke (cutting) end hole—insertion parallel to dural fibres.
- Whitacre/Sprotte (splitting)—side hole, 'pencil point'.
- 25–29G depending on personal preference. Use 22G in an elderly patient with a difficult back.

Suggested doses for spinal anaesthesia

Block height	Volume of solution
Heavy bupivacaine 0.5%:	
T6–T10	2.5–3 ml
T11–L1	2.5ml
L2–L5	2.0ml
S1–S5 (saddle block)	1.0–1.5ml (sitting position)
Plain bupivacaine 0.5% (or levobupivacaine 0.5%):	
T6–T10	Unreliable
T11–L1	2.5–3ml
L2–L5	2.5ml
S1–S5	Not possible to achieve saddle block

Local anaesthetic drugs for spinal anaesthesia
- There is no commercially marketed short-acting intrathecal preparation licensed for spinal anaesthesia within the United Kingdom. Manufacturers advise against the use of lidocaine due to risks of cauda equina syndrome and transient radicular irritation or transient neurological symptoms.
  - Transient neurological symptoms: back pain or dysaesthesia radiating into buttocks and legs. Begins within 24hr of procedure. Usually self-resolving in 3–5d. No neurological sequelae
- Ropivacaine does not have a product licence for intrathecal use.
- Bupivacaine plain or heavy can be used (usually 0.5%).
  - 'Heavy' is hyperbaric and contains 8% dextrose.
  - 'Plain' bupivacaine is isobaric at body temperature.
  - Due to spread in the intrathecal space, heavy solutions can be used to achieve a higher block. Plain solutions will usually produce a lower block height (T12–L1) with consequently less hypotension, under normal conditions.[1]
- See drug additive chart—pp716, 1040.

Clinical tips
- Ideally injection should be at the L3/4 interspace; if there is difficulty go down not up as the level of termination of the conus is variable.
- Accurate surface identification of the L3/4 interspace is difficult—70% of clinicians mark higher.
- A sitting position increases CSF pressure and hence improves CSF flow with fine needles. Also easier to find the midline in obese patients.
- Lateral position offers familiarity of practice and possibility of sedation.
- Often problems are due to too short an introducer and a flexible needle—can use a sterile 19G needle as a longer introducer for most 25G spinal needles.

- The midline approach is conceptually easier, but osteophytes and calcification of the interspinous ligament in the elderly increase the difficulty.
- In the lateral/paramedian approach the lamina acts as a depth gauge; the interlaminar space is preserved in elderly patients.
- Low-dose bupivacaine/levobupivacaine 6–8mg ± fentanyl 10–25μg is possible for day case spinal anaesthesia.

Contraindications
- Relative contraindications:
  - Aortic stenosis/mitral stenosis (profound hypotension—sympathetic block).
  - Previous back surgery (technical difficulty).
  - Neurological disease (medicolegal).
  - Systemic sepsis (increased incidence of epidural abscess, meningitis).
- Absolute contraindications:
  - Local sepsis.
  - Patient refusal.
  - Anticoagulation: see p214/p699/p1058.

Continuous spinal anaesthesia (CSA)—spinal catheters
- Better control over level, intensity, and duration of block.
- Possibly less hypotension: incremental dosing and reduced total dose.
- Recent trend to larger catheters e.g. 20G epidural, 22–24G 'catheter-over-needle'.
- Low incidence of post dural puncture headache in older patients (1–6%).
- This block is indicated for lower abdominal, hip, and knee surgery.
- Technique:
  - Make a dural puncture using your needle of choice (18G Tuohy)
  - The level of insertion should be at or below L3/4
  - Insert a catheter 3cm into CSF and attach a bacterial filter.
  - Inject 1–1.5ml (0.5% plain bupivacaine). Wait 15min and test the block.
  - Inject a further 0.5–1.0ml as necessary or when the level of block decreases by two segments.
- Complications: post dural puncture headache (see p706).

Epidural block
See pp700, 1038

Caudal block
See pp784, 787
Useful in surgery of the perineum in adults
- Adult dose 20–25ml bupivacaine (0.125–0.5%) plain.
- Use a 21G (green) needle or 20G IV cannula.
- Urinary retention is more common in adults.

---

1 Hocking G, Wildsmith JAW (2004). Intrathecal drug spread *British Journal of Anaesthesia*, **93**, 568-578.

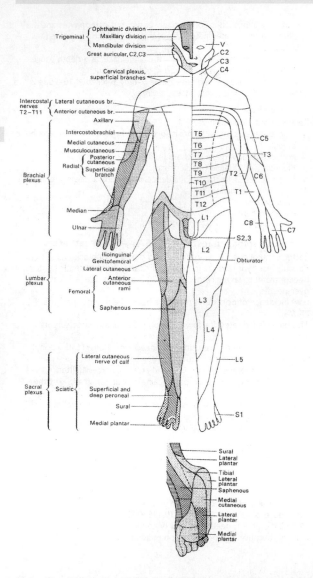

Dermatomes. With kind permission of Oxford University Press.

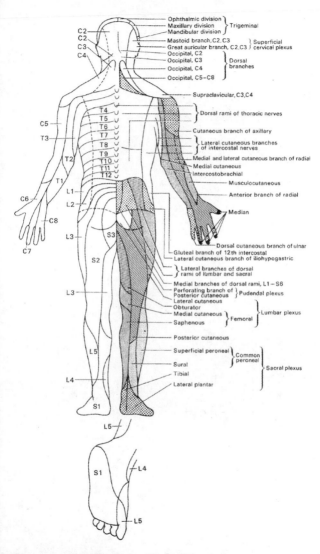

Dermatomes. With kind permission of Oxford University Press.

Chapter 42

Drug formulary

Aidan O'Donnell

See also:

Drug	Description and perioperative indications	Cautions and contraindications	Side-effects	Dose (paediatric)	Dose (adult)
Abciximab (ReoPro®)	Synthetic monoclonal antibody. Glycoprotein IIb/IIIa inhibitor. (Powerful antiplatelet action) Used to prevent ischaemic complications before or during percutaneous coronary intervention	Intracranial or intraspinal surgery (<2yr), trauma or neoplasm. Major surgery. Ongoing haemorrhage. Retinopathy. Can only be given once	Haemorrhage. Nausea and vomiting Chest and back pain. May provoke hypersensitivity		250µg/kg bolus over 1min, then infuse at 0.125µg/kg/ min (max 10 µg/min). Start 10–60min before coronary intervention and continue for at least 12hr
Acetazolamide (Diamox®)	Carbonic anhydrase inhibitor used for acute reduction of intraocular pressure. Weak diuretic	Extravasation causes necrosis	Thrombocytopenia	2–7mg/kg tds	500mg bd
Adenosine	Endogenous nucleoside with antiarrhythmic activity. Slows conduction through AV node. Treatment of acute paroxysmal SVT (including WPW) or differentiation of SVT from VT. Duration 10s	Second or third degree heart block. Asthma. Reduce dose in heart transplant or dipyridamole treatment	Flushing, dyspnoea, headache—all transient	0.05mg/kg, increasing by 0.05mg/kg to max 0.3mg/kg	6mg fast IV bolus, increasing to 12mg at 2min intervals as necessary

Adrenaline	Endogenous catecholamine with alpha and beta action: 1. Treatment of anaphylaxis 2. Bronchodilator 3. Positive inotrope 4. Given by nebuliser for croup 5. Prolongation of local anaesthetic action. 1:1000 contains 1mg/ml, 1:10 000 contains 100µg/ml 1:200 000 contains 5µg/ml	Arrhythmias especially with halothane. Caution in elderly. Via central catheter whenever possible	Hypertension, tachycardia, anxiety, hyperglycaemia, arrhythmias. Reduces uterine blood flow	1–3: IV/IM/IO 0.1ml/kg of 1:10 000 (10µg/kg), ETT 0.1ml/kg of 1:1000 (100µg/kg). Infusion 0.05–1µg/kg/min 4: Nebulisation 0.5ml/kg (up to 5ml) 1:1000. 5. Maximum dose for infiltration 2µg/kg	1–3: IV/IM/ET 1ml aliquots of 1:10 000 up to 5–10ml (0.5–1mg). Infusion 2–20µg/min (0.04–0.4µg/kg/min). 4: Nebulisation 5ml 1: 1000. 5: Maximum dose for infiltration 2µg/kg
Alcohol	See Ethanol				
Alfentanil	Short-acting, potent, opioid analgesic. Duration 10min		Respiratory depression, bradycardia, hypotension	15–50µg/kg over 5min, then 0.5–1 µg/kg/min	250–750µg (5–10µg/kg). Attenuation of CVS response to intubation: 10–20µg/kg
Alimemazine (Trimeprazine)	Sedative antihistamine premed (Vallergan®)		Paediatric	PO: 2mg/kg (over 2yr)	

IV = intravenous. IM = intramuscular. SC = subcutaneous. PO = per os (oral). SL = sublingual. ET = endotracheal. od = once daily. bd = twice daily. tds = three times daily. qds = four times daily. NR = not recommended. Doses are intravenous and dilutions in 0.9% saline unless otherwise stated.

Drug	Description and perioperative indications	Cautions and contraindications	Side-effects	Dose (paediatric)	Dose (adult)
Ametop	See tetracaine				
Aminophylline	Methylxanthine bronchodilator used in prevention and treatment of asthma. Converted to theophylline, a phosphodiesterase inhibitor. Serum levels 10–20mg/l (55–110µmol/l)	Caution in patients already receiving oral or IV theophyllines. Where serum level known aminophylline 0.6mg/kg should increase level by 1mg/l	Palpitations, tachycardia, tachypnoea, seizures, nausea, arrhythmias	5mg/kg over 30min, then 0.5–1mg/kg/hr	5mg/kg over 30min, then 0.5mg/kg/hr infusion
Amiodarone	Mixed class 1C and III antiarrhythmic useful in treatment of supraventricular and ventricular arrhythmias	Via central catheter. Sinoatrial heart block, thyroid dysfunction, pregnancy, porphyria. Dilute in dextrose 5%, not saline	Commonly causes thyroid dysfunction and reversible corneal deposits	25µg/kg/min for 4hr, then 5–15µg/kg/min	5mg/kg over 1–2 hr. Maximum 1.2g in 24hr 300mg slow IV bolus for defib resistant VF
Amoxicillin	Broad spectrum penicillin antibiotic	History of allergy	Nausea, diarrhoea, rash	10–25mg/kg tds. (qds in severe infections)	0.5–1g tds (qds in severe infections)

Aprotinin (Trasylol®)	Inhibits plasmin (responsible for fibrin dissolution) and reduces blood loss in major cardiac/hepatic surgery	Hypersensitivity and phlebitis	2 000 000U (200ml) over 30min, then infusion of 500 000U (50ml) per hour
Atenolol	Cardioselective β-blocker. Long acting	Bradycardia, hypotension, and decreased contractility	0.05mg/kg every 5min—max 4 doses 5–10mg over 10min. PO: 50mg od
Atracurium	Benzylisoquinolinium non-depolarising muscle relaxant. Undergoes temperature- and pH-dependent Hofmann elimination (to laudanosine), plus non-specific enzymatic ester hydrolysis. Useful in severe renal or hepatic disease. Duration 20–35min	Mild histamine release and rash common with higher doses. Flush with saline before and after	Neuromuscular block potentiated by aminoglycosides, loop diuretics, magnesium, lithium, ↓temp, ↓K⁺, ↓pH, prior use of suxamethonium, volatile agents. Store at 2–8°C Intubation: 0.3–0.6mg/kg. Maintenance: 0.1–0.2mg/kg. Infusion: 0.3–0.6mg/kg/hr, monitor neuromuscular blockade

IV = intravenous. IM = intramuscular. SC = subcutaneous. PO = per os (oral). SL = sublingual. ET = endotracheal. od = once daily. bd = twice daily. tds = three times daily. qds = four times daily. NR = not recommended. Doses are intravenous and dilutions in 0.9% saline unless otherwise stated.

Drug	Description and perioperative indications	Cautions and contraindications	Side-effects	Dose (paediatric)	Dose (adult)
Atropine	Muscarinic acetylcholine antagonist. Vagal blockade at AV and sinus node increases heart rate (transient decrease at low doses due to weak agonist effect). Tertiary amine therefore crosses blood–brain barrier	Obstructive uropathy and cardiovascular disease. Glaucoma, myasthenia gravis	Decreases secretions, and lower oesophageal sphincter tone, relaxes bronchial smooth muscle. Confusion in elderly	IV: 10–20µg/kg. Control of muscarinic effects of neostigmine: 10–20µg/kg. IM/SC: 10–30µg/kg. PO: 40µg/kg	300–600µg. Prevention of muscarinic effects of neostigmine: 600–1200µg. Cardiac arrest: 3mg
Augmentin	See co-amoxiclav				
Benzatropine	Antimuscarinic used in acute treatment of drug induced dystonic reactions (except tardive dyskinesia)	Glaucoma, gastrointestinal obstruction	Urinary retention, dry mouth, blurred vision	>3yr 0.02mg/kg repeated after 15min	IV/IM: 1–2mg repeated if necessary
Benzylpenicillin	Broad spectrum antibiotic	History of allergy	Nausea, diarrhoea, rash	25mg/kg qds. 50mg/kg qds for severe infections	300–600mg qds. Higher doses may also be used (up to 2.4g qds)

Drug	Description	Cautions	Side effects	Dose	
Bicarbonate (sodium)	Alkaline salt used for correction of acidosis and to enhance onset of action of local anaesthetics. 8.4% = 1000mmol/l. Dose (mmol) in acidosis: weight (kg) × base deficit × 0.3	Precipitation with calcium containing solutions, increased CO_2 production, necrosis on extravasation. Via central catheter if possible	Alkalosis, hypokalaemia, hypernatraemia, hypocalcaemia	1ml/kg 8.4% solution (1mmol/kg)	Dependent on degree of acidosis. Resuscitation: 50ml of 8.4% then recheck blood gases. Bicarbonation of LA: 1ml 8.4% to 20ml bupivacaine. 1ml 8.4% to 10ml lidocaine/prilocaine
Bretylium	Treatment of resistant ventricular arrhythmias in resuscitation situation only. Class III antiarrhythmic	Phaeochromocytoma. Avoid sympathomimetic amines. May exacerbate arrhythmias due to cardiac glycosides	Severe hypotension, transient hypertension, dizziness, nausea parotid pain	5–10mg/kg over 10–30min (dilute to 10mg/ml in saline or dextrose), then 5–30µg/kg/min	5–10mg/kg over 10min (dilute to 10mg/ml in saline or dextrose). Then 1–2mg/min infusion
Bupivacaine	Amide type local anaesthetic used for infiltration, epidural, and spinal anaesthesia. Slower onset than lidocaine. Duration 200–400min (slightly prolonged by adrenaline) pKa 8.1	Greater cardiotoxicity than other local agents. Do not use for IVRA. Adrenaline-containing solutions contain preservative	Toxicity: tongue/circumoral numbness, restlessness, tinnitus, seizures, cardiac arrest	Infiltration/epidural: maximum dose dependent upon injection site—2mg/kg/4hr recommended	0.25–0.75% solution. Infiltration/epidural: maximum dose dependent upon injection site—2mg/kg/4hr. (2mg/kg with adrenaline). 0.75% solution contraindicated in pregnancy

IV = intravenous. IM = intramuscular. SC = subcutaneous. PO = per os (oral). SL = sublingual. ET = endotracheal. od = once daily. bd = twice daily. tds = three times daily. qds = four times daily. NR = not recommended. Doses are intravenous and dilutions in 0.9% saline unless otherwise stated.

Drug	Description and perioperative indications	Cautions and contraindications	Side-effects	Dose (paediatric)	Dose (adult)
Buprenorphine (Temgesic®)	Opioid with both agonist and antagonist actions. Duration 6hr	May precipitate withdrawal in opioid addicts. Only partially reversed by naloxone	Nausea, respiratory depression, constipation	>6 month. Slow IV/IM: 3–6µg/kg qds. SL: 3–6µg/kg tds	Slow IV/IM: 300–600µg qds. SL: 200–400µg qds
Caffeine	Mild stimulant effective in the treatment of post dural puncture headache. Intravenous preparation available as caffeine sodium benzoate		Insomnia, weakly diuretic, excitation, tachycardia	SCBU: 5mg/kg qds. Prevention of postop. apnoea: 10mg/kg	IV/PO: 300–500mg bd One cup coffee contains 50–100mg Soft drinks may contain up to 35–50mg
Calcium chloride	Electrolyte replacement, positive inotrope, hyperkalaemia, hypermagnesaemia. Calcium chloride 10% contains Ca^{2+} 680µmol/ml	Necrosis on extravasation. Incompatible with bicarbonate	Arrhythmias, hypertension, hypercalcaemia	0.1–0.2ml/kg 10% solution	2–5ml 10% solution (10mg/kg, 0.07mmol/kg)
Calcium gluconate	As calcium chloride. Calcium gluconate 10% contains Ca^{2+} 220µmol/ml	Less phlebitis than calcium chloride	As calcium chloride	0.3–0.5 ml/kg 10% solution (max 20ml)	6–15ml of 10% solution (30mg/kg, 0.07mmol/kg)

Drug	Description	Cautions	Side effects	Paediatric dose	Adult dose
Carboprost (Hemabate®)	Synthetic prostaglandin F₂ used to treat severe post-partum haemorrhage due to uterine atony (after ergometrine and oxytocin failed)	Asthma, diabetes, epilepsy, jaundice, anaemia, glaucoma. Large doses may cause uterine rupture	Fever, bronchospasm. Nausea, vomiting, flushing. May cause cardiovascular collapse		Never give IV. 250µg deep IM or directly into the myometrium. Repeat if needed after at least 15min. Max dose 2mg/24hr
Cefotaxime	Third generation cephalosporin broad spectrum antibiotic	Penicillin sensitivity		25mg/kg tds. 50mg/kg qds in severe infections	1g bd (up to 12g daily in divided doses in severe infections)
Cefuroxime	Second generation cephalosporin broad spectrum antibiotic	10% cross-sensitivity with penicillin allergy		20–30mg/kg tds	750mg–1.5g tds
Celecoxib (Celebrex®)	NSAID with selective inhibition of cyclo-oxygenase II (Cox II) enzyme. Reduced gastric, asthma, and platelet side effects	Hypersensitivity to sulphonamides or aspirin, severe renal impairment, peptic ulceration		NR	PO: 100–200mg bd

IV = intravenous. IM = intramuscular. SC = subcutaneous. PO = per os (oral). SL = sublingual. ET = endotracheal. od = once daily. bd = twice daily. tds = three times daily. qds = four times daily. NR = not recommended. Doses are intravenous and dilutions in 0.9% saline unless otherwise stated.

Drug	Description and perioperative indications	Cautions and contraindications	Side-effects	Dose (paediatric)	Dose (adult)
Cetirizine (Zirtek®)	Non-sedative antihistamine. Relief of allergy, urticaria	Prostatic hypertrophy, urinary retention, glaucoma, porphyria	Dry mouth	PO: 0.2mg/kg up to 10mg	PO: 10mg od
Chloral hydrate	Formerly a popular hypnotic in children	Avoid prolonged use. Caution in elderly, gastritis, and porphyria	Gastric irritation, ataxia	PO: 25–50mg/kg as single dose for sedation (up to 1g)	PO: 0.5–1g nocte
Chlorphenamine (Piriton®)	Sedative antihistamine. Relief of allergy, urticaria, anaphylaxis	Prostatic hypertrophy, urinary retention, glaucoma, porphyria	Drowsiness, dry mouth	<1yr NR. PO: 0.1mg/kg up to 4mg qds	Slow IV/IM/SC: 10–20mg. PO: 4mg 4-hourly
Chlorpromazine	Phenothiazine, antipsychotic. Mild alpha blocking action. Potent antiemetic and used for chronic hiccups	Hypotension	Extrapyramidal and anticholinergic symptoms, sedation, hypotension	0.1–1mg/kg over 20min	Up to 25mg (at 1mg/min diluted in saline to 1mg/ml). Deep IM: 25–50mg 6-8-hourly
Cimetidine	Competitive H₂ histamine receptor antagonist. Reduction of gastric acid	Hypotension and arrhythmias on rapid IV administration. Confusion in elderly	IV/PO: 10–15mg/kg bd	200mg over 2min (diluted in saline) qds. PO: 400mg bd

			Intubation: 150μg/kg. Maintenance: 30μg/kg every 20min. Infusion: 0.06–0.18mg/kg/hr	Intubation: 150μg/kg. Maintenance: 30μg/kg every 20–30min. Infusion: 0.06–0.18mg/kg/hr
Cisatracurium (Nimbex®)	Single isomer of atracurium with greater potency, longer duration of action, and less histamine release. Duration 55min	Neuromuscular block potentiated by aminoglycosides, loop diuretics, magnesium, lithium, ↓temp, ↓K⁺, ↓pH, prior use of suxamethonium, volatile agents. Store at 2–8°C	Enhanced effect in myasthenia gravis, effects antagonised by anticholin-esterases e.g. neostigmine. Monitor response with peripheral nerve stimulator	
Citrate (sodium)	Non-particulate antacid oral premedication. Aspiration prophylaxis			PO: 30ml 0.3M solution
Clomethiazole (Heminevrin®)	Hypnotic sedative used in alcohol withdrawal and status epilepticus. IV preparation no longer available	Caution in elderly	Nasal congestion, confusion, phlebitis, hypotension, coma	PO: 1–2 capsules at night

IV = intravenous. IM = intramuscular. SC = subcutaneous. PO = per os (oral). SL = sublingual. ET = endotracheal. od = once daily. bd = twice daily. tds = three times daily. qds = four times daily. NR = not recommended. Doses are intravenous and dilutions in 0.9% saline unless otherwise stated.

Drug	Description and perioperative indications	Cautions and contraindications	Side-effects	Dose (paediatric)	Dose (adult)
Clopidogrel (Plavix®)	Antiplatelet drug used to prevent myocardial infarction and stroke. (Irreversible antagonism of ADP receptors on platelets)	Liver and renal impairment Stop 7–14d preop	Haemorrhage, abdominal pain, dyspepsia, diarrhoea		75mg PO od. (300mg in acute coronary syndrome)
Clonidine	Selective α_2 agonist. Reduces requirement for opioids and volatile anaesthetics. Enhances epidural analgesia	Rebound hypertension on acute withdrawal of chronic therapy	Hypotension, sedation	3–5µg/kg slowly. PO premed: 4µg/kg. Caudal: 1µg/kg	150–300µg over 5min. Epidural: 150µg in 10ml saline
Co-amoxiclav (Augmentin®)	Mixture of amoxicillin and clavulanic acid. 1.2g contains 1g amoxicillin	See amoxicillin	See amoxicillin	10–30mg/kg tds (qds in severe infections)	600mg–1.2g tds (qds in severe infections)
Cocaine	Ester type local anaesthetic and potent vasoconstrictor. Topical anaesthesia of mucous membranes (nasal passages). Duration 20–30min	Topical use only. Caution with other sympathomimetic agents, halothane, anticholinesterase deficiency. Porphyria, MAOIs	Hypertension, arrhythmias, euphoria	1–3mg/kg topical	4–10% solution. Maximum topical dose 3mg/kg
Co-codamol 8/500	Combination oral analgesic containing codeine 8mg and paracetamol 500mg	See paracetamol		NR	PO: 1–2 tablets qds (maximum 8 tablets per day)

Drug	Description	Cautions/Notes	Side effects	Dose
Co-codamol 30/500	Combination oral analgesic containing codeine 30mg and paracetamol 500mg	See paracetamol. When no strength is specified co-codamol 8/500 is dispensed	NR	PO: 1–2 tablets qds (maximum 8 tablets per day)
Co-codaprin	Combination oral analgesic containing codeine 8mg and aspirin 400mg	As NSAIDs	NR	PO: 1–2 tablets qds (maximum 8 tablets per day)
Codeine phosphate	Opioid used for mild to moderate pain		Nausea, vomiting, dysphoria, drowsiness, constipation	PO/IM: 30–60mg 4-hourly (max 240mg/d) PO/IM/PR: 1mg/kg 6-hourly (max 3mg/kg/d)
Co-dydramol	Combination oral analgesic containing dihydrocodeine 10mg and paracetamol 500mg	See paracetamol	NR	PO: 1–2 tablets qds (maximum 8 tablets per day)
Co-proxamol	Combination oral analgesic containing dextropro-poxyphene 32.5 mg and paracetamol 325 mg	See paracetamol	NR	PO: 1–2 tablets qds (maximum 8 tablets per day)
Cyclizine	Antihistamine, antimuscarinic anti-emetic agent	Caution in severe heart failure	Drowsiness, dry mouth, blurred vision, tachycardia	IV/IM: 1mg/kg up to 50mg tds IV/IM/PO: 50mg tds

IV = intravenous. IM = intramuscular. SC = subcutaneous. PO = per os (oral). SL = sublingual. ET = endotracheal. od = once daily. bd = twice daily. tds = three times daily. qds = four times daily. NR = not recommended. Doses are intravenous and dilutions in 0.9% saline unless otherwise stated.

Drug	Description and perioperative indications	Cautions and contraindications	Side-effects	Dose (paediatric)	Dose (adult)
Dalteparin (Fragmin®)	Low molecular weight heparin used in prevention of venous thromboembolism	Once daily dosing. APTT monitoring not usually required		SC prophylaxis: 50U/kg od	SC prophylaxis: 2500un od (5000U in high risk)
Dantrolene	Direct-acting skeletal muscle relaxant used in treatment of malignant hyperpyrexia and neuroleptic malignant syndrome. 20mg/vial—reconstitute in 60ml warm water and give via blood set	Avoid combination with calcium channel blockers (verapamil) as may cause hyperkalaemia and cardiovascular collapse. Crosses placenta	Skeletal muscle weakness (22%), phlebitis (10%)	1mg/kg repeated every 5min to a maximum of 10mg/kg	1mg/kg repeated every 5min to a maximum of 10mg/kg Usually 2.5mg/kg
Desmopressin (DDAVP®)	Synthetic analogue of vasopressin (ADH) with longer duration of action and reduced pressor effect. Used for neurogenic diabetes insipidus and haemophilia (enhances factor VIII activity)	Caution in hypertension and CVS disease	Hypertension, angina, abdominal pain, flushing, hyponatraemia	IV/IM/SC: 0.4µg/kg. Intranasal: 5–20µg/d PO: 100–200µg tds	IV/IM/SC: 1–4µg/day. Intranasal: 10–40µg/d PO: 100–200µg tds. Haemophilia: 0.3µg/kg (in 50ml saline over 30min IV)

Dexamethasone	Prednisolone derivative corticosteroid. Less sodium retention than hydrocortisone. Cerebral oedema, oedema prevention, anti-emetic	Interacts with anticholinesterase agents to increase weakness in myasthenia gravis	IV/IM/SC: 4–8mg. Cerebral oedema: 4mg qds. Antiemesis 8mg (Dexamethasone 0.75mg = prednisolone 5mg)
		See prednisolone	IV/IM/SC: 200–400µg/kg bd. Cerebral oedema: 100µg/kg qds. Croup: 250µg/ kg, then 125µg/kg qds for 24h. Anti-emetic: 150µg/kg
Diamorphine	Potent opioid analgesic	Histamine release, hypotension, bronchospasm, nausea, vomiting, pruritus, dysphoria	IV/SC: 50µg/kg then 15µg/kg/hr. Epidural: 2.5mg in 60ml 0.125% bupivacaine at 0.1–0.4ml/kg/hr Intranasal: 100µg/kg in 0.2ml saline
		Spinal/epidural use associated with risk of respiratory depression, pruritus, nausea	IV/IM/SC: 2.5–5mg 4-hourly Epidural: 2.5mg diluted in 10ml local anaesthetic/saline, then 0.1–0.5mg/hr Spinal: 0.25–0.5mg
Diazepam	Long-acting benzodiazepine. Sedation or termination of status epilepticus. Alcohol withdrawal	Sedation, circulatory depression	0.2–0.3mg/kg. Rectal: 0.5mg/kg as Stesolid® or may use IV preparation
		Thrombophlebitis: emulsion (Diazemuls®) less irritant to veins	2–10mg, repeat if required

IV = intravenous. IM = intramuscular. SC = subcutaneous. PO = per os (oral). SL = sublingual. ET = endotracheal.od = once daily. bd = twice daily, tds = three times daily. qds = four times daily. NR = not recommended. Doses are intravenous and dilutions in 0.9% saline unless otherwise stated.

Drug	Description and perioperative indications	Cautions and contraindications	Side-effects	Dose (paediatric)	Dose (adult)
Diclofenac sodium (Voltarol®)	Potent NSAID analgesic for mild to moderate pain	Hypersensitivity to aspirin, asthma, severe renal impairment, peptic ulceration	Gastrointestinal upset or bleeding, bronchospasm, tinnitus, fluid retention, platelet inhibition	PO/PR: 1mg/kg tds. Maximum 3mg/kg/day (>1yr)	PO/PR: 25–50mg tds (or 100mg 18-hourly). Maximum 150mg/d
Digoxin	Cardiac glycoside. Weak inotrope and control of ventricular response in supraventricular arrhythmia. Therapeutic levels 0.5–2µg/l	Reduce dose in elderly. Enhanced effect/toxicity in hypokalaemia. Avoid cardioversion in toxicity	Anorexia, nausea, fatigue, arrhythmias	Rapid IV/PO loading: 15µg/kg stat, then 5µg/kg qds, PO: 4µg/kg bd.	Rapid IV loading: 250–500µg over 30min. Maximum 1mg/24 hr. PO loading: 1–1.5mg in divided doses over 24hr. PO maintenance: 125–250µg/d
Dihydrocodeine tartrate	Opioid used for mild to moderate pain		Nausea, vomiting, dysphoria, drowsiness	PO/IM/PR: 0.5–1mg/kg 4-hourly	PO/IM: 30–60mg 4-hourly
Dobutamine	β₁ adrenergic agonist, positive inotrope and chronotrope. Cardiac failure	Arrhythmias and hypertension. Phlebitis, but can be administered peripherally	Tachycardia. Decreased peripheral and pulmonary vascular resistance	Infusion: 2–20µg/kg/min	Infusion: 2.5–10µg/kg/min

Drug	Description	Cautions	Side effects	Dose	Dose
Domperidone	Anti-emetic acting on chemoreceptor trigger zone and peripheral D_2 receptors	Renal impairment. Not recommended for PONV prophylaxis	Raised prolactin. Rarely acute dystonic reactions	PO: 200–400µg/kg 4-6-hourly	PO: 10–20mg 4-6-hourly. PR: 30–60mg 4-6-hourly
Dopamine	Naturally occurring catecholamine with α_1, β_1 and dopaminergic activity. Inotropic agent	Via central catheter. Phaeochromocytoma (due to noradrenaline release)	Tachycardia, dysrhythmias	Infusion: 2–20µg/kg/min	Infusion: 2–10µg/kg/min
Dopexamine	Catecholamine with β_2 and dopaminergic activity. Inotropic agent	Via central catheter. Phaeochromocytoma, hypokalaemia	Tachycardia	Infusion: 0.5–6µg/kg/min	Infusion: 0.5–6µg/kg/min
Doxapram	Respiratory stimulant acting through carotid chemo-receptors and medulla. Duration 12min	Epilepsy, airway obstruction, acute asthma, severe CVS disease	Risk of arrhythmia. Hypertension	1–1.5mg/kg slowly. Infusion: 0.5–1mg/kg/hr for 1hr	Infusion: 2–4mg/min
Droperidol	Butyrophenone related to haloperidol. Neuroleptic anaesthesia and potent anti-emetic. Duration 4hr	Alpha adrenergic blocker. Parkinson's disease	Vasodilatation, hypotension. Dystonic reactions	Anti-emetic: 25–75µg/kg	Anti-emetic: 0.5–2.5mg Neuroleptic anaesthesia: 0.2mg/kg with fentanyl 4µg/kg

IV = intravenous. IM = intramuscular. SC = subcutaneous. PO = per os (oral). SL = sublingual. ET = endotracheal. od = once daily. bd = twice daily. tds = three times daily. qds = four times daily. NR = not recommended. Doses are intravenous and dilutions in 0.9% saline unless otherwise stated.

Drug	Description and perioperative indications	Cautions and contraindications	Side-effects	Dose (paediatric)	Dose (adult)
Edrophonium (Tensilon®)	Anticholinesterase used in diagnostic assessment of myasthenia gravis. 15 times less potent than neostigmine	Short acting (10min)	Bradycardia, AV block	20µg/kg test dose, then 80µg/kg	1mg slow IV every 2–4min. Maximum 10mg Reversal: 0.5mg/kg with anticholinergic
EMLA	Eutectic mixture of 2.5% lidocaine and 2.5% prilocaine. Topical anaesthesia	Absorption of anaesthetic depends on surface area and duration of application. Avoid use on abrasions or mucous membranes	Methaemoglobin-aemia in high doses	NR <1yr	Apply under occlusive dressing 1–5hr before procedure (maximum 60g)
Enoxaparin (Clexane®)	Low molecular weight heparin used in prevention of venous thromboembolism	Once daily dosing and APTT monitoring not usually required		SC prophylaxis: 0.4–0.8mg/kg od	SC prophylaxis: 20mg (2000U) od (40mg if high risk)
Enoximone	Type III phosphodiesterase inhibitor used in cardiac failure with increased filling pressures. Inodilator	Stenotic valvular disease, cardiomyopathy	Arrhythmias, hypotension, nausea	Infusion: 5–20µg/kg/min	Infusion: 90µg/kg/min for 10–30min, then 5–20µg/kg/min (maximum 24mg/kg/d)

Ephedrine	Direct and indirect sympathomimetic (α and β adrenergic action). Vasopressor, safe in pregnancy. Duration 10–60min	Caution in elderly, hypertension and CVS disease. Tachyphylaxis. Avoid with MAOI	Tachycardia, hypertension		3–6mg repeated (dilute 30mg in 10ml saline, 1ml increments). IM: 30mg
Ergometrine	Ergot alkaloid used to control uterine hypotony or bleeding. Syntometrine® = ergometrine 500µg/ml and oxytocin 5U/ml	Severe cardiac disease or hypertension	Vasoconstriction, hypertension, vomiting		IM: 1ml as Syntometrine®. Not recommended IV
Erythromycin	Macrolide antibiotic with spectrum similar to penicillin	Arrhythmias with cisapride, terfenadrine, astemizole	Nausea, diarrhoea	10–25mg/kg qds over 15–60min	500 mg–1g qds over 15–60min
Esmolol	Short-acting cardioselective β-blocker. Metabolised by red cell esterases. Treatment of supraventricular tachycardia or intra-operative hypertension Duration 10min	Asthma, heart failure, AV block, verapamil treatment	Hypotension, bradycardia. May prolong action of suxamethonium	SVT: 0.5mg/kg over 1min, then 50–200µg/kg/min	SVT: 0.5mg/kg over 1min, then 50–200µg/kg/min. Hypertension: 25–100µg/kg, then 50–300µg/kg/min

IV = intravenous. IM = intramuscular. SC = subcutaneous. PO = per os (oral). SL = sublingual. ET = endotracheal.od = once daily. bd = twice daily. tds = three times daily. qds = four times daily. NR = not recommended. Doses are intravenous and dilutions in 0.9% saline unless otherwise stated.

Drug	Description and perioperative indications	Cautions and contraindications	Side-effects	Dose (paediatric)	Dose (adult)
Ethanol	Useful sedative/hypnotic. Has been tried as an intravenous induction agent in doses of up to 44g	Administered as dehydrated absolute alcohol BP	Diuretic effect		2g (2ml) diluted to 5–10% solution in saline or dextrose, repeated as necessary
Etomidate	IV induction agent. Cardiostable in therapeutic doses. Available in lipid	Pain on injection. Adrenocortical suppression	Nausea and vomiting. Myoclonic movements	0.3mg/kg	0.3mg/kg
Fentanyl	Synthetic phenylpiperidine derivative opioid analgesic. High lipid solubility and cardiostability. Duration 30–60min	Reduce dose in elderly. Delayed respiratory depression and pruritus if epidural/spinal	Circulatory and ventilatory depression. High doses may produce muscle rigidity	1–5µg/kg, up to 25µg/kg if postop. ventilation. Infusion: 2–4µg/kg/hr	1–5µg/kg (up to 50µg/kg). Epidural: 50–100µg (diluted in 10ml saline/local anaesthetic). Spinal: 5–20µg
Flecainide	Class 1C anti-arrhythmic agent used for VT, WPW, and 'chemical cardioversion' of paroxysmal AF	Rise in pacemaker threshold. AV block, heart failure, recent MI	Nausea and vomiting Pro-arrhythmic effects, AV block.		'Chemical cardioversion': 2mg/kg up to 150mg (over 15min with ECG monitoring) PO: 200–300mg

Flucloxacillin	Penicillinase-resistant antibiotic active against staphylococci	Hypotension on rapid IV administration	Thrombophlebitis	10–25mg/kg qds	500mg–1g qds slow IV
Flumazenil	Benzodiazepine receptor antagonist. Duration 45–90min	Benzodiazepine dependence (acute withdrawal), resedation if long-acting benzodiazepine	Arrhythmia, seizures	5µg/kg, then up repeat to 40µg/kg. Infusion: 2–10µg/kg/hr	200µg then 100µg at 60s intervals (up to maximum 1mg). Infusion: 100–400µg/hr
Fondaparinux (Arixtra®)	Synthetic pentasaccharide which inhibits activated factor X. DVT prophylaxis after major lower limb orthopaedic surgery	Active bleeding, severe renal impairment, bacterial endocarditis. Caution with spinal or epidural (p1059)	Haemorrhage, thrombocytopenia, oedema, deranged LFTs	NR	SC: 2.5mg od start 6hr postop. Do not give IM or IV. Monitor platelet count
Fosphenytoin	Prodrug of phenytoin. Can be administered more rapidly. Dosages in phenytoin equivalents (PE): fosphenytoin1.5mg = phenytoin 1mg	See phenytoin- monitor ECG/BP Infusion rate: 50–100 mg(PE)/min (status 100– 150mg(PE)/min)	See phenytoin	>5yrs: 10–15 mg(PE)/kg then 4–5mg(PE)/kg daily Infusion rate: 1–2mg(PE)/kg/min	Infusion: 10–15 mg(PE)/kg then 4–5mg(PE)/kg daily Status: 15mg(PE)/kg Can also be administered IM

IV = intravenous. IM = intramuscular. SC = subcutaneous. PO = per os (oral). SL = sublingual. ET = endotracheal. od = once daily. bd = twice daily. tds = three times daily. qds = four times daily. NR = not recommended. Doses are intravenous and dilutions in 0.9% saline unless otherwise stated.

Drug	Description and perioperative indications	Cautions and contraindications	Side-effects	Dose (paediatric)	Dose (adult)
Furosemide (frusemide)	Loop diuretic used in treatment of hypertension, congestive cardiac failure, renal failure, fluid overload		Hypotension, tinnitus, ototoxicity, hypokalaemia, and hyperglycaemia	0.5–1.5mg/kg bd	10–40mg slowly
Gallamine	Long-acting non-depolarising neuromuscular blocker	Impaired renal function (renal excretion)	Tachycardia	1–2mg/kg	Intubation: 1–1.5mg/kg. Maintenance: 0.1–0.75mg/kg
Gentamicin	Aminoglycoside antibiotic active against Gram-negative bacteria. Peak level 6–10mg/l. Trough level <1–2mg/l	Impairs neuromuscular transmission—avoid in myasthenia	Ototoxicity and nephrotoxicity	2mg/kg tds or 5mg/kg/d as a single dose (administered over 5min)	1–1.5mg/kg tds or 3–5mg/kg/d as a single dose (administered over 5min)
Glucagon	Polypeptide hormone used in treatment of hypoglycaemia and overdose of β-blocker. Hyperglycaemic action lasts 10–30min	Glucose must be administered as soon as possible. Phaeochromocytoma	Hypertension, hypotension, nausea, vomiting	<25kg 0.5U (0.5 mg) >25kg 1U	SC/IM/IV: 1U (1mg). β-blocker overdose unresponsive to atropine: 50–150 μg/kg in glucose 5%

Drug	Description	Cautions	Side effects	Dose	Dose
Glucose	Treatment of hypoglycaemia in unconscious patient	50% solution irritant therefore flush after administration		0.5ml/kg of 50% solution; use more dilute solutions	25–50g (50–100ml 50% solution). Can use more dilute solutions
Glyceryl trinitrate	Organic nitrate vasodilator. Controlled hypotension, angina, congestive cardiac failure	Remove patches before defibrillation to avoid electrical arcing	Tachycardia, hypotension, headache, nausea, flushing, methaemoglobinaemia	10–50µg/kg/hr starting dose up to 300µg/kg/hr	Infusion: 0.5–10 mg/hr. SL tabs: 0.3–1mg prn. SL spray: 400µg prn. Patch: 5–10mg/24hr
Glycopyrrolate (glycopyrronium bromide)	Quaternary ammonium anticholinergic agent. Bradycardia, blockade of muscarinic effects of anticholinesterases, antisialogogue	Caution in glaucoma, cardiovascular disease. Unlike atropine does not cross blood–brain barrier	Paradoxical bradycardia in small doses. Reduces lower oesophageal sphincter tone	4–10µg/kg.	200–400µg. Control of muscarinic effects of neostigmine: 200µg for each 1mg neostigmine
Granisetron (Kytril®)	5HT$_3$ receptor antagonist. Anti-emetic. Long-acting	Pregnancy, breast-feeding	Reduces colonic motility. Headache	NR	1mg diluted to 5ml with saline. Give over 30s. Max 2mg/d

IV = intravenous. IM = intramuscular. SC = subcutaneous. PO = per os (oral). SL = sublingual. ET = endotracheal. od = once daily. bd = twice daily. tds = three times daily. qds = four times daily. NR = not recommended. Doses are intravenous and dilutions in 0.9% saline unless otherwise stated.

Drug	Description and perioperative indications	Cautions and contraindications	Side-effects	Dose (paediatric)	Dose (adult)
Haloperidol	Butyrophenone derivative antipsychotic. Useful anti-emetic	Neuroleptic malignant syndrome	Extrapyramidal reactions	NR	IM/IV: 2–10mg 4–8-hourly (max 18mg/d) Anti-emetic: 0.5–2mg IV
Heparin (unfractionated)	Endogenous mucopoly-saccharide used for anticoagulation. Half-life 1–3hr. 100U = 1mg	Monitor activated partial thromboplastin time (APTT). Reversed with protamine	Haemorrhage, thrombocytopenia, hyperkalaemia	Low dose: 50–75U/kg IV then 10–15 U/kg/hr. Full dose: 200U/kg IV then 15–30U/kg/hr	Low dose SC: 5000U bd. Full dose IV: 5000U, then 24 000–48 000U per 24hr infusion
Hyaluronidase	Enzyme used to enhance permeation of injected fluids or local anaesthetics. Treatment of extravasation. Hypodermoclysis: 150U/l	Not for intravenous administration	Occasional severe allergy	Local anaesthetic: 15U/ml	Ophthalmology: 10–15U/ml local Extravasation: 1500U in 1ml saline infiltrated to affected area
Hydralazine	Direct-acting arteriolar vasodilator used to control arterial pressure. Duration 2–4hr	Higher doses required in rapid acetylators. SLE	Increased heart rate, cardiac output, stroke volume	0.1–0.5mg/kg	5mg every 5min to a maximum of 20mg

Drug					
Hydrocortisone (cortisol)	Endogenous steroid with anti-inflammatory and potent mineralocorticoid action (steroid of choice in replacement therapy—active form of cortisone). Treatment of allergy	(hydrocortisone 20mg = prednisolone 5mg)	Hyperglycaemia, hypertension, psychic disturbance, muscle weakness, fluid retention	4mg/kg then 2–4mg/kg qds	IV/IM: 50–200mg qds. Adrenal suppression and surgery; 25mg at induction then 25mg qds PO: 10–20mg/d
Hydromorphone hydrochloride	Opioid used for moderate to severe pain	As morphine	Nausea, vomiting, dysphoria, drowsiness		PO: 1.3–4mg 4-hourly increased as necessary. PO slow release: 4mg bd
Hyoscine hydrobromide (Scopolamine®)	Antimuscarinic sedative anti-emetic agent used as premedication. (L-isomer of hyoscine)	See atropine. Avoid in elderly—delirium	See atropine. Sedation	IV/IM/SC: 10µg/kg	IV/IM/SC: 200–600µg. PO: 300µg qds
Hyoscine butylbromide (Buscopan®)	Antimuscarinic agent used as an antispasmodic (racemic hyoscine)	See atropine	See atropine		IV/IM: 20mg slowly repeated if necessary

IV = intravenous. IM = intramuscular. SC = subcutaneous. PO = per os (oral). SL = sublingual. ET = endotracheal. od = once daily. bd = twice daily. tds = three times daily. qds = four times daily. NR = not recommended. Doses are intravenous and dilutions in 0.9% saline unless otherwise stated.

Drug	Description and perioperative indications	Cautions and contraindications	Side-effects	Dose (paediatric)	Dose (adult)
Ibuprofen	NSAID analgesic for mild to moderate pain. Best side-effect profile of NSAIDs	Hypersensitivity to aspirin, asthma, severe renal impairment, peptic ulceration	Gastrointestinal upset or bleeding, bronchospasm, tinnitus, fluid retention, platelet inhibition	PO: 10mg/kg tds or 5mg/kg qds (>7kg)	PO: 400mg qds
Imipenem	Carbapenem broad spectrum antibiotic. Administered with cilastatin to reduce renal metabolism	Caution in renal failure and pregnancy	Nausea, vomiting, diarrhoea, convulsions, thrombophlebitis	>3 months 15mg/kg over 30min qds (25mg/kg severe infections)	Slow IV (1hr): 250–500mg qds. Surgical prophylaxis: 1g at induction, repeated after 3hr
Indometacin	NSAID analgesic for moderate pain. High incidence of side-effects. Also used for neonatal ductus arteriosus closure	Hypersensitivity to aspirin, asthma, severe renal impairment, peptic ulceration	Gastrointestinal upset or bleeding, bronchospasm, tinnitus, fluid retention, platelet inhibition	Ductus closure: 100–200μg/kg, three doses	PO: 50–100mg bd. PR: 100mg bd
Insulin (Actrapid®)	Human soluble pancreatic hormone facilitating intracellular transport of glucose and anabolism. Diabetes mellitus, ketoacidosis and hyperkalaemia	Monitor blood glucose and serum potassium. Store at 2–8°C	Hypoglycaemia, hypokalaemia	Ketoacidosis: 0.1–0.2U/kg then 0.1U/kg/hr	Ketoacidosis: 10–20U then 5–10U/hr. Sliding scale (p150). Hyperkalaemia (p178)

Drug	Description	Cautions	Side effects	Dose	Dose
Isoprenaline	Synthetic catecholamine with potent β adrenergic agonist activity. Emergency treatment of heart block or bradycardia unresponsive to atropine. β-blocker overdose	Ischaemic heart disease, hyperthyroidism, diabetes mellitus	Tachycardia, arrhythmias, sweating, tremor	Infusion: 1–10µg/kg/hr	Infusion: 0.5–10µg/min. (0.2mg in 500ml 5% dextrose at 2–20ml/min or 1mg in 50ml at 1.5–30ml/hr)
Ketamine	Phencyclidine derivative producing dissociative anaesthesia. Induction/maintenance of anaesthesia in high-risk or hypovolaemic patients	Emergence delirium reduced by benzodiazepines. Caution in hypertension. Control excess salivation with antimuscarinic agent	Bronchodilation. Increased ICP, blood pressure, uterine tone, salivation. Respiratory depression if given rapidly	Induction: 1–2mg/kg IV, 5–10mg/kg IM. Infusion: 1–3mg/kg/hr Caudal: 0.5mg/kg (preservative free only)	Induction: 1–2mg/kg IV, 5–10mg/kg IM. Infusion: 1–3mg/kg/hr (analgesia only 0.25mg/kg/hr).
Ketorolac (Toradol®)	NSAID analgesic for mild to moderate pain. Not licensed for perioperative use	Hypersensitivity to aspirin, asthma, severe renal impairment, peptic ulceration	Gastrointestinal upset or bleeding, bronchospasm, tinnitus, fluid retention, platelet inhibition	Slow IV/IM: 0.5mg/kg up to 30mg qds	Slow IV/IM: 10mg then 10–30mg every 4–6hr (maximum daily dose 90mg, but 60mg in elderly)

IV = intravenous. IM = intramuscular. SC = subcutaneous. PO = per os (oral). SL = sublingual. ET = endotracheal. od = once daily. bd = twice daily. tds = three times daily. qds = four times daily. NR = not recommended. Doses are intravenous and dilutions in 0.9% saline unless otherwise stated.

Drug	Description and perioperative indications	Cautions and contraindications	Side-effects	Dose (paediatric)	Dose (adult)
Labetalol	Combined α (mild) and β adrenergic receptor antagonist. Blood pressure control without reflex tachycardia. Duration 2–4hr	Asthma, heart failure, AV block, verapamil treatment	Hypotension, bradycardia, bronchospasm, liver damage	0.2mg/kg boluses up to 1mg/kg. Infusion: 1–3mg/kg/hr	5mg increments up to 100mg. Infusion: 20–160mg/hr (in dextrose)
Lansoprazole (Zoton®)	Proton pump inhibitor. Reduction of gastric acid secretion	Liver disease, pregnancy	Headache, diarrhoea	PO: 0.3–0.6mg/kg od	PO: 15–30mg od
Levobupivacaine (Chirocaine®)	Levorotatory(s) enantiomer of bupivacaine with reduced cardiotoxicity	See bupivacaine	See bupivacaine	See bupivacaine	See bupivacaine Max dose: 150mg Max/24hr: 400mg
Lidocaine (lignocaine)	Amide type local anaesthetic: 1. Treatment of ventricular arrhythmias 2. Reduction of pressor response to intubation. 3. Local anaesthetic—rapid onset, duration 30–90min (prolonged by adrenaline) pKa 7.7	Adrenaline-containing solutions contain preservative Maximum dose dependent upon injection site— 3mg/kg/4hr (6mg/kg with adrenaline)	Toxicity: tongue/circumoral numbness, restlessness, tinnitus, seizures, cardiac arrest Prolongs action of neuromuscular blockers	1. Antiarrhythmic: 1mg/kg then 10–50μg/kg/min 2. Attenuation of pressor response: 1.5mg/kg 3. Local anaesthesia: 0.5–2% solution	1. Antiarrhythmic: 1mg/kg then 1–4mg/min 2. Attenuation of pressor response: 1.5mg/kg 3. Local anaesthesia: 0.5–2% solution

Drug					
Loratidine (Claritiyn®)	Non-sedative antihistamine. Relief of allergy, urticaria	Prostatic hypertrophy, urinary retention, glaucoma, porphyria	Dry mouth	<2yr NR. PO: 0.2mg/kg up to 10mg od	PO: 10mg od
Lorazepam	Benzodiazepine: 1. Sedation or premedication. 2. Status epilepticus. Duration 6–10hr	Decreased requirement for anaesthetic agents	Respiratory depression in combination with opioids. Amnesia	Status 0.1mg/kg; max 4mg	1. PO: 2–4mg 1–2hr preop. IV/IM: 1.5–2.5mg 2. Status: 4mg IV
Lormetazepam	Benzodiazepine hypnotic sedative premec.	Decreased requirement for anaesthetic agents	Respiratory depression in combination with opioids. Amnesia	NR	0.5–1.5mg 1–2hr preop. (elderly 0.5mg)
Magnesium sulphate	Essential mineral used to treat: 1. Hypomagnesaemia 2. Arrhythmias 3. Eclamptic seizures 4. Severe asthma Magnesium sulphate 50% = 500mg/ml = 2mmol Mg^{2+}/ml. Normal plasma level Mg^{2+} 0.75–1.05mmol/l Therapeutic level 2–4mmol/l	Potentiates muscle relaxants. Monitoring of serum level essential during treatment. Myasthenia and muscular dystrophy. Heart block Magnesium sulphate 1g ≡ Mg^{2+} 4mmol	CNS depression, hypotension, muscle weakness	1. Hypomagnesaemia: 0.2ml/kg 50% solution over 20min 2. Arrhythmias: 0.1ml/kg 50% solution over 20min	1. Hypomagnesaemia: 10–15mg/kg over 20min, then 1g/hr. 2. Arrhythmias/ asthma: 2g (8mmol) over 10min 3. Eclampsia: 4g (16mmol) over 10min then 1g/hr for 24hr (see p746)

IV = intravenous. IM = intramuscular. SC = subcutaneous. PO = per os (oral). SL = sublingual. ET = endotracheal. od = once daily. bd = twice daily. tds = three times daily. qds = four times daily. NR = not recommended. Doses are intravenous and dilutions in 0.9% saline unless otherwise stated.

Drug	Description and perioperative indications	Cautions and contraindications	Side-effects	Dose (paediatric)	Dose (adult)
Mannitol	Osmotic diuretic used for renal protection and reduction of intracranial pressure. 20% solution = 20g/100ml	Extracellular volume expansion, especially in severe renal or cardiovascular disease	Diuresis, ARF, hypertonicity	0.25–0.5g/kg	0.25–1g/kg (typically 0.5g/kg of 20% solution)
Metaraminol (Aramine®)	Potent direct/indirect acting α adrenergic sympathomimetic. Treatment of hypotension. Duration 20–60min	MAOIs, pregnancy. Caution in elderly and hypertensives. Extravasation can cause necrosis	Hypertension, reflex bradycardia, arrhythmias, decreased renal and placental perfusion	10µg/kg then 0.1–1µg/kg/min	0.5–2mg. Dilute 10mg in 20ml saline and give 0.5–1ml increments (increase dilution in elderly)
Methohexitone	Short-acting barbiturate induction agent useful for ECT. Duration 5–10min. 1% solution = 10mg/ml	Porphyria. Premedication reduces excitation at induction	Excitatory phenomenon, hypotension, respiratory depression, hiccups	1–2mg/kg	1–1.5mg/kg. Infusion: 50–150µg/kg/min
Methoxamine (Vasoxine®)	Potent direct-acting α₁ adrenergic sympathomimetic. Treatment of hypotension. Duration 15–60min	Pregnancy. Caution in elderly and hypertensives. Extravasation can cause necrosis	Hypertension, reflex bradycardia, arrhythmias, decreased renal and placental perfusion	10µg/kg increment	1–2mg. Dilute 20mg in 20ml saline and give 0.5–1ml increments (increase dilution in elderly)

Drug	Uses	Cautions	Side effects	Dose (paediatric)	Dose (adult)
Methylene blue (Methylthioninium chloride)	1. Treatment of methaemoglobinaemia. 2. Ureteric identification during surgery (renally excreted). 3. Identification of parathyroid glands during surgery	G-6-PD deficiency. Blue colouration causes acute changes in pulse oximetry readings	Tachycardia, nausea, stains skin	1–4mg/kg slow IV	1–2mg/kg slow IV
Metoclopramide	Dopaminergic anti-emetic which increases gastric emptying and lower oesophageal sphincter tone	Hypertension in phaeochromocytoma. Inhibits plasma cholinesterase. Increases IOP	Extrapyramidal/dystonic reactions (treat with benzatropine or procyclidine)	PO/IM/IV: 0.15mg/kg up to 10mg tds	PO/IM/IV: 10mg tds
Metoprolol	Cardioselective β-blocker	Asthma, heart failure, AV block, verapamil treatment	Causes bradycardia, hypotension, and decreased cardiac contractility	0.1mg/kg up to 5mg over 10min	1–5mg over 10min
Metronidazole	Antibiotic with activity against anaerobic bacteria	Disulfiram (Antabuse®) like effect		7.5mg/kg tds. PR: 125–500mg tds	500mg tds. PR: 1g tds

IV = intravenous. IM = intramuscular. SC = subcutaneous. PO = per os (oral). SL = sublingual. ET = endotracheal. od = once daily. bd = twice daily. tds = three times daily. qds = four times daily. NR = not recommended. Doses are intravenous and dilutions in 0.9% saline unless otherwise stated.

Drug	Description and perioperative indications	Cautions and contraindications	Side-effects	Dose (paediatric)	Dose (adult)
Midazolam	Short-acting benzodiazepine. Sedative, anxiolytic, amnesic, anticonvulsant. Duration 20–60min. Oral administration of IV preparation effective though larger dose required	Reduce dose in elderly (very sensitive)	Hypotension, respiratory depression, apnoea	0.1–0.2mg/kg. PO: 0.5mg/kg (use IV preparation in orange squash). Intranasal: 0.2–0.3mg/kg (use 5mg/ml IV preparation)	Sedation: 0.5–5mg, titrate to effect. PO: 0.5mg/kg (use IV preparation in orange squash). IM: 2.5–10mg (0.1mg/kg)
Milrinone	Selective phosphodiesterase inhibitor used in cardiac failure with increased filling pressures. Inodilator used after cardiac surgery	Stenotic valvular disease, cardiomyopathy	Arrhythmias, hypotension, nausea	50µg/kg over 10min, then 0.375–0.75µg/kg/min. Maximum 1.13mg/kg/d	50µg/kg over 10min, then 0.375–0.75µg/kg/min. 1.13mg/kg/d
Mivacurium	Short-acting non-depolarising muscle relaxant. Metabolised by plasma cholinesterase. Duration 6–16min (often variable). Enhanced duration if low plasma cholinesterase. Antagonised by neostigmine—but avoid giving too early to avoid inhibiting drug metabolism	See cisatracurium. Some histamine release. Avoid in asthma	See cisatracurium	Intubation: 0.15–0.2mg/kg. Maintenance: 0.1mg/kg. Infusion: 10–15µg/kg/min	Intubation: 0.07–0.25mg/kg (doses of 0.07, 0.15, 0.2, and 0.25mg/kg produce block for 13, 16, 20, and 23min respectively). Maintenance: 0.1mg/kg. Infusion: 0.4–0.6mg/kg/hr

Morphine	Opioid analgesic	Histamine release, hypotension, bronchospasm, nausea, vomiting, pruritus, dysphoria	Prolonged risk of respiratory depression, pruritus, nausea when used via spinal/epidural	PO: 0.3–0.5mg/kg 4-hourly. IV boluses: 50–100μg/kg For PCA, NCA, infusion see p782	IV: 2.5–10mg. IM/SC: 5–10mg 4-hourly. PO: 10–30mg 4-hourly. PCA: 1mg 5min lockout. Infusion: 1–3.5mg/hr. Epidural: 2–5mg preservative free. Spinal: 0.1–1mg preservative free
Naloxone	Pure opioid antagonist. Can be used in low doses to reverse pruritus associated with epidural opiates and as depot IM injection in newborn of mothers given opioids		Beware renarcotisation if reversing long-acting opioid. Caution in opioid addicts—may precipitate acute withdrawal. Duration of action 30min	5–10μg/kg. Infusion: 5–20μg/kg/hr. IM depot in newborn: 200μg. Pruritus: 0.5μg/kg	200–400μg titrated to desired effect. Treatment of opioid/epidural pruritus: 100μg bolus plus 300μg added to IV fluids
Naproxen	NSAID analgesic for mild to moderate pain	See ibuprofen	See ibuprofen	PO: 5mg/kg bd (>5yr)	PO: 500mg bd

IV = intravenous. IM = intramuscular. SC = subcutaneous. PO = per os (oral). SL = sublingual. ET = endotracheal. od = once daily. bd = twice daily. tds = three times daily. qds = four times daily. NR = not recommended. Doses are intravenous and dilutions in 0.9% saline unless otherwise stated.

Drug	Description and perioperative indications	Cautions and contraindications	Side-effects	Dose (paediatric)	Dose (adult)
Neostigmine	Anticholinesterase used for: 1. Reversal of non-depolarising muscle relaxant. 2. Treatment of myasthenia gravis. Duration 60min IV (2–4hr PO)	Administer with antimuscarinic agent	Bradycardia, nausea, excessive salivation (muscarinic effects)	50µg/kg with atropine 20µg/kg or glycopyrronium 10µg/kg	1. 50–70µg/kg (maximum 5mg) with atropine 10–20µg/kg or glycopyrronium 10–15µg/kg. 2. PO: 15–30mg at suitable intervals
Neostigmine and glycopyrronium	Combination of neostigmine methylsulphate (2.5mg) and glycopyrronium (500µg) per 1ml	See neostigmine	See neostigmine	0.02ml/kg (dilute 1ml with 4ml saline, give 0.1ml/kg)	1–2ml over 30s
Nimodipine	Calcium channel blocker used to prevent vascular spasm after subarachnoid haemorrhage	Via central catheter. Cerebral oedema, raised intracranial pressure, grapefruit juice. Incompatible with PVC	Hypotension, flushing, headache	Infusion: 0.1–1µg/kg/min	PO: 60mg 4-hourly (maximum 360mg/d). Infusion: 1mg/hr increasing after 2hr to 2mg/hr
Nitroprusside (sodium—SNP)	Nitric oxide generating potent peripheral vasodilator. Controlled hypotension	Protect solution from light. Metabolism yields cyanide which is then converted to thiocyanate	Methaemoglobin-aemia, hypotension, tachycardia. Cyanide causes tachycardia, sweating, acidosis	Infusion: 0.3–1.5µg/kg/min	Infusion: 0.3–1.5µg/kg/min (up to 6µg/kg/min). Maximum dose: 1.5mg/kg (acutely)

Noradrenaline	Potent catecholamine α adrenergic agonist. Vasoconstriction	Via central catheter only. Potentiated by MAOI and tricyclic antidepressants	Reflex bradycardia, arrhythmia, hypertension	Infusion: 0.1–1µg/kg/min	Infusion: 2–20µg/min (0.04–0.4µg/kg/min)
Octreotide	Somatostatin analogue used in treatment of carcinoid, acromegaly, and variceal bleeding (unlicensed use)	Pituitary tumour expansion, reduced need for anti-diabetic treatments	GI disturbance, gallstones, hyper- and hypoglycaemia	SC: 1µg/kg od/bd	SC: 50µg od/bd increased up to 200µg tds. IV: 50µg diluted in saline (ECG monitoring)
Omeprazole (Losec®)	Proton pump inhibitor. Reduction in gastric acid secretion		Headache, diarrhoea	PO:0. 7–1.4mg/kg up to 40mg od	PO/Slow IV: 20–40mg od. Premedication PO: 40mg evening before and morning of surgery
Ondansetron	Serotonin (5HT$_3$) receptor antagonist anti-emetic		Hypotension, headache, flushing	>2yr. Slow IV: 100µg/kg (maximum 4mg) qds	Slow IV/IM: 4mg qds
Oxybuprocaine (Benoxinate®)	Local anaesthetic. Topical anaesthesia to cornea				0.4% solution. 0.5ml eye drops

IV = intravenous. IM = intramuscular. SC = subcutaneous. PO = per os (oral). SL = sublingual. ET = endotracheal. od = once daily. bd = twice daily. tds = three times daily.qds = four times daily. NR = not recommended. Doses are intravenous and dilutions in 0.9% saline unless otherwise stated.

Drug	Description and perioperative indications	Cautions and contraindications	Side-effects	Dose (paediatric)	Dose (adult)
Oxycodone	Opioid used for moderate pain, often in palliative care. IV preparation available: dose 1–10mg 4-hourly		Nausea, vomiting, dysphoria, drowsiness		PO: Oxynorm® 5mg 4-6-hourly increased up to 400 mg/d as required. Oxycontin® 10mg bd, increased up to 400mg/d as required
Oxytocin (Syntocinon®)	Nonapeptide hormone which stimulates uterine contraction. Induction of labour and prevention of postpartum haemorrhage		Vasodilatation, hypotension, flushing, tachycardia		Postpartum slow IV: 5U, followed if required by infusion (30U in 500ml saline at 30–125ml/hr)
Pancuronium	Long-acting aminosteroid non-depolarising muscle relaxant. Little histamine release. Duration 45–65min	Increased heart rate and blood pressure due to vagolysis and sympathetic stimulation. See cisatracurium	See cisatracurium	Intubation: 0.08–0.15mg/kg. Maintenance: 0.01–0.05mg/kg	Intubation: 0.04–0.1mg/kg. Maintenance: 0.01–0.05mg/kg
Pantoprazole	Proton pump inhibitor used to inhibit gastric acid secretion	Liver disease, pregnancy. Renal disease	Headache, pruritus, NR bronchospasm		PO/Slow IV: 40mg od

Paracetamol	Mild to moderate analgesic and antipyretic	Neonates: 10–15mg/kg 6-hourly (5mg/kg if jaundiced). Max 60mg/kg/d	Liver damage in overdose	PO/PR: 20mg/kg 6-hourly. Rectal loading dose 30–40mg/kg (>44 wk post conception)	PO: 0.5–1g qds Slow IV: 0.5–1g qds
Paraldehyde	Status epilepticus			Deep IM: 0.2ml/kg. PR: 0.3ml/kg	Deep IM: 5–10ml. PR: 10–20ml
Parecoxib (Dynastat®)	See celecoxib. Pro-drug of valdecoxib Cox II inhibitor Licensed for acute pain	See celecoxib. Reconstitute with 0.9% saline			IV/IM: 40 mg, then 20–40mg 6–12-hourly (max 80mg/d)
Pethidine	Synthetic opioid: 1. Analgesia (agent of choice in asthma). 2. Postoperative shivering	Seizures possible in high dosage—maximum daily dose 1g/d (20mg/kg/d). MAOI	Respiratory depression, hypotension, dysphoria	IV/IM/SC: 0.5–1mg/kg. Infusion: 5mg/kg in 50ml 5% dextrose at 1–3ml/hr (100–300µg/kg/hr)	IM/SC: 25–100mg 3-hourly. IV: 25–50mg. Epidural: 25–50mg in 10ml saline or LA PCA: 10mg/5min lockout. Shivering: 10–25mg

IV = intravenous. IM = intramuscular. SC = subcutaneous. PO = per os (oral). SL = sublingual. ET = endotracheal. od = once daily. bd = twice daily. tds = three times daily. qds = four times daily. NR = not recommended. Doses are intravenous and dilutions in 0.9% saline unless otherwise stated.

Drug	Description and perioperative indications	Cautions and contraindications	Side-effects	Dose (paediatric)	Dose (adult)
Phentolamine (Rogitine®)	α_1 and α_2 adrenergic antagonist. Peripheral vasodilatation and controlled hypotension. Treatment of extravasation. Duration 10min	Treat excessive hypotension with noradrenaline or methoxamine (not adrenaline/ephedrine due to β effects)	Hypotension, tachycardia, flushing	0.1mg/kg then 5–50μg/kg/min	2–5mg (10mg in 10ml saline, 1ml aliquots)
Phenylephrine	Selective direct-acting α adrenergic agonist. Peripheral vasoconstriction and treatment of hypotension. Duration 20min	Caution in elderly or cardiovascular disease. Hyperthyroidism	Reflex bradycardia, arrhythmias	2–10μg/kg then 1–5μg/kg/min	20–100μg increments (10mg in 500ml saline, 1ml aliquots), IM: 2–5mg. Infusion: 30–60μg/min
Phenytoin	Anticonvulsant and treatment of digoxin toxicity. Serum levels 10–20mg/l (40–80μmol/l)	Avoid in AV heart block and pregnancy. Monitor ECG/BP on IV administration. Porphyria	Hypotension, AV conduction defects, ataxia. Enzyme induction	Loading dose: 15mg/kg over 1hr.	15mg/kg over 1hr (dilute to 10mg/ml in saline), then 100mg tds. Arrhythmia: 3.5–5mg/kg (rate <50mg/min)
Piperacurium	Piperazinium derivative long-acting non-depolarising muscle relaxant. Duration 45–120min	See cisatracurium	See cisatracurium		Intubation: 0.08mg/kg. Maintenance: 0.01–0.04mg/kg

Piroxicam	NSAID analgesic for moderate pain. High incidence of side effects	Hypersensitivity to aspirin, asthma, severe renal impairment, peptic ulceration. Avoid in porphyria	Gastrointestinal upset or bleeding, bronchospasm, tinnitus, fluid retention, platelet inhibition		PO/PR: 10–30mg od
Potassium chloride	Electrolyte replacement (see p176)	Dilute solution before administration	Rapid infusion can cause cardiac arrest. High concentration causes phlebitis	0.5mmol/kg over 1hr. Maintenance: 2–4mmol/kg/d	10–20mmol/hr (max. concentration 40mmol/l peripherally). With ECG monitoring: up to 20–40mmol/hr via central line (max 200mmol/d)
Prednisolone	Orally active corticosteroid. Less mineralocorticoid action than hydrocortisone	Adrenal suppression, severe systemic infections	Dyspepsia and ulceration, osteoporosis, myopathy, psychosis, impaired healing, diabetes mellitus	PO: 1–2mg/kg od. Croup: 4mg/kg then 1mg/kg tds	PO: 10–60mg od, reduced to 2.5–15mg od.

IV = intravenous. IM = intramuscular. SC = subcutaneous. PO = per os (oral). SL = sublingual. ET = endotracheal. od = once daily. bd = twice daily. tds = three times daily. qds = four times daily. NR = not recommended. Doses are intravenous and dilutions in 0.9% saline unless otherwise stated.

Drug	Description and perioperative indications	Cautions and contraindications	Side-effects	Dose (paediatric)	Dose (adult)
Prilocaine	Amide type local anaesthetic. Less toxic than lidocaine. Used for infiltration and IVRA. Rapid onset. Duration 30–90min (prolonged by adrenaline) pKa 7.9	Adrenaline-containing solutions contain preservative. Significant methaemoglobinaemia if dose >600mg	Toxicity; tongue/circumoral numbness, restlessness, tinnitus, seizures, cardiac arrest	NR <6 months	Local anaesthesia: 0.5–2% solution. Maximum dose dependent upon injection site— 6mg/kg/4hr (8mg/kg with adrenaline)
Prochlorperazine	Phenothiazine anti-emetic	Hypotension on rapid IV administration. Neuroleptic malignant syndrome	Tardive dyskinesia and extrapyramidal symptoms	>10kg, PO: 0.1– 0.4mg/kg tds. IM: 0.1– 0.2mg/kg tds	IM: 12.5mg tds. PO: 20mg then 5–10mg tds
Procyclidine	Antimuscarinic used in acute treatment of drug-induced dystonic reactions (except tardive dyskinesia)	Glaucoma, gastrointestinal obstruction	Urinary retention, dry mouth, blurred vision	<2yr: 0.5–2mg. 2–10yr: 2–5mg	IV: 5mg. IM: 5–10mg repeat after 20min if needed
Promethazine (Phenergan®)	Phenothiazine, antihistamine, anticholinergic, antiemetic sedative. Paediatric sedation		Extrapyramidal reactions	>2yr Sedation/premed PO: 1–2mg/kg	PO/IM: 25–50mg

Drug	Description	Cautions	Side effects	Dose	Dose
Propofol	Di-isopropylphenol IV induction agent. Rapid recovery and little nausea. Agent of choice for day stay surgery, sedation or laryngeal mask insertion—can be used for ECT	Reduce dose in elderly or haemodynamically unstable. Not recommended for Caesarean section. Allergy to eggs, peanuts, soya and soybean oil. Caution in epilepsy	Apnoea, hypotension, pain on injection. Myoclonic spasms, rarely convulsions	Induction: 2–5mg/kg. Infusion: 4–15mg/kg/hr. NR induction <1 month. NR maintenance <3yr	Induction: 2–3mg/kg. Infusion: 6–10mg/kg/hr. TCI: initially 4–8µg/ml then 3–6µg/ml (reduce in elderly)
Propranolol	Non-selective β adrenergic antagonist. Controlled hypotension	Asthma, heart failure, AV block, verapamil treatment	Bradycardia, hypotension, AV block, bronchospasm	0.1mg/kg over 5min	1mg increments up to 5–10mg
Protamine	Basic protein produced from salmon sperm. Heparin antagonist	Weakly anticoagulant and marked histamine release. Risk of allergy	Severe hypotension, pulmonary hypertension, bronchospasm, flushing	Slow IV: 1mg per 1mg heparin (100U) to be reversed	Slow IV: 1mg per 1mg heparin (100U) to be reversed
Proxymetacaine (proparacaine)	Local anaesthetic. Topical anaesthesia to cornea	Less stinging than with other eye drops			0.5% solution. 0.5ml eye drops
Pyridostigmine	Long-acting anticholinesterase used in treatment of myasthenia gravis	See neostigmine	See neostigmine	PO: 1–3mg/kg at intervals (4–12-hourly)	PO: 30–120mg at intervals through day (maximum 1.2g/d)

IV = intravenous. IM = intramuscular. SC = subcutaneous. PO = per os (oral). SL = sublingual. ET = endotracheal. od = once daily. bd = twice daily. tds = three times daily. qds = four times daily. NR = not recommended. Doses are intravenous and dilutions in 0.9% saline unless otherwise stated.

Drug	Description and perioperative indications	Cautions and contraindications	Side-effects	Dose (paediatric)	Dose (adult)
Ranitidine	Histamine (H_2) receptor antagonist. Reduction in gastric acid secretion	Porphyria	Tachycardia	IV: 1mg/kg slowly tds. PO: 2–4mg/kg bd	IV: 50mg (diluted in 20ml saline, given over 2min) qds. IM: 50mg qds. PO: 150mg bd or 300mg od
Remifentanil (Ultiva®)	Ultra short-acting opioid used to supplement general anaesthesia. Metabolised by non-specific plasma cholinesterase. Duration 5–10min. Can be used as PCA in labour: 25–75μg bolus 3min lockout (0.5–1.5ml of 50μg/ml) May be mixed with propofol: 125μg/50ml SV, 250–500μg/50ml IPPV		Muscle rigidity, respiratory depression, hypotension, bradycardia	0.1–0.4μg/kg/min	Slow bolus: up to 1μg/kg. Infusion (IPPV): 0.1–0.5μg/kg/min. Infusion (SV): 0.025–0.1μg/kg/min Start at 0.1μg/kg/min and adjust dose as necessary
Rocuronium (Esmeron®)	Rapidly acting aminosteroid non-depolarising muscle relaxant. Rapid sequence induction (avoiding suxamethonium). Duration 10–40min (variable) Intubating conditions within 1min	See cisatracurium	Mild tachycardia. See cisatracurium	Intubation: 0.6–1mg/kg. Maintenance: 0.1–0.15mg/kg. Infusion: 0.3–0.6mg/kg/hr	Intubation: 0.6–1mg/kg Maintenance: 0.1–0.15mg/kg. Infusion: 0.3–0.6mg/kg/hr

Drug	Notes	Side effects	Dose (IV/other)	Dose (PO/other)
Rofecoxib (Vioxx®)	See celecoxib. Recently withdrawn from use	See celecoxib		PO: 12.5–25mg od Acute pain: 50mg od
Ropivacaine	Amide type local anaesthetic agent. Possibly less motor block than other agents. Duration similar to bupivacaine, but lower toxicity pKa 8.1		NR	0.2–1% solution. Infiltration/epidural: maximum dose dependent upon injection site— 3–4mg/kg/4hr
			0.2–1% solution. Maximum dose dependent upon injection site— 3–4mg/kg/4hr	
Salbutamol	β₂ receptor agonist. Treatment of bronchospasm Larger doses now suggested in paeds: 15µg/kg/min over 10min, then 1–5µg/kg/min	Tremor, vasodilatation, tachycardia Hypokalaemia possible	4µg/kg slow IV then 0.1–1µg/kg/min. Nebuliser <5yr 2.5mg, >5yr 2.5–5mg	250µg slow IV then 5µg/min (up to 20µg/min). Nebuliser: 2.5–5mg prn

IV = intravenous. IM = intramuscular. SC = subcutaneous. PO = per os (oral). SL = sublingual. ET = endotracheal. od = once daily. bd = twice daily. tds = three times daily.qds = four times daily. NR = not recommended. Doses are intravenous and dilutions in 0.9% saline unless otherwise stated.

Drug	Description and perioperative indications	Cautions and contraindications	Side-effects	Dose (paediatric)	Dose (adult)
Sufentanil	More potent thiamyl analogue of fentanyl (five times potency). Analgesia. Duration 20–45min	See fentanyl	See fentanyl		Analgesia:10–30µg (0.2–0.6µg/kg). Anaesthesia: 0.6–4µg/kg
Suxamethonium	Depolarising muscle relaxant. Rapid short-acting muscle paralysis. Phase II block develops with repeated doses (>8mg/kg). Store at 2–8°C	Prolonged block in plasma cholinesterase deficiency, hypokalaemia, hypocalcaemia. Malignant hyperthermia, myopathies Increased serum K$^+$ (normally 0.5mmol/l greater in burns, trauma, upper motor neuron	Increased intraocular pressure. Bradycardia with second dose	1–2mg/kg	1–1.5mg/kg. Infusion: 0.5–10mg/min
Teicoplanin	Glycopeptide antibiotic with activity against aerobic and anaerobic Gram-positive bacteria	Renal impairment	Ototoxicity, nephrotoxicity Blood disorders	10mg/kg for 3 doses 12-hourly then 6mg/kg od	IV/IM: 400mg for 3 doses 12-hourly then 200mg od
Temazepam	Benzodiazepine. Sedation or premedication. Duration 1–2hr	Decreased requirement for anaesthetic agents	Respiratory depression in combination with opioids. Amnesia	PO: 0.5–1mg/kg preop	PO: 10–40mg 1hr preop (elderly 10–20mg)

Tenoxicam	NSAID analgesic for mild to moderate pain	Hypersensitivity to aspirin, asthma, severe renal impairment, peptic ulceration	Gastrointestinal upset or bleeding, bronchospasm, tinnitus, fluid retention, platelet inhibition	NR	PO: 20mg od. IV/IM: 20mg od
Tetracaine (amethocaine) (Ametop®)	Ester type local anaesthetic. Topical analgesia prior to venepuncture. Ametop® gel contains 4% amethocaine. (Also available as eye drops, but has temporary disruptive effect on corneal epithelium). Duration 4hr	Apply only to intact skin under occlusive dressing. Remove after 45min. Rapid absorption through mucosa		As adult. <1 month NR	Each tube expels 1.5g (sufficient for area 6 × 5cm)
Thiopental	Short-acting thiobarbiturate. Induction of anaesthesia, anticonvulsant, cerebral protection. Recovery due to redistribution	Accumulation with repeated doses. Caution in hypovolaemia and elderly. Porphyria	Hypotension- Necrosis if intra-arterial	Induction: neonate 2–4mg/kg, child 5–6mg/kg	Induction/cerebral protection: 3–5mg/kg. Anticonvulsant: 0.5–2mg/kg prn

IV = intravenous. IM = intramuscular. SC = subcutaneous. PO = per os (oral). SL = sublingual. ET = endotracheal. od = once daily. bd = twice daily. tds = three times daily. qds = four times daily. NR = not recommended. Doses are intravenous and dilutions in 0.9% saline unless otherwise stated.

Drug	Description and perioperative indications	Cautions and contraindications	Side-effects	Dose (paediatric)	Dose (adult)
Tramadol	Opioid analgesic thought to have less respiratory depression, constipation, euphoria, or abuse potential than other opioids. Has opioid and non-opioid mechanisms of action	Only 30% antagonised by naloxone. Caution in epilepsy. Previously not recommended for intra-operative use. MAOI	Nausea, dizziness, dry mouth. Increased side effects in conjunction with other opioids	1–2mg/kg 6-hourly	PO: 50–100mg 4-hourly. Slow IV/IM: 50–100mg 4-hourly (100mg initially then 50mg increments to maximum 250mg). Maximum 600mg/d
Tranexamic acid	Inhibits plasminogen activation reducing fibrin dissolution by plasmin. Reduced haemorrhage in prostatectomy or dental extraction	Avoid in thromboembolic disease, renal impairment, and pregnancy	Dizziness, nausea	PO: 15–20mg/kg tds	Slow IV: 0.5–1g tds. PO:15–25mg/kg tds
Triamcinolone hexacetonide (Lederspan®)	Relatively insoluble corticosteroid for depot injection. (Epidural unlicensed use) (triamcinolone 4mg = prednisolone 5mg)	Dose depends upon site of injection. Strict asepsis essential. Dilute 20mg/ml solution prior to use		Intra-articular or intrasynovial: 2.5–15mg	Intra-articular or intrasynovial: 2–30mg. Epidural: 40–60mg diluted with local anaesthetic
Trimeprazine	See alimemazine				
Trimetaphan	Ganglion blocking hypotensive agent	Tachyphylaxis with prolonged use	Tachycardia, mydriasis		0.04–0.1mg/kg/min 2–4mg/min

D-Tubocurarine	Intermediate acting non-depolarising muscle relaxant	See cisatracurium. Asthma	See Cisatracurium Hypotension due to histamine release and ganglion blockade	Intubation: 0.3–0.6mg/kg. Maintenance: 0.05–0.3mg/kg
Valdecoxib (Bextra®)	See celecoxib Cox II inhibitor	See celecoxib Postop use after CABG		PO: 10–20mg od (40mg dysmenorrhoea)
Vancomycin	Glycopeptide antibiotic with activity against aerobic and anaerobic Gram-positive bacteria. Peak level <30mg/l. Trough level 5–10mg/l	Avoid rapid infusion (hypotension, wheezing, urticaria, 'red man' syndrome). Reduce dose in renal impairment	Ototoxicity, nephrotoxicity, phlebitis, neutro-penia	>1 month: 10mg/kg over 2hr qds	1g over 100min bd (check blood levels after third dose)
Vasopressin (Pitressin®)	Synthetic ADH used in treatment of diabetes insipidus, resistant vasodilatory shock	Extreme caution in coronary vascular disease	Pallor, coronary vasoconstriction, water intoxication	Diabetes insipidus SC/IM: 2–10U 4-hourly	Diabetes insipidus SC/IM: 5–20U 4-hourly Sepsis 1–4U/hr Shock infusion
Vecuronium	Aminosteroid non-depolarising muscle relaxant. Cardiostable and no histamine release. Duration 30–45min	See cisatracurium	See cisatracurium	Intubation: <4 month 10–20µg/kg, plus increments as required >5 month 100µg/kg	Intubation: 80–100µg/kg. Maintenance: 20–30µg/kg. Infusion: 0.8–1.4µg/kg/min

IV = intravenous. IM = intramuscular. SC = subcutaneous. PO = per os (oral). SL = sublingual. ET = endotracheal. od = once daily. bd = twice daily. tds = three times daily. qds = four times daily. NR = not recommended. Doses are intravenous and dilutions in 0.9% saline unless otherwise stated.

Drug	Description and perioperative indications	Cautions and contraindications	Side-effects	Dose (paediatric)	Dose (adult)
Warfarin	Coumarin derivative oral anticoagulant. DVT prophylaxis: INR 2.0–2.5. DVT/PE treatment, AF, mitral valve disease: INR 2.5–3.0. Recurrent DVT/PE, prosthetic heart valve: INR 3.0–4.5	Pregnancy, peptic ulcer disease. Reduce dose in elderly	Haemorrhage	PO: 0.2mg/kg up to 10mg od for 2d, then 0.05–0.2mg/kg od	PO: 10mg od for 2d then 3–9mg od dependent on INR
Ximelagatran (Parenteral form is Melagatran) (Exanta®)	Oral thrombin inhibitor. DVT prophylaxis after major orthopaedic surgery. Prevention of CVA in AF.	Not yet approved in UK. Coagulopathy or active bleeding. Caution with spinal or epidural (p1059)	Haemorrhage, deranged LFTs. Difficult to reverse		Melagatran 3mg SC 4–12hr postop PO: 24–36mg bd
Zolpidem	Short-acting imidazopyridine hypnotic with little hangover effect	Obstructive sleep apnoea, myasthenia gravis	Nausea, dizziness	NR	PO: 10mg nocte (elderly 5mg)
Zopiclone	Short-acting cyclopyrrolone hypnotic with little hangover effect	Obstructive sleep apnoea, myasthenia gravis	Nausea, bitter taste in mouth	NR	PO: 7.5mg nocte (elderly 3.75mg)

IV = intravenous. IM = intramuscular. SC = subcutaneous. PO = per os (oral). SL = sublingual. ET = endotracheal. od = once daily. bd = twice daily. tds = three times daily. qds = four times daily. NR = not recommended. Doses are intravenous and dilutions in 0.9% saline unless otherwise stated.

Infusion regimes

Drug	Indication	Diluent	Dose	Suggested regime (60kg adult)	Infusion range	Initial rate (adult)	Comments
Adrenaline	Treatment of hypotension	0.9% saline, 5% dextrose	2–20µg/min (0.04– 0.4µg/kg/min)	5mg/50ml (100µg/ml)	1.2–12+ml/hr	5ml/hr	Via central catheter. Suggest 1mg/50ml for initial intra-operative use (or 1mg/500ml if no central access)
Alfentanil	Analgesia	0.9% saline, 5% dextrose	0.5–1µg/kg/min	Undiluted (500µg/ml)	0–8ml/hr	4ml/hr	1–2mg can be added to 50ml propofol for infusion
Aminophylline	Bronchodila-tion	0.9% saline, 5% dextrose	0.5mg/kg/hr	250mg/50ml (5mg/ml)	0–6ml/hr	6ml/h	After 5mg/kg slow bolus
Amiodarone	Treatment of arrhythmias	5% dextrose only	Loading infusion 5mg/kg over 1–2hr, then 900mg over 24hr	300mg/50ml (6mg/ml)	25–50ml/hr then 6ml/h	25ml/hr	Via central line (peripherally in extremis). Max^m 1.2g in 24hr
Atracurium	Muscle relaxant	0.9% saline, 5% dextrose	0.3–0.6mg/kg/hr	undiluted (10mg/ml)	1.5–4ml/hr	3ml/hr	Assess rate with nerve stimulator
Cis-atracurium	Muscle relaxant	0.9% saline, 5% dextrose	0.06–0.18mg/hr	undiluted (2mg/ml)	2–5ml/hr	5ml/hr	Assess rate with nerve stimulator

Alternative regimes for any infusion:
3mg/kg/50ml then 1ml/hr = 1µg/kg/min
3mg/50ml then 1ml/hr = 1µg/min
Rate (ml/hr) = 60 × Rate (µg/kg/min) × wt (kg) ÷ conc (µg/ml)

Drug	Indication	Diluent	Dose	Suggested regime (60kg adult)	Infusion range	Initial rate (adult)	Comments
Digoxin	Rapid control of ventricular rate	0.9% saline, 5% dextrose	250–500µg over 30–60min	250–500µg/ 50ml	0–100ml/hr	50ml/hr	ECG monitoring suggested
Dobutamine	Cardiac failure/ inotrope	0.9% saline, 5% dextrose	2.5–10µg/kg/min	250mg/50ml (5mg/ml)	2–7ml/hr	2ml/hr	
Dopamine	Inotrope	0.9% saline, 5% dextrose	2–10µg/kg/min	200mg/50ml (4mg/ml)	2–9ml/hr	2ml/hr	Via central line
Dopexamine	Inotrope	0.9% saline, 5% dextrose	0.5–6µg/kg/min	50mg/50ml (1mg/ml)	2–22ml/hr	2ml/hr	May be given via large peripheral vein
Doxapram	Respiratory stimulant	0.9% saline, 5% dextrose	2–4mg/min	200mg/50ml (4mg/ml)	30–60ml/hr	30ml/hr	Maximum dose 4mg/kg
Enoximone	Inodilator	0.9% saline only	90µg/kg/min for 10–30min, then 5–20µg/kg/min	100mg/50ml (2mg/ml)	9–36ml/hr	162ml/hr for 10–30min	Maximum 24mg/kg/d
Esmolol	β-blocker	0.9% saline, 5% dextrose	50–200µg/ kg/min	2.5g/50ml (50mg/ml)	3–15ml/hr	3ml/hr	ECG monitoring
Glyceryl trinitrate	Controlled hypotension	0.9% saline, 5% dextrose	0.5–12ml/hr	50mg/50ml (1mg/ml)	0.5–12ml/hr	5ml/hr	
Heparin	Anticoagulation	0.9% saline, 5% dextrose	24 000–48 000U per 24hr	50 000U/50ml (1000U/ml)	1–2ml/hr	2ml/hr	Check APTT after 12hr

			Dose	Concentration	Rate	Rate	Notes
Insulin (soluble)	Diabetes mellitus	0.9% saline	Sliding scale	50U/50ml (1U/ml)	Sliding scale	Sliding scale	
Isoprenaline	Treatment of heart block or bradycardia	5% dextrose saline	0.5–10µg/min	1mg/50ml (20µg/ml)	1.5–30ml/hr	7ml/hr	Induction 0.5–2mg/kg
Ketamine	General anaesthesia	0.9% saline, 5% dextrose	1–3mg/kg/hr	500mg/50ml (10mg/ml)	6–18ml/hr	10ml/hr	
Ketamine	Analgesia	0.9% saline, 5% dextrose	0.2mg/kg/hr	200mg/50ml (4mg/ml)	0–6ml/hr	3ml/hr	With midazolam 2–5 mg/hr
Ketamine	'Trauma' mixture	0.9% saline	0.5ml/kg/hr	50ml mixture (4mg/ml ketamine)	15–45ml/hr	30ml/hr	200mg ketamine + 10mg midazolam + 10mg vecuronium in 50ml
Lidocaine (lignocaine)	Ventricular arrhythmias	0.9% saline	4mg/min for 30min, 2mg/min for 2hr, then 1mg/min for 24hr	500mg/50ml (10mg/ml = 1%)	6–24ml/hr	24ml/hr	After 50–100mg slow IV bolus. ECG monitoring

Alternative regimes for any infusion:

3mg/kg/50ml then 1ml/hr = 1µg/kg/min

3mg/50ml then 1ml/hr = 1µg/min

Rate (ml/hr) = 60 × Rate (µg/kg/min) × wt (kg) ÷ conc (µg/ml)

Drug	Indication	Diluent	Dose	Suggested regime (60kg adult)	Infusion range	Initial rate (adult)	Comments
Milrinone	Inodilator	0.9% saline, 5% dextrose	50µg/kg over 10min, then 0.375–0.75µg/kg/min	10mg/50ml (0.2mg/ml)	7–14ml/hr	90ml/hr for 10min	Maximum 1.13mg/kg/day
Mivacurium	Muscle relaxant	0.9% saline, 5% dextrose	0.4–0.6mg/kg/hr	Undiluted (2mg/ml)	12–18ml/hr	18ml/hr	Assess rate with nerve stimulator
Morphine	Analgesia	0.9% saline	0–3.5mg/hr	50mg/50ml (1mg/ml)	0–3.5ml/hr	2ml/hr	Monitor respiration and sedation hourly. Administer oxygen
Naloxone	Opioid antagonist	0.9% saline, 5% dextrose	>1µg/kg/hr	2mg/500ml (4µg/ml)		100ml/hr	Rate adjusted according to response
Nimodipine	Prevention of vasospasm after SAH	0.9% saline, 5% dextrose	1mg/hr increasing to 2mg/hr after 2hr	Undiluted (0.2mg/ml)	5–10ml/hr	5ml/hr	Via central line. Incompatible with polyvinyl chloride
Nitroprusside (sodium)	Controlled hypotension	5% dextrose	0.3–1.5µg/kg/min	25mg/50ml (500µg/ml)	2–10ml/hr	5ml/hr	Maximum dose 1.5mg/kg. Protect from light

Noradrenaline	Treatment of hypotension	5% dextrose	2–20µg/min (0.04–0.4µg/kg/min)	4mg/40ml (100µg/ml)	1.2–12+ml/hr	5ml/hr	Via central line
Octreotide	Somatostatin analogue	0.9% saline	25–50µg/hr	500µg/50ml (10µg/ml)	2–5ml/hr	5ml/hr	Use in variceal bleeding unlicensed
Oxytocin (Syntocinon)	Prevention of uterine atony	0.9% saline, 5% dextrose	0.02–0.125U/min	30U in 500ml (0.06U/ml)	30–125ml/hr	125ml/hr	Individual unit protocols vary
Phenytoin	Anticonvulsant prophylaxis	0.9% saline	15mg/kg	900mg/90ml (administer through 0.22–0.5µm filter)	Up to 50mg/min	180ml/hr	ECG and BP monitoring, Complete within 1hr of preparation
Propofol	Anaesthesia	Undiluted (10mg/ml)	6–10mg/kg/hr		36–60ml/hr		TCI: initially 4–8µg/ml then 3–6µg/ml
Propofol	Sedation	Undiluted (10mg/ml)	0–3mg/kg/hr		0–20ml/hr		TCI: 0–2.5µg/ml

Alternative regimes for any infusion:

3mg/kg/50ml then 1ml/hr = 1µg/kg/min
3mg/50ml then 1ml/hr = 1µg/min
Rate (ml/hr) = 60 × Rate (µg/kg/min) × wt (kg) ÷ conc (µg/ml)

Drug	Indication	Diluent	Dose	Suggested regime (60kg adult)	Infusion range	Initial rate (adult)	Comments
Remifentanil	Analgesia during general anaesthesia	0.9% saline, 5% dextrose	0.1–0.5μg/kg/min	2mg/40ml (50μg/ml)	5–40ml/hr IPPV. 2–7ml/hr SV	8ml/hr IPPV. 2ml/hr SV	Suggest starting at 0.1μg/kg/min (8ml/hr) then adjust up to 0.25μg/kg/min (20ml/hr) as required
Rocuronium	Muscle relaxant	0.9% saline, 5% dextrose	0.3–0.6mg/kg/hr	Undiluted (10mg/ml)	1.5–4ml/hr	3ml/hr	Assess rate with nerve stimulator
Salbutamol	Bronchospasm	5% dextrose	5–20μg/min	1mg/50ml (20μg/ml)	15–60ml/hr	30ml/hr	After 250μg slow IV bolus
Sodium bicarbonate	Acidosis		[weight (kg) × base deficit × 0.3] mmol	Undiluted (8.4% solution)			8.4% = 1000mmol/l. Via central line if possible
Vancomycin	Antibiotic	0.9% saline, 5% dextrose	1g	1g/500ml	500ml/100min	500ml/100min	
Vecuronium	Muscle relaxant	0.9% saline, 5% dextrose	0.05–0.08mg/kg/hr	Undiluted (2mg/ml)	1.5–3ml/hr	2.5ml/hr	Assess rate with nerve stimulator

Medical gas	State in cylinder	Body colour	Shoulder colour	Cylinder Capacity Type C (litres)	Cylinder capacity Type D (litres)	Cylinder capacity Type E (litres)	Cylinder capacity Type F (litres)	Cylinder pressure when full (×100 kPa)	Critical temp (°C)
Oxygen (O_2)	gas	black	white	170	340	680	1360	137	−118.4
Nitrous Oxide (N_2O)	liquid	blue	blue	450	900	1800	3600	44*	36.4
O_2:N_2O 50:50 (Entonox)	gas	blue	blue & white		500		2000	137	−6[†]
Medical air	gas	grey	black & white			640	1280	137	
Carbon dioxide (CO_2)	liquid	grey	grey	450		1800		50*	30
O_2:CO_2 95:5	gas	black	grey & white				1360	137	
Helium (He)	gas	brown	brown		300		1200	137	−268
O_2:He 21:79	gas	black	brown & white				1200	137	
Water capacity of cylinder (l)				1.2	2.32	4.68	9,43		

*Where the contents are liquid, the pressure is not a reliable method of judging the contents.
[†]Entonox separates into oxygen and nitrous oxide at −6°C—pseudocritical' temperature.
Pressures quoted for full cylinders are at 15°C.
Cylinder colours and contents may vary outside the UK.

MAC values

	MAC in oxygen/air[1] (%)			MAC in 67% N₂O (%)			BP (°C)	SVP (kPa)	Oil: gas part. coeff.	Blood: gas part. coeff.	MW	Bio trans. (%)
	1yr	40yr	80yr	1yr	40yr	80yr						
Halothane	0.95	0.75	0.58	0.47	0.27	0.10	50.2	32.5	224	2.3	197.4	25
Enflurane	2.08	1.63	1.27	1.03	0.58	0.22	56.5	22.9	96	1.91	184.5	3
Isoflurane	1.49	1.17	0.91	0.74	0.42	0.17	48.5	31.9	91	1.4	184.5	0.2
Sevoflurane	2.29	1.80	1.40	1.13	0.65	0.25	58.5	21.3	53	0.59	200	2.5
Desflurane	8.3	6.6	5.1	4.2	2.4	0.93	23.5	88.5	18.7	0.42	168	Minimal
Nitrous Oxide	133	104	81	NA	NA	NA	-88	5080	1.4	0.47	44	0
Xenon	92	72	57	NA	NA	NA	-107.1	5800	20	0.14	131.3	0

Potency (MAC) correlates with oil: gas partition coefficient (hence lipid solubility).
Speed of onset correlates with blood: gas partition coefficient (lower = faster).
SVP = saturated vapour pressure at 20°C, MW = molecular weight, BP = boiling point, biotrans. = biotransformation
part. coeff. = partition coefficient at 37°C, part. coeff. = partition coefficient at 20°C, MW = molecular weight, BP = boiling point, biotrans. = biotransformation

1 Nickalls RWD, Mapleson WW (2003). Age-related iso-MAC charts for isoflurane, sevoflurane and desflurane in man. *British Journal Anaesthesia* **91**, 170–174.

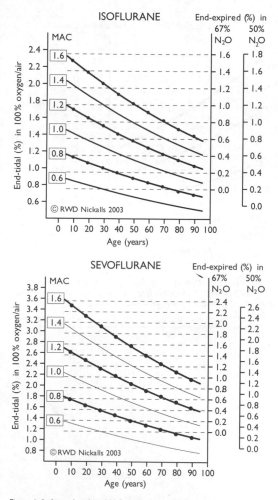

Figure 1–3: Age-related iso-MAC charts for isoflurane, sevoflurane, and desfluran
(courtesy of Dr RWD Nickalls). Reasonable ranges of MAC: SV/LMA 1.2–1.6 M/
IPPV with opiates 1.0–1.3 MAC; IPPV with remifentanil (0.25µg/kg/min) 0.6–0.9

1 Nickalls RWD, Mapleson WW (2003). Age-related iso-MAC charts for isoflurane, s
and desflurane in man. *British Journal of Anaesthesia* **91**: 170–174. http://bja.oxfordj
cgi/reprint/91/2/170.pdf
2 Lerou JGC (2004). Nomogram to estimate age-related MAC. *British Journal of An*
288–291.

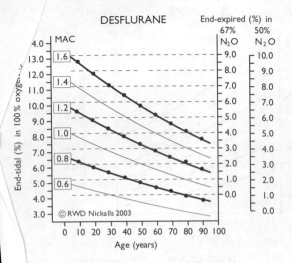

re 1–3: Age-related iso-MAC charts for isoflurane, sevoflurane, and desflurane
rtesy of Dr RWD Nickalls). Reasonable ranges of MAC: SV/LMA 1.2–1.6 MAC;
ith opiates 1.0–1.3 MAC; IPPV with remifentanil (0.25μg/kg/min) 0.6–0.9
Continued

apleson WW (2003). Age-related iso-MAC charts for isoflurane, sevoflurane
cg/n man. *British Journal of Anaesthesia* **91**: 170–174. http://bja.oxfordjournals.org/
2 Ler).pdf
288–29). Nomogram to estimate age-related MAC. *British Journal of Anaesthesia*, **93**,

Antibiotic prophylaxis

Endocarditis prophylaxis[1,2]

Dental, oral, respiratory tract, or oesophageal procedures

Risk	Prophylaxis
High risk	Amoxicillin 2g IV plus gentamicin 1.5mg/kg IV at induction, then amoxicillin 1g IV/PO 6hr later
	If allergic to penicillin vancomycin 1g IV over 120min plus gentamicin 1.5mg/kg IV at induction, or clindamycin 300mg IV over 10min at induction, then clindamycin 150mg PO/IV 6hr later
Moderate risk	Amoxicillin 2g at induction
	If allergic to penicillin clindamycin 300mg IV over 10min at induction, then clindamycin 150mg PO/IV 6hr later

Genitourinary or gastrointestinal procedures

Risk	Prophylaxis
Moderate/High	Amoxicillin 2g IV plus gentamicin 1.5mg/kg IV at induction, then amoxicillin 1g IV/PO 6hr later
	If allergic to penicillin vancomycin 1g IV over 120min plus gentamicin 1.5mg/kg IV at induction

Endocarditis risk

High risk	Moderate risk
Previous endocarditis (highest risk)	Acquired valvular heart disease (rheumatic)
Prosthetic heart valve	Non-cyanotic congenital defects (PDA, Coarct, VSD, ASD)
Mitral valve prolapse with regurg	Other structural abnormalities (HOCM)
Complex congenital heart disease	
Surgical systemic: pulmonary shunts	

Recent exposure to penicillin

If patient has received penicillin during previous month follow recommendations for penicillin allergic.

1 Ramsdale DR, Turner-Stokes L; Advisory group of the British Cardiac Society Clinical Practice Committee (2004). Prophylaxis and treatment of infective endocarditis in adults: a concise guide. *Clinical Medicine*, **4**, 545–550.
2 www.bnf.org

Surgical prophylaxis

Soiling risk	Operation	Bacterial prevalence	IV Antibiotics (usually single dose)
Clean	Head & neck	Oral streptococci/ anaerobes/Staph aureus	Augmentin 1.2g or Clindamycin 300mg
	Hysterectomy	Staph aureus/ anaerobes	Augmentin 1.2g or Cefuroxime 1.5g + metronidazole 500mg
	Cardiac/ vascular/ amputation	Staph aureus/ coagulase negative staphylococci	Cefuroxime 1.5g or Augmentin 1.2g or Vancomycin 1g if penicillin allergic
	Urinary catheterisation/ instrumentation	Previously not catheterised, or uninfected urine	None necessary
		Change of catheter/ recently catheterised	Gentamicin 80mg or Cefuroxime 1.5g or Ciprofloxacin 500mg orally
	Prosthetic joint insertion	Staphylococci including coagulase negative staph	Cefuroxime 1.5g or Vancomycin 1g Prophylaxis may be for 1–3 doses
Intermediate	ERCP (significant sepsis occurs in 0.5–1%)	Gram negatives/ Pseudomonas/ Enterococci	Ciprofloxacin 750mg Orally (will not cover enterococci) or Piperacillin 2g + gentamicin 160mg
	Cholecystectomy		Cefuroxime 1.5g + metronidazole 500mg or Gentamicin 160mg
	'Routine' appendicectomy	Anaerobes	Cefuroxime 1.5g + metronidazole 500mg
	Elective colorectal surgery	Coliforms/anaerobes/ Pseudomonas/ enterococci	Cefuroxime 1.5g + metronidazole 500mg or Gentamicin 3–5mg/kg + metronidazole 500mg
'Dirty'	Often emergency; perforated viscus, peritonitis	Coliforms/anaerobes/ Pseudomonas/ enterococci	Gentamicin 3–5mg/kg + cefotaxime 2g + metronidazole 500mg or Imipenem 0.5–1g + metronidazole 500mg. Continuation therapy needed

Penicillin allergy

- How 'allergic'? What happens (e.g. diarrhoea is not an allergy)? Was it anaphylaxis?
- Check old drug charts—may have had a penicillin in the past without problems. This further strengthens the case against genuine penicillin allergy.
- If penicillin allergy is only a rash, cephalosporins may be used with care—2–5% cross-sensitivity in practice.
- If history of anaphylaxis with penicillin, avoid any β-lactam (i.e. no penicillins, cephalosporins, or carbapenems). Discuss alternatives with microbiologist. Remember vancomycin has no gram negative cover.

Prophylaxis for perioperative aspiration pneumonia

- General tendency to over-treat 'aspiration pneumonia', much of which is due to chemical pneumonitis. Organisms likely to cause infection are from oropharynx, mainly anaerobes, but may include gram-negative aerobes, including Pseudomonas spp in hospitalised patients. If prophylaxis is deemed necessary, choose antibiotics which cover anaerobes:
  - Augmentin 1.2g IV for three doses 8-hourly
  - Clarithromycin 500mg IV for two doses 12-hourly
  - Where gram negative bacteria may be problematic—Cefuroxime 1.5g IV tds ± metronidazole 500mg IV tds.

Chapter 43

Anaesthesia data

James Szymankiewicz

ASA/CEPOD classifications

ASA classification of physical state

Grade	Description
1	A healthy patient with no systemic disease
2	Mild to moderate systemic disease
3	Severe systemic disease imposing functional limitation on patient
4	Severe systemic disease which is a constant threat to life
5	Moribund patient who is not expected to survive with or without the operation
6	A brain stem dead patient whose organs are being removed for donor purposes

For emergency cases the suffix 'E' is used

CEPOD classification

Description of surgery	
Elective	Intervention planned or booked in advance of routine admission to hospital. Timing to suit patient, hospital and staff
Expedited	Patient requiring early treatment where the condition is not an immediate threat to life, limb or organ survival. Normally within days of decision to operate
Urgent	Intervention for acute onset or clinical deterioration of potentially life-threatening conditions, for those conditions that may threaten the survival of limb or organ, for fixation of many fractures and for the relief of pain or other distressing symptoms. Normally within hours of decision to operate
Immediate	Immediate life, limb or organ-saving intervention—resuscitation simultaneous with intervention. Normally within minutes of decision to operate A) Life saving B) Other e.g. limb or organ saving

Breathing circuits

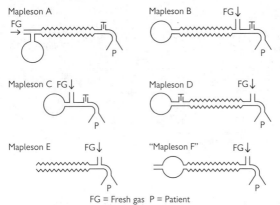

Mapleson A

Mapleson B

Mapleson C

Mapleson D

Mapleson E

"Mapleson F"

FG = Fresh gas P = Patient

Mapleson classification of breathing circuits

Fresh gas flows in anaesthetic breathing systems		
	Spontaneous ventilation	**Intermittent positive pressure ventilation**
Mapleson A (Lack or Magill)	MV (theoretically V_A) 80ml/kg/min	2.5 × MV (200ml/kg/min)
Mapleson D (Bain or coaxial Mapleson D)	2–3 × MV (150–250ml/kg/min)	70ml/kg/min for $PaCO_2$ of 5.3kPa. (40mmHg) 100ml/kg/min for $PaCO_2$ of 4.3kPa (32mmHg)
Mapleson E (Ayre's T-piece)	2 × MV	As Mapleson D. Minimum of 3l/min fresh gas flow
Mapleson F (Jackson Rees modification of Ayre's T-piece)	As Mapleson E	As Mapleson E

MV = minute ventilation; V_A = alveolar ventilation

Pulmonary function tests

In males

Age (yr) Assuming height 175cm	FEV$_1$ (l)	FVC (l)	FEV$_1$/FVC (%)	PEFR (l/min)
20	4.15	4.95	82.5	625
30	4.00	4.84	80.6	612
40	3.69	4.62	76.9	586
50	3.38	4.40	73.1	560
60	3.06	4.18	69.4	533
70	2.75	3.96	65.7	507

In females

Age (yr) Assuming height 160cm	FEV$_1$ (l)	FVC (l)	FEV$_1$/FVC (%)	PEFR (l/min)
20	3.09	3.83	81.0	433
30	2.94	3.68	79.9	422
40	2.64	3.38	77.7	401
50	2.34	3.08	75.5	380
60	2.04	2.78	73.2	359
70	1.74	2.48	71.0	338

FEV$_1$ = forced expiratory volume in 1s; FVC = forced vital capacity; PEFR = peak expiratory flow rate.

Arterial/mixed venous blood gases

	Mixed venous blood gases		Arterial blood gases	
	mmHg	kPa	mmHg	kPa
O$_2$	37–42	4.9–5.6	90–110	12.0–14.7
CO$_2$	40–52	5.3–6.9	34–46	4.53–6.1
N$_2$	573	76.4	573	76.4
pH	7.32–7.42		7.36–7.44	
SaO$_2$	>75%		>99%	

Cardiovascular physiology data

Cardiovascular pressures

	Range (mmHg)	Mean (mmHg)
Central venous pressure (CVP)	0–8	4
Right atrial (RA)	0–8	4
Right ventricular (RV):		
Systolic	14–30	25
End-diastolic (RVEDP)	0–8	4
Pulmonary arterial (PA):		
Systolic	15–30	23
Diastolic	5–15	10
Mean (PAP)	10–20	15
Mean pulmonary artery wedge (PAWP)	5–15	10
Left atrial (LA)	4–12	7
Left ventricular (LV):		
Systolic	90–140	120
End-diastolic (LVEDP)	4–12	7

Derived haemodynamic variables

Variable value	Formula	Normal values
Cardiac output (CO)	SV × HR	4.5–8l/min
Cardiac index (CI)	CO/BSA	2.7–4l/min/m^2
Stroke volume (SV)	(CO/HR) × 1000	60–130ml/beat
Stroke volume index (SI)	SV/BSA	38–60ml/beat/m^2
Systemic vascular resistance (SVR)	80 × (MAP–CVP)/CO	770–1500dyn.s/cm^5
Systemic vascular resistance index (SVRI)	80 × (MAP–CVP)/CI	1860–2500dyn.s/cm^5/m^2
Pulmonary vascular resistance (PVR)	80 × (PAP–PCWP)/CO	100–250dyn.s/cm^5
Pulmonary vascular resistance index (PVRI)	80 × (PAP–PCWP)/CI	225–315dyn.s/cm^5/m^2
Left ventricular stroke work index (LVSWI)	SI × MAP × 0.0144	50–62g.m/m^2/beat
Rate–pressure product (RPP)	SAP × HR	9600
Ejection fraction (EF)	(EDV–ESV)/EDV	>0.6
Mean arterial pressure (MAP)	MAP = CO × SVR	80–90mmHg
Estimated MAP (MAPest)	MAPest = Diastolic BP + $1/3$ pulse pressure	
Cerebral perfusion pressure (CPP)	CPP = MAP–ICP	70–75mmHg

BSA = body surface area; HR = heart rate; MAP = mean arterial pressure; CVP = central venous pressure; PAP = mean pulmonary arterial pressure; PCWP = pulmonary capillary wedge pressure; SAP = systolic arterial pressure; ESV = end-systolic volume; EDV = end-diastolic volume

Respiratory physiology data

Normal values for the oesophageal Doppler

Index		Value
Cardiac output		5l/min
Stroke volume		70ml
Flow time corrected (FTC)		330–360ms
Peak velocity	20yr	90–120cm/sec
	50yr	70–100cm/sec
	70yr	50–80cm/sec

Lung volumes

	Adult (70 kg)
Dead space (V_D)	2ml/kg
Tidal volume (V_T)	7–10ml/kg
Alveolar ventilation (V_A)	70ml/kg/min
Minute ventilation (V_E)	85–100ml/kg/min
Vital capacity (VC)	50–55ml/kg
Respiratory rate (RR)	12–18 breaths/min
Total lung capacity (TLC)	5000–6500ml
Inspiratory reserve volume (IRV)	3300–3750ml
Expiratory reserve volume (ERV)	950–1200ml
Functional residual capacity (FRC)	2300–2800ml
Residual volume (RV)	1200–1700ml

Gas laws

Boyle's law	Pressure is inversely proportional to volume (at a constant temperature)	$P \propto 1/V$
Charles' law	Volume is proportional to temperature (at a constant pressure)	$V \propto T$
Gay–Lussac's law	Pressure is proportional to temperature (at a constant volume)	$P \propto T$
Dalton's law of partial pressure	If a container holds a mixture of gases the pressure exerted by each gas (i.e. the partial pressure) is the same as if it alone occupied the container	

Useful equations

Alveolar gas equation $P_AO_2 = PiO_2 - \dfrac{P_ACO_2}{RQ}$

Where P_AO_2 = alveolar oxygen tension, PiO_2 = inspired oxygen tension, P_ACO_2 = alveolar CO_2 tension, RQ = respiratory quotient

Alveolar volume is the volume of fresh gas reaching the alveoli (V_A)
V_A = tidal volume (V_T) – Anatomical dead space (V_D)

Alveolar ventilation is the amount of fresh gas reaching the alveoli per min (V_A x Resp rate)

Oxygen flux (oxygen delivery) = cardiac output x oxygen content of blood

Oxygen content of blood = (O_2 bound to Hb) + (O_2 dissolved)
(per 100ml) $(SaO_2 \times 1.34 \times Hb)$ $(0.023 \times PO_2)$

Shunt equation

$$Qs/Qt = \dfrac{CcO_2 - CaO_2}{CcO_2 - CvO_2}$$

Where Qs = shunt flow, Qt = total flow, CcO_2 = pulmonary capillary oxygen content, CaO_2 = arterial oxygen content, CvO_2 = mixed venous oxygen content.

Laplace's law for a sphere

Pressure across the wall = 2 x tension/radius

Reynold's number

Predicts whether gas flow is likely to be laminar or turbulent

$$Re = \dfrac{diameter \times velocity \times density}{viscosity}$$

<1000 = laminar flow

>2000 = turbulent flow

Hagen-Poiseuille law

Describes laminar flow in tubes

$$Flow\ rate = \dfrac{Pressure\ difference \times r^4}{length \times viscosity}$$

r^4 = radius to the 4th power

Anion gap

$$(Na^+ + K^+) - (HCO_3^- + Cl^-)$$

normal value 5–12mmol/l

Normal values

Haematology

Measurement	Reference range
White cell count	$4.0–11.0 \times 10^9/l$
Red cell count	♂$4.5–6.5 \times 10^{12}/l$ ♀$3.9–5.6 \times 10^{12}/l$
Haemoglobin	♂$13.5–18.0g/dl$ ♀$11.5–16.0g/dl$
Packed red cell volume (haematocrit)	♂$0.4–0.54l/l$ ♀$0.37–0.47l/l$
Mean cell volume	$76–96fl$
Mean cell haemoglobin	$27–32pg$
Neutrophils	$2.0–7.5 \times 10^9/l$ 40–75% WCC
Lymphocytes	$1.3–3.5 \times 10^9/l$ 20–45% WCC
Eosinophils	$0.04–0.44 \times 10^9/l$ 1–6% WCC
Basophils	$0.0–0.10 \times 10^9/l$ 0.1% WCC
Monocytes	$0.2–0.8 \times 10^9/l$ 2–10% WCC
Platelet count	$150–400 \times 10^9/l$
Prothrombin time (factors I, II, VII, X)	10–14s
Activated partial thromboplastin time (VIII, IX, XI, XII)	35–45s
INR	
Normal	1
Anticoagulation targets: Atrial fibrillation Treatment DVT/PE Prosthetic valve	 2.5 (± 0.5) 2.5 (± 0.5) 3.5 (± 0.5)

Biochemistry

	Specimen	Reference interval
Adrenocorticotrophic hormone	P	<80ng/l
Alanine aminotransferase (ALT)	P	5–35iu/l
Albumin	P	35–50g/l
Aldosterone	P	100–500pmol/l
Alkaline phosphatase	P	30–300iu/l (adults)
Amylase	P	0–180 Somogyi u/dl
α-fetoprotein	S	<10ku/l
Angiotensin II	P	5–35pmol/l
Antidiuretic hormone (ADH)	P	0.9–4.6pmol/l
Aspartate transaminase (AST)	P	5–35iu/l
Bicarbonate	P	24–30mmol/l
Bilirubin	P	3–17μmol/l
Calcitonin	P	<0.1μg/l
Calcium (ionised)	P	1.0–1.25mmol/l
Calcium (total)	P	2.12–2.65mmol/l
Chloride	P	95–105mmol/l
Cholesterol	P	3.9–7.8mmol/l
VLDL	P	0.128–0.645mmol/l
LDL	P	1.55–4.4mmol/l
HDL	P	0.9–1.93mmol/l
Cholinesterase	P	♂5900–12220u/l ♀4650–10440u/l
Cortisol	P	a.m. 450–700nmol/l midnight 80–280nmol/l
Creatine kinase (CK)	P	25–195iu/l
Creatinine (∞ to lean body mass)	P	70–150mmol/l
CRP	P	0–12mg/l
Ferritin	P	12–200μg/l
Folate	S	2.1μg/l
Gamma-glutamyl transpeptidase	P	11–51iu/l
Glucose (fasting)	P	3.5–5.5mmol/l
Glycated (glycosylated) Hb	B	2.3–6.5%
Growth hormone	P	<20mu/l
HbA$_{1c}$ (= glycosylated Hb)	B	2.3–6.5%

Table *contd.*

	Specimen	Reference interval
Iron	S	♂ 14–31µmol/l ♀ 11–30µmol/l
Magnesium	P	0.7–1mmol/l
Osmolality	P	278–305mosmol/kg
Parathyroid hormone (PTH)	P	<0.8–8.5pmol/l
Phosphate (inorganic)	P	0.8–1.45mmol/l
Potassium	P	3.5–5.0mmol/l
Prolactin	P	<450u/l; <600u/l
Protein (total)	P	60–80g/l
Red cell folate	B	0.36–1.44µmol/l (160–640µg/l)
Renin (erect/recumbent)	P	2.8–4.5/1.1–2.7pmol/ml/hr
Sodium	P	135–145mmol/l
Thyroid-binding globulin (TBG)	P	7–17mg/l
Thyroid-stimulating hormone (TSH) NR widens with age	P	0.5–5.7mu/l
Thyroxine (T_4)	P	70–140mmol/l
Thyroxine (free)	P	9–22pmol/l
Total iron binding capacity	S	54–75µmol/l
Triglyceride	P	0.55–1.90mmol/l
Tri-iodothyroinine (T_3)	P	1.2–3.0nmol/l
Troponin T	P	0–0.1ng/l Sample must be taken at least 12hr after symptoms
Urate	P	♂210–480µmol/l ♀150–390µmol/l
Urea	P	2.5–6.7mmol/l
Vitamin B_{12}	S	0.13–0.68nmol/l (>150ng/l)

P = plasma (e.g. heparin bottle); S = serum (clotted; no anticoagulant); B = whole blood (edetic acid EDTA bottle)

Drug levels

Drug		Therapeutic level
Digoxin		0.8–2.0µg/l (1–2.6nmol/l)
Phenytoin		40–80µmol/l
Valproate		60–100mg/l
Lithium		0.4–1.0mmol/l
Theophylline		55–110µmol/l
Gentamicin	Pre dose	<2mg/l
	Post dose	6–10mg/l
Vancomycin	Pre dose	5–10mg/l
	Post dose	20–30mg/l

Useful websites

www.rcoa.ac.uk	Royal College of Anaesthetists
www.aagbi.org	Association of Anaesthetists of Great Britain and Ireland
www.asahq.org	American Society of Anaesthesiologists
www.anzca.edu.au	Australian and New Zealand College of Anaesthetists
www.ics.ac.uk	Intensive Care Society
www.esicm.org	European Society of Intensive Care
www.sccm.org	Society of Critical Care Medicine (USA)
www.anzics.com	Australian and New Zealand Intensive Care Society
www.pedsanesthesia.org	Society for Pediatric Anesthesia
www.vasgbi.com	Vascular Anaesthesia Society of Great Britain and Ireland
www.acta.org.uk	Association of Cardiothoracic Anaesthetists
www.thoracic.org	American Thoracic Society
www.oaa-anaes.ac.uk	Obstetric Anaesthetist Association
www.boas.org	British Ophthalmic Anaesthesia Society
www.das.uk.com	The Difficult Airway Society
www.nasgbi.org.uk	Neuroanaesthesia Society
www.snacc.org	Society of Neurosurgical Anaesthesia and Critical Care
www.alfanaes.freeserve.co.uk/alfahome.htm	Association for Low Flow Anaesthesia
www.sivauk.org	Society for Intravenous Anaesthesia
www.esraeurope.org	European Society of Regional Anaesthesia
www.asra.com	American Society of Regional Anaesthesia and Pain Medicine
www.britishpainsociety.org	The British Pain Society
www.resus.org.uk	The Resuscitation Council
www.aagbi.org/trainee.html	Group of Anaesthetists in Training
www.world-anaesthesia.org	World Anaesthesia Society
www.bja.oupjournals.org	British Journal of Anaesthesia
www.anesthesia-analgesia.org	Anesthesia and Analgesia

Table *contd*

www.bmj.com	British Medical Journal
www.anesthesiology.org	Anesthesiology
www.thelancet.com	The Lancet
www.ebandolier.com	Evidence Based Healthcare
www.cochrane.org	Cochrane Collaboration
www.nice.org.uk	National Institute of Clinical Excellence
www.scata.org.uk	Society for Computing and Technology in Anaesthesia
www.uptodate.com	Internet Based Resource
www.handango.com	Software for PDA
www.anesthesiadoc.net	Online Anaesthesia Resource
www.ccmtutorials.com/index.htm	Critical Care Medicine Tutorials
www.virtual-anaesthesia-textbook.com	Virtual Anaesthetic Textbook
www.ncbi.nlm.nih.gov/PubMed	PubMed
www.eguidelines.co.uk	eGuidelines
www.sign.ac.uk	Scottish Intercollegiate Guidelines
www.frca.co.uk	Anaesthesia UK
www.gasnet.org	Global Anaesthesiology Server Network
www.gmc-uk.org	General Medical Council
www.bma.org.uk	British Medical Association
www.mps.org.uk	The Medical Protection Society
www.the-mdu.com	The Medical Defence Union
www.mddus.com	The Medical and Dental Defence Union of Scotland
www.histansoc.org.uk	History of Anaesthesia Society
www.rcplondon.ac.uk	Royal College of Physicians
www.rcseng.ac.uk	Royal College of Surgeons of England
www.roysocmed.ac.uk	Royal Society of Medicine
www.bnfc.org	BNF for Children 2005
www.bnf.org	BNF

Checklist for anaesthetic equipment

Use this guidance in association with the manufacturer's instructions for checking your specific anaesthesia machine—certain models should not have the common gas outlet occluded (see Check 5)

The following checks should be made prior to each operating session. In addition, Checks 2, 6 and 9 should be made prior to each new patient during a session.

1. Check that the anaesthetic machine is connected to the electricity supply (if appropriate) and switched on.

Note: Some anaesthetic workstations may enter an integral self-test programme when switched on; those functions tested by such a programme need not be retested.

- Take note of any information or labelling on the anaesthetic machine referring to the current status of the machine. Particular attention should be paid to recent servicing. Servicing labels should be fixed in the service logbook.

2. Check that all monitoring devices, in particular the oxygen analyser, pulse oximeter and capnograph, are functioning and have appropriate alarm limits.

- Check that gas sampling lines are properly attached and free of obstructions.
- Check that an appropriate frequency of recording non-invasive blood pressure is selected.

(Some monitors need to be in stand-by mode to avoid unnecessary alarms before being connected to the patient.)

3. Check with a 'tug test' that each pipeline is correctly inserted into the appropriate gas supply terminal.

Note: CO_2 cylinders should not be present on the anaesthetic machine unless requested by the anaesthetist. A blanking plug should be fitted to any empty cylinder yoke.

- Check that the anaesthetic machine is connected to a supply of oxygen and that an adequate supply of oxygen is available from a reserve oxygen cylinder.
- Check that adequate supplies of other gases (nitrous oxide, air) are available and connected as appropriate.
- Check that all pipeline pressure gauges in use on the anaesthetic machine indicate 400–500kPa.

4. Check the operation of flow meters (where fitted).

- Check that each flow valve operates smoothly and that the bobbin moves freely throughout its range.
- Check the anti-hypoxia device is working correctly.
- Check the operation of the emergency oxygen bypass control.

5. Check the vaporiser(s).

- Check that each vaporiser is adequately, but not over, filled.
- Check that each vaporiser is correctly seated on the back bar and not tilted.
- Check the vaporiser for leaks (with vaporiser on and off) by temporarily occluding the common gas outlet. Turn the vaporiser(s) off when checks are completed.

- Repeat the leak test immediately after changing any vaporiser.

6. Check the breathing system to be employed.

Note: A new single use bacterial/viral filter and angle-piece/catheter mount must be used for each patient. Packaging should not be removed until point of use.

- Inspect the system for correct configuration. All connections should be secured by 'push and twist'.
- Perform a pressure leak test on the breathing system by occluding the patient-end and compressing the reservoir bag. Bain-type co-axial systems should have the inner tube compressed for the leak test.
- Check the correct operation of all valves, including unidirectional valves within a circle, and all exhaust valves.
- Check for patency and flow of gas through the whole breathing system including the filter and anglepiece/catheter mount.

7. Check that the ventilator is configured appropriately for its intended use.

- Check that the ventilator tubing is correctly configured and securely attached.
- Set the controls for use and ensure that an adequate pressure is generated during the inspiratory phase.
- Check the pressure relief valve functions.
- Check that the disconnect alarms function correctly.
- Ensure that an alternative means to ventilate the patient's lungs is available. (see 10. below)

8. Check that the anaesthetic gas scavenging system is switched on and is functioning correctly.

- Check that the tubing is attached to the appropriate exhaust port of the breathing system, ventilator or workstation.

9. Check that all ancillary equipment which may be needed is present and working.

- This includes laryngoscopes, intubation aids, intubation forceps, bougies etc. and appropriately sized face masks, airways, tracheal tubes and connectors, which must be checked for patency.
- Check that the suction apparatus is functioning and that all connectors are secure.
- Check that the patient trolley, bed or operating table can be rapidly tilted head down.

10. Check that an alternative means to ventilate the patient is immediately available (e.g. self-inflating bag and oxygen cylinder).

- Check that the self-inflating bag and cylinder of oxygen are functioning correctly and the cylinder contains an adequate supply of oxygen.

11. Recording

- Sign and date the logbook kept with the anaesthetic machine to confirm the machine has been checked.
- Record on each patient's anaesthetic chart that the anaesthetic machine, breathing system and monitoring has been checked.

'Checking Anaesthetic Equipment 3 (2004)' (courtesy of the Association of Anaesthetists of Great Britain and Ireland)

Index

C